Praise for

Laughing Your Way to
Passing the Pediatric Boards™

"While I chose not to go to medical school, I got 'close' — I survived majoring in Biology at Yale and graduated with honors despite all the pre-meds in my major! After all the time and money you've spent on your education, you owe it to yourself to pass your boards the first time and this book can help but only if you read it! Dr. Stu Silverstein knows the value of being prepared and he's darn funny."

—Eric Tyson, Syndicated Columnist; Best-Selling author of **Personal Finance for Dummies** and **Investing for Dummies** (IDG Books)

"As a med student studying pediatrics, I found this prep book to be incredibly helpful for passing the boards. Dr. Silverstein's book is super easy to follow, with each chapter broken down to be clear and digestible. For anyone looking for an affordable pediatric prep book, that is painless and great study material, I highly recommend this one!"

"It's an amazing compilation that slips in bits of humor while you revise for your exams. An innovative way to pull a student out of nodding off. I love the book!"

"This book is awesome. I do credit it to my successful Board study plan. If you only have money for one book, buy this one."

"Great resource and very funny. I was laughing on the first page and recognizing test taking pearls from day one."

Laughing Your Way to Passing the Pediatric Boards, 2022 Edition! ®

The Seriously Funny Study Guide™

"Taking the boredom out of Board Review" ®

By Stu Silverstein, M.D., FAAP

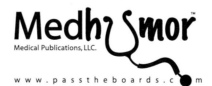

www.passtheboards.com

MedHumor Medical Publications, Stamford, Connecticut

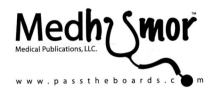

www.passtheboards.com

Published by:

Medhumor Medical Publications, LLC
1127 High Ridge Road, Suite 332
Stamford, CT 06905 U.S.A.

ISBN: 978-1-7320780-7-9

Printed in the United States of America

This book is designed to provide information and guidance in regard to the subject matter covered. It is to be used as a study guide for physicians preparing for the General Pediatric Certifying Exam administered by the American Board of Pediatrics. It is not meant to be a clinical manual. The reader is advised to consult textbooks and other reference manuals in making clinical decisions. It is not the purpose of this book to reprint all the information that is otherwise available, but rather to assist the Board Candidate in organizing the material to facilitate study and recall on the exam. The reader is encouraged to read other sources of material, in particular picture atlases that are available.

Although every precaution has been taken in the preparation of this book, the publisher, author, and members of the editorial board assume no responsibility for errors, omissions or typographical mistakes. Nor is any liability assumed for damages resulting from the direct and indirect use of the information contained herein. The book contains information that is up-to-date only up to the printing date. Due to the very nature of the medical profession, there will be points out-of-date as soon as the book rolls off the press. The purpose of this book is to educate and entertain.

**If you do not wish to be bound by the above,
you may return this book to the publisher for a full refund.**

Publisher:

MedHumor Medical Publications, LLC
Stamford, CT.

President:
Stuart Silverstein, MD, FAAP

Medical Director
Firefly After Hours Pediatrics, LLC
Stamford, CT

President / CEO
MedHumor Medical Publications, LLC
Stamford, CT

Marketing and Customer Support:
Daniel J. Silverstein

Senior Editor:
Lourdes Geise, MD, FAAP
Windrose Health Network, Indianapolis, IN.

Layout Designer:
Antoinette D'Amore, A.D. Design
addesign@videotron.ca

Cover Designer:
Diana Corona
https://dribbble.com/dcoronastudio

Illustrations:
© Medhumor Medical Publications, LLC

Comic Strip Cartoon:
Conceived / Stu Silverstein, MD, FAAP
© Medhumor Medical Publications, LLC

About the Author

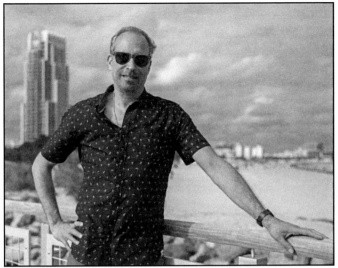

Dr. Stu Silverstein is the founder and CEO of Medhumor Medical Publications, LLC which began with the publication of the critically acclaimed *Laughing Your Way to Passing the Pediatric Boards*® back in the spring of 2000. Word spread quickly that finally there was a book out there that turned a traditionally daunting process into one that was actually fun and enjoyable. This groundbreaking study guide truly "Took the Boredom out of Board review"® with reports from our readers that they were able to reduce their study and review time in half. Those who were taking the exam for the 2nd time not only passed but increased their scores dramatically. We are well into our 2nd decade of helping pediatricians prepare for their boards through fun and innovation.

Our pediatric titles have also been critically acclaimed. Medhumor Publications, LLC has since expanded our catalogue, which now includes Neonatology, Neurology, USMLE and Pediatric MOC Recertification titles.

The concepts of the *Laughing Your Way to Passing the Boards*® and Medhumor Medical Publications, LLC were conceived by Dr. Silverstein. He decided to redirect his years of experience in the field of standup comedy and comedy-writing after he realized the critical need for a study guide that spoke the language of colleagues rather than the language of dusty textbooks. His work as a Standup Comedian and Medical Humorist has been featured in newspapers, radio programs and TV shows, including the New York Times, WCBS news radio in NY City, as well as World News Tonight with the late Peter Jennings.

Dr. Silverstein has also served as a contributing editor for the Resident and Staff Physician annual board review issue and has authored numerous articles on medical humor. He has served on the faculty of the Osler Institute Board Review course, UCLA Pediatric Board Review course and several local board review courses. He is the co-author of "What about Me? Growing up with a Developmentally Disabled Sibling" written with Dr. Bryna Siegel, professor of Child Psychiatry, the University of California San Francisco. Dr. Silverstein is in demand as a lecturer for residency programs on successful preparation for the pediatric board exam.

In addition to writing, lecturing, and expanding the scope of Medhumor Medical Publications, LLC., Dr. Silverstein is the Medical Director for Firefly After Hours Pediatrics, a subacute emergency practice, and is a former Assistant Clinical Professor of Emergency Medicine at the New York Medical College in Valhalla, New York.

The 2022 Edition

In putting together the 2019 edition of *Laughing Your Way to Passing the Pediatric Boards*® we updated and added material based on the content specifications published by the American Board of Pediatrics, the American Academy of Pediatrics, as well as Pediatrics in Review®, the AAP Red Book® and a variety of primary sources and journal articles.

The 2022 edition is completely updated based on the Content Specifications outlined by he American Board of Pediatrics and the American Academy of Pediatrics. We have also included a high yield index to help direct your studying.

This year we have added additional illustrations to help reinforce the important concepts that require visualization.

In addition we have added a new margin icon to the family which points out important information that has been added or dramatically changes since the 2019 edition was released.

We are always humbled and honored to hear from so many board candidates who give us credit for passing this difficult exam. This is even more fulfilling when this praise comes from those taking the exam for the 2nd time.

We hope that this, our 2022 edition will continue to serve those for whom passing the pediatric board exam is the next ticket to be punched. 2020 and the beginning of 2021 has been a rough time and we hope that this book finds everyone healthy and ready to move forward with energy and grace.

—Stuart Silverstein, MD, FAAP
Stamford, CT

This book is once again dedicated
to my wife Guita and
my children, Isra, Daniel, and Ariel
whose very existence gives life meaning
and keeps things in perspective.

Every day they remind me
that it is never too late
to have a happy childhood.

Acknowledgments

I would like to acknowledge Lourdes Geise, MD, FAAP who initially contacted us as one of our readers noting improvement which we could make in our next edition. It wasn't long before we realized that her keen eye for detail and wide fund of knowledge made her an ideal technical and copy editor for updating and revising our titles. We know that much of the improvement in this edition can be attributed to her due diligence while working under a tight deadline without hesitation. This year we have added a panel of colleagues to help update the book , they are all listed in the credit section. Each of you have provided us with fresh feedback and perspective.

The layout and design of our books are the result of the talented, diligent eye and creativity of our layout designer, Antoinette D'Amore. Without Antoinette's assistance, the book you are holding would be a bunch of random uneven paragraphs with no adherence to standard paging and layout.

My son Daniel Silverstein, continues to assist and consult for us regarding content development. Daniel has graduated from the University of Connecticut (UCONN) Storrs with honors earning his BS in Molecular and Cell Biology. He is now starting his first year as a medical student at the Hackensack Meridian School of Medicine. When our first edition was released Daniel was a mere child of 2. Amazing things happen in 20 short years.

My daughter Isra has completed her Psy. D. in clinical psychology from the University of Hartford, and is currently working as a Psychologist in Los Angeles. A special shout-out to my youngest son, Ariel who is now 18 and a graduate of Westhill High School. He is studying business and marketing and has launched a successful merchandising business. That business has grown exponentially and will only grow more now that he is done with high school. It is a pleasure to watch him grow and work hard at school, on the ice and in all endeavors he takes on.

Judy Falbel, our business manager and accountant, has been instrumental in keeping our financial books balanced so we can focus on publishing and producing board review books.

I would like to acknowledge my parents Richard and Beverly Silverstein of Boynton Beach, Florida for their encouragement early on and for instilling in me the importance of diligence and staying the course despite adversity.

I would like to also thank my wife, Dr. Guita Sazan for encouraging me to use my talents.

My friend Darren Kessler is as close to me as a brother, which proves that doctors and lawyers can indeed be close friends. I would like to thank Darren for always encouraging me and reminding me of the big picture when I doubted myself the most. Your ever-present encouragement has been a driving force in more ways than you realize.

I apologize to anyone not listed; it is difficult to remember everyone when facing a deadline to go to press!

Table of Contents

Section A: Successful & Efficient Exam Preparation

Chapter 1

A User's Guide to Laughing Your Way to Passing the Pediatric Boards®

So you've completed high school.[1] That was a proud moment and you have the crème colored tassel dangling from your rearview mirror to prove it. Then came *college* and you graduated Summa Cum (Very) Laude and got your Phi Beta Kappa Key, which opened the door to additional student debt. Then it was off to *med school* and you got the Golden MD or DO degree.

Then you "matched" and were given the opportunity to be available as a *de facto* concierge desk coordinator, while making less per hour than the guy with the strange deodorant fixing the elevators.

All along the way you had to get your "admission ticket" punched by passing a gauntlet of USMLE Step Exams.[2] In doing so, you've proven that you are good at the USMLE Step mental stairmaster machine. Let's face it; if you have made it to this point, you are at the tip of the pyramid. You've graduated from the *23rd grade.*[3]

Therefore, anyone who is reading this has reached the top of the food chain.[4] Just when you thought it was safe, you have to get one more token, one more badge, one more item to add to your CAQH online attestation, one more item on the managed care credentialing application: *change Board Eligible to Board Certified.*

The Liberty Bell Curve !

No big deal for the Standardized Test Veteran? You would think so, but think again. The makers of the test create a bell curve out of a group that is already jammed into the nose cone at the far right of the general population curve. There will be a host of tough questions to separate the greatest test takers from the great, the mice from the murines.

You need to be in the middle of the curve in order to convert the bell curve to the Liberty Bell curve and you are free from the shackles.

Raw Scores, Passing Scores, and Who's Keeping Score?

Raw score is the percentage of questions you answer correctly.

The passing grade is 180 on a scale of 1-300. This is called your scaled score.

However, this does not mean you need to answer 60% of the questions correctly to pass. You will likely need at least 80% or higher to pass.

The International Medical Graduate !

If you are from another country, I don't even want to think about from what grade you are graduating. Chances are you have had to come here and start from scratch, which meant becoming an Intern taking orders from someone half your age and half your experience.

You then had to complete another residency, even though you were Professor Emeritus of Neonatology back in your country of origin. In addition, you had to pass all those standardized exams in a foreign language.

You can get information from the Board directly:

The American Board of Pediatrics
111 Silver Cedar Court
Chapel Hill, NC 27514

Voice: 919-929-0461
Fax: 919-929-9255
www.apb.org

---

[1] With honors
[2] Which you did or you would not be reading this.
[3] Don't bother adding it up, I am correct.
[4] Unless you are the significant other of a Board Candidate, in which case I can assure you that there is nothing interesting here, so just put this down and watch the re-runs of American Idol

There is some allegorical formula and algorithm that calculates your scaled score.

Since the exam can be taken during a 3 day period there are multiple versions of the exam. According to the ABP, the different versions vary in their degree of difficulty. If you are taking a more difficult version you need to get a lower percentage correct to reach the 180 benchmark. The opposite is also true. The easier the exam, the more questions you need to answer correctly to get to the 180 milestone.

We recommend shooting for 80% correct when taking practice exams as a safe margin. You can't control which test you are taking so you might as well assume you will be taking the most difficult version. You should therefore shoot for answering 80% correct. You should answer every question even if it is a guess. You never know if that question will count and you do not lose points for answering incorrectly.

So How Many Pass?

The American Board of Pediatrics only publishes the passing rate for **first time test takers**. This information is updated annually on their website.

The passing rate for first time test takers , between 2016-2020 ranged between 80-90%.

Are you a 2nd or 3rd Timer?

However, this is for first time test takers. If you have taken the exam and failed, this statistic doesn't apply.

If you have failed, the test before, it was either because you didn't study properly, or because you don't take exams well. Either way, this book is especially for you! Unless you change your approach to the exam you are likely to fail the exam again.

If you are taking the exam for a 2nd time you are scored the same way. However, statistically you are more likely to fail. Again, this is especially so if you do not change the way you prepare.

Organizing and Scheduling Your Study

This exam is special. It requires a system for organizing the material so that you can have it at your fingertips when you take the exam. For many folks, anxiety is also a problem so you also need a *system to control anxiety*.[5]

Organizing the Material So That You Remember It Cold

In addition to helping you develop a strategy for organizing your study and controlling your anxiety, this book will show you how to organize and memorize the material with techniques and mnemonics that work. We have included a sample study schedule to help you get started.

We will include:

1. Buzzwords, phrases, and patterns in the question that point to the correct answers
2. Proven memorization techniques and systems that maximize retention and recognition
3. Tips for the exam day
4. Methods that maximize your ability to recognize the graphics and illustrations

Most importantly, you must "study to the test". While studying ask yourself, how might this material be worked into a question format. Always be studying to the exam. This is not about clinical knowledge !

---

[5] We cover this in another chapter, and we don't mean pharmacology.

How to Use This Book

You can go through this book cover to cover, or choose your own order. We suggest you read through the first section first, and then go through the rest of the material in the order you prefer. You can then go through the book again focusing on your weak areas.

Guideposts Along the Way

As you read the book, you will notice pictures in the margin that emphasize important points. These "Guideposts" will indicate a particular category of information.

Guideposts

DEFINITION	*Definition*	This points to a "definition."[6]
PERIL	*Perils*	This alerts you to important information that can trip yo up on the exam. This includes common misunderstandings or traps you can fall into if you do not read the question carefully.
MNEMONIC	*Mnemonic Device*	This indicates a mnemonic that helps make the material impossible to forget.
HOT TIP	*Hot Tip*	"This draws attention to an important clinical point or a "Board Pearl," to help you on potential trouble areas.
MYTH	*Myth*	This signifies a popularly held myth that isn't true. This is a classic trap laid by Board Examiners.[7]
BUZZWORDS	*Key Words and Pattern Recognition*	This describes buzzwords, key phrases and patterns that are pathognomonic for a given condition. By learning this, you will often be able to recognize the answer in the wording of the question itself.
COIN FLIP	*Down to two choices*	This points out minute differences between similar disorders, which are critical to answering many questions correctly.
TAKE HOME MESSAGE	*Take Home Message*	This is the Bottom Line to remember.
TREATMENT	*Treatment*	This points to specific treatments for a given diagnosis or disorder.
VERY BORING MATERIAL WARNING!	*Boring*	Warning! Very boring material. Take a break, splash cold water on your face and walk around the room before reading.
UPDATED & NEW BREAKING NEWS INFORMATION	*Updated Criteria and New Topics*	Material and criteria that has been specifically updated, changed and revised since our last publication in 2019. It also includes topics which have been added since our last publication.

---

[6] Knowing the definition will save you from being tricked. For example, LGA is greater than the 90th %ile. Should they describe a child in the 88th percentile this would NOT be LGA.

[7] For example: Sugar causes ADHD.

On the exam, you may be presented with specific case scenarios. **In these instances, just knowing the material is not enough.** Understanding how you can be diverted from the correct answer and even fall prey because you know <u>too much</u> can often be the difference between passing and failing the exam.

We call your attention to these case studies with the following icons:

	Case Study	Here we will present you with a case study or summarize how they might present a given vignette.
	The Diversion	As is common in most examinations, the test writers try to dissuade you from the correct answer by tripping you up if you are unsure of the subject matter. Here we explain how you might be diverted from the correct answer. The diversion can come in many forms: • **Understatement:** The understatement minimizes information that is key to answering correctly: "Other than ibuprofen, the patient is not taking any medications." • **Abnormal physical findings in a forest of normal findings:** A list of normal findings with the word *hepatomegaly* mixed in, making it easy to overlook. • **Emphasis on diversionary factors:** An example would be implying purpura of the lower extremity is child abuse by noting the child is being raised by a single mother in the first sentence, rather than emphasizing findings consistent with actual diagnosis, Henoch Schönlein Purpura. We use the diversion icon in other areas as well to call attention to material that can be confusing and easily result in choosing incorrect answers.
	Answer Revealed	Here we reveal the correct answer and show you how the correct answer can be deduced by carefully teasing out the important information and filtering out the diversionary material.

Chapter 2

What ? Me Worry ! ?
Alleviating Exam Anxiety

The Boards Vs Clinical Practice

It's the Boards' World—We Just Live In It

Passing the Boards requires a different set of skills than being a good clinician. You can be a great clinician and fail the boards if you do not prepare correctly or if you have poor test taking skills. On the other hand, you can be a master test taker, pass the Boards, and be a mediocre clinician. I'm sure you've never encountered anyone like this.

- Organized planning and study will get you 1/3 of the way to passing the exam
- Good solid focused test taking strategies is another 3rd.
- Of course, the remaining 1/3 piece of the puzzle is having the information at your fingertips, and we cover this in the main section of this book.

Anxious Over Being Anxious

We are frequently approached by readers who feel that they know the material well, have used some memory techniques, retain the material in long-term memory, and yet still fail the exam. Often this is a result of test taking anxiety. This is truly a pity!

It is a pity because anxiety is a physiological reaction, nothing more. And its effects can be reversed. Our anxiety response has more to do with a perceived threat than how well we are or aren't prepared.

- **Motivational speaker Zig Ziegler defines** "FEAR" as *"False Evidence Appearing Real,"* and this could apply to anyone taking the Boards.
- One can also define **FEAR** as *"Fluids Electrolytes And Residency."*
- We have recently heard it can also mean **F** Everything And Relax.

Extreme Anxiety is as Useless as a Stethoscope Around a Psychiatrist's Neck

When I performed standup comedy in clubs, I got to know many comedians and saw them in action backstage. We all needed some anxiety to get us going, to give us that "edge" on stage. Some would get very anxious; others wouldn't get anxious at all.

What I noticed most was that the level of anxiety was independent of talent and prep time they had put into their routine.[1] I would see very talented comics become nauseated, and some with virtually no talent—folks who would make the old guy in Pawn Stars seem electrifying by comparison—walk out confident that they were funny. The same applies to those taking the Board Exam.

Do not mistake your anxiety as an indication of your ability to pass:

You need to counter the physical response of stress and anxiety. No matter what your level of preparedness, excess anxiety will only work against you. You need only a little anxiety to get your blood going. Stretching before the exam would be a good idea. However, this should be done at home before leaving for the exam.

Everyone who takes the Pediatric Board exam experiences anxiety. *Some of you experience anxiety about not experiencing anxiety,* and that can make anyone anxious—even those claiming that they experience no anxiety.

The Anxiety Channel

Let's face it; some anxiety is good and even necessary. Without anxiety, you wouldn't have any motivation to turn away from binge watching *Lupin* on Netflix®, and study hypoparathyroidism. Too much anxiety, however, and you feel like the resident who snapchatted photos to the Pediatric Department Chairman instead of his significant other after 3 hour liver rounds.

Anxiety Level

←——————————————————————————————→

Watching highlight reels on The Curling Channel.	Discovering that the discretionary photos you intended to post on Snapchat® were posted on your LinkedIn® account

HOT TIP

Take systematic steps to reduce anxiety. Consider meditative recordings, progressive relaxation, aromatherapy, download a mindfulness meditation app.

If You Think You Will Fail, You are Right!
If You Think You Will Pass, You are also Right!

What do all of these quotes have in common?

Henry Ford once said,

> *"If you think you will succeed you are correct. If you think you will fail you are also correct."*

Your Mother once said,

> *"You're not going out to play until you finish your homework!"*

My friend the ophthalmologist's mother once said:

> *"Stop fooling around with those darts, you're not going to be happy until you take someone's eye out"*

---

[1] This is very similar to parental anxiety in the practice of pediatrics. One can rarely use a parent's anxiety as a gauge for the severity of a child's disease. Some parents are frantic over an ear infection while others are unfazed over a child with signs of meningitis.

What they have in common is this: They were all correct.

You need to stop negative self-talk in its tracks and your self-talk must be about passing. The first step is to envision yourself passing. You cannot begin taking the steps to pass unless you do this first!

If you send this message to your subconscious, it will find the means to pass the exam!

24 Hours to Go!

 Do Not...do NOT...and in case you missed it the first two times, DO NOT study the day before the exam. I would even say do not (DO NOT) study 2 days before the exam.

The Big Day!

The day of the exam, you want to wake up and do whatever it is that gets you pumped up and energized. For some it means music, for some it means no sound at all and. The one thing you should NOT do is study some more.

There is really nothing you will learn in the hour before the exam that will be the difference between passing and failing. What **could be** the difference is a stressed out fatigued brain vs. a rested one. *The material has to marinate.*

Dressed to Kill and Eat for Skill!

The word out there among test taking gurus is to avoid taking caffeine before the exam. Well, **if you drink coffee every day, this is not the day to quit.** Some additional nutritional tips can come in handy:

- Sugar and other forms of junk are not a good idea.
- Enjoy a well-balanced breakfast with fruits.
- Have a few peeled fruits available.
- A multivitamin in the morning as long as you take it with food.

Feel free to take some extra Vitamin B12 and Folic Acid. Both are good for the nerves and get flushed out the kidneys during times of stress and high caffeine intake.

Warning, do not take vitamins or supplements on an empty stomach!

Stretch and do whatever it takes to relax. Make sure you have a sweater in case the person in charge of the Prometric® Center has untreated hyperthyroidism and is as clammy as a Chef on *Hell's Kitchen*.

On the other hand, you want to have something very light in case the heat is turned up to the temperature of a mosh pit on the equator.

Prometric® Center

Prometric® Power

You will most likely be taking the exam at a Prometric Center®. This has its own set of issues.

My personal experience with this situation is limited to the Pediatric MOC exam. I wish I had been advised on steps I could have taken to make this experience more pleasant. Here is my advice on the process based on that experience.

Have You Made a Reservation?

So I went through the registration process for the local Prometric® center. I thought I was set. However, as the day of the exam approached, I wondered why I had not received any e-mail confirmation. I had gone "retro" and registered by phone to make sure I was doing it correctly. That was a mistake! It turns out they wrote down my e-mail incorrectly and registered me for a site halfway across the state. **We recommend that you confirm your reservation early**.

I had to register for another date to take the exam at a site closer to my home. This error would have been a much larger issue with the Certification Exam, since you only have a 3 day window within which you can take the exam.

GPS = Get to Prometrics Sooner

It is good advice when they say allow a lot of time to find the Prometric® Center. Chances are Murphy's Law will be in effect and there will either be traffic, or worse, construction, the car in front of you will be the driver who is lost without a GPS, AND the address of the center will be invisible on YOUR GPS. This is what happened to me. The test center was located in an unmarked building in an industrial park. Waze® kept informing me that I had arrived at my location, which was an intersection between 2 dump trucks and a freestyle axe throwing tavern.

You might want to take a cab to the exam. Uber®, Lyft® or just have a friend drive you. You don't need the added worry about finding parking, having enough gas or or dodging off target axes!

Getting through the Door !

You should plan on arriving 30 minutes early to avoid any added anxiety. If you are the type of person that feels that arriving early is lost time and live in the fast lane, consider this down time to be a chance to relax. However, do not use this time to study! Use this time to just relax to get in a positive mindset.

When you finally arrive, your experience will be similar to going through airport security without the wand scan. You will be given a locker and informed that you have to empty your pockets. **I suggest you bring some ibuprofen with you in case you get a headache. I sure wish I had. If you take prescription medication remember to take that with you as well.**

Everyone you know should be aware that you are taking an all day exam and inaccessible. This is probably the most important exam in your career to date. Nobody should be expecting you to respond to texts, e-mails and definitely not responding to calls.

Turn it Off !

After the exam I was informed that the phone I left in my locker rang and buzzed as texts and calls came through. They could have told me to turn the phone off or put it on vibrate mode but they didn't. You should put your phone in airplane and do not disturb mode. If not now, then when?

Keeping the Train of Thought on Track despite the Click Clack

When you finally sit for the exam, you will likely be in a room full of exam takers in their own cubicles. While it is theoretically quiet, it really isn't. These are individuals taking all sorts of exams. Some are taking the LSAT, the SAT, the BACE (Bowling Alley Certification Exam), or the DNR exam. Some of these exams require lots of data entry and the constant Click Clack Moo® might derail your ability to keep your focus. Those of you who are easily distracted by a symphony of gum smacking in B Minor will need to find a way to filter out the noise.

I wish I had brought along foam earplugs . While they DO provide you with over the ear headphones, they are the hard plastic over the ear headphones from the early 1970s. They have plastic edges that have the potential to permanently deform the shape of your head without fully blocking sound.

They did filter out some noise if you don't mind the painful distraction of the hard edges cutting grooves into your outer ear. Consider foam ear plug inserts or the over the ear air mufflers used at firing ranges.

Again, we suggest you bring light clothing with a zip up jacket. You never know if it will be too hot or too cold there.

You won't need a calculator because there is an on-screen calculator there for you to summon up during the exam.

Time for Questions !

The exam consists of approximately 350 Questions divided by 4 sections. The questions are evenly divided. Each section is 1 hour and 45 minutes and consists of approximately 85 questions.

You will need time for instructions, the optional tutorial, and the survey at the end, plus review of the honor code. **All told this will be a 9 hour day.**

Once you close out a section you cannot go back and change an answer. **Therefore if an answer in section 1 is revealed later in section 2, it won't help you!**

You have an optional 15 minute breaks between sections. You will be given a 60 minute lunch break between sections 2 and 3. DO NOT STUDY DURING LUNCH!

That may sound daunting but be thankful you are not taking the 2 DAY, 9 hour a day exam that was in place for your pediatric ancestors including yours truly!

Navigating the Mouseclicks

While you no longer have to worry about lining up the grid and filling in the circles with a number 2 pencil, there are other pitfalls waiting to trip you up.

During each question set, you are given a **warning** when you have **an hour** remaining and then when you have **30 minutes remaining**. This was the case on the recertification exam, and the specifics might be different on your exam. **You should know where you should be at 15 minutes, 30 minutes etc. so you are not caught by surprise in the end.**

The Hold Button is On !

There is a hold button for questions you are not sure of or just want to come back to later. I suggest that you answer all the questions you are sure of first, and place the ones you are not sure of on hold to come back to later. **You need to make sure you release the hold button when you come back to answer the question! In order to enter an answer you must first "release the question".**

I made the mistake of not realizing this. I went back and entered answers to these questions and thought I was done. However, when I looked at the main menu the questions were still listed as incomplete. Fortunately, I had time to spare.

There is a tutorial on the ABP website to familiarize yourself with the format of the test. We strongly encourage you to take advantage of that.

Of Course I am going to Read the Question!
I'm a Doctor Dammit !

When we say, "read the question," we are not merely stating the obvious. This means pay close attention what they are asking. Key words in the last sentence of the question are very important.

Words like **"least," "most," "first,"** "etiology," "diagnosis," "treatment" and especially **"except"** are important to note before moving on to the listed choices.

Chapter 3

Time Management in a Bottle

You cannot possibly go into this test without preparation. If you are taking this exam for the 2nd, 3rd, ...*nth* time, then past methods, by definition, will not work.

If you actually have a job, family, friends and hobbies, then over the next few months there will certainly be things that you would prefer to do besides memorizing the the clinical features of Alport syndrome.

Better Late Than Never

If you are reading this and actually are a few weeks away from the exam, and are a good memorizer, then some of the memorization techniques are still better than memorizing and cramming without any method at all.

Sprint vs. Marathon Running

"By failing to prepare, you are preparing to fail."
— Benjamin Franklin

Was this you in College?

- ❑ "I pulled an all nighter and passed. Whooooo !!!!!"
- ❑ "We Passed...Quadruple Mocca Latte Espresso and me."
- ❑ "I work better under 1,000 PSI pressure."
- ❑ "Did we give up when the Germans bombed Pearl Harbor?" – John Belushi in *Animal House.*

While these methods worked well in college and maybe even in med school, they will not work for this exam unless you were among the select few who studied during residency in lieu of eating.

If you procrastinate, you will find yourself at the 11th hour with too little time to adequately prepare. This is a **Marathon** you are preparing for, not a sprint. You must take steady *small* steps to prepare for the big event.

Artificial Intensity

Somebody once said:

" If it wasn't for the last minute nothing would ever get done"

Some of us need the "adrenaline rush" to get going and motivated, yet leaving studying to the last month is not going to work. On the other hand, without deadlines most of us won't be productive and other more pleasant activities will take over.

You need to find a way to trick the brain into believing there is a deadline. This will create the adrenaline rush many of you need to get unpleasant tasks done.

The solution is a compromise called *"mini-deadlines."* Mini-deadlines means breaking the Boards into smaller subcategories, making the project less formidable. If you set strict deadlines for completing each category, you get the benefit of working "under the gun."

- First, break the Boards into the subspecialties outlined in this book.
- Next- Break these into smaller subcategories.
- Divide your study week so that you put in at least 2 hours a night, 3 nights a week.
- Schedule this as you would schedule any appointment and you will stick to the plan.
- Next, schedule the topics you will study and review in each of these "appointment slots". This will ensure that you are not short at the end of the program.
- Allow some blank spots in between and for the last few weeks in case you underestimate the amount of time a given topic actually takes. In fact, *add 20% to the time you think it will take to cover a subcategory.*

Identify what material you do not like to study or is less "crammable." These are the subjects with which you should start. You have more energy early on and if you leave the topics that are of more personal interest to you for later, your interest will be maintained longer. Subjects like Fluids and Lytes, which really cannot be memorized and require you to think through and learn the physiology, should be done first. It is difficult to go over this material when you are anxious and pressed for time. And this is an important part of the exam.

When the Going Gets Boring!

You need to set up an actual study schedule. Set it up as if you had patients scheduled and have no choice but to show up. The actual schedule needs to be organized by you. You may be tempted to say that setting up a study schedule is a waste of precious time. You're wrong! In fact, you can't afford NOT to take the time.

This system gives you the advantages of advanced organized study along with the rush and thrill of cramming at the last minute. After all, if you "have to" get through Cardiology, it will be difficult to study when the *"going gets boring."*

Strike While the Iron is Cold

Yes you read that correctly. There are topics that you find more challenging and boring. Do these first . By striking while the iron is cold it will be easier to study the hotter , more interesting material later.

Gas Expands to Fill the Void

If you take a small amount of gas and put it into a large container, it will fill the entire space. We tend to do the same thing with our time.

If we have a lot of time, or we *perceive* that we have a lot of time (for example, 3 months to get ready for the boards), then less stressful activities will look more enticing. You'll say things like "I wonder how many likes I got on that photo of me on the beach on Instagram® in the past 3 minutes."

That is why this proven method works. You won't be sidetracked from a 2-hour *appointment* to "study thyroid disease." Again, the key is to trick the brain into believing there is a deadline to falsely create a sense of urgency.

As a result of this organized study, you will actually have *more time to do the things you enjoy,* **with half the guilt.** Heck, if you are one of the fortunate souls whose main source of joy and pleasure is studying calcium metabolism, you are in even better shape.

Each time you get through a topic you will feel empowered and the feeling is cumulative.

The 80/20 Rule:

In the *2018 edition of "Laughing your way to Passing the Pediatric Boards®"* we have focused on the material outlined in the most recent content specifications of the American Board of Pediatrics.

There is a core set of material that they have to test, and 80% of the material will come from these topics with 20% at most coming from new or updated material.

The 80/20 rule can apply to board preparation as follows:

- 80% of the exam will derive from the core material
- Spending 80% of your time on this material will improve your score 20%
- Make your study time 20% more efficient and you will retain 80% more material.

Think of the the 80/20 rule as you begin preparing for the exam. Knowing the core material cold will put you in a great position to pass.

Zebras may not be common in clinical practice, but they are very common "on the Boards"! However, there are only some zebras you need to know and these zebras are well represented in the core material we cover. Leave the Albino Zebras to those clustered around the 99th %ile.

Chapter 4

Board Games: Successful Test Taking Strategies

So, we've now walked you from signing up for the exam to getting to the Prometrics® Center. Now you've made it to sitting in front of the monitor for the test. The entire pre-season has led up to this, and now we're going to take you right into the end zone.

Don't Miss the Hidden Clues

You are allowed to use scratch paper and make notes. As you go through the questions we suggest you make notes. You will of course need to leave these notes behind, since you are not allowed to take notes out of the exam.

For any vignette, we suggest that you list out and write down in bulleted format:

- Pertinent negatives and positives in the history
- Abnormal physical findings and normal physical finding that you think are relevant[1]
- Abnormal labs and normal labs that you think are relevant
- Key words at the end of the question that tell you what they are specifically asking

HOT TIP When studying you are learning patterns based on descriptions. Therefore it is important to put "numbers" into "words." This pertains to vital signs and lab values especially. For example, if the heart rate is elevated, you shoult write "tachycardia" on the scratch sheet. If the chloride value is low write down "hypochlroremia."

Easy to Forget the Basics, But Don't

The basics are often forgotten. Unfortunately, this can result in careless errors negating all your hard work and focus.

Read the Question

When we get to a standardized exam we are told to "read the question." This is such a cliché that most of us glaze over when we hear it, since who *isn't* going to read the question? However, it is critical advice when you realize that reading the question means focusing on what they are really asking. Once again, this is often found in the last sentence.

HOT TIP Carefully note key words like "**except**," "**most**," "the cause," and "**most likely**" best accomplish this. By paying close attention to this, you will avoid careless errors.

---

[1] For example, if they list a newborn who is cyanotic and tell you he has no murmur, that's a pertinent negative.

Tripping on the Slippery — <u>Except</u> for Rocks

We are trained to look for the correct answers. When the question contains words like "except," "not," or "least," take more time with the question. Most questions have you look for the "correct" choices, and your mind is trained that way and is going to look for "correct" choices automatically.

If you are tired or it is late in the exam, *it is easy to get sloppy and choose one of the "correct" choices when the question is* **asking you to pick the incorrect choice.** Take the extra time to be careful when going through this type of question. Mentally cross out the "correct" choices as you read through the choices.

Know Your Own Way

Some folks like to read the question first; others like to read the choices first. Personally, I like to read the questions first and jot down the words I think are important and then read the answers. The other way, I find myself tricked by the traps and decoys they leave in the answer. Others swear by reading the answers first.

Best to try both methods while taking practice questions and see which works better for you.

Invest in Rest

We've said this before, but it bears mentioning again: do not study the day before and, if possible, do not study 2 days before the exam. This will pay off. If you have organized your study and treated it like the marathon it is, then anything you study during the last day will be counterproductive. Your brain needs to recharge and the information has to "marinate." Think of it as a muscle—you would not want to lift weights just before an athletic competition, and the same applies here.

THE FOUR FACES OF ABP: QUESTION FORMATS

FIVE ITEM MULTIPLE-CHOICE: With 5 choice MLQs there is one real answer and four distractions called "choices." Your job is to not be thrown off by the distractors that are carefully placed there by professional test writers and their collaborators.

One approach is to eliminate the answers you know are not correct, in order to avoid distraction. This will increase the chances of "guessing" the correct one if you are not sure. Other techniques are:

❑ Ignore the choices and read the entire question first.

❑ Come up with your own answer before looking at the choices.

❑ Compare each choice with what you thought it should be.

❑ Follow your gut reaction even if you don't know why.

Even if the correct answer jumps up at you, take the extra minute to read over the other choices. You might be surprised to find a "better" and therefore "BEST" answer.

Once again, it is especially important to read the question carefully when the answer jumps out at you. The question could be asking ' Each of the following is true EXCEPT "

In this case 2 choices will jump out at you as being correct but the one " incorrect " answer is the correct one.

If you find yourself between two answers that seem correct, look for the word or phrase that might make it "second best." Recheck the last sentence of the question to make sure you have read the question correctly.

If you are truly in the dark, choices which contain terms like "Always" and "Never" are usually not the correct answer.

Length sometimes does matter !

They need to get in a lot of information to have it be correct, and as a result the longest answer is often the correct one. Try this with your practice questions and see if it works. It often will.

CLINICAL Vignettes FOLLOWED BY SEVERAL QUESTIONS: Here they provide you with a volume of facts and data that would make even the most patient person's eyes glaze over from boredom. They may even give you the diagnosis and ask questions related to it.

Often they want you to:

- ❏ Come up with "the next step"
- ❏ Figure out something with the disorder or the inheritance pattern
- ❏ Determine treatment and management

By using solid memory techniques like the ones in this book, you will have the details locked in and linked to each other.

HOT TIP

Here's where jotting down the important points really comes in handy, by making pertinent pieces of information stand out and come together.

Multiple Guessing

Remember, there is no penalty for wrong answers. There will be questions to which you just have no clue. Statistically, you will get 20 -25% correct if you pick the same choice each time you are making a "wild guess." My favorite is B or C. You decide which is your favorite, but be consistent, and choose the same letter each time you are making a wild guess, ahem... **"educated choice"**.

Know When to Hold Them !

If you are truly stumped, and think it would help you to marinate some more and come back to the question later, then feel free to use the HOLD button. **But don't forget to "unhold" the question before walking away from the exam.**

PERIL

If you have a difficult time with the first three questions, don't panic. Take a deep breath and put them on hold and do the next questions. You will find those questions that you know cold. Slam-dunk a few of those to get your confidence back.

HOT TIP

Not only will you get your confidence back (which will allow you to go back to those initial difficult questions in a better mental state), but you may also find the key to the answer in questions found later in this section of the exam. Yes, this does happen.

Once you have ansered a few questions correctly the difficult questions won't be as daunting.

PERIL

During your review, change the answers only if you are **sure** you chose the wrong answer. Your instincts are usually correct when taking an educated guess. You can test this in the practice questions you take.

Finish Line

If you finish before the allotted time, do you just keep reviewing and reviewing? The answer is no! You should simply review 1-2 times and then close out the section and leave.

However, if you are confident enough to leave early, go ahead! This will allow you to take a break and possibly finish the exam earlier in the day, reducing the risk for the end of the day energy drop.

If you leave early, use the time to rest. Do NOT look up the answers during lunch and torment yourself. Your brain will serve you better if you rest it during the lunch break.

If there happen to be colleagues who are also taking the exam at your center, don't chit chat with them about the questions. This never helps anyone and usually just heightens anxiety.

Gotten Down to the Core

There are a few key principles that one needs to know. These are the facts, clinical principles and specific pieces of information that the Boards expect you to know.

There are also some general rules, e.g., "the least invasive test" is often the answer, "the child is normal; do nothing" is often the answer, etc. Going in with these rules will often score big points on the test.

If the words include "*grandmother has told parents*" the answer will, more likely than not, be "reassurance." **In general, "reassurance" is often the correct answer.**

Phrases and Mazes: Answers Found in Questions

Often the key to the answer can be found embedded in the question. This is because there are only so many ways to *classically* describe a disorder.

Therefore, becoming familiar with these hot phrases, buzzwords and keywords will allow you to pick up on the answers immediately. (How many ways can you describe a child with Henoch Schönlein Purpura or Rocky Mountain Spotted Fever?) We note some of these important keywords, buzzwords and classic pathognomonic patterns. Often these pathognomonic descriptions are the key to answering the question correctly.

Compass Points to Passing

The following principles can serve as a compass to help through the fog of anxiety or difficulty that you may encounter while taking the exam.

1. No Cutting Edge Here

If there is some raging controversy going on, it will not be tested on the exam. If there is, it is probably an experimental question for those who get their jollies from writing test questions. Recent developments will not appear on the test either. In general , the focus should be on the 80% of the basic core material you need to pass the exam.

2. Zebras and Geezers

Often, if there is a bizarre polysyllabic disorder that you read about in the *Accta Taurus Excretia*[2], it may very well be the correct answer.

3. That's "Mr. Vitamin A" To You

You will have to know the formal names for all vitamins and viruses. You will not see **Vitamin A** listed anywhere in the answer. Instead you will see **retinol**. What, you wanted them to make it easy for you?

4. Bus Full of Hemophiliacs

You will have to be familiar with the complications of common disorders and typical treatments of common diseases. This is more important than knowing about uncommon disorders.

5. Know Where You Come From

Just because you have never seen a case of Measles, Mumps, Rubella or CHICKENPOX, it doesn't mean they are not going to appear on the Boards. These, plus nutritional deficiencies, are all common occurrences on the Boards.

6. The Generalist is Always Right (Almost)

Calling in a consultant or a surgeon is often the wrong answer on the Boards. Choose this only if you are sure it is the correct answer. The one exception is the ophthalmologist, which is usually the correct answer. Likewise, again, the less invasive the test, the more likely it is going to be the correct answer.

7. Waiting to Develop

Often they have a mother come to the office complaining about a child's lack of development, compared to one of her other children. Again, the correct answer is often to "reassure the mother" unless there are real specific developmental delays described.

8. Déjà Vu All Over Again

You will be sitting there taking the test. You will put down an answer to question 18 that you are not quite sure of, and suddenly there you are on question 28, and the answer to 18 is right there in the wording of question 28.

You are not imagining things; this often happens. I am not sure if this is deliberate or coincidence, but it does happen. Unwrap it when it does: it is a gift. Of course, you might have to resist the temptation to shout out DAMMIT. That is because you just found the answer to question 17, from Section 1 and you are now at the end of Section 2. You won't be able to correct the error. These things happen.

Clinical Case Scenarios/Vignettes

This is a potentially intimidating part of the exam, but it need not be if you follow a few strategies to "tame" the "jungle of information" they throw at you.

---

[2] Latin for Journal of BS.

Steps to Simplify the Question

1. The disorders here are presented in their "classic" presentation. Follow the bouncing buzzwords that are sprinkled throughout our text , and often the diagnosis will jump out at you.

2. The labs and physical findings are all there for a reason. They are there to rule in or rule out something. Rarely there may be information deliberately left there to divert you from the correct answer. A careful read of the question and the other information will help prevent you from being tricked.

   Put abnormal labs into words on your scratch pad. For example, if a low serum sodium is one of the labs, write down hyponatremia.

3. Sometimes they have you read a lengthy diatribe. You're so proud that you have recognized the buzz words and identified the diagnosis, and then in the last sentence they tell you the diagnosis you just came up with and the following three questions are just "related" to the diagnosis. So why did they have you read the question? I don't know. But here is a solution:

If you see a lengthy clinical scenario taking up a half a page, read the last sentence to see if the diagnosis is sitting there. If so, read the question just in case, but you will be able to read it much faster already knowing what the diagnosis is.

Again, some folks suggest that you read the choices first. We don't usually recommend this since it may cause you to be tricked by the "distractors" they place there for you. Remember, often they are asking something you know cold, but it is foggy with a smokescreen of misinformation, numbers and data. Once you note the important points and put them into "words" on your scratch pad, the answer will be obvious and all your hard studying will work for you. **We cannot overemphasize the importance of "putting numbers into words".**

If you get distracted and deceived, you will be led down the primrose path to the wrong diagnosis. The traps will be laid in the phrasing of the question and the wrong choices will be there like landmines.

You will then order the wrong diagnostic test and come up with the wrong treatment. This is where knowing the key descriptive word or phrase is critical.

Our *Volume 3 QA : Vignettes* title walks you through this process with dozens of sample questions.

If you have studied the limited number of case scenarios in each specialty, the correct answer will become a reflex that only involves your spinal cord; you might even be able to check your neocortex at the coat check.

8 Simple Steps for Each Question

1. Free up the Facts with a Flashilight

Remember, one of the best ways to approach a dangerous and tricky situation is with a flashlight. In this case the flashlight is writing down important points on scratch paper and putting numbers and lab findings into words. This will enable you to add up the clinical facts with minimal distraction.

This technique serves two purposes.

One, you are **making important pieces of information stand out**. This allows you to go back and filter out irrelevant information that doesn't help or distracts you from identifying the correct diagnosis.

Two, there are pieces of information that **seem irrelevant** but are very relevant. These pertinent negatives are **windows** to the correct answer. Most of the points in the question are there for a reason; don't discount them unless you are certain that they are there as a deliberate distraction.

Going through this process will help you methodically distinguish the relevant from the irrelevant. It will also, by force of habit, help you identify the importance of seemingly irrelevant material.

 This is often where the key to the answer lies.

This extra step may seem time consuming at first, but if you do this on practice questions it will be second nature on the exam, and in the end it will help you better focus on the questions, making them a fun puzzle to solve, and will save you time and energy.

2. Analysis Leads to Paralysis

Often the question is simpler than you think. Over-reading and looking for tricks is how you can turn a slam-dunk into a missed lay-up. Too many of these can turn the tide to a failing grade. This is how fellows in pediatric cardiology, for example, can often end up with this section cardiology being their lowest score.

3. Read the Whole Question

On the other hand, even if you are sure of your answer, read the whole question to make sure you are not missing a better choice.

4. Down to Two Choices

Often you will be down to 2 choices. You will have to choose one as being more correct. They might ask, "What is the first thing you should do in clinical practice?" In clinical practice it seems like you would be doing them all first but on the Boards, you must make a choice. This is the gray zone, which is where the real thinking goes in. At this point, pay attention to the following:

❑ Is one choice more invasive?

Board Case: Choosing Between 2 Correct Choices

An example of being faced with 2 seemingly correct answers is the following scenario. They could present a clinical description of a small tension pneumothorax. It was easy to eliminate choice C, which was to order a Head CT.

Invariably you were down to B (insert a chest tube) and D (administer oxygen). You had to pick the "best choice" and the "first" thing you should do.

If you follow the checklist, you would come up with "administer oxygen," which is the correct choice. (If you overanalyze trying to see if they want to know that you know it IS a pneumo-thorax they are describing, you might be tempted to pick chest tube.)

Administering oxygen is the least inva-sive, and giving it may make the chest tube unnecessary. No harm is done, since you are administering oxygen while prepping for the chest tube, which is what you would do in "real life" anyway.

❑ Is there any harm in choosing one treatment over the other and will it impact outcome if you try it first?

❑ Consider what would absolutely be done first in clinical practice.

5. The Devil is in the Details

Pay attention to certain details like gender. Often this will give you a clue. For example, if the patient is a female, it is unlikely to be an **X-linked disorder**. If they describe the patient as coming from a certain ethnic group, they are not being politically incorrect; they are trying to point you to the diagnosis. Likewise, pay attention to the age of the patient. A 3-year-old with upper airway stridor is more likely to have croup than a teenager returning from a weekend snowboarding.

If they describe a patient who is visiting or immigrating from a **developing nation**, the answer will often be a **chronic condition** that has gone undiagnosed (e.g., sickle cell disease) or a disease that is rare in the US due to **immunization**. This disease may be common in other parts of the world, because of perceived or real inconsistent immunization practices outside the US. The same would apply for parents who they note are "against immunizations."

6. Put Numbers into Words

When you study the clinical descriptions, you are memorizing terms like "microcytic anemia," "febrile" "tachycardia," "tachypneic," "neutropenia," and "cyanotic mouth breathing drone."[3]

The main point is that you are memorizing the descriptions and not the numbers and the data. This is why it is important to actually write down in words what they are describing. Write it down in the scratch pad. Again we cannot emphasize this enough.

For example, if you note that the platelet count is low, you should write down "thrombocytopenia". If the respiratory rate is high, write down "tachypnea." In doing so, the picture they are drawing will come into focus.

7. Eliminate the Incorrect Choices

Eliminate all the wrong choices as you encounter them.

8. Move it Along: Nothing to See Here

Don't be afraid to move on if you have no idea what the answer is. Place these questions on hold but remember to release and answer the question later.

Another reason to not spend a lot of time on these bizarre questions: they may be experimental questions for the sheer enjoyment of the professional test writer or they may be thrown out due to a technicality. It would be a pity if you spent a lot of time on something like this.

---

[3] Oh sorry, the last one is a description of my college roommate who failed pre-med and is now in charge of auditing claims for a major insurance provider.

Final Word

Remember, most folks who fail are within 10-15 questions of passing. Following these test-taking techniques can often be an important deciding factor in answering these pivotal 10-15 questions correctly and thus the difference between passing and failing.

Section B: Pearls and Perils: Specific Core Facts and Details

Humorously Coded for Easy Memorization and Long Term Memory

Chapter 5

Research and Statistics
The Numbers Games

Safely Navigating the Minefields of Sensitivity and Specificity

Even though you will probably never be a bench scientist or personally engage in clinical trials, you will be required to know the basics of biostatistics and answer some questions on biostatistics on the exam.

You will be called upon to distinguish between sensitivity and specificity. In all likelihood, this will take place at a time in the exam when you yourself have been completely numbed and desensitized, to the point that you can't even distinguish light from dark. However, keeping a few basics in mind will help keep all this straight so you can get these predictable questions answered correctly.

We have heard from readers that the traditional explanation of sensitivity and specificity can be mind blowing no matter how many times they go through it. You are not alone! Before reading each of the explanations below, we provide the following mine-sweeping analogy to create a visual, more intuitive and less abstract, model. Pardon the violence, but we hope it helps. Harsh images also makes this easier to remember.

We will explain sensitivity and specificity in three ways:

(1) visual narrative

(2) equation

(3) table forms to bring these points home.

We believe that this model should help you understand the rest of the material since you can always go back to the visual narrative analogy to help avoid the minefield of confusion we have all encountered in keeping this straight.

Sensitive Mines

Imagine you are monitoring a minefield to determine the number of enemy combatants that are blown up by using the number of explosions you hear in the distance.

In the first case, you place mines that are **very sensitive** that go off regardless of the weight of the person or even animal that triggers the explosion. In this instance, if there are no explosions, then you know that no enemy combatants crossed. Therefore it is a very discriminant test. For example, a diagnostic test with a sensitivity of 100% has **no false negative results**. **Therefore the negative test results are reliable** (true negative).

However, since small animals could trigger the explosion, **positive results are not as reliable**. Therefore a highly sensitive test can have **lots of false positives** if it catches the wrong stuff, too. In this example, where a true positive means that soldiers triggered the mines, 5, for example, explosions triggered by rabbits would all be false positives.

This is why **sensitive tests are good screening tests.** A negative test rules out a disease but a positive test doesn't necessarily rule in the disease. An example would be ANA to screen for lupus. A negative ANA virtually rules out lupus. But a positive ANA just means further testing is needed to distinguish lupus from other disease that can cause or "trip" a positive ANA mine.

Still having trouble ? Just remember this, highly SeNsitive tests have reliable **T**rue **N**egatives (TN) with low **F**alse **N**egatives (FN). A positive screening test is not necessarily worrisome - it could have just "caught the wrong stuff" (these are the false positives!).

Sensitivity: the real deal

The probability that a test will correctly identify a True Positive (TP) result when used on a population with the disease (positive cases).

Looking at the ANA screening test again, a highly sensitive ANA screen will catch all patients with lupus. But remember, because highly sensitive tests can **also** "catch the wrong stuff," not all patients with a positive ANA screen will have lupus (i.e., false positives).

Calculating sensitivity: True Positives divided by the total number of all patients with the disease, including those *correctly* tagged positive (TP), and those *falsely* tagged negative (FN) on a test (True Positives + False Negatives).

$$\text{Sensitivity Formula:} \quad \frac{TP}{TP+FN}$$

In a test with high sensitivity, **negative** results can RULE OUT disease since there are very few false negatives. But a positive test result **may or may not be reliable.** Therefore, a test that is seNsitive could be a good screeNing test. Negative results are likely truly negative, so you can cease and desist further workup.

Remember, **N**egative results are reliable in seNsitive tests.

Specific Mines

Using the minefield analogy again here, let's assume the average soldier weighs more than 70 kg. We then set the mines to detonate at 70 kg or more. These are **specific** thresholds for detonation. In this case, rabbits and other small animals won't trigger the mines. Therefore, the number of explosions is **very specific** in helping you determine the number of soldiers who cross the field.

Still having trouble? Remember, sPecific tests have reliable **T**rue **P**ositives (TP) with low **F**alse **P**ositives (FP).

Since positive results are reliable, **a specific test can be used to determine treatment.** A positive urine culture would be an example of a specific test for a UTI, where treatment can be based on a positive result.

We believe that this model should help understand the rest of the material since you can always go back to this visual analogy to help avoid the minefield of confusion we have all encountered in keeping this straight.

While a positive result is very reliable, false negatives can occur. For example, if one soldier weighing less than 70 kg crosses the field, there would be no explosion. **A soldier getting away "without getting caught" by detonation represents a false negative result**. However, there are very few soldiers weighing less than 70 kg, and therefore one would expect very few false negatives.

Specificity: the real deal

The probability that a test will correctly identify a True Negative (TN) result when used on a population without disease (negative cases).[1]

Looking again at the example for urine culture, a clean-catch urine culture is highly specific and will catch all patients with a UTI grown on specific media. But remember, because a highly specific test on specific bacterial media can "miss" growth of other less frequent infectious causes (such as viruses), not all patients with a negative culture are actually infection-free (i.e., false negatives).

Calculating specificity: True Negatives divided by the total number of all patients without the disease, including those correctly tagged negative (TN), and those falsely tagged positive (FP) on a test (True Negatives + False Positives).

$$\text{Specificity Formula:} \quad \frac{TN}{TN+FP}$$

In a test with high specificity, there are very few false positives; so positive test results would be reliable. Positive results in highly specific tests can RULE IN disease. However, negative results aren't always reliable, as the test may "miss" some patients who fall outside the set threshold (false negatives). Highly speCific tests are therefore great **Confirmation tests** to verify the presence of disease.

Remember, Positive results are reliable in sPecific tests.

High sPecificity is good for confirming Positive disease.

Physicians may prefer tests with high specificity over those with high sensitivity in very important scenarios, where a false positive misdiagnosis would have consequences.

> ## The minefield of Positive Predictive and Negative Predictive Value
>
> A test with good positive and negative predictive values would be sensitive enough to minimize false negatives and specific enough to minimize false positives.
>
> In our landmine analogy this would translate to a mine that is sensitive enough to pick up all movement, and specific enough to distinguish human from animal movement.

---

[1] False positives: those tagged "positive" on a test even though they don't actually have the disease. True negatives: healthy patents who were correctly tagged "negative" for disease.

Positive Predictive Value (PPV)[2]

The probability that someone who tests positive actually has the disease and is not a false positive. This is usually much more important to clinicians than sensitivity or specificity (or it should be).

The higher the positive predictive value, the higher the reliability of a positive result.

PPV looks at the **reliability of a positive test** - how well a test actually identifies positive cases. Basically, it tells you how worried your patient should be with a positive result.

Calculating PPV: True Positives divided by all positive test results (True Positives + False Positives).

PPV Formula:
$$\frac{TP}{TP+FP}$$

Highly sensitive tests such as the ANA screen would NOT have a good positive predictive value since they are associated with a high false positive rate.

PPV is **directly** correlated with **prevalence** - the percentage of a population with disease at a given point (snapshot) in time. **Positive predictive value is most useful when the prevalence is high.** As prevalence increases, PPV increases. As prevalence falls, PPV falls.

For example, the positive predictive value for mammogram screening would be higher when limited to women over 40 rather than women of all ages.

The higher the positive predictive value, the higher the reliability of a positive result.

Negative Predictive Value (NPV)

The probability that someone who tests negative is actually disease free and is not a false negative.

NPV looks at the **reliability of a negative test** - how well a negative test result identifies patients with no disease.

The higher the NPV, the higher the reliability of a negative result.

Calculating NPV: True Negatives divided by all negative test results (True Negatives + False Negatives).

NVP Formula:
$$\frac{TN}{TN+FN}$$

In contrast to PPV, NPV is **inversely** correlated with prevalence. That is to say, NPV is most useful when the prevalence of disease is low. **As prevalence increases, NPV falls. As prevalence falls, NPV increases.**

For example, the negative predictive value of newborn sickle cell screening is higher when you test all infants in the US and not just African American infants.

---

[2] Not to be confused with Positive Pressure Ventilation or Pay Per View.

The table below shows an overview of sensitivity, specificity, PPV and NPV for the visually inclined. Memorizing this will earn you a few easy points on the exam.

	Positive Disease	Negative Disease	
Positive Test	True Positive (TP)	False Positive (FP)	**PPV:** TP/(TP+FP)
Negative Test	False Negative (FN)	True Negative (TN)	**NPV:** TN/(TN+FN)
Sensitivity: TP/(TP+FN)		**Specificity:** TN/(TN+FP)	

The Null Hypothesis and whether to Accept or Reject Mr Null's Proposal

Are we proving the null hypothesis or rejecting the null hypothesis when research confirms our results? Are you left with a giant null in your head when you think about this? Good. So are we - which is why we are here to help.

Null must have been a cynic. The null hypothesis basically claims that the results obtained are **due to chance alone**, and not due to the variables being studied.

In other words, the null hypothesis represents the cynic claiming that your intervention is not significant and is only a result of chance.

Therefore, the ideal goal of research is to be able to prove that the results are **not due to chance**, and reject the null hypothesis.

Rejecting the null hypothesis basically means the study results are "statistically significant."

P Value

The P value is one of the most misunderstood values, especially by clinical physicians who do not care to do research ever!

The P value represents **the chance that the null hypothesis was rejected in error**. Therefore it represents the odds that that **Null was correct and the results were due to chance** and not attributed to the studied variables. Obviously, you'd like Mr. Null to be very wrong and P value to be very small in order to find true cause and effects.

For example, a P value <0.01 means there is a less than 1 % chance that the null hypothesis was rejected in error and that the results are due to chance alone.

For purposes of the exam:

- P<0.05 is significant enough to reject the null hypothesis (i.e., "statistically significant")
- P<0.01 is even more significant enough to reject the null hypothesis (i.e.,"highly significant")

 The lower the P value, the more significant the study.

Type I and Type II errors

A **Type I error** is what we think of as a big OOPS - that we thought something was significant (or different, or better) when it really wasn't. That is, we **rejected the null hypothesis in error**.

 Therefore the probability of a Type I error is the same as the P value!

 Basically, the results of the study were mistakingly labeled as significant. The effect of the intervention was overestimated.

Type I error = 'I" screwed up with my study!

A **Type II error** is just the opposite of a Type I error- where we **rejected the null hypothesis** in error. Here, we determined that the findings **occured by chance**, and accepted the null hypothesis when in reality, they should have been attributed to the studied variables, and therefore statistically significant.

Basically, the results of the study were **mistakingly labeled as insignificant**, when there was actual strong evidence to support the study. **The effect of the intervention was underestimated.**

Obviously, in most cases of clinical medicine, a Type I error is worse than a Type II error. (Remember primum non nocere).[3]

Data analysis

Validity in research addresses whether an instrument or test actually measured what it intended to measure. Does a pacifier thermometer really give you the same reading as the rectal thermometer? **Internal Validity (IV)** reflects accuracy and **External Validity (EV)** reflects generalizability. There cannot be EV without IV. If a test is not accurate, it does not matter if it is generalizable.

Reliability refers to the consistency or repeatability of scores. If you did it again, with the same individual, would the same results be obtained? It may or may not be valid (like with the pacifier thermometer example).

---

[3] Latin phrase which means "First, do no harm."

Intention to Treat (ITT) analysis insists that all patients remain in the original groups to which they were initially randomly assigned in the study. You have to decide your "intention" at the beginning of the study and stay there, you can't change your mind and move the individuals to another group "mid-stream."

This helps maintain the power of the study because if patients could be moved to another group as the study progresses, the benefits of the original randomization process would be lost and bias would creep in.

The **Number Needed to Treat (NNT)** is defined as the number of patients that you would need to treat to prevent one additional adverse effect.

Example: Is it worth treating ear infections, when you realize that most ear infections resolve on their own? The number needed to treat would represent the number of children that you would have to start on antibiotics in order to prevent one complication. So if your complication is mastoiditis, how many kids with ear infections would need to be treated to prevent one episode of mastoiditis? Clearly, depending on your group (i.e., healthy 10 year olds vs HIV-positive toddlers), the NNT changes.

 Calculating NNT:

- Requires you to know the **Absolute Risk Reduction (ARR)** for the study treatment
- **ARR** = (rate in untreated group – rate in treated group); or (rate in treatment A - rate in treatment B)
- **NNT = 1/ARR**

These equations work best when used in **randomized controlled trial** settings where we are comparing 2 treatment groups; or a treatment versus control group. The whole point is to work with the more effective group that will lead to less adverse event outcomes as a result.

In the above example, let's say the incidence of developing the complication of mastoiditis in patients with acute otitis media treated with amoxicillin is 15% (i.e., 0.15), and untreated control groups is 65% (i.e., 0.65). We can then calculate ARR using only the difference (without any positive or negative value signs):

ARR = (rate in untreated group - rate in treated group) = [0.65-0.15] = 0.50. Therefore, NNT = 1/ARR = 1/0.50 = 2. So, we would need to treat 2 people for acute otitis media in order to avoid 1 adverse event of mastoiditis.

Reading and Interpreting Results

 Incidence - the number of newly diagnosed cases of a disease in a given period of time.

Prevalence - the total number of cases of disease (in %) existing in a population at a given time ("snapshot").

Standard deviation - a measure of the spread of individual values around the mean or average value.

The **standard error** describes how accurate the sample mean value used in the analysis is compared to the "true" population mean value. It stands to reason then, that the closer the sample mean is to the "true" mean, the more accurate the study results are.

Example: If you are trying to determine the average height of 10 year old girls in the U.S., then your study individuals should have a range of heights that are representative of the general population, because you obviously cannot study the entire population of the U.S.

The **confidence interval** (CI) is a measure of the reliability of your result. It consists of a range of values in which you are confident that the true population result will be found. In some instances, the true population result may be missed altogether.

Example: In the example above, if you choose your study cohort from an elementary school in California that serves mostly an underprivileged Mexican population, the results would likely not be representative of the general population of the U.S.

In applied practice, confidence intervals most commonly used are at the 95% confidence level (i.e., the level at which you are 95% confident that your result lies within the true result of the general population).

Greater levels of variance within a population yield larger confidence intervals, and therefore less precise estimates of the measure.

"**Statistically significant**" means that the results obtained are likely related to the intervention, and therefore have a small probability of occurring by chance alone.

"Statistically significant" does not automatically imply clinical importance.

Although this measures a chance of association or causality, it does not measure strength of association or clinical importance. For example, a quiet NICU leads to a decrease in premie heart rate. Is this decrease clinically important? That is a whole separate question: Does it happen? Yes. Does it matter? Who knows ?

The **pre-test probability** is your best estimate of the probability that a condition is present before you start diagnostic testing. The diagnostic test result will help you establish your **post-test probability** of the suspected condition. For example, how likely do you think the diagnosis of strep throat is before you see the rapid Strep test result?

You may get confused between Positive Predictive Value (PPV) and pre-test probability. I know that I did! **The PPV applies to a test. The pretest probability applies to a condition.** What is the probability a condition exists before you even run the test?

The **Likelihood Ratio (LR)** of a test is the likelihood that a person who has the condition (i.e., strep throat) will have a positive test result (i.e., positive rapid strep test). The LR indicates by how much the result of the test will raise or lower your pretest probability and get you closer to the post-test probability.

Remember, a test's sensitivity and specificity come into play here. Suppose you see a patient with sore throat. You are 80% certain she has strep throat after the history and physical, but before the rapid strep test. When you run the rapid strep test, how does your 80% change if the test is positive? How about if the test is negative? Keep in mind that positive and negative rapid strep test results are not 100% diagnostic.

• L.R. > 1 increases the probability that the condition is present.

• L.R. < 1 makes the condition less likely.

The **Absolute Risk (AR)** of developing a condition is calculated by dividing the number of patients who develop disease by the total patients exposed.

$$AR = \frac{(+)\ \textbf{disease patients}}{\textbf{total patients (in \%)}}$$

The **Relative Risk (RR)** compares the probability of an outcome in the exposed group to the probability of the outcome in an unexposed group. For example, what is the relative risk of UTI in a circumcised infant vs an uncircumcised infant?

$$RR = \frac{\textbf{EXPOSED patients (disease/total)}}{\textbf{UNEXPOSED patients (disease/total)}}$$

The **Odds Ratio (OR)** represents the *o*dds of an outcome in one group compared to the odds of that outcome in another group. For example, what are the odds of developing a UTI in a circumcised infant vs. an uncircumcised infant?

$$OR = \frac{\textbf{CASES (exposed/unexposed)}}{\textbf{CONTROLS (exposed/unexposed)}}$$

		OUTCOME	
Exposure		Cases	Controls
		UTI	No UTI
Circumcised (exposed)		a	b
Uncircumcised (unexposed)		c	d

A R = a/(a+b)
R R = [a/(a+b) / c / (c+d)]
OR = [a / (a + c) / b / (b + d)]

Make sure to go over this chart a few times with real numbers to understand these concepts well.

Let's assign numbers to the table above, where

    a= 5,
    b= 95,
    c= 200, and
    d= 800.

We can now use this information to calculate each ratio:

- AR = a/(a+b) = 5/(5+95) = 5/100 = 0.05 = 5% chance of getting a UTI if a boy is circumcised.
- RR = [a/(a+b) / c/(c+d)] = 5/(5+95) / 200/(200+800) = (5/100) / (200/1000) = 0.25, meaning that a circumcised boy is 0.25 times as likely as an uncircumcised boy to get a UTI. Alternatively, an uncircumcised boy is 4 times more likely to get a UTI than a circumcised boy.
- OR = [a/(a+c) / b/(b+d)] = [5/(5+200) / 95/(95/800)] = (5/205) / (95/895) = 0.23, which are the odds of developing a UTI in the circumcised group. Therefore, the odds of developing a UTI are reduced by 77% with a circumcision.

Studying Studies

 Even though most of us are not enrolled in an MD/Ph.D program and will only be reading review articles and other CME activities to remain current, not sifting through original studies questioning their validity, we are nevertheless expected to know the nuts and bolts of setting up a study, analyzing the results and interpreting their validity.

This is in addition to keeping up with a busy practice and understanding the Affordable Care Act better than the representatives who drafted it and are, in the end, exempt from the law they passed anyway.

We will try to keep this staggeringly painfully bone-dry topic simple and easy, cooking it all down to digestible nuggets that will keep you sufficiently nourished on the exam.

"Best practice" in medical care is derived from "**evidence-based**" care, key word being **evidence**. And just like in *Law and Order*, some evidence is stronger than other evidence, and some is not really evidence at all but opinion, and some was planted to throw you off the track. To paraphrase George Orwell from A*nimal Farm*, some evidence is more equal than others.

You are expected to understand the following validity hierarchy. They are listed in order from BEST to not-so-best.

- Systematic reviews, Meta-analysis
- Randomized, controlled trials
- Cohort Studies
- Case-control studies
- Cross-sectional studies
- Case studies/Case reports
- Expert opinions/Editorials

Systematic reviews/Meta-analyses are discussed in detail at the end of the chapter.

Randomized Controlled Trials

Randomized Controlled Trials (RCTs) are considered the **gold standard** of research designs. Study participants are assigned randomly to one treatment or another (or no treatment).

A major strength of RCTs is the minimalization of confounding variables by making the baseline groups equivalent. They are also usually "blind" to both the participants and those administering the study (aka, "double-blind" studies).

A RCT therefore reduces both expectation (or performance) bias by patients and ascertainment bias by study interpreters regarding the results. Limitations of this study are usually the cost and time required.

Cohort Studies

Cohort studies involve comparison of a group (or cohort) with an exposure to a control group without an exposure. The cohorts can be analyzed in two ways:

1) **prospective cohort studies**, which follow both groups over time as an ongoing process to evaluate for a future outcome, or

2) **retrospective cohort studies**, which **trace both groups through previously collected medical records/data from a starting set-point at an earlier time,** to investigate associated risks for a certain outcome. These are also known as "historical cohorts."

An example for a prospective cohort study: you wonder if exposure to violent video games causes children to become violent. To study this, you might choose a group of boys who play violent video games, and another group of boys who have never been allowed to play violent video games, and compare the rates of violent actions (bullying episodes, fight suspensions, etc) between the two groups.

Advantages of cohort studies include clearly-set time intervals from exposure to outcome; which allow for calculation of the rate of disease in exposed and unexposed individuals. These also allow us to study multiple outcomes.

Limitations of these studies are large sample size required and the long time necessary for the study. They are relatively expensive, and many subjects may be lost to follow up due to the length of time required for the study to be completed..

Case-control Studies

Case-control studies are useful when you only have a **small** sample size, a long latency period, or a rare outcome. You start with patients with the disease ("case") and patients without the disease ("control"), and then check for exposure to risk factors.

In contrast to cohort studies, case-control studies begin with a known outcome of each group, and retroactively evaluate exposure. For example: is MMR vaccine linked to autism? You would start with a group of children with autism (cases) and without autism (controls). You would then see how many got the MMR vaccine **before developing autism symptoms**, and how many didn't.

Advantages of case-control studies are that they allow for the study of multiple risk factors, are quick to conduct, are relatively inexpensive, and require fewer subjects than a cohort study. A significant limitation is the risk of confounding variables.

Cross-sectional Studies

Cross-sectional studies are observational, and are great at looking at associations between two measured factors at one point in time (i.e., "snapshot" time interval). They do not look at measures over time. **Limitations include the risk of confounding variables, and that the results cannot be used to infer causality.**

An example of a cross-sectional study would be to check the heart rates of walkers on the day of a fundraising walk to benefit the homeless (or in some parts of the country, those too poor to upgrade their smart phone annually).

You could then separate these heart rate results by gender, age, height, weight, religion, hair color, political orientation, or whatever you want; and try to make associations (i.e., people with red hair run higher heart rates than people with blond hair); but all you know is the heart rate of that population on that specific day. And just because you see an association, you cannot conclude from this that the red hair is the reason for the higher heart rate. Correlation doesn't mean causation.

Case Reports

Case reports and **anecdotal reports** are based on **individual outcomes**. They are limited because they may have many confounding variables.

For example, you note that one child's wheezing resolved after a dose of phenobarbital for his seizure disorder. Another child's wheezing resolved after he reached the 2nd level of the Legend of Zelda®. Does this mean we should start considering these as treatments for wheezing? Most teenagers would say yes to Zelda!®

At best, you could say that a case report presents an interesting possibility that someone might want to design a study on in the future.

Longitudinal Studies

Longitudinal studies involve studying the same group of individuals over an extended period of time. For example, do people who walk one mile every day lower their resting heart rate over time? do teens who play combat video games have the same cardio benefits as those who walk a mile every day?

Reviewing Review Articles

Systematic Review

A **systematic review** uses a well-defined approach to locate and summarize articles related to a clinical question. It requires:

1. A specific clinical question,
2. A thorough search for studies,
3. A clear explanation for which studies were considered and which were not, and
4. A descriptive results section summarizing the findings.

Meta-analysis

A **meta-analysis** pools all the statistical results collected from a group of articles. A meta-analysis should meet all 4 criteria for a systematic review, **plus**:

A. Present a summary statistic using data from all of the included studies,
B. Report whether combining all the statistics was even possible, and
C. Assess for publication bias, meaning that some studies were not published but would have affected the data.

Because both systematic reviews and meta-analyses are large-scope reviews that evaluate data from multiple published studies; they **have the highest validity** (although meta-analyses are better). However, heterogeneity in data collection, analysis and interpretation of each included study makes these designs difficult to generalize.

In addition, these reviews are limited by the concept of "garbage in, garbage out," meaning that your conclusions are based on data collected outside of your control. If the data was not correct, then your conclusions will not be correct.

Chapter 6

Sketches about Ethics

You can expect to be tested on questions on medical ethics. Since passing can often come down to just a few questions here and there, familiarity with some basic concepts can be the difference between passing and failing. In this chapter, we present the key information that will allow you to navigate these questions, successfully turning them into low hanging fruit.

To Treat or Not to Treat: That is the Question

Family values

It is important to know that there is no **ethical difference** between withholding or later withdrawing treatment.

Doctor vs. Parent

The opinion and guidelines of the family prevail over your opinion as the physician. The only exception is when **the interests of the child** in your opinion differ from the parent/guardian's opinion. In cases where there is a conflict, resolution would require the opinion of an ethics committee.

Disabuse in cases of Abuse

Of course if a child is the victim of nonaccidental trauma (a.k.a. child abuse), the parents (if they are the perpetrators) will not be considered to have the child's best interest in mind. Clearly their decisions will be, pardon the pun, disabused in favor of the doctor. When considering suspension of treatment in cases of child abuse, an alternate guardian would be appointed or the hospital ethics committee would be involved.

Guess Who's Coming to DNR

In general, once again, the family's decisions should determine when and how to implement DO NOT RESUSCITATE (DNR) orders.

Interventions during surgery

In situations when a child has DNR orders in place and the child is going in for a surgical procedure, it would be difficult for the surgical team to determine if they can implement a certain intervention during

Advance Directives

Advanced directives are written documents that describe the wishes of the family regarding the elements of advanced care planning. This would include end-of-life care.

Palliative care of course comes into play with the diagnosis of a life threatening condition or situation. This would focus on the physical, social, psychological and spiritual needs of the child.

the surgery. For example could they resolve a surgical complication such as hypoxia or an arrhythmia? Without that ability, most surgeries, would not be worth the risk.

In such instances, temporary suspensions to the standing DNR orders would be appropriate. These are referred to as "beneficial interventions" or "required reconsiderations".

These routine "beneficial interventions" or "required reconsiderations" should be planned in advance and be very specific.

If the treatment is indicated and cannot be obtained any other way, you are the patient's advocate and are to hold to that duty despite any financial disincentives.

Not so Crucial Services

On the other hand, families may wish to obtain treatments and services that the pediatrician feels are not helpful and it is made clear in the question that the treatment is not essential. In that case, it would be appropriate to decline advocating for these services. However, you are expected to explain to the family why you are not willing to advocate for these services.

> ### Limiting Limited Resources
>
> Important points to keep in mind when answering questions on allocation of health care include:
>
> - Rationing of healthcare is a fact of life the question is where and how (duh!)
> - Taking cost into consideration is not unethical, in fact on a global level it is very ethical
> - NICU costs are disproportionately high and there are approaches which can help ration that care appropriately

Tricky NICU: Imperiled Newborns

All treatment decisions are based on the newborn's best interest, factoring in parental wishes. In the end, the newborn's best interest overrides parental wishes. Again, when these are at odds, the decision is made through the ethics committee.

You can be presented with various scenarios including

> A) **Treatment is clearly futile, and yet the parents wish to continue treatment** – in this case the correct decision is to override the parents with the help of the hospital ethics committee or other resources.
>
> B) **The best interests are not clear but the parents wish to withdraw care** – In this situation, where the effectiveness of treatment is unclear, it is appropriate to defer to the parents authority.

Withdrawal must be based on **the best long term interests** of the infant. Watch for hints that the issue is the staff growing weary of the futility of care but the treatment is not necessarily futile.

Regarding extreme prematurity, the gold standard question is the percentage of survival with *maximal care* rather than on gestational age alone.

Organ transplantation and donation

Dead Donor Rule – stipulates that the removal of both paired/vital organs or one non paired vital organ cannot precede or cause death.

Watch for a question where it is not clear that the donor was declared dead by universally accepted standards. Monty Python fans can recall the "bring out your dead" scene where the person about to be placed in the cart declares "I'm not dead yet"!

Cardiorespiratory Death is considered to be a controversial definition of death.

A DNR order cannot factor in the DONOR status of the patient - The decision to withdraw or withhold treatment must be made independent of the organ donation status of the donor patient or potential benefits to the organ-receiving patient.

Maternal-Fetal Conflicts

You will likely be asked at least one questions where the maternal and fetal benefits are in conflict.

You are expected to know that the autonomy and bodily integrity of the mother is critical and must be honored. Consider this in answering any question that poses maternal –fetal conflict of interest.

You could be presented with a scenario where a Cesarean section is recommended for *variable* decelerations and the mother refuses. You would be expected to reinforce the need for the section while validating the mother's concerns and confirming your support for her decision.

Since variable decelerations are not necessarily life threatening, there is wiggle room allowing for the mother's wishes to be honored.

Threats of legal coercion including intervention by the courts, will be the wrong answer regarding a Cesarean section.

Rights During Pregnancy

An important concept is that pregnant women have the same rights to make medical decisions as those who are not pregnant.

Brain Death Defined

There is enough confusion over what constitutes brain death to render one comatose after sifting through the definitions.

You may nevertheless be asked to answer mindless questions on brain death and it will be useful to learn the following basics

Consciousness - involves wakefulness and awareness of self and environment.

Coma – Patients in a coma lack wakefulness and also lack awareness of self and environment.

Vegetative State – Patients in a vegetative state lack awareness but do have wakefulness.

Conditions that can mimic brain death must be treated or excluded. This would include correction of metabolic derangement, intoxication and hypothermia.

Autonomy

Basically autonomy in pediatrics is graded with age and development.

 Parents have authority and NOT autonomy over their children.

Beneficence and Nonmaleficence

No, these are not the godmothers in *Sleeping Beauty*, they are the other two guiding principles in Ethics, besides Autonomy.

Beneficence is the duty of the physician to act in the best interest of the patient.

Nonmaleficence is the duty to do no harm.

Therefore you could be presented with a mother who needs to be treated for depression or newly diagnosed cancer.

In this case the correct course would be to **help the mother make the decision** based on best evidence and the specifics of the situation. Options could include deferment of treatment or termination of the pregnancy[1] to begin treatment.

In any questions regarding conflict of maternal-fetal interest, discussion of all aspects and respecting the woman's decision are key. This would include a woman suffering from depression or other mental illnesses, which should not detract from respecting the mother's wishes. Of course it might require more clarification, but the main point is the mother's wishes are always of tantamount importance.

What about underage mothers?

All states either allow the minor mother to make all decisions for her newborn, or or have no policy on the matter. Any concerns brought forth, perhaps by the medical team or the teen's mother, would be resolved by family court.

The Age of Assent

An important principle you can be tested on is assent. Although children cannot make decisions on their own and consent to treatment, they should participate in the decisions. In other words they should be made to feel important and empowered even if they are not in complete control of the final decision.

Assent basically equals willingness to accept treatment. Unlike consent, it is not mandatory, it is just preferred.

The following should be considered when approaching questions on this topic

- The child's input should be solicited
- The child should be helped to gain an age-appropriate understanding of the situation
- Be honest in telling the child what to expect regarding treatment
- Try to understand the factors that influence the child's conclusions

In cases where treatment is not essential, or in cases of non-therapeutic research, the child's assent should be an important consideration in the parent's consent.

If a culture does not traditionally factor in a child's opinion, this should be respected and not outright rejected.

In situations where treatment is crucial or lifesaving and will be undertaken regardless of the child's assenting to the plan, the child should be told this and his opinion not requested.

> ### No Shots for Me! It's my religion!
>
> When answering questions regarding parental refusal to vaccinate (for religious or other reasons) the correct answer will center on the use of open communication to discuss and understand vaccine refusal or hesitancy
>
> Vaccine refusal does not meet criteria for medical neglect and parents should be allowed to refuse vaccines without concern for being reported to child protective services. Vaccines, at least at the time of publication, cannot be forced by court order.
>
> In other situations where the treatment is likely to prevent substantial harm, the child's right to treatment outweighs parental religious freedom.

---

1 They could only present you with a first trimester termination rather than a later stage pregnancy, since the mother could not elect something in and of itself that is an ethical dilemma.

Screening Through the Screens of Newborn Testing

Passively-Permitted-Not-Quite-Mandatory Newborn Screening

Newborn screening is not mandatory. However, by doing nothing, parents are **giving passive permission**. Opting out of newborn screening requires their actively signing a waiver.

In determining whether a disease should be included in newborn screening, the disease should

- Have a significant deleterious effect on the child
- Have effective treatment available if diagnosed early
- Have a screen that is acceptable to the population[2]

Keep this in mind if you are asked about a disorder that is being considered for inclusion in newborn screening.

Blinded by the Screen

Newborn screens are not diagnostic. False positives are common and only a trigger for more definitive testing.

We just told you that false negatives should be low, but they are NOT zero. Some cases WILL get missed by screening. So be careful. You may be presented with a patient who has a classic presentation of a metabolic disorder that was negative on a newborn screen. Don't be tricked into believing a negative screen completely rules out the disease. The correct answer will center on working up the disorder regardless.

Reflexive referral for genetic counseling, especially for only a positive newborn screen without confirmation, will never be the correct answer.

"Correcting" Ambiguous Genitalia

Ambiguous genitalia is being replaced by the more general term "disorders of sex development".

For the purposes of the exam, it is important to note that determining which gender to raise the child should be a multidisciplinary approach.

---

[2] This is included in the Wilson and Büngner 1968 WHO report for those who really must know.

PERIL

Before implementing irreversible genital surgery, the possibility of gender change in adulthood should be factored in and the surgery should be reversible if possible. Likewise fertility should be preserved if possible.

Risk-benefit principles apply here and you are expected to be open and honest when dealing with parents. In addition, when the child gets older, the child should be told of the medical condition gradually and based on the child's developmental level. Their condition should not disclosed as a shocking surprise in adulthood.

Integrating Complementary, Alternative, and Conventional Treatment

Do you know the difference between integrative, complementary and alternative treatments? I didn't think so! Well you will need to know this difference and a bit more for the exam.

We will of course integrate all of that for you right here.

DEFINITION

Conventional medicine is intended to be based on knowledge of safety and efficacy obtained from randomized, controlled trials. It excludes all treatments that are not supported by such studies and evidence.

DEFINITION

Alternative medicine are treatments that are outside of conventional treatments, and include chiropractic treatment, herbs, bioelectronics remedies, and nutritional therapy.

DEFINITION

Complementary medicine uses both alternative treatments as well as conventional treatments.

DEFINITION

Integrative medicine blends conventional medicine and alternative therapies for which there is some evidence of safety and effectiveness.

PERIL

There is a very fine difference here between complementary and integrative. Integrative would include things that were once considered to be alternative but are now considered evidence-based, such as omega-3 rich fish oil and probiotics.

UPDATED & NEW BREAKING NEWS INFORMATION

You could be presented with a child with a chronic illness where the parents want to include alternative, integrative and / or complementary medical therapy.

After factoring in the safety of these treatments you have to also consider patient autonomy and parental authority when answering these types of questions.

DEFINITION

Some herbs and vitamins can interfere with the metabolism and elimination of medications, for example St. John's Wort and garlic. This could very well be include in a question where a medication isn't as effective as it had been in the past.

What is the correct approach to patients using non conventional treatment?

- Risk-benefit rules apply whether discussing conventional or non - conventional treatment.
- Courts won't interfere with the use of alternative treatment unless it is life threatening or coupled with refusal to use conventional treatment.
- Medication that is less effective than proven conventional treatments should not be used *instead* of these proven conventional treatments.
- IF a physician is not comfortable with the alternative treatment, then transfer to another physician who is comfortable, would not be inappropriate.

The Enchantment of Enhancement Therapy

Regardless of the specific enhancement therapy mentioned, you are expected to counsel parents on the importance of individualism and happiness being independent of extrinsic factors. In other words, being the tallest and brightest doesn't lead to happiness which is intrinsic not extrinsic.

This is of course philosophical but it is the correct philosophy on the boards.

The Growing use of Growth Hormone

The conditions for which growth hormone is FDA-approved include *Turner syndrome, chronic renal insufficiency* and *Prader-Willi syndrome.*

Non growth hormone deficient idiopathic short stature is also an FDA-approved indication. It's effectiveness and positive psychosocial impact is debatable. The cost can also be substantial.

Research and Children

Informed Consent

Informed consent has three aspects

1) Information about the proposed research,
2) Assessment of participant's understanding and decision making capacit
3) Signing of the consent document.

Minors younger than 7 must have consent from their guardians or proxies.

Children who are 7 or older, in addition to consent from their guardian, must also "assent" to the participation. This I because 7 is the age of (you guessed it) assent.

Healthy children cannot participate in studies that involve more than minimal risk.

Children with a condition or disorder can participate in studies that pose "more than" minimal risk if there is potential benefit to them from the study. This would include an experimental treatment where there are no other known proven-effective treatments.

If there is no direct benefit, then the study could be appropriate only if there is a "minor" increase over minimal risk.

These are the buzz words that will likely be used in the question. While they are subjective in the real world, they will be absolute on the boards.

Chapter 7

Patient Safety and Quality Improvement

Medical Errors

The failure to complete a planned action as intended, or the use of a wrong plan to achieve an aim.[1] **A medical error does not need to result in harm to the patient.**

Active errors occur at the point of interface between humans and a complex system, for example ordering the wrong medication or overriding an alert.

Latent errors are less apparent problems within a system that contribute to adverse events, like lack of an alert, or a nursing shortage).

Medication Error

A medication error is **the most common type of medical error**. As you should realize, it is an error that involves medication.

This includes errors in ordering, transmission of e-scripts, preparing, labeling or administering the medication.

Preventing Medication Errors

You are expected to be familiar with, and can be tested on, important steps that can be implemented to reduce medication error including:

- **Current Medications:** Identifying current medications the patient is on including OTC and herbal medications.
- **Staying away from Nuts:** Including drugs and foods as well as the specifics of any reactions in the allergy list. When patients are allergic to nuts are they supposed to stay away from people that are considered to be nuts? Sorry couldn't resist.
- **Doctor's handwriting** – this is the same admonition to school children since the inception of hieroglyphics and is becoming less relevant in the age of EMR but for purposes of the boards this is still relevant.
- **Avoid obscure and confusing abbreviations** – "when it doubt write it out" is the old maxim i.e. write out "daily" instead of "QD" and write out "units" instead of "U".

---

[1] These are defined by the Institute of Medicine (IOM).

- **No Weight Poor Fate** - for obvious dosing purposes, a weight must be obtained for all pediatric patients.
- **Dewey Decimal Manners: Zeroes Go First** – zeroes precede and never follow numbers that involve decimals. For example, 0.5 is acceptable, but 5.0 is not acceptable since it can be confused with 50.
- **What's this for?** – For medications that sound alike, the diagnosis should be included in prescriptions and verbal orders. Imagine a child with ADHD being prescribed Methadone instead of Methylphenidate. On the other hand a drug seeker being prescribed Lodine® (an NSAID) instead of Codeine might not be a bad thing, but you see the point and what you could be tested on.

Adverse Events

An adverse event is **an injury caused by medical management** rather than by the underlying disease or condition. By definition, an adverse event **causes harm** to the patient.

Most medical errors do not lead to an adverse event! Likewise, many adverse events are not caused by medical errors, but by **unexpected complications** of the planned medical management.

Most medical errors are a consequence of system based issues. Therefore, focus should be on system improvements and solutions rather than individual blaming or reprimanding.

Adverse Drug Event

An adverse drug event (ADE) is **an injury resulting from the use of a drug**.

An adverse drug event may be due to a **medication error**, but it could also be due to an **unforeseen reason** such as an unknown drug allergy.

Near Miss Event

This is a potential adverse event where a medical error places a patient at risk for injury **without actually resulting in injury**.

They could describe **2 situations** on the exam that would be considered to be near miss events.

- Intercepted
- Non intercepted

> **Era of No Errors !**
>
> You might be asked to choose methods that reduce or even prevent medication errors. These include the following:
>
> 1) Keep your pharmacist close by and involved
> 2) Computerized order entry (does anyone actually use handwritten prescription pads anymore?)
> 3) Education and inclusion of team members
> 4) Pre-Printed standard order sheets
> 5) Medication administration based on bar codes

With an **intercepted error,** the error is noted before it gets to the patient. For all intents and purposes, it never happened. You prescribe 4,000 mg amoxicillin twice a day for a toddler and the pharmacist calls you to see if you have lost your mind! You confirm that you still have a functioning neocortex but are using a new EMR to comply with meaningful use. You correctly prescribe 400 mg and no harm no foul to the patient.

A **non-intercepted error** as you can guess, is an error that reaches the patient.

It **may or may not cause injury.** If you prescribe amoxicillin to a toddler who has a documented amoxicillin allergy, and the toddler takes it but has no adverse effect, it would be considered a non-intercepted error that caused no harm.

Sentinel Event

An unanticipated actual or potential **death or serious physical or psychological injury** as a result of medical care.

"Never Events"
A serious reportable event is an error in medical care that is identifiable, preventable, and has serious consequences for the patient. They are also called "Never Events" because they should never happen in a hospital, such as wrong-side surgery.

Not all sentinel events are a result of medical error but **all sentinel events require root cause analysis (RCA)** to search for improvements in the system.

Children are not Just Little Adults[2]

The risk for ADEs is 3 times higher in hospitalized children than adults.

Weighted Errors

As anyone taking this exam and reading this book knows, medications doses are **weight specific** for children. This can be hard on anyone, but especially on non pediatricians in a setting that is not accustomed to caring for children.

Root Cause Analysis
Root Cause Analysis (RCA) is a **structured method** used to analyze serious adverse events and find **system problems** (latent errors) to prevent incidents from recurring.

On a similar note, watch for questions involving compounding **adult prepackaged medications** for children. This is a common cause of dosing error.

---

[2] But some adults are just big babies.

Nicks in the NICU

 Even in the NICU where, by definition, the care is centered on infants, medication error is a high risk. Do not assume that medication error isn't a factor just because they are describing a situation in a NICU setting.

Parents Is People Too!

Yes the grammar is incorrect. This is to point out that medical errors can occur outside of the hospital and doctor's office.

When presented with a patient with an adverse reaction, read the question carefully and pay particular attention to descriptions of:

- Parents or caregivers who **do not speak English well**[3]
- Use of **home folk or traditional remedies** interacting with prescribed medications

First Do No Harm

You are expected to understand and answer questions on the impact of medical errors on pediatric patients. We have put together some important information that will help you approach such questions without being the victim of your own errors on the exam.

M and M of Medical Errors

The mortality and morbidity of medical errors in pediatric patients has thankfully come under focus over the past 10 years.

Some important statistics to keep in mind:

- Adverse events occur in 1% of pediatric hospitalizations
- 60% of these events are preventable

The rising ADE rates may reflect an increased ability to detect rather than an actual increase in the incidence of these events. Therefore make sure you read the question carefully.

Follow the Money Trail of Medical Error

The estimated cost of medical errors in the US is believed to be $37 billion each year. That is a lot of student loan repayment.

---

3 Did you know that ONCE is eleven in Spanish? SO ordering a medication ONCE A DAY could be a big problem.

Medical errors increase the length of stay and Medicare and Medicaid are beginning a trend of not reimbursing to correct these errors. Of course "government money see, private money do" and private insurance companies will soon be doing the same.

This issue will likely find its way to the boards.

Just the Facts:
Detecting and Reporting Events

Let's face it, nobody wants to be called out for, or even admit to, making a medical error. Nobody wants to be a whistleblower. However, this isn't what's best for patient outcomes and *this* is the take home message when answering any question on the boards dealing with this issue.

Like the crowd witnessing a mugging waiting for someone else to call the police, most medical errors likely are unreported. It is very likely that known statistics are an underestimation.

After a medical error is identified, the correct answer would note that there should be a discussion, to review the error and find solutions. That discussion should take place as soon as possible.

Barriers to Reporting

You are expected to be aware of the barriers to reporting medical errors and correctly answer questions on the subject. Some of these barriers include:

- Not wanting to be blamed
- Not wanting to appear to be incompetent
- Not wanting to be the whistleblower
- Fear of Litigation
- Fear of Hierarchy and Retribution

Responsible and Effective Reporting

Many people complain about the effectiveness of random searching at the airport vs selective and strategic searching.[4] The same applies here, randomly auditing charts for medical errors would waste resources and will likely be unfruitful.

Smoking Gun and Triggering

One method you could be tested on is **"triggering"** which is basically a smoking gun technique. For example, auditing all charts where the use of a drug to reverse sedation could identify an adverse drug event involving a sedative.

---

[4] This is just a metaphor please not emails about the pitfalls of profiling.

Blameless Reporting and Immunity

Blameless reporting is a trend whose goal is to increase reporting for the common good. This coupled with **immunity** when it comes to litigation and **counseling and debriefing services** for those who do come clean are considered to be a growing trend of win -win strategies for health care providers, eh, doctors, as well as patients.

Shift Happens! Full Disclosure and Sheltering the Storm

You will likely be facing questions dealing with medical errors that have occurred and how to share these with patients. They expect you to know about *shifting* approaches to common thinking regarding disclosing errors to patients and their families.

When choosing the correct answer, you are expected to **be totally transparent** with the patient/ family in disclosing **why** it happened, how it will **impact** them, and **steps being taken to prevent such an error from happening again**.

While fear of litigation is why such conciliatory and appropriate action might not be taken, it has been shown to **reduce litigation** and **decrease settlement amounts** when it does take place.

Apologizing would likely be correct on the exam. There is a movement toward preventing such apologies from being used in legal proceedings as an admission of wrong doing or demonstration of liability.

The negative impact on doctors who make medical errors is also becoming increasingly recognized, **Suspending judgment of competence** and **providing support through debriefing** would also likely be correct on the exam.

If you are asked for the most effective way to reduce medical errors, the correct answer will likely be something along the lines of open communication.

It's all about a culture of safety. The key is considered to be an open exchange of information between all team members, as well as attention to details. Open communication with family members would also be considered an important factor in reducing medication errors.

Man and Machine

Medical errors are often a combination of Man and Machine.

Machine

Computerized forced screen formats do reduce medication errors. They do so in obvious ways such as eliminating **handwriting** issues. Weight-based calculators with pediatric lightning rod **overdose alarms** also help reduce dosing errors. Some systems include **alerts** for drug **interactions** and drug **contraindications** based on diagnosis.

A similar alarm fatigue occurs in EMRs where drug-drug interactions occur with such high frequency that they start to become ignored. When this happens, fatal interactions may occur.

Alarms are set to call attention to abnormal findings (HR, RR, oxygen levels, etc), but alarm fatigue occurs when alarms are set off with such high frequency that they start to be ignored. In this case, the solution might be to reset the alarm trigger point.

Man (and Woman)

 Of course, computers make mistakes.[5] Therefore human maintenance is in order.

Having a pharmacist on **inpatient rounds** and requesting **order reviews** by pediatric pharmacist specialists are recognized strategies for reducing pediatric medication errors.

The answer to any question on what your attitude should be when a prescription error is brought to your attention should be that you are very **thankful** and **gracious** for their bringing it to your attention.

Having lists, "cheat sheets", and mnemonics during patient handoffs during change of shift decreases the risks of miscommunications and leads to less errors of things being missed or left out.

Closed loop communication, where the receiver summarizes and repeats the information received, also helps reduce miscommunication.

---

[5] Technically computers DON'T make mistakes but the programmers may have made mistakes.

Chapter 8

Growth and Development

Physiologic Growth

A child's growth pattern is a good indicator of his or her general health. It is imperative that you use growth charts to monitor linear growth and weight gain.

The following are some important facts and numbers to keep in mind when distinguishing between normal growth and abnormal growth — which is an area fertile for getting tripped up on the exam through deception.

Weight

The average birth weight (50th percentile) for a full term newborn is 3.25 kg.
The average newborn loses up to 10% of birthweight and regains it by 2 weeks of age.

- Birthweight: **doubles** by 5 months, **triples** by 1 year
- Men's weight triples during their first year of marriage, especially if they become fathers for the first time that year

Some infants may not regain their birthweight until 3 weeks of age. Therefore, if you are presented with an infant younger than 3 weeks who has not regained their birthweight, the correct answer is to reassure and re-evaluate in one week.

However, this would only apply if you are not given any other information in the history. If there are hints and suggestionsof underlying disease such as poor feeding and/or heart disease look for and is consistent with those diagnoses

Length

The average birth length (50th percentile) for a full term newborn is 50 cm. 50/50 in length.
Easy to remember.

Birth length is:
- **1.5 x by age 2**
- **2 x by age 4**[1]
- **3 x by age 13**

The growth rate is 20 cm/year in the first year of life; then 5-6 cm/year until the start of puberty.
Birth size is impacted more by maternal factors and in utero conditions than genetic growth potential.

---

[1] Did you know that at 2 years of age, you are half your adult height? Really!

An infant may cross percentiles in the first 12-18 months as the genetic, hormonal and environmental factors start to overcome the maternal factors.

However, shifts across **two or more percentile lines** on the growth curve after age 2 years of age are uncommon and most likely represent an abnormality of growth.

Remember that **chronic diseases** have a significant effect on linear growth velocity

Head Circumference

Normal head circumference at birth for a full term newborn is 35 cm.

Head growth is:
- **1 cm/month for the first 6 months**
- **0.5 cm/month from 6-12 months**

Big Heads

We are not talking about Kanye West's swollen ego here. We are talking about **macrocephaly** and **hydrocephaly** and how to distinguish between them. Let's start with definitions.

Macrocephaly

Macrocephaly is a head circumference of **2 standard deviations (SD) above the mean** or above the **97th percentile for age.**

If they describe an infant with an increasing head circumference but make a point to mention normal development, the first thing you should do is **measure the parents' heads.**[2] Parents with big heads usually have kids with big heads; this is normal familial macrocephaly.

> ## Big Bad Head
> **Irritability**, or **lethargy, poor appetite, persistent vomiting, a bulging fontanelle, impaired upward gaze (sundowning),** and **other neurological findings** in an infant with a rapidly enlarging head would tell you that you are dealing with hydrocephalus.

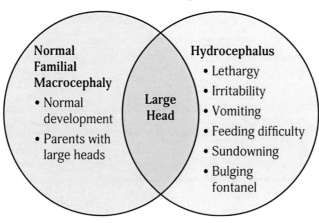

---

2 Tell them you would like to buy them a Stetson cowboy hat for National Texas Appreciation Day.

Small heads

DEFINITION

Microcephaly is a head circumference of **more than 2 SD below the mean** or **below the 3rd percentile for age**.

Primary microcephaly- infants born with heads below the 3rd percentile who remain "below normal." This is caused by a number of genetic conditions and in utero infections.

Acquired microcephaly- infants with a normal head circumference at birth, who later develop heads below the 3rd percentile. Causes include perinatal or postnatal insults (i.e., asphyxia; as well as genetic, metabolic, infectious and toxicology factors).

PERIL

If you are presented with an infant whose head circumference decreases, while the weight and height remain normal, there needs to be a cause.

Failure to Thrive

Here it is: Failure to Thrive (FTT) - the one section you thought you knew and could skip studying. It used to be thought that FTT was due to "organic" causes (i.e., underlying medical conditions) or "non-organic" causes (i.e, non-medical conditions); and you were done.

But NOOOOO, that is "old school". FTT is now considered "a physical sign that a child is receiving inadequate nutrition for optimal growth and development" and the investigation into the root cause(s) begins.

DEFINITION

There is no one single definition of FTT. However if you are presented with any of the following on the exam, FTT is likely what they are getting at:

- Weight is below the 5th percentile for age
- Weight that drops down two major percentile channels
- Weight less than 80% of the ideal weight for age
- Weight below the 5th percentile on the weight-for-length curve.

HOT TIP

Remember that there are specific growth charts for children with certain genetic conditions like Down, Turner, and William's syndrome. Children should be compared to these "normals" before their growth is considered abnormal. This could be an important factor on the exam.

PERIL

It is normal for infants and toddlers to change percentiles up to two percentile channels up or down **between birth and 2 years of age**.

Short, long and Dysmorphic

COIN FLIP

You will need to determine the likely cause of a measurement discrepancy as follows:

Inadequate Caloric Intake – Weight will drop initially, followed by decreased length and sparing head circumference.

Endocrine disorders – Presents with short stature with normal or elevated weight.

Chromosomal abnormalities – Microcephaly and dysmorphic feature.

Chronic medical conditions – Weight and height fall together.

Feeding FTT

Most cases of FTT are due to *nonorganic factors*. Sophisticated tests and labs are *not the first steps to be taken*.

Evaluation of the diet is the first step. If this has already been done, then look at the mother/child interaction (with a focus on feeding technique).

It's Organic

Organic causes of FTT include:

- Chronic renal failure
- Thyroid and other metabolic disorders
- Disorders leading to inadequate absorption
- Disorders leading to inadequate utilization

In these cases, however, there would have to be something in the presenting history to suggest these as the causative factors.

Watch for signs in the history that would suggest a change, such as a new caretaker assuming care of an infant. In this case, *improper mixing of formula* might be the reason behind the failure to thrive.

Normal Developmental Milestones

For many of us, remembering the details of the normal developmental milestones is about as exciting as deleting spam emails. Unfortunately, on the Boards, you will be expected to identify a child's age by their developmental milestones. Knowing this cold will be worth several points on the exam, perhaps the few points that stand between you and a passing grade.

I have found the most effective way to do this is to raise a child. However, at this point, unless you are a PGY-1 preparing for the boards in advance, there probably isn't enough time to conceive and raise a few kids before the exam.[3]

It is important to remember these milestones both using *months* and *years*. As you can see, much of the first year is spent growing and developing gross motor skills, while fine motor, language and social skills (one hopes) are the focus thereafter.

When encountered with a scenario that may indicate milestones between ages; look at the milestone that is MOST ADVANCED to guide you to the patitent's closest age.

> ## Making up for Lost Time
>
>
>
> - 28 wk GA infant who is now 2.5 months old, really 38 wk GA, would be expected to have the milestones of a full term newborn, not of a 2-month-old.
> - You no longer have to factor in the prematurity after age 2 years.

Developmental Milestone Mnemonics

The following are some mnemonics that should help keep the sometimes confusing milestones straight.

2 Month Old can...

- Follow mom in both directions (i.e., visually track) → **2 months = 2 sides**
- Lift head (with 45 degree lag) and chest while prone → **2 months = 2 parts**
- Smile (social/reciprocal) and coo → **2 months = 2 social cues; "coo" rhymes with "2"**

---

[3] It is, however, fair to use your friends' kids as examples!

4 Month Old can...

- Grasp and shake a rattle; scratch and grab clothes
- Laugh and squeal; place objects in mouth
- Pull to sit; in tripod positon; roll front to back
- FULL head lift (90 degrees, no lag) while prone; bears weight on forearms
- Bears weight on STIFF LEGS while held upright

Picture a number 4 as a rattle.

6 Month Old can...

- Sit WITH support; "raking grasp" (i.e., radial/palmar grasp)
- Object transfer (i.e., transfer a cube from one hand to another)
- Roll in BOTH directions (front to back; back to front)
- LOW crawl (on belly)
- Bounce on a high chair; bang objects, babble

Change the word "six" to "sit" → **"sit month olds can sit."**

Change the number "6" to the letter "b" → "**b** months old can **b**ABBLE, **b**OUNCE, **b**ANG OBJECTS, **b**ELLY CRAWL; roll in **b**OTH DIRECTIONS.

9 Month Old can...

- Sit WTHOUT support
- Pull up to stand (imagine the number "9" standing up)
- Easily get scared (i.e., "stranger anxiety")
- Bang 2 blocks; clasp 2 hands;
- PLAY: "patty-cake," "peek-a-boo"
- Say "mama" and "dada" **non-specifically; turn to their name**

Picture a "scared" baby calling out "mama" non-specifically in a crowded room since he has separation anxiety and can't find her. When he finally gets to her, he grabs onto her skirt, pulls up and stands.

1 Year (12 Month Old) can...

- Walk with ONE hand held; point with ONE finger
- Cruise; take their 1st steps (ONE step at a time)
- Say "mama" and "dada" **specifically**, and ONE other word

Baby, do the Jerk!

All about those **reflexes**, and when they **disappear...**

- Stepping reflex: 1-2 months
- Palmar reflex: 3-4 months
- Fencer (asymmetric tonic clonic) reflex: 3-4 months
- Rooting reflex: 4 months
- Moro reflex: 3-6 months
- Plantar reflex: 8-9 months
- Parachute reflex: starts at 8-9 months, *persists for life!*

The "Scissor Grasp"

Develops at 6-8 months.

When my baby turns...

- To sound @ 4 months
- To voice @ 6 months
- To name @ 9 months

- HIGH crawl (on hands and knees)
- MATURE pincer grasp (between tips of thumb and index finger)
- Object permanence (i.e., crawl to last place object was seen)

1 year olds are all about the ONEs

15 Month Old can...

- Walk well; CRAWL upstairs with hand held
- Stoop down to recover objects; drink from cup held solo; stack 2 cubes
- Follow 1-step commands (without gesture)
- Know 1 body part; know 4-6 words

18 Month Old can...

> **21 Month Olds**
> - Know 30-50 words

- Walk fast; fall sometimes; WALK upstairs with hand held
- CLIMB onto furniture and sit down; throw a ball casually
- Take off SMALL clothing items (hat, gloves, socks)
- Turn pages of book (3 at a time); feed self MESSY (with spoon); stack 4 cubes
- Know 1-4 body parts; know 10-25 words (all very similar to the average 18 *year* old)

2 Year (24 Month Old) can...

- Run well; broad jump (2 feet wide apart); walk upstairs while holding rail (2 feet on each step)
- Open/close cupboards; take off ALL clothing items
- Kick a ball; throw a ball overhand; PARALLEL play (next to peers); **say their 1st name**
- Feed self WELL (with spoon); know 6 body parts; stack 6 cubes; DRAW SCRIBBLE LINES
- Know 50-100 words with 50% intelligibility; make 2-3 word sentences (short phrases)

3 Year Old can...

- Walk upstairs with **alternating** feet; walk downstairs 2 feet on each step
- Ride a **tri**cycle (**3** wheels); hop on foot **3** times; DRAW A CIRCLE; stack 8-10 cubes
- Put on large buttons; wash hands on own; PRETEND play (imaginary friends)
- Name 1 color; use a crayon; count to 4; know pronouns (he/she/it); ask questions (why?)
- Speak in **3**-word sentences with 75% intelligibility; answer **3** questions: **their name (1st and last)**/ age/sex

3 year olds are all about the 3's

4 Year Old can...

- Walk both upstairs and downstairs with alternating feet
- Read a tumbling E chart (vision screen); tell stories; ask more questions!
- Play hide-and-seek; change rules of game (cheat!); pretend play + COOPERATIVE play (with peers)
- Speak in **4**-word sentences with 100% intelligibility; DRAW A SQUARE (**4** sides); draw **4** body parts
- Identify opposites (which is easy to remember since they practice them all the time. You say "yes," they say "no." You say "wear your red coat," they say "blue." You get the picture.)

Rule of 4s

- Recite a **4**-word sentence
- Identify **4** primary colors

- Draw a square (**4** sides)

- Build a gate out of blocks (picture a #**4** as a gate)
- A stranger will understand **4/4** of what they are saying

- Count to **4**
- Draw a **4**-part person ("stick figure")

- Balance on 1 foot for **4** seconds

Say my name

- 2 years - say their 1st name
- 3 years - say their 1st and last name
- 6 years - write their 1st and last name

---

5 Year Old can...

- Walk backwards heel-to-toe; skip; tie a knot; draw a 6-part person
- Know multiple colors (think of the "rainbow"); count to 10
- Correctly grab a pencil; write out letters; DRAW A TRIANGLE

Dance with me

- 2 years - jump (broad)
- 3 years - hop
- 5 years - skip, walk back

These are all skills required for school. Picture a child trying to avoid school by walking backwards.

6 Year Old can...

- Ride a bicycle; know directions - right vs. left
- Count to 100; **write 1st and last name**; DRAW A DIAMOND

Know thy shapes

- 2 years - SCRIBBLE LINES
- 3 years - CIRCLE
- **3-4 years - CROSS**
- 4 years - SQUARE
- 5 years - TRIANGLE
* 6 years - DIAMOND

Language Skills

The following will make it quite easy to keep language development straight. It might even allow you to get the question right without even knowing the other parameters.

They often ask how much of what a child says is intelligible at different ages. The following chart should help:

Age	% of what they say is intelligible
Age 2	2/4 = 50% intelligible
Age 3	3/4 = 75% intelligible
Age 4	4/4 = 100% intelligible[4]
Pediatric Intern	1/3 intelligible
PGY 2	2/3 intelligible
PGY 3	3/3 (100%) intelligible
Chief Resident	I better try to sound intelligible
Chairman	What's intelligible?
Professor Emeritus	2/4 = 50% intelligible

Stuttering

HOT TIP

Stuttering can **be normal up to age 3 or 4**. It often disappears once vocabulary rapidly increases. Therefore, this is one of those cases where "normal and reassurance" is often the correct answer.

Persistence **beyond preschool age** would require referral for evaluation. Other indications for referral would be: if stuttering persists for more than 6-8 weeks, if there is marked parental concern, or if there are associated symptoms of child stress such as facial tics.

Language Deficits

A **hearing evaluation** is the first thing to do with any language delay, and is often the answer on the Boards, especially if they mention a history of TORCH infections, hyperbilirubinemia, meningitis, or NICU stay.

Chronic hearing loss, including hearing loss due to chronic otitis media, not only impacts language development, it can also impact emotional development, as well as the ability to read. Hearing loss that begins after 5 has less of an impact than hearing loss that occurs before then.

PERIL

Although it may seem counterintuitive, the most important intervention for language development in an infant with a congenital hearing loss is family involvement, including non-verbal communication. Family use of both verbal and nonverbal communication has been shown to have the most positive impact on language acquisition in children with hearing loss.

---

[4] Which is everything, for those who have difficulty with fractions.

This is considered to be more important than specific formal interventions.

A bilingual home, and older children speaking for the child **do not explain language delays**.

Developmental screening tests

Systematic monitoring "structured surveillance" of a child's development using standardized screening tools has been proven to identify delays children much more often than open-ended questions to parents or physician observation alone ie, "unstructured surveillance".

The AAP currently recommends:

- universal post-partum mood disorder screening in the first year after birth
- general structured developmental screening at 9, 18, and 24-or-30 months
- autism specific screening at 18 and 24 months
- social emotional screening whenever a screening instrument is abnormal
- kindergarten readiness screening at 4 years
- social-emotional/ mental health/ psychosocial function screening at every health supervision visit from ages 5 to 18 years
- substance abuse-specific screening at every health supervision visit throughout adolescence.

> ### Early Intervention /
> ### A Good IDEA
>
> Infants and children under age 3 identified with developmental delays will benefit from early intervention, so the answer in Boards will always be REFER.
>
> Part C of IDEA covers early intervention services for children under age 3 years. The goal of this program is to allow children to reach their developmental cognitive potential. Programs must be family-based and culturally sensitive.
>
> The Individuals with Disabilities Education Act (IDEA) outlines guidelines for the education of children in the United States who have developmental delays or other problems that may interfere with learning.

Like it or not, you will be required to know or be familiar with some developmental screening tools. Below are the most popular ones:

General Developmental Screens:

For Parents (Subjective)

- Ages and Stage Questionnaire (ASQ)
  - 5-60 months; gross/fine motor, expressive/receptive language, problem solving, social/ emotional milestones
- Child Development Inventories/Review
  - 3-73 months; major milestones above
- Parents' Evaluation of Developmental Status - Developmental Milestones (PEDS-DM)
  - 0-8 years; major milestones above

For Providers (Objective)

- **Bailey Neurodevelopmental Screen (BINS)**
  - Premies at 3-24 months; neurodevelopmental functioning and skills
  - Assess tone, movement, symmetry, imitation, language
- **Denver Developmental Screening Test II (DDST-II)**
  - 1-72 months; assess suspected developmental delay

Specialized Developmental and Mental Health Screens:

- **Modified Checklist for Autism in Toddlers (MCHAT)**
  - 18 months & 24 months; by parents
- **Pediatric Symptom Checklist (PSC)**
  - 11+ years; by parents
- **Vanderbilt Assessment Scale**
  - 6-12 years; by parents and teachers
- Connors Comprehensive Behavioral Rating Scale (CBRS)
  - 6-18 years; by providers
- Patient administered questionnaires
  - PHQ2/9: 12+ years; screen for depression
  - GAD7: 13+ years; screen for anxiety

> ### 3D Developmental Deviation
>
> There are 3 ways development can go astray. They can be remembered as the 3Ds of Developmental Deviation:
>
>
>
> **D**ELAY in development
>
> **D**EVIATION in the order of skills acquisition or an **atypical** patterns of development
>
> **D**ISSOCIATION where different areas of development advance at different rates.

Chapter 9

LLC: Disorders of Cognition, Language, and Learning

Clinical functioning is paramount for disorders in cognition, language, learning and neurodevelopment.

Intellectual Disability[1] (ID)

DEFINITION

Impairment of general mental abilities that impair adaptive functioning in conceptual, social, and practical domains.

HOT TIP

There is a **decreased emphasis on IQ**, although IQ is generally around 70 or below.

You are expected to know how to go about identifying the possible etiology of intellectual disability. This prevents unnecessary testing and allows for appropriate management.

This includes

> **History** – delayed milestones, FTT (failure to thrive), exposures consistent with known diagnoses.
>
> **Family history** – look for history of stillborn infants, miscarriages, or consanguinity.
>
> **Physical exam** – looking for dysmorphism or unusual features.
>
> **Genetic testing** – there are genetic causes of intellectual disability.
>
> **Imaging studies** – would be limited to those with features that warrant them, i.e. micro/macrocephaly. MRI is the imaging study of choice.

PERIL

In the absence of seizures, an EEG is not indicated.

PERIL

Metabolic screening is not indicated in the absence of physical findings or history that support the testing.

Genetics is the most common cause of intellectual disability; however, other causes to consider are **perinatal infections** or prenatal exposure to **teratogen**s.

#1 Preventable ID

The most common **preventable** cause of intellectual disability is **congenital hypothyroidism**.

Genetic ID

Down syndrome is the most common **genetic** cause of ID.

Fragile X

Fragile X is the most common **inherited** disorder known to cause I.D.

Family history is crucial; if you are presented with a question where they note a family tree full of "uncles with learning problems," they may be presenting an x-linked disorder such as Fragile X.

Alcohol

The most common **teratogen** causing intellectual disability is alcohol.

PERIL

Children with fetal alcohol syndrome who have IQs in the normal range are not out of the woods; they can still have neurobehavioral deficits. They are at increased risk for psychiatric disorders as well.

---

[1] Formerly known as mental retardation.

Degrees of Intellectual Disability

• Severe intellectual disability is usually picked up at a younger age.

• Up to 85% of all cases of intellectual disability fall in the mild range. Mild intellectual disability is usually picked up at a later age, often at the time of entry into school.

HOT TIP Visual impairment may result in delay of motor development.

Language

Language development in young children is often a better gauge of cognitive function than gross motor development.

PERIL

Even an infant with profound hearing loss may demonstrate normal "language" development until 6-9 months, right up to where babbling does not progress to definite "mama" and "dada".

DEFINITION

Speech and Language skills are defined as a disability if they are at 2/3 or below what is expected for the child's age. If there is no standard test then a standard score of 70 or lower would qualify as a disbility.

HOT TIP

A child with a speech and language delay would need a general developmental screen to rule out other developmental delays. Even if the issue is resolved, the child needs to be monitored for language based learning issues including reading difficulties.

PERIL

In addition, a formal audiology evaluation is indicated.

Adaptive Functioning

The level and severity of impairment is determined by the anticipated level of adaptive functioning. This is what determines the level of care that will be needed and what needs to be planned for.

TAKE HOME MESSAGE This isn't always aligned with intellectual ability.

Consonant Counseling

If you are presented with a child younger than 6 years who is having difficulty pronouncing certain consonants, reassurance is all that is needed.

Autism Spectrum Disorder (ASD)

DEFINITION

As of the most recent DSM, autism is now **a spectrum**, encompassing an array of function. The diagnosis is still made **clinically**, with no single definitive diagnostic test.

DEFINITION

Diagnosis of Autism Spectrum Disorder involves

A. persistent deficits in social communication and social interaction across contexts, not accounted for by general developmental delays and

B. presence of restricted, repetitive, stereotyped behavior, interests and activities.

COIN FLIP

An important component of autism, and one that distinguishes it from other causes of language delay is the **lack of eye contact and lack of social engagement**. It would be important to know about the child's **interactions with other family members**.

Delayed and atypical language, along with odd interests and activities, may distinguish autism and autistic spectrum disorders from intellectual disability. **Good social interaction** for the most part rules out autism.

PERIL

A **hearing test** is an absolute MUST in any child undergoing evaluation for speech delay, even if you think the diagnosis is autism.

Children with autism are at increased risk for several medical conditions. These include seizures GI disorders sleep disturbance motor disorders obesity as well as pica. Additional comorbidities could include ADHD, anxiety and depression.

HOT TIP

When presented with a **behavioral change** in a child with autism, **medical conditions** should be ruled out first, for example constipation, ear infection, constipation, or possible injury that went unnoticed.

Struggling in School

Some reasons a child may struggle in school include:
- Speech/language impairment
- Learning Disability
- Borderline IQ/ "slow learner"
- Intellectual disability
- Autism Spectrum Disorder
- Medical conditions
- Behavioral/ Mental Health
- Environmental/ Social
- Sleep disturbances

Learning Disabilities (LD)

HOT TIP

Read the family history carefully checking for others with speech, language, learning, or even behavior problems like ADHD, which may be a clue to specific disorders such as Fragile X syndrome.

PERIL

A child can have a **learning disability** with normal or even superior **intelligence**.

Having a learning disability means there is a gap between the **expected (age appropriate)** and the **observed** performance in one of the following areas:

- *Listening*
- *Speaking*
- *Reading*
- *Writing*
- *Reasoning*
- *Math skills*

LD Red Flags

Some of the specific red flags you may be presented with include delay in speech and language development, as well as:

- Inability to recognize letters and numbers by the end of kindergarten
- Speech delay in a preschooler
- Inability to read simple words by the end of the first grade.

On Grade Retention

Grade retention is not a frequent recommendation anymore because:

- Temporary academic gains are not sustained.
- It does not improve student outcomes.
- Does not address LDs and other factors for school failure.

If you are presented with a child **younger than 7** who reverses letters such as "**b**" and "**d,**" do not be quick to make a diagnosis of dyslexia or another learning disability. This can be a **normal finding** up to age 7.

Early intervention is the key; delay in recognizing learning disabilities may result in repeated academic failures, which often negatively impacts a child's school motivation. The earlier a learning disorder is discovered, the easier it is to implement methods that help the child overcome or compensate for the disability.

Medications and Medical Conditions

Read the history carefully for medical conditions, keeping in mind that **anticonvulsants** and **antihistamines** can alter school performance.

Watch for signs of **depression** as an underlying cause of poor school performance. On the other hand, poor school performance may lead to depression. You might have to distinguish the chicken from the egg.

Children with learning disabilities are at increased risk for **behavioral** and **mood disorders** in general.

Learning disabilities are **not outgrown**.

Engagement in **extracurricular activities** may be important for the **self esteem** of a child with a learning disability. In addition, **special tools** that help a child overcome a specific learning disability are to be encouraged and used; this may include private tutoring, resource room help, etc.

Unless there is a profound inability to read the letters on a page, the most commonly-encountered ophthalmological disorders generally do not impact reading ability. Gimmicks like tinted eyeglasses and eye gymnastics will be incorrect choices to improve reading ability (no matter how cool the described exercises are).

If you are presented with a child who is having difficulty in classes such as history or social studies, they may describing a child with difficulty reading or with short term memory problems.

Intelligence and Performance Testing

IQ Tests

The validity of IQ tests can be influenced by:

- social/ cultural biases within the standardized tests
- linguistic differences between the child's native language and the test
- level of motivation during test taking

- level of rapport between examiner and test taker
- emotional state during test taking
- developmental disability (ASD/ CP)
- developmental impairment interfering with test taking (fine motor or visual delays)

HOT TIP

The predictive validity of IQ tests increases with age. In general, IQ does not crystallize until 7-9 years of age, so do not refer children for IQ testing under that age.

Achievement Test

Achievement tests distinguish between I.Q. (potential) and achievement (actual) intellectual performance.

PERIL

Achievement testing can be influenced by many factors (which may be included with the history you are presented), including:

Genetics, cultural or language bias, emotional and/or psychosocial factors, as well as ability to focus and pay attention.

Sub test profile scores are more important than overall test scores on IQ tests such as the Wechsler Intelligence Scale for Children (WISC-IV), since the subtest scores allow for more detailed information on the child's difficulties.

If you are presented with a patient with below normal scores on an achievement test despite a normal IQ, they are probably pointing you toward a **specific learning disability**.

School accommodations

Individualized Educational Program (IEP) are plans devised for students who qualify for special education based on the 13 specific disabilities in the IDEA.

Parents can request evaluation for disabilities by the school under the IDEA and school is required to respond to their request with whether they agree to evaluate or not. Parents may then appeal.

Visual Impairment

Children with visual impairment require certified **mobility specialists** and teachers trained in educating children with visual impairments.

School Failure

When presented with a child with school failure, first consideration should be given to a **medical history, educational history, physical exam, including vision and hearing screens family history,** and **emotional issues**.

Once this is all out of the way, tests can be **implemented**.

If you are presented with a patient who is experiencing school failure, read the question carefully in order to avoid your own exam failure.

Watch for signs of underlying medical conditions, such as asthma, inflammatory bowel disease, or neurological disorders such as Tourette syndrome and seizures.

Watch for psychosocial issues, including divorce or a recent move.

Definitions

Individuals with Disabilities Education Act: (IDEA) requires special education for children with disabilities and provides funding for appropriate public education for children from age 3-22 and appropriate early interventions for children younger than 3.

DEFINITION

It federally mandates public schools to evaluate and accommodate children with 13 specific disabilities, modify the curriculum to the child's individual needs in the "least restrictive environment", and provide related services (PT, OT, psych, transportation).

Americans with Disability Act (ADA): Prohibits discrimination child care centers and from discriminating against children with disabilities. This would include children with gastrostomy tubes if that is included in the question.

Section 504 of the Rehabilitation Act - prohibits discrimination on the basis of disability in programs that receive federal funding. It affords equal access to free appropriate public education for school aged children and reasonable accommodations in college

---

[2] Including ID, S/L impairment, ASD, LD, DD, ADHD, and medical disabilities.

Transition Plans

At age 14, an Individualized Transition plan is incorporated into the IEP to plan for a student's future as an adult, addressing such issues as the age at which s/he leaves school and what career path might be appropriate. The individual and the parents should be encouraged to participate in this planning.

Chapter 10

Behavior and Mental Health

Much of what you will see in general pediatrics practice is behavior-related. Because of this, behavioral and mental health issues have emphasis on the boards.

Behavioral Concerns

Maternal Infant Bonding

Maternal infant bonding is important immediately after birth.

 If you are asked which is more important to do in the **first hour of life** and offered choices of

    1) vitamin K administration,

    2) erythromycin eye drops, or

    3) maternal-infant skin-to-skin contact,

The correct answer would be **skin-to-skin contact**.

Colic

Colic **starts at 3 weeks of age** and **ends at 3 months of age** and is defined as crying more than **3 hours per day**, more than **3 days per week**, for more than **3 weeks** for no apparent reason. Colic was initially thought to be due to GI symptoms, but is now felt to be **multifactorial**.

Remember that colic is a diagnosis that is **based on history**. The physical exam rarely shows anything, and there are **no labs** that confirm the diagnosis.

 These ages even hold true for premature infants.

A typical presentation would be crying episodes in an **otherwise healthy infant**. The crying usually **starts suddenly** and tends to be around the **same time every day**, usually evening time. These babies cry

> ### The Crying Game
>
> Anyone with an infant should know that they are in for the crying game. You must be familiar with normal crying patterns of infants.
>
> **Birth – 6 weeks** – up to 2 hours a day can be normal
>
> **6 weeks and beyond** – 3 hours a day can be normal

harder and **longer** than non-colicky babies, and tend to **draw up their legs, tense their abdomens,** and **arch their backs,** so parents think they are in pain.

TREATMENT

The correct management is to **reduce parental frustration** by having another caretaker take over. **Support and reassurance** are the most important interventions. Medications (even gas drops) and changing formula are rarely going to be the correct answers on the exam.

MNEMONIC

Correct answers usually include the "S"s: **s**waddling, **s**hushing, **s**winging, **s**ucking (pacifier), and **s**trolling away. Probiotics (Lactobacillus reuteri) could be a correct answer.

> ### Reasons to Cry
> Know that infants who cry excessively are at increased risk for child abuse.

CASE STUDY

You are presented with a mother who is beside herself because her 2 month old infant "cries continuously." The infant typically cries 2 hours in the early morning around 5 AM, and around 1 hour at night, usually around 1 AM. What should the parents do?

THE DIVERSION

The diversion here is the timing. Anyone can relate to the frustration of an inconsolable infant crying for an entire hour at 1AM and then another 2 hour cycle at 5AM. The timing of the crying is the diversion. Your choices will include thickening formula, acetaminophen, antacids, and single malt whiskey nipples (for the parents). If you go for any of these diversionary answers, you might be the one crying for 3 hours a day.

ANSWER REVEALED

When you are presented with a crying infant, add up the *total hours crying*. **If it equals only 3 hours, this is normal and nothing more than "parental reassurance" is needed.**

Temper Tantrums

TAKE HOME MESSAGE

Most children have temper tantrums at some point in their lives. This is especially common in toddlers. If tantrums are caused by frustration with a task, redirecting them or distracting them before the tantrum can occur is a useful strategy. A consistent daily routine is helpful for most children this age.

Parents should be advised to **ignore tantrums if possible,** unless the child is in danger of harming himself/herself. The child should be allowed to calm down in a safe place. Physical restraint is not usually a good idea because it may increase the child's frustration.

Breath-holding Spells

The typical presentation is a toddler who is **angry, frustrated** or **in pain**. It can occur between the ages of 6 -18 months. It is involuntary. The child then cries and then:

- **Simple Breath-holding spell** – the child becomes pale or cyanotic
- **Complex Breath-holding spell-** the child then continues to cry until he/she is unconscious

Occasionally it can progress to a **hypoxic seizure with a postictal period**. However, this is still considered a breath-holding spell, not a seizure disorder.

The best management is behavioral modification. It is also important to reassure parents that the breath-holding, and even the seizure, are not harmful in any way, to avoid parents fearing the spells and giving in to their child's demands to avoid them at any cost.

> ### Anemia and Breath-Holding Spells
>
> There is an **association** between **iron-deficiency anemia** and the incidence of breath-holding spells.
>
> Anemia is **not** considered to be the actual cause of breath-holding spells, but treatment of the anemia often reduces the frequency of breath-holding spells.
>
> This is a minor difference in the wording, and you need to read the question carefully to see what they are asking. Serum iron and ferritin levels could be correct answer.

Setting Limits with Toddlers

A golden rule of behavior management is to **praise** a child's desirable behaviors and **ignore** undesirable behaviors if possible. When a child displays undesirable behaviors, the parent or caregiver should **withdraw all attention**. This is called **extinction**. Initially the behavior may worsen (which is called an **extinction burst**), but if the parent can endure, the behavior should decrease in frequency.

Time out and other forms of Discipline

You could be tested on the appropriate way to manage a behavioral problem with different age groups, including the following:

Time Out - This is time out from negative behavior; sort of a penalty box, for you hockey fans out there. This works best for age 1 and up. Time-out should last **one minute per year** of the child's age.

Time In -This is **positive feedback**, where a parent makes reassuring contact when a child is engaging in appropriate behavior, thus establishing positive reinforcement.

Token Economy – Where the child receives a "token" for positive behavior. This is most effective and appropriate for ages 3-7 years and the preferred strategy for children with ADHD.

Self-Stimulation

Head Banging

HOT TIP
If you are presented with a **neurologically-intact** child **who is younger than 5 years old** exhibiting head-banging behavior, especially around bed time, it is considered **normal** and **no intervention** is necessary.

PERIL
If they present you with a toddler with language delay, poor eye contact, and head banging, don't automatically assume a diagnosis of autism. They may describe other signs of **neglect** such as missed pediatrician appointments, which will clue you into child neglect being the actual diagnosis.

If they present a child **older than 4**, or signs and symptoms of **developmental delay**, then that is your clue that this falls outside the range of normal head-banging behavior.

Thumb Sucking

The best **initial intervention** for thumb sucking in a **toddler** is **redirecting** so they need their thumbs for another activity, and **positive reinforcement (praise)** when the child is not engaging in thumb sucking.

PERIL
Active measures should not be undertaken until the age of 4, since it is likely to be something the child will outgrow. Most thumb sucking is considered to be harmless and no intervention is indicated, especially on the boards.

Prolonged thumb sucking beyond age 4 can lead to dental problems, including malocclusion.

Biting Behavior

Biting may be considered a normal behavior (as a reaction to frustration) up to age 3.

The correct management is for parents to redirect, remove any positive reinforcement, and/or place the child in time out. A simple and neutral verbal scolding of "No biting" should accompany the redirecting.

It should be pretty obvious here that a choice on your test that says "Bite the child back" would be the wrong answer.

Masturbation

CASE STUDY
You are presented with a preschool or school age child who is masturbating. They will then ask for the most appropriate intervention.

THE DIVERSION
They could throw in misleading information in the history, like the mother travels a lot on business, or the parents are divorced and the child was with the father over the weekend.

ANSWER REVEALED
Masturbation in children is considered normal to a certain extent - they may also include something in the history regarding vulvovaginitis, recurrent UTI, or the use of bubble baths — all of which would increase sexual self-stimulation behavior in children. However, if they were to describe a child imitating sexual activity, this would not be a normal finding.

Figuring out Fears and Phobias

A **fear** is age-appropriate discomfort over a situation that is realistic within the context. A **phobia** is anxiety that is excessive based on the potential danger posed, after accounting for age and developmental level. By definition, a phobia needs to interfere with daily function for at least 6 months.

Phobias may be managed through **desensitization** via gradual controlled exposure to the feared situation or object. Alternatively, **cognitive behavioral techniques** (where the child is shown how to reframe the situations triggering the phobia) may be useful.

Medications will not likely be the correct answer, since effectiveness of medications for phobias has not been well-studied as of the time of publication of this book. By about 8 years of age they have developed a conscience and insight that aligns their behavior with societal norms and expectations.

Adolescent Parents

Most of the information on this subject that you may be tested on is common sense, but it is still worth emphasizing here.

Teen parents typically do not stay together very long. **Unrealistic expectations** may contribute to misinterpretation of age-appropriate behavior. For example, a 15 month old eating with their hands and making a mess might be misinterpreted as insubordination. Situations such as this may result in inappropriate punishment.

In general, involvement of the teen father is beneficial to the child, but it can be very dependent on the nature of his relationship with the mother.

Children's Anxieties

In young children, separation anxiety disorder and specific phobias are more common.

In adolescents, social anxiety disorder is more common.

School Phobia

School phobia occurs more frequently when there is only one caretaker (for example, a single mother). The best way to deal with it is to have mom go to the school with the child and wean the amount of time spent there.

Separation anxiety can be a normal developmental stage in preschool children.

Pure truancy may be a component of oppositional defiant disorder.

Resilience

Resilience is the ability to withstand, adapt to and recover from disappointments and hardships.

It is fostered with a strong and stable relationship with at least one responsive and nurturing adult. It can be a parents, teacher or even a coach. Providing opportunities to make decisions and develop coping strategies is key.

Mental Health Concerns

Post Traumatic Stress Disorder

You need to be familiar with the signs and symptoms associated with post traumatic stress disorder, or PTSD, which includes rape-trauma syndrome.

The typical presentation is of a teenage female who, weeks to months after experiencing a sexual assault, presents with **chronic pains, recurrent nightmares, fears of being alone, diminished interest in school,** and/or **decreased appetite.**

Attention Deficit Disorders

Core symptoms

❏ Inattentiveness
❏ Impulsivity
❏ Hyperactivity only in ADHD, not in ADD

DEFINITION

These symptoms must be **present before age 12,**[1] and present in **2 or more settings**. The symptoms must **impair functioning**, be present for **at least 6 months**, and not be explained by another condition.

The **ADHD-predominantly hyperactive** "presentation" (previously referred to as "subtype") affects males more than females. **ADHD-inattentive presentation** is more common among girls.

While it is often diagnosed upon entering school, there is usually retrospective evidence of symptoms during the toddler and preschool years as well (e.g., sleep disturbance, behavioral concerns).

TAKE HOME MESSAGE

60-80% of children diagnosed with ADHD continue to meet the criteria for diagnosis at adolescence and adulthood.

Studies have shown that maternal tobacco and/or alcohol use, as well as lead exposure, low birthweight, prematurity, and IUGR all increase the risk of ADHD.

PERIL

Symptoms can be easily repressed in the office setting, especially at the initial visit. Since the office visit itself constitutes a novel and therefore "stimulating" experience, it may not even represent an *active* repression of symptoms.

ADHD or something else?

In practice, ADHD is quite distinctive, and conditions in the differential rarely cause ADHD symptoms. Once again, this is the Boards' world and we just live there, so **on the Boards, items on the differential often DO cause ADHD symptoms.**

COIN FLIP

Absence seizures may present similarly to ADHD- inattentive presentation. However, history alone can often rule it out, and ordering an EEG may not be the correct answer. The buzzwords for absence seizures are **"suddenly stops speaking"** and then **"snaps out of it and comes to."** They may describe odd movements like **"twitching of eyelids or lips."** Remember, absence seizures can be induced through **hyperventilation**; ADHD cannot.

COIN FLIP

Depression and **anxiety** may be in the differential; either may result in "inattention" and/or "acting out behaviors." When there is no past history of inattention or depression, think of **substance abuse**, especially in teens.

---

[1] Previously, the cutoff for diagnosis was age 7.

Ruling Out Organic Causes of ADHD-like Symptoms

HOT TIP

Ruling out organic and medical conditions that can mimic ADHD is critical on the Boards. Often the labs and data in the question already do this, but not always.

The following must be considered:

❏ Visual or hearing deficits

❏ Lead toxicity

❏ Hyperthyroidism and hypothyroidism

❏ Previous neuro damage, either by infection or trauma

❏ Medications on board (They could slip that in) Phenobarbital may have cognitive effects, including ADHD-like symptoms. Antihistamines may also do this.

TAKE HOME MESSAGE

Don't forget to consider "the bigger picture" of conditions like Fragile X, Fetal Alcohol Syndrome, and WIlliams Syndrome which may present with ADHD but bring along many other symptoms as well.

BUZZWORDS

If they describe classic ADHD, look for clues in the question that they are getting at something else. For example, if they add "lethargy," "abdominal pain," or "poor appetite," they could be hinting at **lead toxicity**.

TREATMENT

The best proven treatment modalities are a combination of pharmacological and behavioral therapy or pharmacotherapy alone **(primarily stimulants)** but it is important to allow families to add their own complementary methods as long as they are not harmful to the child.

PERIL

Families will often seek out **alternative treatments** for ADHD and other chronic illnesses. Most complementary/alternative strategies to treat ADHD have not been proven in terms of efficacy.

Stimulants

PERIL

These medications should be used with caution in small children and those with **heart conditions, seizures, and on certain psychiatric medications**.

BUZZWORDS

Side effects of stimulants are kind of obvious since they are stimulants and include insomnia, weight loss, anorexia, rash, GI complaints, tachycardia, BP elevation, palpitations and arrhythmia, headaches, restlessness, and visual disturbances. Abnormal liver function and hair loss have also been reported.

ADHD Comorbidities

Approximately 65% of children with ADHD may have a **coexisting condition** such as oppositional defiant disorder, conduct disorder, anxiety disorder, mood disorder, learning disorder, or social immaturity. Substance abuse is a risk factor especially in adolescens who are untreated.

The Heart of the Matter

PERIL

Despite previous concerns, an EKG is NOT indicated prior to starting stimulant and/or other medications for ADHD.

It is important to consider cardiovascular risks in children with preexisting cardiac conditions, but in children **without preexisting cardiac conditions**, the actual risk of sudden death or ventricular arrhythmia is not significantly higher than in children who are NOT taking stimulants and/or other medications for ADHD. .

Stimulants may worsen or improve **anxiety**.

Use of stimulants may **increase the serum concentrations of TCAs and seizure meds**. Hypertensive crisis may ensue if used in the presence of **MAO inhibitors**.

Stimulant medication will improve attention in children (and adults) who do not have ADHD. Therefore, improved symptoms on stimulants is not diagnostic of ADHD.

Stimulant medications may **unmask tic symptoms** in children who are predisposed to tic disorders such as Tourette syndrome. However, stimulants do not cause Tourette syndrome.

The isolated appearance of motor tics while on stimulant medications is usually transient; this is not a contraindication to the use of stimulants.

Stimulant medication use after school is often necessary to complete homework. The administration of medication outside of the school setting may provide an opportunity for parents to observe for any adverse effects.

Nonstimulants

Nonstimulants which may be used in ADHD managements include **atomoxetine** (Strattera®) which is a norepinephrine reuptake inhibitor, and **clonidine** (Kapvay®) and **guanfacine** (Intuniv®) which are alpha adrenergic agonists.

Atomoxetine may not be administered within 2 weeks of MAO inhibitors and is to be used with caution in patients with **cardiac conditions** or with **concurrent albuterol therapy**. Increased risk of **suicidal thinking** has been reported so close monitoring is indicated, especially in preteen boys.

Common side effects of atomoxetine include GI symptoms, poor weight gain, fatigue, dizziness, mood swings, aggression and severe liver injury. It should be administed at bedtime because it is **sedating**. Stimulant mediations and atomoxetine increase BP, clonidine and guanfacine (central sympatholytics) can decrease BP.

Depression

The most important thing is to **distinguish normal variation from true blue** depression. In addition to the usual signs - somatization, withdrawal, appetite changes, and falling grades - **acting out may be a sign of**

Fading Fads and Assessing CAMs

Parents of children with developmental concerns, behavioral problems, or autism may sometimes turn to complementary and alternative medicine to help their child. Here are some things to keep in mind:

The Feingold diet has not been shown to be beneficial in managing ADHD or learning disabilities.

Likewise, sugar restriction has not been shown to be beneficial in managing or treating ADHD or other behavioral disorders.

However, sugar or candy should not be used as a reward for good behavior.

Megavitamin therapy has actually been shown to increase disruptive behavior, and certainly has no role in managing learning disabilities or behavioral problems.

For purposes of the boards, complementary or alternative medicine solutions for autism and other developmental disorders have not been proven to be effective. This includes sensory integration therapy, eye exercises, chelation therapy, or hyperbaric oxygen chambers.

---

depression. However, it is important to keep in mind that adolescents may have mood swings without being depressed. If symptoms are interfering with daily functioning and are beyond the limits of normal, depression is likely.

Parental depression increases the risk for depression in children, both from a genetic and environmental perspective. Children with **chronic illnesses** are at increased risk for depression, especially those taking glucocorticoids and immunosuppressive agents. Mood swings in depression are more intense and persistent and accompanied by other symptoms. This can include weight change, increased energy or increased sleep. Watch for a description of declining academic or athletic interest or performance.

Keep in mind that comorbid conditions such as **anxiety, ADHD,** or **substance abuse** may be present in pediatric patients with depression.

If medication is needed, fluoxetine is usually the first-line agent.

Fluoxetine

Fluoxetine is a selective serotonin reuptake inhibitor (SSRI) antidepressant. It is also contraindicated in patients taking **MAO inhibitors**. Use with caution in children on **diuretics** and with **liver** or **kidney disease**.

Common **side effects** of SSRIs include headache, insomnia, GI upset and weight loss. It **inhibits** the CYP 450 system so **concomitant drug levels may increase**.

Amitriptyline

Amitriptyline is a tricyclic antidepressant (TCA). It is contraindicated in children with **seizures** and **severe cardiac disorders** and in patients who have used **MAO-inhibitors**[2] in the last 14 days.

It must not be abruptly discontinued in those who have been taking high doses for prolonged periods of time. It is metabolized by the **CYP 450 system**.

Common **side effects** of amitriptyline include sedation, urinary retention, constipation, dry mouth, dizziness, drowsiness, liver enzyme elevation and arrhythmia. Monitor **EKG, BP** and **CBC** at the start of therapy and with dose changes. It may discolor the urine (blue/green).

Depressing and Alarming Antidepressants

Several classes of medications may be used as antidepressants in children and adolescents but most carry a **"Black Box Warning"**.

This warning emphasizes that antidepressants may in fact worsen depression (sounds backwards right?) and **increase risk of suicidality**. This requires careful monitoring when these meds are started or the dose is changed.

If mania is noticed after starting an antidepressants, the medication should be discontinued immediately and bipolar disease should be considered.

Antidepressants for Kids

Fluoxetine is the only FDA-approved medication for the treatment of depression in children and adolescents, although **citalopram** or **sertraline** could also be correct answers on the exam.

---

[2] Who are all these evil "MAO inhibitors" that we need to avoid? They include the antidepressants phenelzine, tranylcypromine, isocarboxazid, moclobemide, pargyline, procarbazine, and selegiline. I for one don't think I've ever had to manage a patient on a single one of those drugs. Have you? Regardless you can have patients on the boards taking these medications.

Psychotherapy

Cognitive behavioral therapy (CBT) is considered to be the most effective psychotherapeutic treatment for depression in children and adolescents. If medication is needed, fluoxetine is usually the first-line agent.

The most effective psychotherapy for depression in adolescents is interpersonal (address relationship and communication problems) and cognitive behavioral therapy (reframing negative thoughts and changing behaviors to improve mood).

Suicide

One suicide in a community can have a domino effect. The reasons for this are controversial, but the amount of media attention in the community is thought to have a role in increasing the risk of multiple suicides.

Screening for suicidal ideation by asking a depressed teen about suicidal thoughts would likely be a correct choice on the exam. It does not "put the idea in his/her head." Dismissing a suicidal gesture that "seems" to be superficial would also not be a correct choice. A "gesture" undertaken alone (with no rescue available) should be especially concerning.

Risk Factors for suicide:

- Substance abuse
- Loss of a loved one
- Family discord
- Social isolation
- Availability of firearms
- Previous suicide attempt
- Family history of suicide
- Native American teens and Hispanic females
- Underlying mood and anxiety disorders

Females engage in **self harming behavior** more often than males. However, **males** are more likely to **die of suicide**.

Concerns for suicide include:

- revealing suicidal thoughts on social media, being preoccupied with death in drawings, play, music and media.
- suicide in adolescent is impacted by the contagion effect; when reported by the media and is followed by a cluster of peer suicides.
- decline in self care, grades, or performance along with withdrawal or delusions are suggestive of psychosis.

Normal Rebelliousness or More?

You will be expected to distinguish adolescent rebellious behavior which is appropriate for their developmental phase from pathological features of Oppositional Defiant Disorder (ODD) and Conduct Disorder (CD).

ODD involves exactly that: **opposition**. These kids display negativistic, defiant, disobedient, and hostile behaviors and flat-out refuse to do what they are told. They have **little respect for authority**. In general **"ADD kids can't, and ODD kids won't."**

For a typical presentation of a child with a **conduct disorder**, they would have to describe severe behavioral concerns (such as lying, stealing, setting fires, or cruelty to animals) that **impinge on the basics right of others** or **violate major age-appropriate social rules** and are consistent over the course of at least 6 months.

> ### DDMD
> Disruptive dysregulation mood disorder is a new diagnosis that involves persistently irritable mood with severe temper outbursts that occur 3 or more times a week.

Treating these behavior disorders involves a **team approach**, including management of comorbid conditions such as ADHD or depression if present. The entire family may be involved in behavior therapy, and structured parent training programs may be beneficial.

Obsessive Compulsive Disorder (OCD)

Think OCD if they describe children or teens engaging in intensely driven, seemingly pointless repetitive behaviors (**compulsions**) along with recurrent thoughts and worries (**obsessions**). OCD is **a form of anxiety**, and the anxiety is relieved by the behaviors.

OCD is partly genetic and partly environmental, some believe **immunoreactive**, ie. may be due to infection in a susceptible individual.

> ### PANDAS
> PANDAS stands for **Pediatric Auto-immune Neuropsychiatric Disorders Associated with Streptococcal infection**. OCD may be one of these neuropsychiatric disorders.

- OCD consists of obsessions and compulsions that consume typically > 1 hour/day and are functionally impairing.
- Cognitive Behavioral Therapy (CBT) is the first line treatment, second line is SSRIs (fluoxetine, sertraline, fluvoxamine).
- Comorbidities include tic disorders, anxiety disorders and ADHD.

Psychotic Disorders

These patients have **hallucinations** (seeing or hearing things that are not really there) and/ or **delusions** (a belief a persons holds as

> ### Canabis Psychoticus
> Cannabis exposure has been found to produce transient psychotic states in 10-15% of users.

true despite absence of proof). Examples of delusions are being watched by aliens or having superpowers. **Schizophrenia** is one psychotic disorder that may begin in childhood.

The cornerstone of treatment is **antipsychotic medication**, but affected children require **extensive support and counseling** as well. They often stop taking medication as soon as they feel well, thinking symptoms will not recur.

Bipolar Disorder (BPD)

A **major depressive episode** may be the initial presentation of BPD. Those patients may **start antidepressants and become manic**. Manic symptoms include disruptive behavior, decreased need for sleep, racing thoughts manifested as "flight of ideas", elation, hypersexual behavior, and grandiose thinking.

Patients with BPD have a high rate of **coexisting ADHD and psychiatric disorders** such as anxiety, conduct disorders, substance abuse, and ODD.

> ## Bipolar and the Family
>
> **Family history** is the biggest predictor of developing bipolar disorder.
>
> The disorder is felt to be due to **both genetic and environmental factors**: genetically susceptible children being raised in a dysfunctional home and being victims of emotional traumas during a time of crucial CNS maturation.
>
> Years of anxiety, sleep disorders, mood disturbances, and adjustment issues may precede the onset of bipolar disease.

Aggressive Behaviors

Aggression is a type of **disruptive behavior** and may include temper tantrums, hitting, biting, stealing, and defiance of authority. When these behaviors are temporary, they may be considered normal. When they form a pattern over time, or are inappropriate for age, they are considered a psychiatric disorder.

Risk factors for aggressive behaviors include:

- neglect
- psychological maltreatment that destroys a child's sense of self and personal safety
- family history of aggressive behavior including incarceration and use of physical discipline
- exposure to violence in the media, including movies and video games
- lead poisoning

Parent management training (such as using positive reinforcement) and **cognitive behavior therapy** are the most effective treatments. Comorbid conditions such as ADHD, depression, mood disorders, and anxiety may benefit from medication.

Sleep Disorders

Disrupted or insufficient sleep may have deleterious effects on cognition, regulation of affect, attention, overall health and quality of life as well as secondary effects on parental functioning.

The extinction technique for treating behavioral insomnia involves putting the child to bed drowsy and waiting progressively longer intervals before checking on the child; intervals lengthened over 2 weeks until the child falls asleep independently.

Fading technique involves temporarily moving the bedtime to the current sleep-onset time and gradually advancing it to the desired bedtime over the next few weeks

Conversion Disorder

- also known as functional neurologic symptom disorder.
- recent stressors identified with or without a secondary gain.
- neurologic symptoms are present which are not consistent with recognized pathophysiology of medical conditions.
- neurologic disorder, panic disorder and dissociative disorder may occur with conversion disorder.

PNES (psychogenic non epileptic seizures)

- forward pelvic thrusting
- side to side head or body movements
- closed eyes resistant to opening
- lack of post ictal confusion.

Chapter 11

Psychosocial Issues

Toilet Training

75% of children will have full bladder and bowel control by age 36 months. Positive reinforcement (praise/rewards) is preferred over punishment-based reinforcement, which rarely works.

Enuresis

Nocturnal Enuresis

Primary nocturnal enuresis (PNE) refers to enuresis in a child who has never been dry on consecutive nights for 6 months. This may only be diagnosed **after age 5**.

Secondary nocturnal enuresis (SNE) refers to those who start wetting after being dry 6 months.

The initial workup consists of a history, physical exam, and **urinalysis**.

- **Enuresis alarms** are by far the most effective strategy for curing nocturnal enuresis. However, they require intensive effort and may take 3-4 months to work.
- **15% of cases** of enuresis per year will **resolve with no intervention**.
- Non-organic causes of enuresis are related to **small bladder, excessive fluid intake before bed,** and **deep sleeping**.

Treatment of nocturnal enuresis involves **behavioral modification** including limiting nighttime fluids 2 hours before bedtime, limiting dairy products 4 hours before bedtime, and double voiding prior to going to bed.

Overflowing SUDS

The following are some organic causes of enuresis to consider. Look for clues in the question.

SUDS = Envision a child with enuresis who is urinating soapsuds instead of urine. This will help you recall organic causes of enuresis.

Sickle cell trait
Urinary Tract Infection or Anomaly
Diabetes
Seizure or **S**acral (Lumbar-sacral)

Secondary Nocturnal Enuresis (SNE)

Consider the following:

- severe snoring and sleep disruption
- urinary tract infection or diabetes
- constipation
- stress: moves, divorce, abuse, etc

Desmopressin (DDAVP)

If they were to present desmopressin as a treatment option for PNE, be aware that the FDA advises **not to use it in the intranasal form** due to risk of severe hyponatremia and seizures.

It is acceptable to use it in **tablet** form nightly for 6 months and then stop it for 2 weeks to see if the problem has resolved. Relapse after resolution is common with desmopressin.

Diurnal Enuresis

 If you are presented with a patient with **diurnal enuresis** after a period of daytime continence, the most likely diagnosis is behavioral, ie. waiting too long to head to the restroom, or psychological, i.e. stress or abuse.

Diurnal enuresis cannot be diagnosed prior to age 3.

Just in case it's not behavioral, check a UA and consider **UTI, diabetes mellitus, diabetes insipidus, or kidney disease.**

Stool withholding

Usually stool is withheld because it is perceived or has been experienced as **painful**. This results in larger more painful stools, and a vicious cycle ensues.

In older children, laxatives are often used. The premature discontinuation of laxatives often leads to recurrence of stool withholding.

In the absence of constipation since infancy, a workup for Hirschsprung's disease is inappropriate.

Stooling tie with UTI

Chronic constipation may be associated with UTIs because of stasis and urinary retention.

Reacting to Family Stressors

Divorce and Coparenting

A child's response to divorce is developmental stage-dependent. The same holds true for a child's response to an illness in the family.

Somatization and regression of developmental milestones are typical responses to divorce and other stresses.

As a result of the increase in joint custody arrangements, **involvement of divorced fathers** in their children's lives has increased.

However, the impact of joint custody can result in **increased conflict between parents,** which often has a negative effect on the children.

Consistency, structure, and routine help children adjust to the divorce, both in the short and in the long term.

Children of divorce may have more difficulties with intimate relationships, including marriage, as adults. They may have increased conflict in the workplace as well.

> **Bouncing Back**
>
> After the immediate adjustment to a significant life stressor, such as death or divorce, 75% of children recover within 2-3 years, unless new stresses keep appearing.

Age-based response to divorce:

Age	Typical Response to Divorce
Toddlers (2-3 years)	Commonly develop separation anxiety.
Pre-school (4-5 years)	Regression of the most recently obtained developmental milestones.
Early School Age (6-8)	Overt grieving, fears of rejection, guilt, and fantasies that the parents will get back together.
Late School Age (9-12)	Anger at one or both parents. Open mourning of the loss of the safety and structure of an intact family.
Teenagers	Depression and acting out. More likely to be romantically and sexually active. Suicidal thoughts and ideation are also possible responses. PERIL Teenagers might fake indifference, but **true indifference will never be the correct answer**.

(No) Divorce from Reality

When answering questions on divorce best to use common sense, therefore all correct answers will be consistent with

- Maintaining structure and routine
- Both parents should be involved in their care
- Encourage meaningful relations with both parent
- Schedules should be predictable and structured

Death in the Family

A child's response to a death in the family will depend on the age of the child, as outlined in the table below. The response is **similar to that of divorce, since both involve a loss**.

Age of Child	Response to Death in the Family
Pre-schoolers	May **confuse death with sleep** or believe that death is only **temporary**. They may also blame their thoughts or actions for the death as a result of **"magical thinking"**. **Regression** of developmental milestones is common. **Acting out** and **tantrums** are also possible.
School-Age	**Somatic complaints** are very common, as well as **sleep disturbances** and **decreased school performance**. May develop a **morbid fascination with death**. They figure out their **own mortality**.
Teenagers	Of course, **acting out** is a possible reaction. Acting out is always a possibility with teenagers, and can never be the wrong choice on the exam. May ask **"Why not me?"** and/ or **"challenge mortality"** and take more risks.

PERIL Lack of mourning or the appearance of coping well on the surface should never be taken at face value - "no additional intervention" will never be the correct choice for a child mourning a death.

HOT TIP **Loss of appetite** is common in all age groups; however, overt failure to thrive is not a common result. There are also unique factors to consider for each individual situation/relationship with the deceased.

Untimely Death

Important caveats to consider when answering questions related to death and grieving in children include:

- Don't be ambiguous
- Be honest
- Use age appropriate language.

Chronic Illness and the Family

Grief Reaction to a Child with a Disability

A possible initial sequence of reactions is as follows:

Shock and fear

Denial and disbelief

Sadness and anger

Acceptance

HOT TIP Initially, a parent may not want to see the child, or may postpone contact after birth by not feeding the child. The correct response is to encourage contact and promote bonding to help work through the fear. Parents may require time to fully comprehend the situation and/or mourn the loss of a "normal" child.

The following factors are considered to be **protective for siblings** of children with chronic disabilities:

- Larger family size
- Female siblings and older siblings are at higher risk for negative outcomes due to their parentification
- Financial resources serve to buffer negative impacts
- Intact families with harmonious relationships help decrease negative effects

Grief stages

Kubler-Ross described 5 stages of grief. These can apply to death, divorce, or even losing at your March Madness brackets. These are:

1. Denial
2. Anger
3. Bargaining
4. Depression
5. Acceptance

Each stage can take any length of time, the stages do not necessarily proceed in order, and an individual can bounce back between the stages.

Extracurricular activities

Extracurricular activities, such as sports and music, may help improve school performance, with the caveat that over-scheduling can have a detrimental effect.

Cain and Abel

When it comes to sibling rivalry, with or without disabilities, the goal is to have the siblings learn to **resolve their conflicts on their own**. Parents need to step in when physical or verbal abuse occurs. In those cases, the goal is still to enable them to resolve the conflicts on their own.

Transplant Transitions

Although recipients of liver and kidney transplants in childhood initially go through a growth spurt, they typically do not attain their genetic potential regarding adult height.

Poor compliance is a known problem with adolescents who have received transplants.

There are important psychosocial consequences that go along with receiving an organ transplant. Some of this is due to the side effects of immunosuppressive medications, which may include short stature and/or obesity.

One of the most important interventions that can help the family cope better is to **increase home resources**.

In general, the scenario of a **mother and father responding differently** to a child born with a disability is to be expected, and no intervention is necessary unless there is a clear detriment to the child.

Parents who are **health care professionals** and have to use home equipment such as oxygen do not cope better than non-health care professionals.

Home monitors are believed to have a role in apnea management in certain patient populations. However, studies show that they tend to increase parental hostility and depression.

Risk Factors for Abuse and Neglect

Child abuse risk factors can be divided into 4 broad categories

1. External factors
2. Parenting skills
3. Vulnerability of the child
4. Psychological factors

Other forms of domestic violence often occur in addition to child abuse.

Also note that abuse may occur in foster care.

External Factors

External factors that increase the risk for abuse include

- Poor housing
- Multiple young children
- Social isolation
- Family discord

Parental Skills

- Unwanted parenthood
- Unexpected parenthood
- Unrealistic expectations
- Parent abused as a child

Vulnerability of the child

Children who are **hyperactive** are at increased risk for being abused.

HOT TIP

Children with **disabilities** and those born **prematurely** are also at higher risk for abuse.

Psychological factors

TAKE HOME MESSAGE

Alcoholism or **drug abuse,** as well as **parental mental illness,** all increase risk for child abuse and neglect.

Parents who were **abused as children** are at high risk for repeating the pattern.

Unrealistic expectations of the child, as well as **parental depression,** are additional risk factors.

PERIL

Sibling rivalry and siblings hitting each other is rarely an explanation for serious injury. If this is the explanation given in the history, they are trying to tell you the injury was non-accidental.

The gender of the child, parental education, and employment status are not important risk factors for child abuse.

HOT TIP

You need to be familiar with infant feeding patterns, which may reflect deeper mother/ infant relationship problems. These include:

- Feeding the child or infant to quiet them down
- Propping the bottle at bedtime

If you are asked a question about the most important intervention, addressing the individual feeding issues are not the most important interventions. **Psychosocial intervention** is the most important intervention.

Violence and Child Abuse

Intimate Partner Violence (IPV)

IPV, in addition to inactivated polio vaccine, now stands for *intimate partner violence* which used to be called domestic violence.

Mandatory Reporting Requirements

Reporting ANY concern for abuse (physical, sexual, or neglect) is absolutely mandatory in all 50 states. If abuse is implied in the question reporting it will be the correct answer.

Intentional Ingestion

Ingestion that would be unusual for the child's developmental stage may not be accidental.

Consider intentional ingestion or abuse if, for example, an infant ingested alcohol. A scenario such as this could represent a parent's attempt to sedate or stop the infant from crying.

When to screen for IPV

Screening for IPV is recommended as part of routine encounters, but is particularly crucial in cases of children with frequent non specific symptoms including stomach and headaches. Screening mothers only if they are depressed or anxious is a less reliable criterion. And remember, it's not just mothers who are victims of intimate partner violence.

The questions in the screen should be specific rather than general.

"Do you feel Safe at home?" Is an example of a general question.

"What happens when you and your partner disagree?" Would be an example of a more specific question.

As a mandated reporter, even if you only suspect that the parent or guardian is a victim of abuse with no evidence or suspicion of child abuse, you must report the suspected violence because the children are likely being exposed to it.

If the child is older than 3 and verbal, it is best to ask the questions with the child outside the room.

As with ANY suspected abuse, it is NOT a good idea for you to interview the child. Leave that to the authorities.

Children who are exposed to intimate partner violence are:

- At risk for physical injury
- Likely to be aggressive with their peers
- Prone to separation anxiety as toddlers
- At risk for school failure as adolescents as well as risky sexual behavior

They are not at risk for being shy and withdrawn. They are more likely to be aggressive. Infants may cry a lot and be resistant to comforting. Toddlers may exhibit extreme separation anxiety.

Medical Child Abuse

This was previous referred to as Munchausen Syndrome by Proxy and it is is diagnosed when a child's symptoms are **created or invented by a caretaker**, usually the mother.

 The diagnosis should be considered in cases with

- unexplained persistence or recurrence of symptoms
- the child appears healthier than the history or labs indicate
- symptoms are unusual to an experienced physician
- symptoms do not occur when the child is separated from the reporting caretaker
- symptoms have only been witnessed by the perpetrator
- the reporting caretaker refuses to leave the child's side
- negative work ups do not reassure the perpetrator
- the reported history is confusing and convoluted
- and the children have seen many doctors and subspecialists without cause found for symptoms

The **mothers** who inflict the injuries in MSBP may suffer from Munchausen syndrome themselves (self-inflict symptoms for attention) and usually have a more extensive medical background than expected. They often have histories of emotional and physical abuse, neglect, drug and alcohol dependence, or suicide attempts. The **father** is usually passive and distances himself from the situation.

Physicians, although trying to help, are usually the ones responsible for most of the harm done to these children, and most of the harm to the children actually occurs in the hospital.[1]

Once confronted, the parent will usually remove the child from the provider's care. The provider should gather all the medical records available for detailed review and the case should be **reported to CPS**. The child should be **removed from the parent** to see if the symptoms resolve. Videotaping visits in the hospital might be helpful.

---

[1] MSBP is also referred to as "Medical Child Abuse".

Over time, these children are at risk for **developing chronic invalidism** and accept the "illness" resulting in an inability to lead a "normal" life.

These children will **need long-term counseling**.

Somatization Disorders

A somatization disorder is a physical symptom that is **un**intentionally produced, but it has **no physiological explanation.**

If a family member has a chronic physical illness, those children display more somatic symptoms.

The rate of somatization is higher among lower socioeconomic groups.

Conversion disorder – symptoms are incompatible with anatomical and medical logic

Hypochondriasis – preoccupation with illness, frequently in the context of previous illness

Malingering – presenting with false or exaggerated symptoms, often with a motive

Dysmorphic disorder – despite evidence to the contrary, the patient perceives themselves as being ugly or undesirable

Somatic delusions – belief that something is medically wrong and may take on psychotic dimensions, i.e., their pancreas has wings.

If you are presented with a patient with prolonged "effortless and painless" vomiting, rumination syndrome is a likely diagnosis.

Rumination syndrome - effortless and painless vomiting for 2 months, in the absence of an identifiable organic cause.

Treatment is Cognitive Behavioral Psychotherapy.

CASE STUDY

A 15 year old female presents with a sudden loss of sensation in her left leg; she reports that she cannot feel anything in the entire leg. There is no history of trauma, and the neurologist has signed off on the case because the neurological exam is normal. Her grandfather recently died of natural causes, and her parents proudly tell you how wonderfully she has coped and accepted his death like an adult. What is the best explanation for the paralysis of her leg?

THE DIVERSION

You may be smart enough to not go for the neurological choices such as Guillain Barré syndrome, tethered cord, or metastatic disease involving the spinal cord. So you will then be down to two choices, depression and conversion disorder. Conversion disorder seems a bit farfetched and depression is unlikely since she is coping so well, but a mild depression would be expected. If you went down that path you might be depressed to learn you got the question wrong, and you might have a conversion disorder involving your writing hand.

ANSWER REVEALED

Remember: the teen that has "gone through a loss with no problems" does not exist, despite what the parents say. Depression wouldn't explain the physical findings described. The correct answer is conversion disorder. Pick this answer on the exam, and you will be well on your way to converting "board eligible" to "board certified," and, ultimately, "recertified."

PERIL

We often hear that asthma, eczema, and a variety of other disorders have "psychological components to them." Psychosomatic illnesses tend to be exacerbated during times of stress.

There is a double-edged sword to doing an extensive workup in the case of psychosomatic illness, since ordering tests can reinforce the perceived seriousness of the symptoms. You as the physician are expected to overcome your own anxiety and resist the urge to order every test known to man. This will be important if you are presented with a patient who is clearly presenting with a psychosomatic illness or conversion disorder. Ordering tests and studies with obvious psychosomatic illness or converstion disorder will be incorrect.

TREATMENT

Treatment of psychosomatic illness involves recognizing and explaining to the family that **the symptoms are real,** but there is **no organic basis** for them.

The key is **addressing the stress or anxiety** that has led to the symptoms.

HOT TIP

Positive feedback is important. It is also important to **remove secondary gain**, such as missing school.

If weakness is a component of the presentation, limited physical therapy may help.

Somatizations of Stress

"Geez, you know I am really stressed out and I could sure use a nap and some time off." This is not something children will say when they are stressed out. They will complain of, and feel, somatic pain, such as a headache, chest pain, diarrhea and/or abdominal pain. As age increases, so do symptoms of fatigue and insomnia.

In the face of recurrent abdominal pain, you are expected to know that a psychosocial history is important. By definition, the seriousness of the problem is related to its interference with everyday life (which, in the case of children, often includes school attendance).

In addition, school may be a factor in causing the recurrent pain.

If the pain persists on weekends, absence from school is unlikely to be a secondary gain factor.

Once again, remember that children may react to stress by somatizing and/or regressing. **Their perceived ability to have some degree of control over the situation is an important component.**[2]

Watch for signs of **parental anxiety** and how they themselves are dealing with stress (the question may clue you in to this).

Primary Pain Disorders

These were previously known as functional pain disorders. They are due to a variety of factors that are not necessarily medical / organic. These include cultural and psychological factors. These are important considerations even when physical causes are a factor.

The correct answer will be a multidisciplinary approach.

Acetaminophen and ibuprofen (NSAIDs in general) are first line pain meds.

Codeine and tramadol are to be avoided since their unpredictable pharmacokinetics leads to underdosing or overdosing.

Media Influence

The following are the known harmful effects of TV (and now also Internet use and video games) on children:

- Trivializing violence and blurring the distinction between reality and fantasy
- Encouraging passivity at the expense of activity, unless you consider nimble button pushing to be activity
- Television definitely **increases aggressive behavior,** and influences the **toys** played with and the **cereals** eaten

Some important facts to know are that, on average:

- "Screen time" (TV, computer, video game time) takes up more time than school
- Only the time spent sleeping exceeds the number of leisure hours spent on "screen time"

It is recommended that television watching be limited to **2 hours/day**, preferably with the parents watching as well.[3] Children **younger than 2** should **not** watch TV at all.[4]

---

[2] Just like adults, I suppose.
[3] Although there is only so much of "Courage the Cowardly Dog®" one can watch in one sitting.
[4] This is to be factored into any question on the subject. Clearly for anyone who actually has children, I am not sure how practical such an edict is in the real world.

Rock-A-Bye Baby

Sleep Patterns

During a normal sleep cycle, newborns sometimes experience arousal but are not fully awake. Parents may mistake this for the infant being awake, and arouse them from sleep.

Infants should be able to establish a **day/ night schedule** by **2 months of age**.

If the infant is not adjusting to a day/night sleep cycle, the correct management is to keep them awake more during the day so they will be more tired at night.

By **4 months of age**, infants should be capable of **sleeping through the night**.

A **1 year old** should be sleeping **13-14 hours a day**. As opposed to the parent of a 1 year old, who sleeps an average of 13-14 hours a week.

In order to avoid an infant being dependent on the presence of a parent to go back to sleep when they arouse during the night, it is best to put the baby to bed **sleepy but awake** so they learn how to soothe themselves when awake.

"Sleep training" (where the parents let the baby cry before going back into the bedroom) can begin to take place between **4-6 months of age**.

Night Terrors vs. Nightmares

In both cases the child will appear agitated.

Night Terrors

They occur during the **first third of the night**. There will often be a **family history**. This occurs in **boys** more often than in girls.

They will exhibit **distinctive physical findings**: deep breathing, dilated pupils, and sweating with rapid heart rate and respiratory rate. They can also **become mobile**, which may result in an injury.

When they awaken, they will have **no recall of the episod**e.

Most children stop having night terrors by adolescence (when they begin to experience other issues, of course).

The treatment goal is to make sure the **environment is safe** so they do not injure themselves during the night terror. In addition, **pre-waking** the child before the time they usually have the night terror, usually "breaks the cycle".

Intervening during a night terror may be counterproductive and worsen the child's agitation.

Nightmares

These occur during the **last third of the night**. They can be **woken easily,** and they will **recall the nightmare**, often quite vividly. They are not mobile and, therefore, at no real risk for physical injury.

Sexual Orientation

You are expected to understand issues around sexual orientation and gender identity as they develop in childhood and adolescence. The following are some important points to consider when answering questions on this subject on the boards:

- **Sexual orientation is biologically-based.** Influence of adverse life events has not been substantiated.
- Homosexual teens and young adults are at higher risk for **substance abuse, suicide, dropping out of school,** and **being homeless.**

> **Sexual Orientation**
>
> Sexual orientation is determined by mid-adolescence.
>
> There is growing evidence for the bio-logical/genetic/hormonal basis for sexual orientation. One thing to remember for the Boards is that there is no evidence for parental influence or various adverse life events "causing homosexuality."

Sexual orientation is **not a choice.**

Sexual activity is a choice.

Same sex experimentation, especially in early adolescence, is **not a harbinger of homosexuality.**

International Adoption

You are expected to be aware of the physician's role in international adoption.

Before the adoption takes place, the pediatrician should assist the family in **reviewing medical records,** including information about the biological parents.

This information **may be inaccurate**; therefore the medical history should be taken with a grain of salt.

Anticipatory guidance is another role that the pediatrician may play. Included in this should be the advice that **the period of transition and attachment may take up to a year.**

After the adoption takes place, the pediatrician should do a **developmental assessment** of the child and recheck **every 3-4 months** during the first year. **Hearing and vision screening** should be done at the first visit.

Immunization records should be verified. .

Routine blood tests, including **CBC, lead level,** as well as **Hepatitis B, HIV,** and **syphilis** testing are recommended.

If the adopted child is from an area that is endemic for hepatitis C, **hepatitis C serology** should be measured.

TB testing should take place regardless of whether or not they received BCG vaccination (they may actually write this out formally as Bacille Calmette-Guérin). **A positive test should always be addressed** and not automatically attributed to previous BCG vaccination.

Children in Foster Care

Here are some of the important points you might be tested on regarding children in foster care and the role of the pediatrician:

- Children in foster care use more mental and general healthcare resources when compared to others in the same socioeconomic strata.
- The AAP recommends that children in foster care receive more frequent routine evaluations than their peers.
- All children entering foster care require baseline behavioral, mental, and developmental evaluations.
- The pediatrician should communicate directly with the caseworker to facilitate ongoing care, even after the child has been reunited with his/her family.
- A health care *screen* should be performed within 72 hours of placement in foster care.
- A *comprehensive health assessment* should be done within 30 days of entry into foster care
- At court hearings for child abuse, children are represented by *a law guardian* who may be a trained volunteer (Court Appointed Special Advocate or CASA) or an actual attorney.
- Whenever possible, there is a preference to place children with relatives rather than in non-relative foster homes.
- **Reunification of the family** is always the primary goal of Child Protective Services as long as the child is in a safe environment. Having children "adopted out" is an option only if reunification efforts fail.

Vulnerable Child Syndrome (VCS)

When a parent exhibits anxiety over the child being **more vulnerable than other children**.

These parents **overprotect** the child, do not set age-appropriate limits on behavior, and bring them to the doctor, especially the emergency room, for even minor ailments.

Risk factors for VCS

- there is a history of serious illness or injury, even during the pregnancy
- the child reminds the parent of a special someone who died unexpectedly
- the mother has a history of threated abortion, multiple spontaneous abortions, stillbirths, or fertility issues

It is important to provide **anticipatory guidance** to these parents when the risk factors are noted in order to try and prevent VCS. It is crucial to remember to be careful with the words that are used regarding a child's condition. Words like "superinfection" mean one thing to a doctor, but a "super" infection is a super scary thing to a parent.

Providers must uncover **the source of the parent's anxiety**, since many times the parents are unaware of the subconscious connections they are making between the current concerns and past events.

It is important to **actively reassure them** about their child's normal health, growth, and development. Regular scheduled appointments to discuss concerns may be of significant help initially, and may be weaned as parents feel less anxious.

Human Trafficking

Sadly this is becoming an increasingly important topic in the field of pediatrics and fair game on the exam as well.

Human trafficking is defined as the provision, obtainment, recruitment, transportation and/or harboring of a person for physical or sexual services.

This is done through the use of coercion, fraud or force for the purposes of involuntary slavery or servitude.

Risk factors

Although children and adolescents of all ethnic and economic backgrounds can be victims, there are certain factors that increase the risk including:

- Female gender
- Native American ethnicity
- Identifying as LGBTQIA+
- History of illicit substance use/abuse
- History of sexual abuse
- Previous involvement with child protective services
- Housing issues (living in a group home, foster care, orphaned, homeless)

Clinical Red Flags

There are additional clinical, psychological red flags to monitor for:

- While victims can seek medical attention for a variety of reasons, watch for a description of multiple ER visits, recurrent sexually transmitted infections (STIs).
- Unusual tattooing is another telltale sign, which sadly is a form of tagging and tracking.
- Watch for the description of an overbearing " friend" or " relative" who accompanies the patient to visits.

Guidance regarding human trafficking is to be included in anticipatory guidance.

Calling the National Human Trafficking resource center (1-88-373-7888) would be a correct response if it is included among the choices on the exam.

Chapter 12

Nutrition Fruition

Fat Soluble Vitamins

Being familiar with the clinical presentations of the important vitamin toxicities and deficiencies is worth spending time on because it will certainly be worth several points on the exam. They will likely describe patients with classic symptoms. They will most likely be identified by their **formal names**, which you must link somehow to the vitamin letter. Fortunately, you've come to the right place because we have already done this for you.

The only vitamins that are not fat-soluble are vitamins B and C. Fat-soluble vitamins are the ones that come in the gelatin tablet with the oil in the center.

 The fat soluble vitamins can be remembered with the acronym **FAKED** (Fat-soluble - AKED).

Vitamins on a First Name Basis	
Vitamin	**Formal Name**
Vitamin A	Retinol
Vitamin D	Has many forms and variations which are way too boring to bog down this nice table. It gets to sit in its own "Teak Table on the deck" on the side.
Vitamin E	Tocopherol Just remember it as **"Toke-of-E-rol"** to remember it as vitamin E.
Vitamin K	Phylloquinone To help remember that the formal name of vitamin K is phylloquinone, remember the term **"File-O-Kanines:"** Picture a file cabinet full of dogs that are shaped like the letter "K." This will jog your memory that **phylloquinone is vitamin K**, if this is what they call it.

Water Soluble Vitamins

The water-soluble vitamins include the **B vitamins** (all of them) and **vitamin C.**

Vitamins on a First Name Basis	
Vitamin	**Formal Name**
Vitamin B$_1$	Thiamine There only 1 so it's MINE
Vitamin B$_2$	Riboflavin "Ri-BOTH-flavin" Both=2
Vitamin B$_3$	Niacin
Vitamin B$_5$	Pantothenic Acid Change to Pentothenic acid
Vitamin B$_6$	Pyridoxine Pyrido6ine
Vitamin B$_9$	Folate If a fool comes late it is benign (B$_9$)
Vitamin B$_{12}$	Cyanocobalamin
Biotin	Biotin (only has a formal name but is considered to be a **B** vitamin). This is easy to remember since biotin, a B vitamin begins with the B.
Vitamin C	Ascorbic Acid

Vitamin Deficiencies and Toxicities

Vitamin	Deficiency	Toxicity
Vitamin A (Retinol)	**Worldwide, vitamin A deficiency is the most common cause of blindness in young children.** With the formal name retinol so similar to "retina," it is easy to link this to blindness. Vitamin A deficiency can also lead to dryness of the eyes (AKA **xerophthalmia**), and **nyctalopia** (a fancy word for night blindness, but the word you are likely to see on the exam).	Vitamin A intoxication can result in intracranial hypertension (i.e. **pseudotumor cerebri**). MNEMONIC Picture a giant **A** like a big hat causing intracranial pressure.
Vitamin B$_9$ (Folate)	Large tongue and **macrocytic anemia**. Watch if they mention that the children are on **goat's milk**.	Irritability. See box labeled "Macrocytic Anemias."
Vitamin B$_{12}$ (Cyanoco-balamin)	**Macrocytic anemia. Pernicious anemia** (due to poor absorption secondary to decreased intrinsic factor).	Expensive electric urine, but harmless.
Vitamin C (Ascorbic Acid)	Besides **bleeding gums** and **scurvy** (remember the stories of Columbus), they might also describe **leg tenderness and poor wound healing**. HOT TIP Also consider in children with highly restrictive diets (either by parental choice or by other conditions like autism, financial limitations) with refusal to walk.	Vitamin C is well tolerated even in large doses. However, it is escorted out the door through the kidneys, so **excessive mega doses can cause oxalate and cysteine nephrocalcinosis** (also known as kidney stones). HOT TIP It is one of the agents that can **trigger a hemolytic crisis** in a patient with **glucose-6-phosphate dehydrogenase deficiency**.

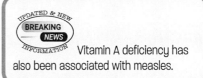

UPDATED & NEW **BREAKING NEWS** INFORMATION Vitamin A deficiency has also been associated with measles.

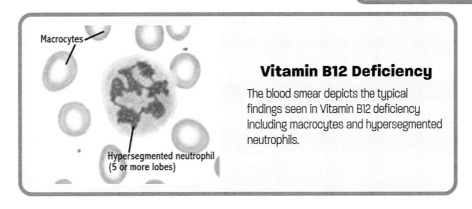

Macrocytes

Vitamin B12 Deficiency

The blood smear depicts the typical findings seen in Vitamin B12 deficiency including macrocytes and hypersegmented neutrophils.

Hypersegmented neutrophil (5 or more lobes)

Vitamin	Deficiency	Toxicity
Vitamin E (Tocopherol)	Vitamin E deficiency may present as **hemolytic anemia in preemies.** Vitamin E deficiency in older children is characterized by **neuropathies, peripheral edema, thrombocytosis, and muscle weakness** but would have to be severely prolonged to cause symptoms.	Vitamin E toxicity is controversial and they should not ask, but if they do, **liver toxicity** is the answer.
Vitamin K (Mr. Phylloquinone to you)	Vitamin K deficiency results in **hemorrhagic disease of the newborn.**[1] HOT TIP **Breast fed babies are particularly vulnerable** because breast milk does not contain much vitamin K.	Vitamin K toxicity is not often an issue and is never really tested on the exam.

MNEMONIC

Picture the E as a fork puncturing the red cells and all the muscles and nerves causing everything to explode and leading to the **triple E of vitamin E deficiency**: Edema, Erythrocyte explosion (hemolytic anemia), and Elevated platelet count.

PERIL

Isotretinoin, used to treat acne in teens, is an analog of vitamin A. So if they present you with a teen on Isotretinoin with symptoms of a brain tumor, think **Vitamin A toxicity and pseudotumor cerebri.**

CASE STUDY

You are presented with a toddler who is noted to be quite yellow.

THE DIVERSION

Buried in the question is the fact that this is a child who has eaten many foods rich in beta carotene,[2] such as carrots, sweet potatoes, and apricots.

The child may be described as "looking" yellow but will not be described as being icteric.

However, the sclerae and oral mucosa are not yellow. This is the key to answering the question correctly.

ANSWER REVEALED

The child is carotenemic, not jaundiced or icteric, and therefore no further evaluation is necessary.

However, the decoy answer, "get a serum bili," is not correct.

Macrocytic anemias

B12 and Folate deficiency both lead to macrocytic anemia.

These deficiencies may be seen in patients noted to be on an exclusive vegetarian and/or vegan diets.

BUZZWORDS

On the exam you can be presented with you will see it in breast-fed infants of mothers who are adhering to vegetarian /vegan diet.

Macrocytic anemia can also be seen in celiac disease, cystic fibrosis, inflammatory bowel disease and short gut syndrome (as with NEC) due to poor absorption.

---

1 For more detail, see HemeOnc chapter.
2 Beta carotene is converted to vitamin A (retinol) by the body, and is therefore a precursor to vitamin A.

Vitamin D

The Faces and Phases of Vitamin D

Just when you thought it was going to be easy, in walks vitamin D, along with all its aliases and accomplices. D has different numbers and each has its own name.

Vitamin	Formal Name	MNEMONIC Mnemonic
Vitamin D_2	Ergocalciferol	It has 2 Cs in the name; therefore, D_2.
Vitamin D_3	Cholecalciferol	It has 3 Cs in the name; therefore, D_3.
25-hydroxy vitamin D	Calcidiol, which is hydroxylated in the liver.[3] This is the primary storage form.	There is only one liver; therefore, only one number.
1,25 hydroxy-calciferol[4]	1,25-dihydroxycholecalciferol is formed in the kidney. **Its friends call it calcitriol. It is the active metabolite of Vitamin D.** MNEMONIC Calci-TRY-ALL tries to help the body by increasing calcium absorption in the gut and releasing it from the bone into the blood.	There are 2 kidneys, therefore, 2 hydroxy groups.

HOT TIP D is the only vitamin known to be converted to a hormone form. There is no dietary requirement when the child is sufficiently exposed to UV sunlight.

BREAKING NEWS INFORMATION Obesity is a risk factor for Vitamin D deficiency.

HOT TIP If the answer comes down to checking the Vit D level, you must be specific. The correct answer will be to **measure the 25-hydroxy Vitamin D level** because this is the primary storage form of Vitamin D.

PERIL Vitamin D deficiency can be seen in patients on antiacids, seizure medications, and corticosteroids. Watch for any of these being described in the history.

BREAKING NEWS INFORMATION More recent recommendations are to supplement all infants whether breast or formula-fed from the first few days of life until age 2.

TAKE HOME MESSAGE Traditional Vit D supplementation is 400 IU per day for infants who are primarily breast-fed.

BREAKING NEWS INFORMATION More recent recommendations are to supplement all infants whether breast or formula-fed from the first few days of life until age 2.

---

[3] 25-hydroxy vitamin D (25 (OH) D3).
[4] 1,25 dihydroxy vitamin D (1,25 (OH)2 D3 or 1,25 (OH)2 D as it is referred to in the illustration of Vitamin D and Calcium Metabolism.

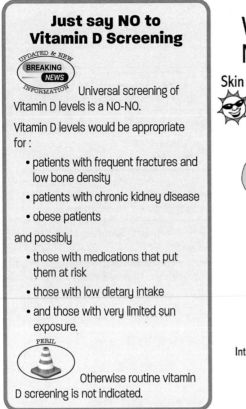

Just say NO to Vitamin D Screening

Universal screening of Vitamin D levels is a NO-NO.

Vitamin D levels would be appropriate for :

- patients with frequent fractures and low bone density
- patients with chronic kidney disease
- obese patients

and possibly

- those with medications that put them at risk
- those with low dietary intake
- and those with very limited sun exposure.

Otherwise routine vitamin D screening is not indicated.

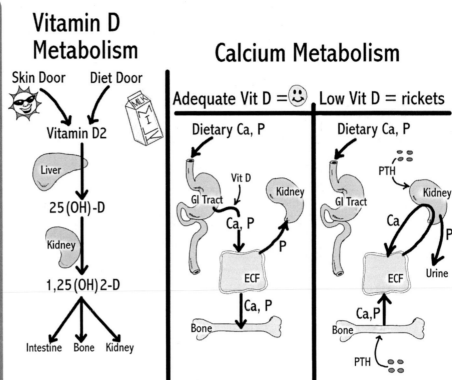

Vitamin D Excess

Vitamin D excess results in disturbances in calcium metabolism, specifically **hypercalcemia** and **hyperphosphatemia**. In addition, it will produce non-specific signs such as **nausea, vomiting, and weakness**.

The more specific findings include **polyuria, polydipsia, elevated BUN, nephrolithiasis**, and **perhaps renal failure**. It can also be **fatal**.

Symptoms of polydipsia, polyuria, and poor growth are **similar to diabetes**. Diabetes and vitamin D both have "**D**." In addition, vitamin D toxicity and diabetes can both result in kidney failure.

D-Toxing

Vitamin D toxicity results in the excess mobilization of calcium and phosphorus from bones and deposition into soft tissue. It is treated with **hydration**, correction of **Na and K depletion, and Lasix®**.

Nutritional Needs

Caloric Needs

Caloric Requirements should be easy to remember. It is similar to calculating fluids:

- ❏ 100 kcal/kg (1st 10 kg)
- ❏ 50 kcal/kg (next 10 kg)
- ❏ 20 kcal/kg (any more kgs.)
- ❏ 1500 kcal for the first 20 kg, then 20 kcal/kg for each additional kg

Caloric intake for children is based on body surface area

The optimal caloric intake is based on a child's body surface area. This of course varies from child to child.

PERIL

The RDA (recommended daily allowance) is only a starting point for estimating the caloric requirements in children.

CASE STUDY

A 3 year old child whose caloric intake is consistent with the RDA is at the 5th percentile for weight.

THE DIVERSION

The question specifically notes that the child is taking the recommended daily caloric intake, with all other clinical criteria within normal limits. What steps can be taken to have the patient gain weight appropriately?

ANSWER REVEALED

The correct answer will be to increase the child's caloric intake. This is because this particular child's caloric requirements exceed the RDA. You need to know that the RDA is a ballpark figure for the general population, which may not apply to any particular patient.

Nutrition Fruition in the Newborn Period

Nutrition is a fairly large part of the exam. They love to ask detailed questions on the differences between formula and breast milk, formula and whole milk, whole milk and 5% fruit juice, fruit juice and scotch, blended scotch and single malt scotch – well, I got carried away there, but you get the picture.

PERIL

Remember that both term and preterm infants require 100-120 kcal/kg/day. Of course, a preterm infant's requirement is closer to 120 and a large term infant's requirement is closer to 100.

However, if you were faced with a choice that states, "both term and preterm infants require 100-120 kcal/kg/day to grow," it would be correct.

Protein Requirements

Premature infants require 3.5 g/kg per day in order to achieve growth and weight gain close to that expected in utero.

Full Term infants, on the other hand, grow well with protein intakes of approximately **2.0 to 2.5 g/kg per day** for the first 6 months.

Fat Storage in the Premature

Preemies have lower levels of fat storage and may have difficulty maintaining appropriate body temperature. Because of this, they expend more energy in heat production that term babies. Premature infants also require more energy for organogenesis and to develop fat stores.

All of this increases nutritional and energy requirements in comparison to term babies.

Catching up

Catch up growth in preemies occurs during the first 2 years.

They should attain corrected height for age by age 2.

Dietary Protein Loading up the Kidney

The infant's kidney cannot handle the same osmotic load as an adult during times of stress, even if:

- an infant is receiving adequate nutrition
- there are no increased insensible water losses
- there is no evidence of renal failure

They can still lose weight due to renal fluid loss as a result of increased solute load.

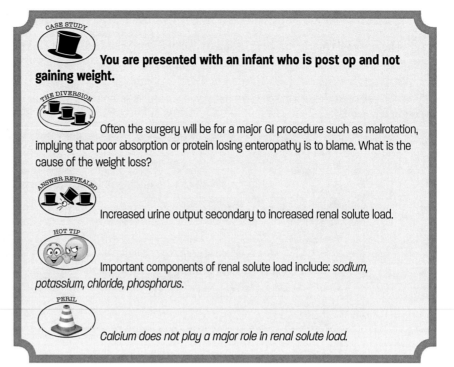

CASE STUDY **You are presented with an infant who is post op and not gaining weight.**

THE DIVERSION Often the surgery will be for a major GI procedure such as malrotation, implying that poor absorption or protein losing enteropathy is to blame. What is the cause of the weight loss?

ANSWER REVEALED Increased urine output secondary to increased renal solute load.

HOT TIP Important components of renal solute load include: *sodium, potassium, chloride, phosphorus.*

PERIL *Calcium does not play a major role in renal solute load.*

Formula for Success

Fluoride

Commercially available formula does not have adequate fluoride. This must be obtained from outside sources, such as drinking water.

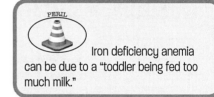

PERIL Iron deficiency anemia can be due to a "toddler being fed too much milk."

Ironing out the Need for Iron

You will be expected to iron out fact from fiction regarding iron fortified formula. The recommended concentration of iron in iron fortified formula is **12mg/L**.

PERIL **Iron supplementation is not routinely required at birth** since full term babies have adequate iron stores. It would, however, be required for those at high risk (e.g., LBW, preterm) in supplement form before 6 months of age, even in breast fed babies. Infants who receive more than 50% of their calories from breast milk need iron supplementation, **starting around 4 months of age**.

PERIL Low iron formula 1.5mg/L is not to be used. It will always be the incorrect choice.

MYTH Iron fortified formula does not cause constipation. This is a trap often laid on the boards so beware.

> **CASE STUDY**
>
> **An infant around 5-6 months of age who is on iron fortified formula (12mg/L) presents with constipation. How would you manage this problem?**
>
> **THE DIVERSION**
>
> The question casually mentions that the infant is on iron fortified formula, 12mg/L. Here they are capitalizing on the myth that iron fortified formula causes constipation. One of the choices is to switch to "reduced iron fortified formula 1.5 mg/L."
>
> **ANSWER REVEALED**
>
> Do not change to low iron formula - this is incorrect.
>
> - *Do not dilute the formula, this has nutritional consequences*
> - *Do not change to whole milk*
> - *Adding cereal will make the constipation worse*
> - *The correct answer* **will be to add fruit juice, to increase the osmotic load.**

Formula Intolerance

DEFINITION

Formula intolerance also goes under the alias of "adverse reaction to formula," and therefore allergy is just one form of formula intolerance.

COIN FLIP

You are expected to know the differences between milk protein allergy (IgE-mediated), milk intolerance (non IgE-mediated), and lactose intolerance.

Keeping Allergies Straight

Remember, with bona fide milk allergy there is a significant cross reactivity with soy-based formula. Therefore, elemental formula will be the correct answer.

Both milk protein allergy and milk intolerance can cause rash, vomiting, and irritability (see GI Section).

Milk Protein Allergy is due to an IgE-mediated response, and presents with rash, vomiting, and irritability.

Lactose intolerance can cause irritability, but not vomiting or rash.

Lactose intolerance can be due to secondary lactase deficiency. This can occur following a GI infection, such as rotavirus.

BUZZWORDS

This may be presented as an infant with bloating and worsening diarrhea after formula is reintroduced into the diet following an episode of viral gastroenteritis.

PERIL

Secondary lactose intolerance can occur following any GI infecion. This would include viral, parasitic or bacterial infection.

Holding off on lactose-containing formula in a very young infant could be appropriate until diarrhea resolves. However, holding off on breastfeeding would not be the correct answer, even if lactase deficiency is hinted at in the question.

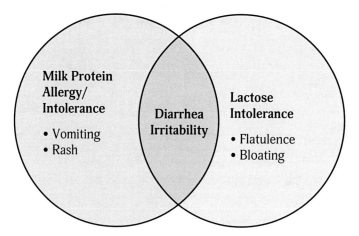

Milk Protein Allergy/Intolerance
- Vomiting
- Rash

Diarrhea Irritability

Lactose Intolerance
- Flatulence
- Bloating

PERIL

Infants fed "non traditional" formula will suffer from nutritional deficiencies, especially on the boards, so watch for this description in the history.

Protein hydrolysate formula is indicated in infants with:
- Allergy to intact milk protein
- Allergy to soy protein

FPIES (Severe Milk Protein Intolerance)

FPIES is actually "food protein-induced enterocolitis syndrome," which is way too convoluted to include in the title heading. This is a **non IgE-mediated** intolerance.

BUZZWORDS

FPIES typically presents in the first 6 months with repeated emesis and either **heme positive stools** or **hematochezia** along with a normal abdominal exam.

PERIL

Even though this is primarily due to cow milk intolerance, it can affect breast fed infants as well, because cow milk protein ingested by the mother can get into the breast milk.

It may also present after starting solid foods, such as rice cereal and oatmeal.

HOT TIP

Switching to soy formula will not be the correct answer since the symptoms frequently continue on soy formula. Therefore, the correct answer would be to switch to a **protein hydrolysate formula, or to completely eliminate the implicated protein from the mother's diet.**

BREAKING NEWS

These infants may progress to altered mental status and shock and be admitted to rule out sepsis, but be afebrile. After discharge, they go home, get exposed to the offending agent again, and get readmitted. Watch for this classic history.

Nutritional Deficiencies

Essential Fatty Acids

This will be described as **scaly dermatitis**, with **alopecia** and **thrombocytopenia**.

Treatment would be with **IV lipids**, with a focus on **linoleic acid** and **linolenic acid** which are essential fatty acids.

Since this can easily be confused with other rashes, consider a diagnosis of a fatty acid deficiency when presented with this pattern. Think of a thin fish with **scales coming off** (scaly rash) that turn into platelets (**low platelet count**) and, of course, the fish is then **bald** (alopecia).

Zinc Deficiency

This is also known as *acrodermatitis enteropathica,* an inherited condition where **zinc is not absorbed well**.

Breast milk contains a protein which facilitates zinc absorption, so if you are presented with an infant with the above findings who was **recently weaned from breast-milk**, zinc deficiency is the most likely cause.

A typical presentation is an infant who has an **extensive eczematous eruption, alopecia,** and is **growing poorly**. The lesions are typically **around the mouth** and perhaps in the **perianal area**.

Picture a **RED SINK (ZINC)** replacing a **mouth (perioral dermatitis)**. The drain of the sink is **clogged with hair**, to help you link this to **alopecia**.

It is **autosomal recessive**.

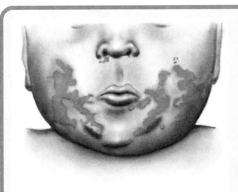

Acrodermatitis Enteropathica

The drawing illustrates the characteristic skin lesions include a periorificial and acral vesiculobullous eruption leading to scaly, sharply demarcated crusted plaques.

Acrodermatitis enteropathica is due to zinc deficiency. The deficiency can be due to nutritional deficiency or a congenital form is due to a defect in zinc absorption.

Manifestations of the disease typically present when the affected infant is weaned from breast feeding.

To distinguish this from eczema, acrodermatitis enteropathica has **no lichenification**. (Lichenification is a classic word associated with eczema).

CASE STUDY

A 7 month old girl who was weaned from breast-milk one month ago now presents with facial dermatitis, including a similar rash on the hands and feet. In addition, the baby has been less energetic, with diarrhea and thin hair. The most likely cause of this is:

THE DIVERSION

The question suggests that this is due to milk allergy or milk intolerance.

ANSWER REVEALED

The correct answer is zinc deficiency. The key is to not fall for the diversionary implication of milk allergy. The pattern described, especially the thin hair coupled with the fact that the child was recently weaned from breast milk, is consistent with zinc deficiency.

Copper Disorders

Menkes Kinky Hair Syndrome

Menkes Kinky Hair Syndrome, an **X-linked disorder**, is due to both **low serum copper** and **low serum ceruloplasmin;** however, the **tissue copper level is high**. They may show **twisted hairs (pili torti)**.

 Picture kinky hairs as **hands grabbing pennies**, to remind you that it is due to copper deficiency.

Wilson's Disease

BUZZWORDS

They will describe "liver deterioration" (i.e. **jaundice, large liver**) along with acute signs of **neurological deterioration**.

This is because of **deposition of copper in the liver and brain**. Also affected are the **eyes** (the classic **Kayser Fleischer rings**) and the kidney. **Visual deficits do NOT occur.**

It is diagnosed by liver biopsy. Ceruloplasmin levels are low, but not diagnostic.

Tracing it Back to the Hospital

Deficiencies of various other trace minerals (eg, magnesium, chromium) are generally limited to hospitalized patients with increased metabolic demands and underlying conditions like malnutrition, malabsorption, short bowel syndrome, significant burns, or dependence on TPN. Therefore you should only consider these deficiencies when presented with a hospitalized patient.

Nutritional Needs of the Premature

Preemies with RDS

If the mother of a preemie wants to breast-feed, the correct management is to have the mother pump so the milk is available for the infant. Breast-feeding can then begin when the baby is ready.

Vitamin D

The vitamin D requirements are higher in premature infants.

Vitamin E

Preterm infants taking formula high in polyunsaturated fatty acids must have vitamin E supplementation **to avoid hemolysis.**

Too Young to Absorb Fat

Premature infants have a **decreased amount of bile acids,** which makes it **difficult for them to absorb long chain triglycerides** and **fat-soluble vitamins.**

Fat Facts

Difference in preterm and full term ability to digest fat:

Most fats require bile salt emulsification so are absorbed less efficiently in premature babies; they can lose up to 20% of ingested fat through the stool.

Preemie Formula – **50%** of **total fat** is from **medium chain triglycerides** which are water soluble and do not require bile salt emulsification.

Mature Breast Milk – **12%** of the **total fat** content is **medium chain triglycerides.**

Breast milk does not contain or need a high amount of medium chain triglycerides because of its high absorptive abilities. Breast milk contains sufficient **linoleic and linolenic acids,** which are both essential (long chain) fatty acids.

Phosphorus and Calcium

Premature infants have poor phosphorus and calcium intake which may lead to osteopenia and rickets. They require supplementation, but **since calcium and phosphorus are poorly absorbed in the gut of preemies, large amounts must be given.**

Inadequate phosphorus (often secondary to prolonged parenteral nutrition) in the very low birthweight preterm infant may result in **demineralization of bone.**

Inadequate calcium can also lead to bone demineralization.

> ### Hind is Higher
> HOT TIP
> The **H**ind milk (the milk at the end of the feeding) is **H**igher in fat (and therefore calories).

This may occur after 1 month of TPN. Typical lab findings would include normal serum calcium and phosphorus. However, **alkaline phosphatase** will be elevated.

If **excessive phosphorus** is provided to a very low birthweight infant, it can lead to **hypocalcemia, tetany, and seizures.**

Breast: Better Than the Rest

Breast milk is good for virtually every reason. The AAP suggests **exclusive breast-feeding until at least 6 months**, and continued use of breast milk up to 12 months.

Supplement with water? The answer they want is "No!"

Colostrum vs. Mature Milk

There are a variety of differences between colostrum (the first few days of breast milk) and "mature" breast milk. Try to remember the following mind numbing facts for the exam!

Arachidonic acid (AA) and **Docosahexaenoic acid (DHA)** – decrease in mature milk. This is true for mothers of premature babies as well. This is important for neurologic development.

Zinc – Same as with AA, and is needed in premature infants especially to prevent skin lesions, poor wound healing, and decreased immune function.

Ergo-cholecalciferol – low levels in colostrum, which increases the risk for rickets.

The colostrum over the first few days postpartum is higher in protein, especially because of the high levels of immune globulins, including secretory IgA. This provides initial protection against infection. It is **yellow in color**, primarily because it is **high in carotene**.

	Colostrum	Mature Milk
Protein	More (2.3 g/dL)	Less (1.2 g/dL)
Fat	Low (1.7 g/dL)	High (4 g/dL)
Lactose	A bit less (6 g/dL)	A bit more (7g/dL)
Energy Content	Less (49 kcal/dL)	More (69 kcal/dL)

Breast Milk vs. Cow's Milk

Breast milk contains more lactose and is, therefore, sweeter.[5]

Cow's milk contains a significantly **higher** amount of **phosphorus** than human milk. The infant kidney cannot get rid of it fast enough,

---

MNEMONIC

BAD BREAST

Contraindications to breast-feeding

Bad Bugs (CMV, HIV, TB, HSV lesions on breast)
Antithyroid Meds
Drugs (amphetamines, cocaine, PCP)

Bad Bugs (CMV, HIV, TB)
Radioactive (Gallium, iodine, technetium-99) and Cytotoxic Drugs (cyclosporine, cyclophosphamide, doxorubicin, and methotrexate)
Errors of Metabolism, Galactosemia, PKU, Urea Cycle Defects (in the baby)
Anti–biotics and Anti–seizures (Meds like Flagyl® and Diazepam)
Sulfonamides
Tetracycline

---

[5] Makes you wonder how they know this. Anyone drinking breast milk shouldn't be verbal enough to describe it!

and since phosphorus and calcium hate each other, when one goes up the other goes down. The result is **hypocalcemia**. Remember that hypocalcemia can occur if they describe an infant on cow's milk prior to one year of age.

"Hypo - cow – lcemia."

When Breast Isn't Best

There are times when breast-feeding is contraindicated, and this is very much fair game.

Metronidazole - It is important to note that Flagyl® (metronidazole) is the most effective treatment of *Trichomonas vaginalis*; however, it is contraindicated with breast-feeding. Therefore, mothers taking this drug must stop breast-feeding during treatment.

Diazepam – is sufficiently concentrated and absorbed by a breast-feeding infant to cause him/her to be shlogged. Therefore, it is contraindicated. Any medication with sedative effects can make its way into breast milk.

Don't be fooled into picking **candidiasis**, **contact dermatitis**, **fibrocystic breast disease**, or **mastitis**. Breast-feeding, if properly managed, *can* continue with each of these conditions.

> ## Who's Nursing Who?
>
> Lower breastfeeding rates are seen among
> - lower socioeconomic groups, especially non-Hispanics
> - less well-educated women
> - young and single women
> - women returning to the workplace
>
> Support from fathers and maternal grandmothers has been shown to increase breastfeeding rates.

Breast Milk vs. Formula and Cow's Milk

They love to ask the differences that nobody remembers. Keeping your curds and whey straight will keep the spider away.

	Human Milk	Cow Milk	Milk-based Cow Formula	Soy-based Formula
Protein	70% Whey 30% Casein Human milk is WHEY better	20% Whey 80% Casein	20-100% Whey 0-80% Casein	100% Soy
Major carbohydrate	Lactose	Lactose	Lactose	Corn syrup or sucrose
Fat	Human milk fats	Butterfat	Vegetable oil	Vegetable oil

Iron

While breast milk is lower in iron, it has **a higher "bioavailability"**.[6]

---

[6] Iron in breast milk is absorbed better than iron in formula.

Watch how they ask the question. If they ask which contains more iron, the answer will be formula. However, if they ask which is a better source, or which results in better absorption, the answer will be breast milk.

Lactose and Calories

Both standard formula and breast milk are **lactose**-based and have the caloric content = 20 kcal/ounce = 20 kcal/30cc = 0.67 kcal/cc.

Protein

Cow's milk is higher in protein content (roughly 3% vs. 1%).

Although cow's milk contains more protein than human milk, this is a case of quality over quantity. The protein quality differs between cow and human milk, as outlined in the previous table.

For very low birthweight infants, the goal is to prevent negative nitrogen balance. This is best done by starting amino acids as soon after birth as possible. This can be prevented with amino acid intake as low as 1.0 - 1.5 g/kg/day.

Fat Content

Cow's milk is roughly 3-4% fat, and human milk varies with Mom's diet (similar to cow's milk).

Antibody

High concentrations of IgA and other antibodies present in breast milk, protect against infectious disease, including local GI immunity.

Lactose-derived oligosaccharides inhibit bacterial adhesions to mucosal surfaces, therefore reducing the risk of bacterial infection. This is the case with both colostrum and mature milk.

"Lactose" derived: picture bacteria that "lack toes" to adhere to mucosal surfaces.

Early Feeding of Solid Foods

You could be presented with a grandmother pushing for early introduction of solid foods,[7] while the mother is perfectly happy exclusively breast-feeding for the first 6 months of life. Aside from fueling the rivalry with grandma again, there are other good reasons for not introducing solid foods too early.

Feeding solid foods such as cereals to breastfed infants before 4-6 months of age increases the likelihood of gastrointestinal infection. In addition, low amylase levels in the infant gut make it more difficult to digest solid foods.

---

[7] "Back in my day, we started Hamburger Helper® at 2 weeks," is a common claim.

> ## Subtraction by Addition
>
> Enhancing the caloric content of formula is not always good.
>
> When mixing formula, adding more powder than is indicated will increase the protein load, which stresses the kidneys. Because of this, lipid and carbohydrate supplements are available.
>
> *Adding carbohydrate* supplement can lead to diarrhea.
>
> *Adding lipid supplement* may increase the risk for diarrhea or delay gastric emptying.
>
> The bottom line is, anything that increases the caloric content beyond 30 kcal/o will be incorrect.

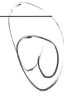

 The introduction of solid foods does not help an infant sleep through the night.

Commercial Baby Foods vs. Home Prepared Foods

For home-prepared foods, several precautions are necessary:

- Foods should be cleaned and pureed so there are no solid chunks inadvertently left behind.
- Food should be fully cooked
- Served fresh or frozen for later
- No salt, seasoning and, of course, no honey should be added

You might be tempted to believe that home prepared foods reduce the risk for food allergies, but once again, Grandma is wrong, and this is not the case.

Obesity

Overweight is defined as a BMI between the 85th and 95th percentiles for age and gender.

Obesity is defined as a BMI greater than the 95th percentile for age and gender.

Obesity due to **exogenous** sources[8] does result in the child being **tall with advanced bone age**. If they are "fat" due to endocrine/genetic (or **endogenous**) reasons, they are usually **short with delayed bone age**.

Genetic causes such as Prader-Willi also cause obesity. Genetic causes can also include short stature, but also tend to include developmental delay and dysmorphic features. Watch for this in the history.

Endocrine causes of Obesity
- Hypothyroidism
- Cushing syndrome
- Growth hormone deficiency

HCG. You gain weight when you are pregnant and your HCG is positive

It's a Medical Thing!

The most common metabolic explanation (and what all mothers and grandmothers want to hear) would be hypothyroidism. However, overweight children who have an otherwise-normal physical exam, normal linear growth, and normal development, DO NOT require testing for the cause of the obesity, only for the consequences: diabetes, liver disease, hyperlipidemia, etc.

---

[8] Commonly known as overeating.

Extreme Zumba and Treatment of Obesity

How many nutritionists does it take to change a light bulb? Answer: Just one, but the bulb has to want to be changed.

The same applies to the lifestyle changes needed to treat obesity. The child and the family have to recognize a problem and want to change. **Weight loss recommendations must include the entire family!**

It is a 3-pronged approach, including **changing diet, increasing exercise, and modifying behavior**.

Diet has to be changed without impacting growth. This may be easier if snacks and sugary drinks are eliminated first.

Exercise regimens are most effective when combined with dietary changes.

Modifying behavior includes support inside and outside the family.

Since the roots of obesity can be found in childhood, **the best obesity therapy available for children is prevention**.

Consequences

Obesity is not just a cosmetic issue. With obesity, there are loads of health risks involved. The list is long and includes such items as **depression, avascular necrosis of the hip, diabetes, hypertension, cardiac disease**, and **osteoarthritis** secondary to the strain on joints, especially those of the lower extremities.[9]

Any child who is noted to be drinking **a lot of diet sodas** (high phosphoric acid content) is at high risk for osteopenia. If the child has been treated with **steroids**, the risk is even higher. The best way to reduce the risk for fractures would be **vitamin D and calcium supplements**.

Nutritional Deficiencies – Kwashiorkor and Marasmus

These are not common in the US, but are popular on the Boards, in refugee camps, and at communes everywhere. You will need to be able to distinguish the two.

Kwashiorkor

This is strictly a **protein** deficiency. That is why they will depict a child with a "**pot belly**" from starvation. Other physical signs may include **pitting edema, rash, thin/frail hair, pallor, and overall thin appearance**.

The edema part is easy enough, because low protein would result in less intravascular oncotic pressure, causing edema. As for the name—kwashiorkor—think of it as "**squash-I-or-kor**." Squash is low in protein, so if that's all you ate, you would be protein-deficient.

---

[9] Also known as the legs.

Marasmus

This is a **general nutritional deficiency.** Therefore, the hallmarks are **muscle wasting without edema.** They are **underweight** and their **hair is normal**.

Remember "More-asmus" since they have MORE problems than Kwashiokor.[10]

What is <u>NO</u> <u>G</u>OOD about NG Feedings?

Whenever possible, **enteral** feedings are preferable to **parenteral** feedings.

Here it is very important to read the question.

If they ask what is the **most common complication** of nasogastric feeding, the answer is **diarrhea**.

The diarrhea is rarely severe enough to cause dehydration.

The second most common complication is **GE reflux**. If elemental formula is used, this risk is reduced considerably.

If they ask what the most **severe** complication is, the answer is **vomiting with aspiration**. This is why it is important to read the question and know the details cold.

Also, remember **ostomy feedings** can result in **wound infections**.

Refeeding Syndrome

Physical and lab findings that are a result for **overly aggressive nutritional treatment of malnourished patients**.

Make a note of this possibility when you are presented with a patient with anorexia, kwashiorkor, marasmus, chronic malnutrition, chronic alcoholism, prolonged fasting, prolonged IV hydration, or any chronic diseases that is associated with nutritional deficiency.

A few days after the refeeding regimen begins, the patient develops signs of **muscle weakness, fatigue,** and **abnormal electrolytes**.

The solution would be to correct the electrolyte deficits and restart the refeedings at a rate that provides about **50% of the targeted kcal/ kg/ day,** with vitamin and trace mineral supplements to meet age-appropriate recommended daily intakes.

Basically slow and steady wins the race and the key is to advance energy and volume intake slowly.

> ### Recheck those Refeeding Labs!
>
> The following can be seen with refeeding syndrome:
> - hypokalemia
> - hypophosphatemia
> - hypomagnesemia
> - hyperglycemia
>
> They can also have cardiac complications due to hypokalemia, sodium (and fluid) retention, as well as B1 (thiamine) deficiency.

---

[10] There can also be a combination of the two, but they will most likely expect you to recognize one or the other and that one is usually Kwashiorkor, since its features are the most distinctive.

Bolus or Continuous — Which is Better?

- **Infants who have gastroesophageal reflux** may respond better to continuous feeds and gain weight better. After a short period of continuous feeds, the vomiting and reflux may stop. They can then tolerate regular PO bolus feedings.

- **Children with Crohn's disease** may need continuous NG feedings, which is helpful in reversing growth failure and inducing remission.

- **Children with malabsorption syndrome** also do better with continuous feedings.

- **Continuous is better for infants who have congenital heart disease.** These infants have increased nutritional demands, and often experience delayed gastric emptying and early satiety. Therefore, bolus feedings can lead to malnourishment and delay of corrective surgery. They need to get fattened up as quickly as possible.

 Bolus is better for infants with oral motor discoordination, as long as there are no gut responses, gastric residuals, or evidence of malabsorption or dumping syndrome.

Bolus is also more convenient for mobile toddlers and children, although they can get continuous feedings at night to increase calories.

> **TPN Risks**
>
> PERIL
> Use of TPN is associated with:
> - catheter sepsis, occlusion
> - cholestasis
> - cholelithiasis
> - electrolyte abnormalities
> - hepatitis
> - hyperglycemia
> - hypertriglyceridemia
> - osteopenia
> - vitamin deficiencies
>
> Cholestasis risk increases with increased lipid content.

Parenteral feedings

HOT TIP
Parenteral feedings **via a central line** are indicated as follows:

- When enteral or oral feedings cannot be administered for 7 days or more.
- When partial oral feedings and standard peripheral IV either cannot meet nutritional requirements or will be needed for prolonged periods of time.
- Whenever possible, some enteral feedings should be maintained, otherwise infants may lose the will and/or ability to feed orally.
- Prolonged periods without enteral nutrition also leave the GI mucosa more vulnerable to infection.

Nutrition in Specific Conditions

Liver Disease

HOT TIP
Patients with liver disease have decreased delivery of bile acids, resulting in **malabsorption of fat-soluble vitamins** such as A,D,E, and K. This is especially the case with **cholestatic disease**. An example of the potential consequences could be an **increased risk for rickets**.

If ascites or portal hypertension is an issue, **fluid restriction** is in order. This means a more concentrated formula (and these formulas can be pretty repulsive), so sometimes NG or gastrostomy feedings are a necessary option. Maintaining adequate caloric intake is crucial to reduce the risk for growth failure.

Heart Failure

Patients with heart failure need to have their caloric intake increased while **restricting fluids**. The solution is to **increase the concentration of the formula**, which increases caloric density without increasing fluid, resulting (hopefully) in appropriate weight gain. These children are often also on diuretics to balance the tendency for fluid overload.

Renal Disease

Patients in acute renal failure tend to be malnourished. In these children, **70% of calories should come from carbohydrates**, and lipids should comprise less than 20%. Protein intake may be up to 0.5 – 2 g/kg/day. Infants in renal failure require **low phosphorus formula**.

Malignancies

Meeting the nutritional needs of children with malignancies is important to their response to treatment. Children with adequate nutrition at the onset of treatment may have reduced risk for infection and reduced severity of chemotherapy side effects.

Neurologically Impaired Patients

Neurologically impaired pediatric patients are at higher risk for GERD and are more prone to ill effects when fundoplication surgery is implemented.

Wound Healing

Adequate caloric intake, especially protein, is essential to wound healing. Vitamins C, A, zinc, and iron are especially important.

Food Allergies

Severe diet restriction in response to multiple food allergies will likely be the wrong answer, due to the **nutritional hazards of diet restriction**. In infants, for example, substituting rice milk for standard formula may result in vitamin D, calcium, protein, and fatty acid deficiency.

Calcium and vitamin D deficiency may occur in older children restricting dairy intake in response to lactose intolerance.

The AAP recommends early introduction (ie. 5-11 months of age) of peanut products for patients at high risk for peanut allergy (i.e. those with severe eczema or known egg allergy).

Cystic Fibrosis

Poor pancreatic function leads to intestinal **protein and fat malabsorption.** These children are at risk for deficiency of the **fat-soluble vitamins D, E, A, and K.**

Better nutritional status in these patients correlates to better lung function. These patients almost always require supplementation of calories to maintain adequate growth during childhood.

Burns

Early and aggressive nutritional support in burn patients significantly reduces their resting energy expenditure and helps **minimize protein catabolism** and weight loss.

A **high carbohydrate diet** is needed because of the relative inability of the burn patient to use fat. They also need **increasing amounts of calcium and magnesium** to maintain normal serum levels.

Chapter 13

Preventive Pediatrics

Prevention is a big part of general pediatrics, so proper guidance and knowledge in this area is emphasized on the Boards. The nice part is that there are a few basic facts that are asked year after year.[1] Of course there are ongoing changes to the immunizations schedule reflected in our revisions.

Immunizations

DTaP and Tdap and the use of Td

The DTaP vaccine is given at 2, 4, 6, 15-18 months[2] and at the kindergarten visit. All pertussis vaccines currently used in the U.S. are acellular[3].

Take that DTaP

DTaP, Td, Tdap, and DT - sneaky! The rules and nomenclature have changed at dizzying rates.

Many of these changes are due to the increased risk for pertussis both in older children and adults, and the young'uns they may infect.

Below you will find much of the important information in digestible format.

The **Tdap** has a little "p" which is less pertussis antigen and a little "d" which is less diphtheria antigen than the DTaP.

Adolescents

Adolescents 11-18 years old should receive a single dose of Tdap. This should preferably be given between the ages of 11-12 years.

HOT TIP

Tdap, meningococcal and HPV vaccines <u>may be given</u> to adolescents during the same visit.

Catch-up Immunizations (diptheria, tetanus, and pertussis style)

Children ages 7 – 18

- **Tdap** should be substituted for a **single dose** of Td in the catch-up series. If it IS substituted, it counts as the Tdap booster and another one is not needed at age 11y.

> ### Age Counts
>
> Immunizations are based on postnatal age, even for preemies. Therefore, you do not adjust the immunization schedule for prematurity.

> ### Td or not DT
> ### That is the Question !
>
>
>
> The Td vaccine is the booster, similar to Tdap.
>
> The DT vaccine is the variant of DTaP vaccine given to small children who can't handle the aP component.

---

[1] For example, the most effective way to prevent drowning is a fence around the pool.
[2] The 4th dose can be given as early as 12 months of age, provided 6 months have elapsed since the 3rd dose was given.
[3] That's why there a little "a" in front of the P". It does not stand for "and".

DTaP is not indicated for children aged 7 or older. It's too much "P" for them. However, if DTaP were to be given in error to a child older than age 7, it **would** count as the adolescent Tdap booster.

DTaP starts with "D for Diapers"; Tdap starts with "T for Teens". More accurately older than 7 and heading toward the teen years.

Also D comes before T in the alphabet. Children are given DTap before Tdap.

Contraindications

Serious allergic reaction. These cases should be referred to an allergist to confirm the allergy and to assess the need for possible desensitization.

Encephalopathy within 7 days of receiving pertussis-containing vaccine (not a contraindication for Td, however).

There must be no other identifiable cause for the reaction.

Deceptively fine for giving Tdap and DTaP

The following conditions might easily be misconstrued as contraindications or precautions for administering Tdap. However, it is safe to administer this vaccine when indicated.

- History of **extensive limb swelling** (that was not part of an arthus reaction) after administering the vaccine
- **Stable neurological conditions,** including well-controlled seizures and cerebral palsy
- **Brachial neuritis**
- **Contact allergy to latex gloves**
- **Pregnancy/breast-feeding**
- **Immunosuppression**
- **Current minor illnesses** including antibiotic use

Anone with a history of pertussis, should still receive *routine Pertussis* immunization since previous infection does not provide sufficient immunity.

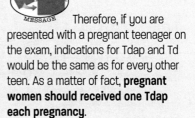

Tap Dancing in Pregnancy

It is important to note that **pregnancy is not a contraindication for Tdap or Td.**

Therefore, if you are presented with a pregnant teenager on the exam, indications for Tdap and Td would be the same as for every other teen. As a matter of fact, **pregnant women should received one Tdap each pregnancy.**

Close family contacts and caregivers of newborns should be immunized for pertussis because there is known waning immunity with pertussis vaccination.

Wound Management

Puncture Wounds

Pseudomonas aeruginosa is likely in **p**lantar **p**unctures through **tennis shoes.**

Puncture wounds with increased risk of infection include those:

- that involve the forefoot
- with puncture through shoes
- in patients with underlying diabetes

and prophylactic antibiotics should be considered in these situations.

Clean wounds

TIG (tetanus immune globulin) would **not** be indicated for clean wounds under any circumstances.

If the immunization status is **unknown**, or a child has received **less than 3 tetanus vaccines**, they need to receive a tetanus vaccine.

If more than **10 years** has passed since the last vaccine was given, then a **booster** is indicated.

Dirty wounds

If you are presented with a patient who sustained a **dirty wound** and they have received **less than 3 tetanus vaccines** or the history is **unknown**, then a **tetanus vaccine and TIG** are indicated.

If **more than 5 years** has past since the last tetanus vaccine was given, a **booster** is indicated.

When tetanus toxoid is indicated, adolescents age 11-18 should receive **a single dose of Tdap** rather than Td if they have not received a previous Tdap. However, if the adolescent received Tdap in the past or if Tdap is not available, then **Td** can be given instead.

If TIG is indicated but not available, then **IV immune globulin (IVIG)** is given.

What is "Dirty"?[4]

Dirty wounds would include those with risk of contamination from feces, dirt, or saliva or those resulting in severe injuries such as in the case of burns, frostbite, or crush injuries.

Haemophilus influenzae b (Hib)

The Hib vaccine has greatly reduced the incidence of invasive disease caused by Hib, including meningitis and epiglottitis.[5]

Depending on the vaccine, the recommended primary series consists of 3 doses given at 2, 4, and 6 months of age, or 2 doses given at 2 and 4 months of age, each with a booster at 12-15 months.

DTaP Combination Vaccines

Some important considerations for the DTaP-IPV-Hib and DTaP-IPV-Hep B combination vaccines are:

- **They cannot be used for those 7 years old or older.** They are only approved for the primary series, and **not to be used as the booster dose** at kindergarten or later.

- **They cannot be used prior to 6 weeks of age**, and therefore cannot be used for the birth dose of hepatitis B vaccine.

---

[4] It's hard to define, but you know it when you see it.
[5] Of course, the incidence of epiglottitis on the board exam is as high as it has ever been.

Hepatitis B Vaccine

Hepatitis B infection is a major cause of liver disease, including **hepatocellular carcinoma**. To head the disease off at the pass, all children receive immunization against hepatitis B.

In 1/3 of cases of Hepatitis B, no identifiable risk factors are identified.

The first dose is typically given at birth (prior to discharge from the nursery), the second dose at 1-2 months, and the third dose 6-18 months after the first dose.

If you are presented with ANY child or adolescent who has not been completely immunized, you should begin or complete the 3-part series.

> Children are at risk for Hepatitis B at the following turning points:
> 1. **Intrapartum**
> 2. **Early childhood** (household contacts or group care facilities)
> 3. **Adolescence** (sexually transmitted and IV drug use)

The only **absolute contraindication** to Hepatitis B vaccination is **severe allergic reaction** to a prior dose. Being pregnant and/or having an autoimmune disease (e.g., SLE) are NOT contraindications, and these individuals can be vaccinated.

If the mother is infected with hepatitis B **(HBsAg positive)** or has **unknown hepatitis status**, the newborn should also receive **hepatitis B immunoglobulin in the first 12 hours of life in addition to the routine immunization**.

HBIG should be given at a different location than the HepB vaccine.

Infants born to HBsAg positive mothers should have their **post vaccination status** verified by serologic testing (HBsAb POS and HBsAg NEG at 9-18 months of age.

Other **high risk groups** should also have serologic testing done to confirm immunity after the Hep B vaccine series. These include **immunocompromised patients, hemodialysis patients,** and those whose jobs place them at high risk, such as **health care workers and prostitutes.** That is a curious linkage, to say the least.

Hepatitis B vaccine in Preemies

Even preemies **weighing less than 2 kg** need to receive the Hep B vaccine **within 30 days of life or before discharge**, whichever is first.

The birth vaccine in infants weighing less than 2 kg does not count toward completion of the series.

Post-exposure prophylaxis

This would apply, for example, after exposure via a needle-stick or contaminated blood transfusion.

Infants and other unvaccinated folks	They get HBIG (just to be sure), and start the Hep B series.
If they received full series and are antibody positive (+)	They are fine and need nothing more.
If they received full series and are antibody negative (-)	Pretty much considered unvaccinated, so they are treated as such; they get **HBIG and full revaccination**.
Unknown immunity	Pretty easy: test for antibody (HBsAb). If negative, give HBIG and start series.

Hepatitis A Vaccine

All children in the U.S. **should receive the vaccine at age 1 year**.

It is administered in **2 doses**, at least 6 months apart (preferably the same brand).

Immunocompromising conditions are *not* a contraindication for receiving the hepatitis A vaccine. Contraindications to the Hepatitis A vaccine include hypersensitivity or allergic reaction to the vaccine components, including **aluminum hydroxide** and **phenoxyethanol**.

There are specific recommendations for children **traveling to areas that are endemic** for hepatitis A. If they are <u>less than 12 months of age</u>, they should receive **passive immunization with immune globulin**. If they are <u>older than 12 months</u>, they should receive the **hepatitis A vaccine**. This should be done four weeks prior to departure if possible (two weeks at the very least).

Meningococcal Vaccine

The MCV4 vaccine provides protection against **A, C, Y and W-135** strains. The B strain is covered by a separate "Men B" vaccine, recommended but not quite mandatory yet.

You can remember these strains by the YWCA acronym, and even stand up and do your own version of The Village People's song if you need a little break.

Routine Immunization for Meningococcemia

Routine immunization against meningococcemia with the **MCV4** vaccine is indicated for the following:

1) Pre-adolescents at the 11-12 year visit.

2) Booster at age 16

Special Considerations

MCV4 primary series is also recommended for children as young as 2 months of age, **but only in special circumstances such as:**

- with immunocompromising conditions such as **HIV, persistent complement deficiency, and functional or anatomic asplenia** (including sickle cell disease).

- any time there is a community outbreak attributable to a vaccine serogroup

- **traveling** to regions where meningococcal disease is prevalent such as the "meningitis belt" in sub Saharan Africa and Saudi Arabia.

 High risk children will continue with boosters for life.

Synchronized Syncope!

BREAKING NEWS — Syncope is common after vaccination, especially in adolescents and young adults. Syncope after vaccination is not a contraindication to future vaccination.

Human Papilloma Virus Vaccine

Gardasil® and Cervarix® are the trade names for the vaccine

The current recommended age for HPV vaccination is recommended in males and females at age 11-12 but can be given as early as 9 years of age.

This provides protection against anal cancer as well as vaginal warts.

If the vaccine is given before age 15 (even a single dose), only a two dose series is required.

If series is started at 15 years or older, a 3 dose series is required.

For all dose series, the first and final dose must be 6 months apart.[6]

 Vaccination is **not** considered to be a substitute for routine cervical cancer screening. Therefore, vaccinated females should go through cervical cancer screening according to recommended schedules.

Measles, Mumps, and Rubella (MMR)

Since the introduction of the MMR vaccine, the incidence of measles, mumps, and rubella have decreased by 99%!

The following points are worth remembering:

- The first dose of the vaccine is given between 12-15 months of age

- A second dose is traditionally given at school entry at 4-6 years of age, but may be given anytime at least 28 days after the first. This additional dose enhances immunity among nonresponders and does NOT serve as a booster.

---

[6] HPV Vaccination can be given into adulthood, usually up to 26 years old, but CAN BE given up to age 45.

Timing is everything

Infants **between ages 6 and 11 months** during an epidemic situation or traveling to a part of the world where measles is endemic would need to be immunized. This would be considered short term immunization, and they would need to resume the regular immunization schedule for MMR at the appropriate age (meaning that such an infant would **receive three doses of MMR**).

MMR may not be given within 4 weeks of other live vaccines, including varicella and live intranasal influenza vaccines. Live vaccines **can be given together** or in a combined vaccine.

Up to 15% of kids who receive MMR will develop a **high fever** (>103) that occurs within 12 days after vaccine administration and lasts 1-2 days.[7] 5% also will develop a **rash** during the same time frame. The correct answer will be **reassurance** if you should be presented with such a scenario on the exam.

Contraindications

The **absolute contraindications** to **MMR** administration are:

(1) Severe allergic reaction to a vaccine component, neomycin, or gelatin

(2) Pregnancy in the patient

(3) Severely immunocompromised (e.g., chemotherapy, AIDS)

The following are **NOT contraindications**:

(1) Positive TB skin test

(2) Concurrent TB skin testing

(3) Pregnancy in the mother or other close contact

(4) Breast feeding

(5) Immunodeficiency in member of household

(6) Egg allergy

(7) Mild or asymptomatic HIV infection CD4 >15% OK

(8) Non life threatening reaction to neomycin

(9) History of seizure (slightly increased risk for this, but not a contraindication)

Withholding the vaccine for mild reactions is a common myth. Don't fall for this trap on the exam.

> ## Just say NO to live vaccines in Pregnancy!
>
> Although there have been no documented cases of birth defects secondary to vaccines, MMR and varicella vaccines are contraindicated in pregnant women; **however, therapeutic abortion is not medically indicated when the vaccines are given accidentally to a pregnant woman.**

> ## MMRV Defer to MMR and V
>
> MMRV vaccine has been associated with a higher rate of **febrile seizures** in children **12-23 months of age**. Therefore, the separate MMR and Varicella vaccines are preferred in this age group.
>
> In addition, **MMRV is contraindicated in children with HIV infection.**

---

[7] This risk is increased with MMRV.

A PPD can be placed **WITH MMR** with no mitigation of its effect. However, a PPD should not be placed within a 4-6 week period **AFTER** MMR has been given.

Varicella Vaccine

The varicella vaccine is given routinely between ages 12 - 15 months. A booster is given upon entry into kindergarten between ages 4-6 years. Any older child who has not had chickenpox should also receive the vaccine series.

The **contraindications** to varicella vaccination are:

(1) Pregnancy

(2) Prior allergic reaction to the vaccine

(3) Substantial suppression of cellular immunity (e.g., severe AIDS, bone marrow transplant, or solid organ transplant)

According to the CDC, the following are **NOT contraindications** to varicella administration:

(1) Pregnancy in the recipient's mother or other household contacts

(2) Mild or asymptomatic HIV infection CD4 >15% OK

(3) Immunodeficiency in household contact

Post-exposure Prophylaxis

VariZIG and Acyclovir may be considered after exposure to varicella in the following situations:

- **Immunocompromised children** with no previous varicella infections or immunizations
- **Pregnant women** without immunity
- **Hospitalized preemies of 28 or more weeks of gestation whose mom lacks immunity**
- **Hospitalized preemies of less than 28 weeks gestation regardless of maternal status**
- **Newborn infants** if mother contracted varicella **5 days before to 2 days after birth**

Administration of **varicella vaccine** within 72 hours and possibly up to 120 hours after varicella exposure may prevent or modify disease and should be considered in susceptible children 12 months of age and

HIV and Live Vaccines

The following is the protocol for administering live vaccines in HIV positive patients.

Measles Vaccine is indicated for those who are:

- **Symptomatic** but not severely immunocompromised
- **Asymptomatic**

As mentioned in the box in the previous page, **they should NOT receive the MMRV.**

Varicella Vaccine

Children with HIV are at increased risk from complications from varicella. Therefore, they should only receive the vaccine if their CD4 counts are high enough.

Influenza Vaccine

Inactivated influenza vaccine is indicated in these patients and **NOT the Live Attenuated Influenza Vaccine** (LAIV or FluMist®).

VariVax® and Aspirin

Patient on chronic aspirin therapy should **avoid aspirin for 6 weeks** post-vaccination because of the risk of Reye syndrome.

Chemotherapy and live vaccines

Inactivated vaccines are usually OK to be given during chemotherapy as long as they are not given during induction or consolidation. Because of the immunodeficiency resulting from chemotherapy, however, **live-virus vaccines usually are withheld for a minimum of 3-6 months after chemotherapy has ended.**

One exception is **varicella immunization** which IS given to children **in remission of ALL** because the risk of natural varicella disease outweighs the risk associated with the live-attenuated vaccine virus.

older if there are no contraindications to vaccine use. A second dose should be given at the age-appropriate interval after the first dose.

Pneumococcal Vaccine

HOT TIP The CDC recommends that all children **younger than 5 years receive the pneumococcal conjugate vaccine** (Prevnar®, PCV-13).

It is administered at 2, 4, 6, and 12-15 months with catch-up recommended for all children 5 years and younger.

23 Valent Salute PPSV23

The PPSV23 is NOT recommended for healthy children because it is less immunogenic than PCV-13 (does not work as well), but it covers more serotypes, so it is reserved for children at higher risk for pneumococcal infection.

Children from groups A, B, and C listed in side table all need PPSV 23 vaccine at (or after) age 2 and at least 8 weeks after PCV-13.

Children from group A receive another PPSV23 5 years later.

No more than 2 doses of PPSV23 are recommended for children.

Pneumo Cuckoo

HOT TIP The only contraindication for receiving pneumococcal vaccine is a **serious allergic reaction** to a component of the vaccine.

Polio Vaccine

IPV (Inactivated Polio Vaccine) is the only poliovirus vaccine available in the United States. For those old enough to recall, there is now no sugar cube or sweet elixir, it's now just needles.

VERY BORING MATERIAL WARNING! The last reported case of wild-type polio occurred in 1979. Since 1986, all other cases of polio acquired in the United States have been **vaccine-associated paralytic poliomyelitis (VAPP)** occurring in vaccine recipients or their contacts and attributable to oral poliovirus (OPV) vaccine. Implementation of an all-IPV vaccine schedule in 2000 essentially ended the occurrence of VAPP cases in the United States.

Administration of IPV vaccine results in seroconversion in 99% to 100% of recipients after 3 doses. Immunity probably is lifelong. So Polio should now be relegated to the dustbin of history along with the iron lung provided everyone gets immunized.

Who's at Risk? Who's Immunocompromised

If you go through the criteria of who who gets which vaccine when, it is convoluted enough. But when you need to also differentiate those who are immunocompromised from those who are simply "at risk" your eyes start to glaze over. At least mine did.

We will reference these groups by A , B and C for purposes of the text.

Group A: Immunocompromised children with anatomic or functional asplenia, sickle cell disease, HIV infection, malignancy, transplant recipient and any immunodeficiency.

Group B: CSF leaks and cochlear implants.

Group C: Chronic heart or lung disease, chronic renal failure or nephrotic syndrome, and diabetes mellitus.

Children 6-18 years of age in Groups A and B who have NEVER received a PCV-13 should receive a single dose of the vaccine because they are at increased risk of invasive pneumococcal disease.

 TAKE HOME MESSAGE Or you could just remember this as any kid who sees a specialist for a serious disease.

Four doses of IPV vaccine are recommended for routine immunization of all infants and children in the United States.

The first 2 doses of the 4-dose IPV vaccine series should be given at 2-month intervals beginning at 2 months of age (minimum age, 6 weeks), and a third dose is recommended at 6 through 18 months of age.

Doses may be given at 4-week intervals when accelerated protection is indicated.

 The final dose in the IPV vaccine series should be administered at 4 years of age or older regardless of the number of previous doses; but 6 months must have elapsed after the last dose.

Rotavirus

After the previous form of rotavirus vaccine was caught in a scandalous relationship with intussusception, a new and improved more honest rotavirus vaccine has appeared on the scene.

Infants in the United States routinely should be immunized with **3 doses of RV5 vaccine administered orally at 2, 4, and 6 months of age or 2 doses of RV1 vaccine administered orally at 2 and 4 months of age**.

The first dose of the rotavirus vaccine should not be given after 15 weeks of age.

Once the series has been started, it needs to be completed by 8 months of age.

If the first dose is administered inadvertently after 15 weeks, then the remainder of the series should still be administered on schedule.

Contraindications

The rotavirus vaccine is contraindicated in infants who had a severe hypersensitivity reaction or allergic reaction to previously administered doses.

Severe combined immune deficiency (SCID) and **history of intussusception** are contraindications for use of both rotavirus vaccines.

Special Considerations

Infants who have rotavirus gastroenteritis

Infants who get mild rotavirus gastroenteritis should still complete the 3-dose schedule. This is because initial infection only confers partial immunity.

> ### Solid organ transplantation and Immunization
>
> Inactivated vaccines should be given at least 2 weeks before transplantation and live vaccines should be given at least 1 month before transplantation for better response before immuno-suppression.
>
> They will likely not get any more live vaccines after transplant. They will restart the inactivated vaccine schedule 6 months after transplantation.

However, infants with **moderate to severe** gastroenteritis should not get the vaccine until clinically improved.

Infants with mild illness

Children with mild illnesses or low grade fever can get the vaccine.

Underlying GI disease

Infants with underlying GI disease who **are not receiving immunosuppressive treatment** should receive the vaccine.

Prematurity

Premature infants can receive the vaccine as long as they are at least 6 weeks of age and are to be **discharged from the nursery.** They also need to be "clinically stable."

Immunocompromised or pregnant household contacts

Immunocompromised household contacts would **not be** a contraindication to vaccine administration. Likewise, pregnant household contacts would **not be** a contraindication to vaccine administration.

Regurgitation of the vaccine

Infants who spit up or vomit the vaccine should just continue with the series. **No re-administration is necessary.**

Hospitalization after vaccination

If an infant receiving the vaccine has to be hospitalized, no precautions beyond universal precautions are necessary.

Immunocompromised infants

The benefits and risks should be weighed in determining whether the vaccine should be administered to immunocompromised infants.

HIV infants usually DO get the Rotavirus vaccine; SCID infants DO NOT.

Influenza

Annual immunization is indicated for:

- All children between 6 months and 18 years.
- Caregivers in or out of the house for children with high risk conditions or children under age 5.

Roto Rotation

PERIL

They could ask you if rotavirus vaccine can be given to children living with pregnant mothers and/or household members that are immunocompromised. Yes, these children should still receive the vaccine, but at risk caregivers should be instructed to avoid handling the child's diapers for 4 weeks after vaccination.

MNEMONIC

CAPE: Think of the influenza vaccine as providing a cape of protection for the following high risk groups.

Chronic metabolic disorder or renal problems and **C**ardiac disease
Asthma and **A**cquired immuno-suppression)
Pulmonary disorder
Empty bladder (renal problems)

Inactivated Influenza Vaccine (IIV) is administered IM and approved for children 6 months and older.

Live attenuated influenza vaccine (LAIV) is a nasal spray approved for healthy children 2 years of age and older.

Children 6 months through 8 years of age should receive 2 doses of the vaccine **the first year they receive the flu vaccine**. The second dose should be administered at least 4 weeks after the first dose.

Children 9 years of age and older need only one dose of vaccine each season.

It is also highly recommended that medical personnel receive the annual influenza vaccine to limit spread of the disease. That means you!

HOT TIP
Since infants cannot receive influenza immunizations until 6 months of age, the only way to protect them is to ensure that their caretakers and household contacts receive the influenza vaccine. This is commonly referred to as "**cocooning**".

Egg Allergy, and Avoiding Egg on your Face

MMR

MYTH
The current MMR preparation does *not* contain enough egg cross-reacting proteins to be an issue.

Yellow Fever

COIN FLIP
Yellow fever, on the other hand, is the only vaccine that has enough egg protein to worry about an allergic reaction, including anaphylaxis. All these patient should see an allergist before receiving the vaccine.

Influenza

HOT TIP
Inactivated Influenza vaccines (IIV) do not contain enough egg to trigger an allergic reaction in most children with an egg allergy.

Patients with a history of anaphylaxis to eggs[8] should have their flu vaccine administered and monitored by a provider capable of recognizing and treating severe allergic conditions.

Foreign Travel

Foreign Vaccinations for Foreign Vacations

You will be expected to know how to obtain information about immunizations for patients and families traveling to foreign countries.

The **CDC website** has information per travel, and many areas now have specialized **Travel Clinics** that you may refer your patient and family to for appropriate immunization. The specifics may not come up on the boards since this is information that changes all the time.

Flu High Risk

For post-exposure prophylaxis, high risk children should be given antiviral chemoprophylaxis.

PERIL
High risk for influenza complications includes kids less than 2 yo, children with preexisting heart or lung disease, and immunocompromising conditions.

Penning Instructions for the Epi Pen

Some important facts on epi pens:

• Epi Pen Junior is for patients weighing 30 kg or less

• They can lose their potency within 6 months of the expiration date

• It should be administered in the outer thigh, not through clothes

• They should be kept at room temperature; therefore, they should not be stored in cars

• A minimum of 3 pens should be prescribed: one for the child, one in an obvious place in the house, and one for the school or baby-sitter

---

[8] There are egg-free versions if the caregivers are refusing to vaccinate due to the minuscule egg risk.

Rabies

There are two rabies vaccines approved for use in the U.S. One is a human diploid cell vaccine and the other is a purified chicken embryo cell vaccine.

If you are presented with a patient with a documented egg allergy and needs the rabies vaccine, the non-chicken embryo vaccine[9] would be the correct answer.

CASE STUDY

You are presented with parents who refuse to immunize their children.

THE DIVERSION

You will be tempted to pick choices that include threatening the parents, or scaring them with a Youtube® video. Other incorrect diversionary choices could include calling them bad parents and rolling your eyes as you roll them out of your practice.

ANSWER REVEALED

Even if you have actually agreed with these other choices, the correct answer would include any combination of the following:

1. Inquire about their specific concern and address it non-confrontationally, providing written materials to support your information whenever possible.

2. Ask them to think about it and invite them to discuss it at their next visit.

3. Advise them to always notify medical providers of their child's underimmunized status during ill visits, especially to the Emergency Room.

4. Have them sign a refusal form that lists the risks of not vaccinating their child.

HOT TIP

They must sign it with each subsequent well child visit, which can actually be persuasive. Nothing like signing on the dotted line to make the knees a bit weak.

Getting through the Screen Door

Cholesterol Screening

Current Screening Guidelines:

Children 5-9 y: Obtain fasting lipid profile only if there is a family history of hyperlipidemia, a parent with dyslipidemia, any other risk factors, or a high-risk condition (see below).

Children 9-11 y: Obtain universal[10] cholesterol screening.

Risk Factors for Hypercholesterolemia

- BMI above 85th percentile
- Poor diet, including too many or too few calories

> **Screen at 3**
> Universal blood pressure screening should begin at age 3.

---

[9] Because chicken embryos live in ... eggs. Palm to head!
[10] "Universal" really means "no thinking required". Check cholesterol regardless of family history or risk factors.

- Chronic steroid medications
- Anticonvulsants
- Beta blockers
- Alcohol abuse
- Chronic diseases – liver, renal, hypothyroidism

Although it might seem counterintuitive, **anorexia nervosa** is a risk factor for hypercholesterolemia.

Risk factors associated with Cardiovascular Disease

- Family history
- Age
- Gender
- Poor Nutrition/ diet
- Physical inactivity
- Tobacco use
- Hypertension
- Hyperlipidemia
- Overweight/ Obesity
- Diabetes mellitus
- Metabolic syndrome
- Elevated inflammatory markers
- Perinatal factors

> **Anticipating Anticipatory Guidance Questions**
>
> You need to be familiar with the importance of providing anticipatory guidance on the following topics at well visits
> * stairway safety
> * use of recreational equipment
> * preventing animal bites
> * appropriate use of topical insect repellants
> * Internet safety
> * limiting TV time

Injury and Illness Prevention

Childproofing the home should be discussed. This is best done at the **6-month visit, before the child is mobile.**

Eclipsing the Sun

Type of UV light	Timing of Risk	The Skinny
UV A	Constant throughout the day **A** is constant **A**ll day	• Drug induced photosensitivity reactions • Also contributes to the problems listed for UVB
UV B	Varies: Strongest from 10AM through 5PM **B** is strongest during **B**usiness hours **B** is **B**ad (though neither UV is good)	• Skin aging • Sunburn • Skin Cancer

The A and B of ultraviolet sunlight

HOT TIP

80% of a person's sun exposure occurs before age 20, or the first 2 decades of life. Using sun screen in the pediatric population may reduce the risk by 80%.

Sunscreen Shots

- Sunscreen with an SPF of at least 15 should be used
- Physical sunscreens block out both UVA and UVB
- It should be applied 20 minutes before sun exposure
- Applying less than optimal amounts reduces the SPF rating

> ### Sunshine and summertime skeeters:
>
>
>
> Sunscreen should be applied, and allowed to dry, *before* applying insect repellent.
>
> Both should be washed off after the child returns inside.

Dueling Airbags and Car Seats

You will need to know the appropriate car seat to use based on weight, height, and age.

UPDATED & NEW
BREAKING
NEWS
INFORMATION

Children should remain rear-facing until they exceed the height and weight of their (convertible or all-in-one) car seat, whether that is 3 or 4 years of age.

The determining factor is weight not age.

At that point they may transition to a forward facing seat with a 5 point harness.

Since these recommendations vary by state and change all the time, it is unlikely to be tested but we have included it just in case there is a general question on the subject.

In general, the parents should follow manufacturer's recommendations for instillation as well as height and weight maximum.

HOT TIP

The middle seat is the safest seat. Children should not be sitting in the front seat until at least age 13, regardless of weight or height.

HOT TIP

Rear facing infant car seats should be positioned at a **45 degree angle**.

> ### Well Stated !
>
> Don't expect many questions about car seat specifics, these recommendations change often and may vary by state. In general, the parents should follow manufacturer's recommendations for instillation as well as height and weight maximum.

Bicycle Safety

Some important facts that you are expected to know regarding bicycle safety:

- Most bicycle deaths and injuries occur in children younger than 15 years
- Bicycle helmets are worn by less than 10% of children riding bicycles
- Bicycle helmets reduce serious injury by 85%
- 75% of deaths are due to head injuries
- Reflectors are required on pedals, tire sidewalls or rims, and the front and rear of the bicycle

You need to be familiar with bicycle safety facts in case you are asked a question that over or underestimates these facts. For example, they may ask you to pick the correct fact from a list of facts which all seem correct.

They might, for instance, include in the list that bicycle helmets reduce serious injury by 65%, that 25% of bicycle fatalities are due to head injuries, that reflectors are required on bicycle tires, or some similar seemingly illogical statement.

The correct answer in this case would be the simple statement regarding reflectors on tires. *When presented with a list of answers with percentages and numbers, look closely at the answer without the numbers. It could be the correct one.*

Firearms in the Home

Some important facts and statistics you are expected to know:

- Safety mechanisms, including trigger locks, may reduce unintentional injury (although this is not proven).
- More than 90% of suicide attempts with a gun are fatal
- Simply living in a home with a gun increases a person's risk of gun-related violence

Even though the official word is that trigger locks "may" reduce risk, **choices that include definitive statements such as "handguns can be safely kept in the home as long as there is a trigger lock in place" will be <u>incorrect</u>**. Locked and unloaded is the key (with ammunition stored and locked in a separate location). In addition, it is recommended that the gun have high trigger pressure to fire, in order to reduce the risk of a child firing a household gun.

Burn Prevention

Know that **hot liquid burns** are the most common burns in the home.

Remember that **sharp demarcation burns** increases the suspicion for child abuse, a.k.a. nonaccidental trauma.

Water heaters should be set at **120 degrees°F**.

Drowning Prevention

 Drowning is more common in **warm weather months**. Peaks are at **preschool age** and **late teens**.

Age-dependent facts

- Infants are most likely to drown in a **bathtub**
- Children younger than 5 are most likely to drown in a **residential pool**
- Adolescents are most likely to drown in **fresh water**
- Above ground pools are less likely to cause drowning
- Drowning is higher among **African American males**
- **Males** account for 75% of all drownings

> ### Floating Your Boat Safely
>
> 90% of boat-related drowning incidents occur in people not wearing life jackets.
>
> The best way to prevent this is ... you guessed it... all individuals aboard a boat should be wearing a **life jacket**.
>
> Additional causes of death and injury while boating include:
> - Carbon monoxide poisoning
> - Fractures and laceration
> - Head injuries
>
> Many of these accidents involve **alcohol**.

The following is an important fact to commit to memory. The AAP recommends a **4-sided fence around the pool, with a self-locking and self-latching gate**. This is the most effective preventive measure for preventing drowning in children.

A fence around the yard (with one side being the back door of the house) is NOT good enough, in real life or on the Boards.

Infant and toddler swimming lessons are fun social events, but **ineffective** when it comes to preventing drowning. Swimming lessons are recommended for children 4 and over but they do not drown-proof children.

Whether home pool, lake, boat or bathtub, the most important safety measure to prevent pediatric drownings is **adequate supervision**, specifically "touch supervision" for young nonswimmers.

Additional recommendations include swimming in locations with lifeguards, CPR training, and use of personal flotation devices.

Tobacco Risks

 Infants whose mothers smoked cigarettes during pregnancy are an increased risk of:

- Preterm birth, IUGR, and low BW
- SIDS
- Wheezing and asthma
- Behavior and attention problems that extend into adulthood

Some important points to be familiar with regarding tobacco use in teenagers are:

- Addiction occurs after **exposure to a small amount of nicotine**
- Certain respiratory sequelae may be seen in the teen years
- School-based education programs aimed at smoking prevention are effective if they focus on **role playing refusal skills** and provide information on the **health impact**
- **Nicotine replacement therapy** is not approved by the FDA for use in adolescents. Therefore, before using this treatment, you must first document that quitting is unlikely to be achieved without assistance, and you must feel confident that the adolescent will use it appropriately. Remember: first do no harm!
- If nicotine replacement fails to stop smoking, then bupropion when combined with counseling is an approved option

Evaluating EVALI

In 2019, the CDC published that ˍ30% of high school students reported using tobacco products (in any form). E-cigarettes and "Vaping" have become increasingly popular in adolescents. These can cause EVALI (E-cigarette vaping associated lung injury) or a severe respiratory illness with cough and shortness of breath and may resemble pneumonia or other viral illnesses.

Indoor Air Pollution

Common exposures may cause breathing or respiratory problems in poorly-ventilated environments. This may include wood fires/stoves, cigarette smoke, hairspray, cooking spray, or other potentially harmful chemicals.

First Aid Considerations

The treatment of choice for a child experiencing an **anaphylactic reaction** is epinephrine. If the question asks for contraindications for epinephrine, there are none. After administration, the next stop is the ER.

You might be questioned on the correct technique for **tick removal**. This consists of grabbing the tick at the skin line with fine tweezers and removing with steady upward traction applied.

Chapter 14

Yellow Snow & Other Environmental Toxins

Risk of Toxicity in Children

You are expected to understand that children are at increased risk from toxic exposures as compared to adults. This starts in utero and continues by virtue of their **smaller size**, which makes them **more vulnerable to an equivalent toxic exposure**. In addition, children of course place more non-food items in their mouths than most adults and are, therefore, at increased risk for exposure to toxic agents in the environment.

Children are also at increased risk for the manifestations of latent toxicity effects over the course of their lifetime as compared to adults.

Placenta Percenta

The placenta is not perfect at protecting the fetus from toxic substances. Specifically, it **blocks cadmium**, but **allows for the transfer of lead**, and even **enhances passage of mercury**.

PCBs and **insecticides** can also cross the placenta easily due to their lipophilic nature and low molecular weight.

Food and Water

Even food and drinking water may be the culprits, especially on the boards. You are expected to know that water may contain *E. coli, cryptosporidium,* and mercury. Food, especially if not handled correctly, may contain a lot more.

Active Decontamination

Activated Charcoal

- The appropriate dosing is typically is 0.5 to 1 g/kg, up to an adult dose range of 25 to 100 g.

When used in patients **at risk for respiratory depression**, such as those who have ingested **phenobarbital, intubation should be done as well**. The charcoal is then served with an **NG tube** and a wide variety of surgical tapes and Surgilube®.

> **Exit Here**
>
> Cathartics, such as magnesium citrate and sorbitol, can be given to expedite exit of the ingested substance and to reduce enterohepatic excretion.

While it may seem obvious, **charcoal cannot be given with antidotes**, because it would interfere with the absorption of the antidote. One exception to this is **N-acetylcysteine**, since it is given in such large quantities.

Remember the mnemonic **CALM** to remember those toxic substances which are "calmly" removed **without charcoal**.

Charcoal is a poor choice for:

- Cyanide
- Alcohol/alkaline ingestion/kerosene
- Lithium
- Heavy Metals

> **Syrup of Ipecac**
>
> It is safe to assume that syrup of ipecac will ALWAYS be the incorrect treatment on the boards.

Gastric Lavage

Gastric lavage is **no longer recommended** for most ingestions. The risks outweigh the benefits.

Its use is reserved for **potential life-threatening ingestions** that have occurred **within 60 minutes** of seeking medical attention.

Toxidromes

Even though you are expected to know specific agents and their treatment, remember that most treatment is **supportive**. With any question, if they ask "what should you do first?" the answer is to **address the A-B-Cs** and search for the specific cause later.

Securing the airway will be the correct answer any time you are presented with an unstable patient.

> **Overdose Underquote**
>
> Remember: when presented with an overdose victim, the drug they have allegedly taken may not be accurate, especially if the drug is placed in "quotes." It could also be a combination of drugs.

Acetaminophen Ingestion

The initial manifestations of acetaminophen toxicity occur in the first 24 hours and include **anorexia, nausea,** and **vomiting**.

In cases of **significant toxicity**, the **liver enzyme levels rise** significantly during a latent phase that lasts 1-4 days.

In **severe toxicity**: following the latent phase, **jaundice and liver tenderness** will develop.

> **The Seat of Acetaminophen**
>
> An acetaminophen **overdose** is diagnosed by a history of ingestion of 140 mg/kg or more.
>
> Acetamoniphen **toxicity** is diagnosed by the level in the nomogram.

The most important predictor of outcome regarding acetaminophen toxicity **is the level taken 4 to 10 hours post ingestion.**

Treatment

It is very common to be **asymptomatic initially,** with liver toxicity presenting later on. Therefore, immediate discharge from the ER when the person is asymptomatic will always be the wrong answer.

- If it has been less than 4 hours since ingestion, the **first step** is to reduce absorption with **activated charcoal.**

- **Second step** -- Obtain an acetaminophen level **4 to 24 hours post ingestion,** and plot level on the published nomogram to determine risk for hepatoxicity.

If it has been determined that **more than 140 mg/kg has been ingested,** then **N-acetylcysteine** can be given without obtaining levels (especially if it would delay initiation of treatment longer than 10 hours after ingestion). N-acetylcysteine prevents the accumulation of toxic metabolites of acetaminophen by replenishing the depleted glutathione stores.

A 17 yo female was seen in the ER 2 days ago for acetaminophen ingestion. Her acetaminophen level 4 hours post ingestion was 250 mcg/mL. She was given an appropriate dose of N-acetylcysteine. Her LFTs today were unremarkable. What is her prognosis?

You might be deceived into believing that, even though the 4 hour level was in the toxic range, the fact that the N-acetylcysteine was given immediately and that her LFTs are normal indicates that the patient is out of the woods. If you pick an answer based on this logic, both you and the patient will still be in the woods.

LFTs can be normal 2-3 days after ingestion, even in cases of severe overdose. The transaminase levels may not rise until 3-4 days after ingestion.

Salicylate Ingestion

Toxic ingestion can include not only aspirin, but also medications that contain salicylates, so look for clues in the question such as **"wintergreen" odor on breath.** Another clue in the history might be tinnitus.

It is unlikely that you will be asked directly how salicylate toxicity occurs, but it helps to understand the treatment. First, it directly activates the medulla causing **hyperventilation and respiratory alkalosis**. The metabolites in the cells cause uncoupling of the oxidative phosphorylation pathway leading to an increase in **anaerobic metabolism and metabolic acidosis**.

Management

- The initial treatment is **activated charcoal**
- **Sodium bicarbonate** (to alkalinize the urine) is required to correct metabolic acidosis.
- Ensure that **hypokalemia** is addressed and consider **glucose** even if not hypoglycemic.

Remember to always **calculate the anion gap** when presented with acidosis and values for Sodium, Potassium, Chloride, and Bicarb. They might not come out and tell you the toxic ingestion but they might give you the elctrolytes and expect you to do the math!

Anion gap = Sodium – (Chloride + Bicarb).

> The anion gap would be elevated in salicylate poisoning.

Fever is consistent with toxicity, so be careful not to follow the "sepsis" tree when they give other clues consistent with salicylate toxicity.

Ibuprofen Ingestion

Most children will be **asymptomatic**, but on the boards they will at least have **nausea and vomiting**.

Management of ibuprofen overdose is primarily **supportive**.

> **You are presented with a teenager who has ingested a fistful of ibuprofen pills as a suicide gesture. Her vital signs are stable and she is otherwise fine physically. You are asked for the most appropriate next step in managing this patient.**
>
> Among the possible diversions could be the obligatory diversion of ipecac, which you should immediately avoid the way you would actually avoid ipecac itself; the same goes for gastric lavage. The most absurd diversion of all would be an ibuprofen level, which doesn't exist.
>
> Of course, it is the "risk for co-ingestion tree" that you should be climbing. The correct answer will therefore be a level for another drug, such as salicylate or acetaminophen levels.

Methanol Toxicity

Once upon a time, rubbing alcohol consisted of methanol. However, it also exists in the board world as well as the real world in the form of **windshield washer fluid, cooking fuel, perfumes,** and **antifreeze** for your car.

Clinical presentation could include **abdominal pain** and **vomiting, inebriation, severe metabolic acidosis, increased anion gap,** and **CNS depression.**

There might not be immediate signs of toxicity (as in the case of a child acting drunk after ingesting ethanol). However, do not be fooled by the innocent presentation in the history. This is a Trojan horse toxicity. Methanol gets broken down to formic acid and formaldehyde, which can wreak havoc, especially on the liver and the optic nerve (leading to **blurred vision, "snow field" vision, and edema of the optic disk**).

This is one of the rare cases where **administration of ethanol** to a minor might be appropriate. In this case, ethanol serves as an **alcohol dehydrogenase antagonist**, slowing the conversion of methanol to formaldehyde.

Another agent that accomplishes the same thing with less toxicity would be **4-methypyrazole (4-MP)**. However, as of this printing it has only been approved in Europe (but if it does make its way to the exam, it will likely be a correct choice).

Additional treatment would include **sodium bicarbonate** to help counter formic acid.

Ethylene Glycol

Ethylene glycol (aka anti-freeze) toxicity occurs in 3 phases.

Patient presents with **a drunken appearance**, with **no odor** of alcohol on the breath, and a **large anion gap**.

> **Phase 1:** Nausea, vomiting, tachycardia, hypertension, metabolic acidosis, and calcium oxalate crystals in the urine leading to hypocalcemia
>
> **Phase 2:** Coma and cardiorespiratory failure, due to acidosis and hypocalcemia
>
> **Phase 3:** 1- 3 days, renal failure due to acute tubular necrosis, with the patient needing dialysis

> **CASE STUDY** You are presented with a patient who is lethargic, ataxic, and has vomited. Lab values will include a low serum bicarb level and an elevated anion gap.[1] At this point, you will have to decide if it is ethanol or ethylene glycol toxicity.
>
> **THE DIVERSION** They drop confusing hints in the question to trick you into believing that ethanol is the culprit.
>
> **ANSWER REVEALED** The key is to look for clues in the question, such as the child being seen alone in the garage. Assuming there isn't a fully stocked bar in the garage, ethylene glycol is the likely culprit. If they throw in something about crystals in the urine, then there really is no diversion at all.

Treatment

Fomepizole works by preventing the breakdown of ethylene glycol to its toxic metabolites (oxalic acid and glycolic acid).

Organophosphates

A typical presentation would be a toddler who is **lethargic**, in **respiratory distress**, and is sweating and wheezing. They often hint at exposure to **insecticides** by mentioning that the child was **in a backyard shed**.

Picture a "leaky farmer" that is crying, drooling, sweating, vomiting and urinating. The farmer aspect will also help you remember that it is an insecticide.

The mechanism of action is by **inhibiting acetylcholinesterase**, and therefore the effect is due to acetylcholine overload. Therefore the effect of organophosphates are **cholinergic**.

The classic mnemonic is SLUDGE:

Salivation/Sweating
Lacrimation
Urination
Defecation or Diarrhea
Gastrointestinal
Emesis

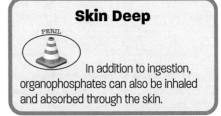

Skin Deep

PERIL In addition to ingestion, organophosphates can also be inhaled and absorbed through the skin.

Insecticides can be insidious in the environment and can have a long term impact on children's health, particularly on brain development. **Unwashed fruits and vegetables** would be one important source. In addition, children are more likely to be exposed in general due to behavioral factors.

---

[1] Remember to calculate the anion gap each time you are presented with a serum sodium, bicarb, and chloride.

Cholinergic effects are broken down into 2 categories, **muscarinic** and **nicotinic**. You need to know how each is managed.

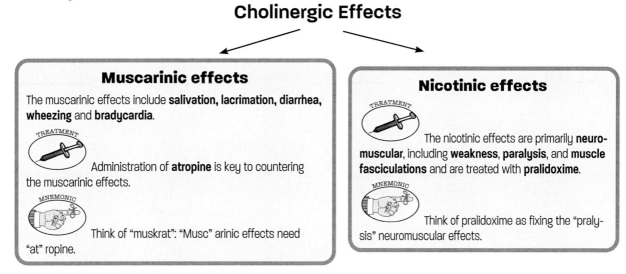

Cholinergic Effects

Muscarinic effects

The muscarinic effects include **salivation, lacrimation, diarrhea, wheezing** and **bradycardia**.

Administration of **atropine** is key to countering the muscarinic effects.

Think of "muskrat": "Musc" arinic effects need "at" ropine.

Nicotinic effects

The nicotinic effects are primarily **neuro-muscular**, including **weakness**, **paralysis**, and **muscle fasciculations** and are treated with **pralidoxime**.

Think of pralidoxime as fixing the "praly-sis" neuromuscular effects.

Tricyclic Antidepressants (TCA)

Medications with anticholinergic side effects include tricyclic antidepressants (TCAs), mydriatic agents, and antispasmodics. Watch for a clinical history of a member of the household taking one of these medications. This would suggest an accidental ingestion of one of these medications.

Here the key will be "**anticholinergic signs**" (like dry mouth, dry mucous membranes) and mydriasis (which you know are dilated pupils). The same symptoms for antihistamine overdose are "**blind as a bat**," "**red as a beet**," "**hot as a hare**," "**dry as a bone**," and "**mad as a hatter**,"[2] "**full as a flask**," and "**bloated as a toad**."

If they present a patient suspected of ingesting TCAs, with the anticholinergic signs described above, watch for **hypertension** and **tachycardia**. Within 24 hours they may develop **dysrhythmias**.

The most important parameter to measure is **EKG monitoring** for **widened QRS complex**. Widening QRS complex is treated with **sodium bicarbonate boluses**. Repeat until the QRS duration is less than 100 msec. Cardiac meds are NOT indicated.

Activated charcoal is the method of choice for decontamination.

The 3 Cs of Managing TCA toxic ingestion

Charcoal decontamination

Clinical management levels are *not* indicated

Cardiac is where the money is

Beta Blocker Ingestion

A child who has ingested a beta blocker will present with a **depressed sensorium** and **bradycardia**, as well as **hypotension**, and perhaps **diaphoresis**.

---

[2] How mad is a hatter anyway?

A child suspected of ingesting a beta blocker would need to be observed **on a monitor**.

Treatment for symptomatic beta blocker ingestion (bradycardia, hypotension) is with **glucagon**.

Carbon Monoxide Toxicity

The key is **sudden flu-like symptoms** (headache, dizziness, nausea, vomiting, fatigue, weakness and confusion) in a patient who is **afebrile**, with a **supple neck**. They may describe **symptoms in other family members**, including the **recent death of a small family pet**. Hopefully you won't also be expected to know how to treat the family pet.

If they were in a house fire, they might give you some signs such as **singed nasal hairs**, **charcoal-stained clothes**, and **carbonaceous sputum**, or **hacking** and **heaving** like Lindsay Lohan walking out of rehab.

Carbon monoxide works by competitively binding hemoglobin thus leading to lower oxygen carrying capacity in the blood. CO has a much higher affinity for hemoglobin than oxygen.

Although obtaining **carboxyhemoglobin levels** is a crucial initial first step, **symptoms do not always correlate with carboxyhemoglobin levels**.

In addition, **cherry red mucous membranes** was previously believed to be a key factor in making the diagnosis, but it is now considered to be too insensitive a sign. Make sure this is not one of the choices you select when asked about important diagnostic criteria.

Oxygen saturations are completely unreliable in this setting. Oxygen saturation will be normal because it does not distinguish between carboxyhemoglobin and oxygenated hemoglobin.

In routine cases, administering **high flow 100% oxygen** would be the correct answer. Hyperbaric oxygen treatment is controversial.

CASE STUDY

You are presented with a patient who is lethargic, confused, and in respiratory distress, emphasizing a *normal pulse oximetry reading*. What is the best treatment?

THE DIVERSION

You may be thrown by the normal pulse oximetry reading and believe that administering 100% oxygen is not the correct answer. You better check your own pulse, since this would be another question you would be answering incorrectly if you fell for this trick.

ANSWER REVEALED

If they describe a patient suffering from carbon monoxide poisoning, then 100 % oxygen would be the correct answer indeed. Pulse oximetry may be normal even in severe CO poisoning. Don't be fooled by a normal pulse oximeter reading.

If there is no improvement with 100% O_2, then carbon monoxide poisoning is not the correct answer. Consider cyanide poisoning (not for you, as a diagnosis).

Cyanide Poisoning

Cyanide poisoning presents in a similar fashion to CO poisoning BUT with a failure to respond to O_2. It works by interfering with aerobic metabolism resulting in metabolic acidosis.

Any smoke exposure can cause cyanide poisoning.

Beware of **smell of almonds**, which has been associated with cyanide poisoning.

The most recently FDA-approved treatment for cyanide poisoning is **hydroxocobalamin**. However, previously **sodium thiosulfate** or **nitrate** were used, so if those show up on boards they may be correct choices as well.

Compliments to the Alternative Chef

Remember to ask about the intake of complementary or alternative medicines in the investigation of potential ingestions.

Chlorine

Ingestion of chlorine, ie. household bleach, a.k.a. "Clorox"® may not require much intervention, and discharge from the ER can be the correct answer since the concentration of hypochlorous acid is low.

The Masquerade Party of Toxicology: Managing Unknown and Multiple Agents

You are expected to know specific points in managing patients who might have ingested multiple agents and/or situations where the agent is unknown.

- First steps (as always) are the **ABCs** of patient stabilization, before anything else.
- Look in the history for hints of **environmental exposures**, such as family members taking medications that could explain the presenting symptoms.
- **Labs**, in addition to drug testing, would focus on **acid/base status, glucose concentration**, and **anion gap**
- **Acetaminophen** and **salicylate** levels should be obtained when multiple agents are suspected or unknown. This would include intentional ingestion.

When unsure, consider starting with an acetaminophen level, salicylate level, ethanol level, urine toxicology screen, complete metabolic panel, and an EKG.

Out of It

For patients with profoundly depressed mental status, an immediate glucose check and an empirical dose of naloxone are recommended.

Caustic Substances

Initial symptoms following ingestion of a caustic substance include **coughing, crying, drooling, difficulty swallowing, and chest pain.**

Gastric lavage is contraindicated with caustic substance ingestion.

If you are presented with a patient who is **symptomatic** after ingesting a caustic substance, **endoscopy** should be implemented in **less than 24 hours** to determine the presence and severity of esophageal burns.

The presence or absence of oral lesions is **not predictive** of esophageal injury.

Alkaline Ingestions

Typically with ingestion of **dishwasher detergent** or **drain cleaner,** the impact is immediate, leading to **burns of exposed tissue,** or oral/esophageal burns. These patients typically present with **drooling, dysphagia,** or **emesis.**

This leads to **deep liquefaction necrosis** of the affected tissues, leading to **ulceration** and **perforation** as potential complications.

Additional findings could include **vomiting** (with **hematemesis**), as well as **stridor** or **wheezing.** Watch for signs of **burns on the face, hands,** or **chest.**

This is why even small amounts of alkali substance can cause significant damage. The toxicity is primarily via direct contact with skin and mucosa; systemic signs will rarely be part of the presentation on the boards.

Activated charcoal is not indicated; it will not absorb alkali, and will inhibit endoscopic examination.

Alkali substances

Alkali substances tend to **injure the esophagus** and may even lead to esophageal perforation.

Acidic substances

In addition to the esophagus, acidic substances **can injure the stomach,** since they are not neutralized as alkali substances are.

"Whipped Oven Cleaner"

Watch for the description of a child who was exposed to a common household cleaning substance that could be mistaken by a child as food, i.e., scented floor cleaners or foam oven cleaner spray bottles that could be confused with whipped cream or edible cheese in a can. Although it would be debatable how appetizing the latter would be to a child.

Endoscopy End Game

Even though esophageal burns can be present in an asymptomatic patient, endoscopy is not indicated, especially on the boards.

However, observation for 6 hours to await presentation of symptoms would be appropriate. If asymptomatic after 6 hours, endoscopy would not be indicated.

If they present you with a patient who has wheezing or stridor in this setting, airway stabilization and/or protection would be indicated as well.

Environmental Exposures

Lead Exposure

CDC and AAP recommend universal screening if >27% of housing was built before 1950 or prevalence of levels 10 or greater in 12% or more of children 12-36 months of age. Refugee children 6m-16y of age should be screened on arrival and 3-6 months post re-settlement.

There is no "safe" lead level so the only normal value is 0. Any positive level deserves a thorough history and physical exam at minimum.

Lead levels as low as 10 mcg/dL can result in **cognitive deficit**, and should therefore be followed.

Lead levels at **70 mcg/dL or higher** would require **chelation therapy**.

Lead Levels	Report/Confirm	Intervention
5-14 mcg/dL	Report to state department and confirm with venous sample within 3 months	Environmental history; screen for iron sufficiency; developmental screening
15-44 mcg/dL	Report to state department and confirm with venous sample within 4 weeks	Same as above plus Consider Xray if pica
45-70 mcg/dL	Report to state department and confirm with venous sample within 48 hours	Same as above plus outpatient chelaton (oral succimer) if asymptomatic. Admit if significant CNS or GI symptoms
>70 mcg/dL	Report to state department and confirm with venous sample immediately	Hosptalize for whole bowel irrigation if lead visible on Xray; parenteral chelaton (IM dimercaprol followed by IV edetate calcium disodium)

While a capillary sample is adequate for screening purposes, it is not acceptable to base treatment on this. The lead level needs to be confirmed with a **venous sample**.

CASE STUDY

A 15-month-old presents with an elevated lead level. The parents have been doing kitchen, bathroom, and home equity loan renovations. What is the most likely cause of the child's lead poisoning?

THE DIVERSION

You will be tempted to pick choices like "pica" or "lead plumbing," especially since the kitchen and bathroom have plumbing that will be exposed. That is the decoy, because if you pick lead plumbing your score will plummet like a lead sinker on a fishing trip.

ANSWER REVEALED

The correct answer is *household dust*. Lead can be absorbed both through the GI and respiratory tracts; therefore, children are at high risk for absorption of lead through household dust during home renovations.

Where is the Lead?

Know that the most important current source of exposure to lead is **lead-based paint in older houses**.

Children either **eat the paint chips** or are exposed to **house dust** or **soil**.

Other sources of exposure to lead include **glazed ceramics, storage battery casings, bullets, cosmetics, leaded glass, jewelry,** and **farm equipment**.

PERIL

Watch for home remedies, such as *azarcon* or *greta,* both of which can lead to elevated serum lead levels. These are powders containing lead that are given as home remedies for GI symptoms or teething.

> **Leading the Way to Diagnosing Lead Poisoning**
>
> Symptoms and signs of lead poisoning include:
> - Headache
> - Irritability
> - Constipation
> - Lethargy
> - Microcytic anemia
> - Burton's lines on teeth
> - Lead lines on x-ray

Iron Ingestion

Toxic ingestion is defined as **40 mg/kg of elemental iron**, but symptomatic patients even with lower ingestions should be treated.

Presentation occurs in 4 phases:

Phase 1: Within 6 hours, vomiting (often hemorrhagic), diarrhea, and abdominal pain develop.

Phase 2: Decreased GI symptoms and deceptive improvement for the next 6-24 hours

Phase 3: Multisystem effects
- Metabolic acidosis
- Coagulopathy
- Cardiovascular collapse

Phase 4: GI obstruction due to scarring and strictures

Management consists of serum iron levels **4 hours post ingestion.**

Serum iron > 350, WBC > 15,000 and **glucose > 150** are seen with severe iron ingestion.

In a symptomatic patient, **an abdominal film** should be done to identify iron tablets which have not yet been absorbed. Additional lab studies should include electrolytes, aminotransferases, CBC, and coagulation studies.

Indications for **chelation** would include **severe symptoms**, as well as the following findings:

- anion gap acidosis,
- serum iron concentrations of greater than 500 mcg/dL (89.5 mcmol/L),
- a significant number of pills visible on abdominal film

With **deferoxamine** chelation treatment, the urine turns **a pink-red color** when the serum iron level exceeds the serum iron binding capacity. Treatment can be stopped when there is adequate clinical improvement and/or **the urine is no longer pink.**[3]

Activated charcoal absorbs iron poorly, and is not indicated for iron ingestion. Syrup of ipecac is, of course, no longer indicated either.

> ### Itty Bitty Teensy Weensy
> Remember that both iron deficiency and lead toxicity lead to microcytic anemia. Might as well check levels for both if you see it.

Mercury

Even though thermometers no longer contain mercury, children are still at risk for environmental exposure. Mercury can be inhaled or ingested, primarily through **consumption of fish** and drinking of **contaminated water**.

Mercury exposure is **not** a high risk during home renovations.

PCBs (polychlorinated biphenyls)

PCBs are synthetic hydrocarbons that are pervasive in the environment and can be concentrated in certain foods.

High exposure to PCBs during fetal development can lead to low birthweight, **dark pigmentation of the skin, early eruption of teeth, acneiform rash,** and **can ultimately be fatal.**

PCB can cause **P**igmentation and rash, **C**utting teeth prematurely, and **B**irthweight that is low.

There are also **long term neurodevelopmental consequences.**

---

[3] Fill in your own Rose Wine joke.

Bioterrorism

Varicella vs. Smallpox (Variola) lesions

Not only do most of you feel terrorized just taking the boards, but elements of bioterrorism are starting to creep their way onto the boards as well. They expect you to distinguish between varicella and smallpox lesions.

Smallpox	Varicella
• Begins in the **face and extremities** • Leaves Scars • Lesions are all in the **same stage** of development	• Begins **centrally** and spreads peripherally • Scarring is rare • Lesions are in **varying stages** of development

 In addition to the general signs of **fever** and **headache**, smallpox may present with **delirium**.

Anthrax

Virtually all cases are **the cutaneous form** of anthrax, which is all you need to know for the boards. The incubation period is less than 2 weeks.

The lesion starts out as a **pruritic papule**, similar to a routine insect bite, that progresses to a central bullous lesion that becomes necrotic, forming an **central black painless eschar**. This is classic for anthrax, and should be easy to identify if a lesion is described as such on the exam. The surrounding tissue is **swollen and red**. There is **no associated tenderness**. The eschar **falls off** in 1- 2 weeks.

Systemic signs including **adenopathy, fever, malaise,** and **headache** also may be present. However, these are vague symptoms; the key to answering questions related to anthrax correctly will be the cutaneous signs outlined above.

Foreign Body Ingestion

3 Coins in the Fountain

Coins are the most commonly ingested foreign bodies in children.

- 95% will pass from one end to the other within 4-6 days
- All coins in the **proximal esophagus** should be removed by **endoscopy asap.**

All coins in the **middle - lower esophagus** should be observed for **12-24 hours** if asymptomatic, followed by endoscopy if the coin does not pass beyond that point. Once an object **reaches the stomach**, it may be observed for passage. Prokinetics are NOT recommended.

If you are asked how to proceed with an asymptomatic child who is suspected of swallowing a coin, always order PA and lateral Xrays. Do not be reassured by the fact that the child is asymptomatic. Always order Xrays.

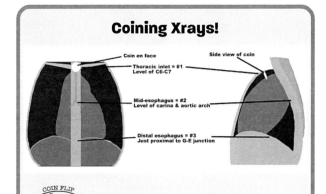

Coining Xrays!

When the coin is in the esophagus you will see the coin face on in the PA film. You will see the coin's edge on the lateral film. Note on the film where the mid esophagus is and where the distal esophagus is.

Coins **in the trachea** are the reverse.

This should help you if they show you an x-ray with an ingested coin and ask you if it's in the esophagus or the trachea.

Breaking Bad Bad Bad Ingestions

There are 3 ingested objects that cannot be ignored, not even long enough for you to check your Fantasy Football scores on your phone.

Coins will be homogenous on X-ray to differentiate it from button batteries, which will have a surrounding halo.

Button disc batteries

Think of this if they describe a child playing with a **TV remote** or **hearing aid** who is suddenly now **having difficulty swallowing** or **is throwing up**.

Any button battery in the esophagus needs to be removed immediately.

Administration of 1 tsp of honey every 15 minutes until X-ray is completed is now a recommendation to try to lessen the damage until removal.

Once battery is in the stomach, it need only be removed if it remains there after 48 hours. Monitor with serial Xrays every 3-4 days until the battery is passed.

Note that it is only **button batteries** that are a problem. Regular batteries like AA, AAA, etc, tend not to be an issue if they make it past the esophagus without causing obstruction.

CASE STUDY

A 3 year old who is completely asymptomatic is brought into your office. The baby-sitter noticed him chewing on a camera 3 days ago. She even brought the camera in to take a picture, but noticed that the camera does not work; the battery lid is open and there is no battery. What is the best next step in managing?

THE DIVERSION

Since they emphasize that the child is asymptomatic, watching and waiting may seem to be the most logical choice vs. charcoal, repeat CXR in a week, or the seemingly gruesome chore of sifting through the stool until the battery is located (and then reinstalling it in the camera). All of these are incorrect.

ANSWER REVEALED

In this case, the correct answer violates the least invasive rule. Here the correct answer will be immediate endoscopy to remove the battery if it is still located in the esophagus, and observation only if has passed into the stomach or below.

Sharp and pointed objects

TAKE HOME MESSAGE

Sharp and pointed objects pose a risk for **perforation**, especially if **longer than 4 to 6 cm**.

Endoscopic removal will most likely be the correct answer whether in the esophagus or further.

Magnets

Magnets may cause perforation if **more than one are ingested** and they attract to each other across bowel walls.

HOT TIP

Inpatient observation for all magnet ingestions will be the correct answer. If "Stay clear of airport security checks" is one of the choices, that could be correct too. And I suppose staying away from the MRI suite would be correct too.

Where's the Beef?

Meat impaction is the most common cause of obstruction in adolescents and adults. The majority of patients have underlying esophageal pathology, like eosinophilic esophagitis.

Refer for endoscopy if it does not pass spontaneously. Do not give meat tenderizer.

Chapter 15

Born Yesterday: Neonatology

Neonatal medicine involves virtually every other area of Pediatrics, including Genetics, GI, Neurology, and Infectious Disease. This chapter will focus on these subjects within the context of the neonatology section of the General Pediatric Boards.

Antenatal Screening

Alpha-fetoprotein (AFP)

Remember, AFP measurement is only a screen, which will need additional studies, including ultrasound, to confirm suspected findings.

HOT TIP

"Incorrect dates" could be the correct explanation for an elevated AFP; therefore, consider incorrect dates as a potential answer. In fact, the most common reason for elevated AFP levels is inaccurate dating of the pregnancy.

High AFP

MNEMONIC

To help remember some of the associations with increased AFP, think of the word **RAIN** (rain elevates the levels of reservoirs, including the AFP reservoir).

> Renal (Nephrosis, Renal Agenesis, Polycystic Kidney Disease)
> Abdominal Wall Defects
> Increased number of fetuses/ Incorrect Dates
> Neuro (Anencephaly and Spina Bifida)

Low AFP

This is mainly associated with chromosomal abnormalities like **Trisomy 21** or **Trisomy 18**.

Neonatal Resuscitation

In the first 60 seconds of an uncomplicated delivery, the infant should be dried, warmed, the airway should be opened and bulb suctioned, and the infant should be dried and gently stimulated to breathe.

Just Right

The AAP recommends the delivery room be 22-26 °C for term deliveries and thermoregulation of all newborns between 97.7-99 °F (36.5-37.5 °C).

If meconium is noted in the amniotic fluid, routine intubation is no longer recommended, as there is no clear evidence of its benefit.

Delayed cord clamping for more than 30 seconds is now recommended for all vigorous term and pre-term newborns who do not require resuscitation at birth because it is associated with less need for transfusion for anemia after birth as well as decreased risk of intraventricular hemorrhage and necrotizing enterocolitis. Risks include higher bilirubin levels and risk of jaundice requiring phototherapy.

Assess respirations: if there is apnea, gasping, or HR<100, begin positive pressure ventilation (PPV) with 21-30% O_2.

If after 30 seconds,

- HR<60 → begin chest compressions
- (CC) >100/min → intubate
- (100% O_2) → if have not already done so, start ECG monitor.

If after 30 seconds, HR is still <60, administer IV epinephrine, consider fluid resuscitation, and continue PPV and CC.

> **Resuscitation Real Pearls**
>
> The most important part of newborn resuscitation is effective ventilation.
>
> An increase in the newborn's HR is the most sensitive indicator of positive response to each resuscitative step.
>
> Remember that during initial neonatal resuscitation, the goal saturation varies depending on minute of life.
>
> 1 minute = 60-65%
>
> 3 minute = 70-75%
>
> 5 minute = 80-85%
>
> 10 minute = 85-95%

Apnea

Apnea is defined as **not breathing for greater than 20 seconds**. Less than that would be considered **periodic breathing**.

The causes of apnea include:

- **A**bnormal metabolism (hypoglycemia, hypocalcemia, anemia, maternal medications)
- **P**DA and other cardiac causes
- **N**eurological (seizures, intracranial hemorrhage, apnea of prematurity)
- **E**pidemiological/Infectious (sepsis, pertussis, RSV and other respiratory infections)
- **A**bnormal swallowing/GERD

When apnea is due to the absence of a signal from the CNS, this is **central apnea**.

 Apnea of prematurity is a type of central apnea. Apnea of prematurity cannot be diagnosed before other causes are ruled out, since it is **a diagnosis of exclusion**.

If there is another cause of the apnea, they will have to provide you with a hint of that cause. This may include **sepsis, medications, profound anemia, or an electrolyte abnormality**.

Apnea of prematurity is treated with **caffeine** or **theophylline**, much the way the apnea of boredom is treated in those preparing for the boards.

Primary vs. Secondary Apnea

Primary Apnea

The post delivery pattern of primary apnea is **gasping**, with increased depth and rate of respiration, followed by apnea. At this point, if **blow-by oxygen and stimulation** are given, there should be a good response.

Primary apnea can be reversed with oxygen and/or tactile stimulation.

Secondary Apnea

If primary apnea does not resolve, there will be another round of gasping, followed by more apnea. This is secondary apnea. Oxygen and stimulation won't work in this case. **Positive pressure ventilation is needed.**

Unfortunately, **primary apnea can occur in utero,** and it is difficult to determine if the newborn is experiencing primary or secondary apnea. Therefore, all apneic newborns who fail to respond to tactile stimulation and remain apneic **30 seconds** after delivery, **require positive pressure ventilation**, under the assumption that they are experiencing secondary apnea.

Around **60 mm Hg pressure** is needed to inflate the lungs for the first breath.

Transient Tachypnea of the Newborn (TTN)

TTN refers to tachypnea in otherwise healthy infants and is **caused by retained fetal fluid**. TTN is seen more commonly in infants **delivered by C-section**.

X ray findings in an infant with TTN will show **fluid in the interlobar fissures** and **increased interstitial pulmonary markings**.

TTN is a diagnosis of exclusion, presenting within the first few hours with, of course, **tachypnea, retractions, nasal flaring**, and **grunting**. Respiratory rate is **greater than 60**. It typically resolves within 72 hours. TTN is unlikely to be the correct answer if the clinical course worsens with time.

Respiratory support, NPO status and **close monitoring** are in order.

Once symptoms are improving, feedings can be started. Feedings should be advanced slowly until the respiratory rate falls below 60 beats/minute.

Respiratory Distress Syndrome (RDS)

RDS is a result of **deficient surfactant** in the lining of the alveoli. Surfactant levels gradually increase until 33-36 weeks gestation, after which there is a surge. If an infant is born prior to this point, he/she will be surfactant deficient and therefore suffer from RDS.[1]

RDS is also known as **"Hyaline Membrane Disease"** because the cellular debris that covers the terminal bronchioles in RDS forms a hyaline membrane — whatever that might be!

The typical presentation of RDS would include **tachypnea, nasal flaring, and expiratory grunting,** as well as **retractions. Cyanosis could be a part of the picture as well.**

Chest x-ray would include **granular opacifications,** and **air bronchograms,** with obscure heart and/or diaphragm borders. The classic description is a **ground glass appearance.** Be sure to look at a classic image to compare this symmetric appearance with the asymmetries seen in meconium aspiration.

If symptoms persist beyond 3 days, a **PDA** could be a complicating factor. In addition, the x-ray findings of **pneumonia secondary to Group B Strep** are often indistinguishable. Therefore, they will have to note something in the history, such as prolonged and progressively worsening symptoms despite respiratory assistance.

Other coexistent conditions can **worsen RDS.** These may include hypoglycemia, hypocalcemia, anemia, and acidosis. Extremes of temperature can be complicating factors in the history as well. In addition, **hypoglycemia** can mimic RDS.

When **hyperbilirubinemia** co-exists with RDS, the threshold for *kernicterus is <u>lowered</u>.*

RDS or GBS Pneumonia

As you know, the CXR will be of no help. Group B strep pneumonia and RDS are indistinguishable. Likewise, non-specific clinical signs like tachypnea, grunting, and respiratory distress are no help. One reliable sign of sepsis in the newborn period is the ratio of bands to total neutrophils; if greater than 0.2, sepsis or pneumonia is more likely. Remember to consider calculating this ratio when the CBC values are given.

In addition, the mention of temperature instability in the infant is a good clue to a diagnosis of GBS pneumonia.

---

[1] Surfactant is needed to keep the alveoli opened during expiration. Imagine trying to breathe in and out of a balloon that collapsed each time you took a breath rather than remaining partially inflated.

Risk for RDS

The risk for RDS **is increased** with:

• Infants of diabetic mothers

• C-section delivery

• Birth asphyxia

The risk for RDS **is decreased** with:

• Prolonged rupture of membranes

• Prenatally administered steroids

Seeing it Coming/Prenatal Tests

If enough time is available before delivery, **prenatal steroids** can help decrease the risk for RDS in premature infants.

Venting and other treatments for RDS

Mechanical ventilation is usually indicated for a pH lower than 7.2 and pCO_2 greater than 60 in infants with RDS (and/or respiratory failure of any cause). Air leaks are more common in infants because of the use of uncuffed ET tubes.

Exogenous surfactant, high frequency ventilators and ECMO[2] are also used when indicated. The goal of treatment is to maintain pO_2 between 50-70 mm Hg and a pCO_2 40-55mm Hg.

Exogenous Surfactant

Once a diagnosis of RDS is made, administration of surfactant is considered within 2 hours of delivery. However, if the baby is <30 weeks, or is otherwise at risk for RDS, therapy should be prophylactic. Once a diagnosis has been made, surfactant administration is termed "rescue."

Clinical improvement is expected as follows:

- Decreased oxygen requirement
- Reduced inspiratory pressure
- Improved lung compliance

Make sure you read the question carefully: decreased pulmonary compliance and increased inspiratory pressure would not be an expected improvement with surfactant. **Decreased inspiratory pressure** and **increased pulmonary compliance** would be.

Pulmonary interstitial emphysema (PIE) can account for some deterioration in infants with RDS on ventilators. This is essentially air leaking into the interstitium, and often precedes a full-blown pneumothorax.

Twins

In general, monozygotic twins are at higher risk for complications because they share a chorion AND an amnion.

B twins are at higher risk for developing respiratory problems than are A twins.

ECMO Okay

You are expected to know the eligibility criteria for ECMO or extracorporeal membrane oxygenation.

ECMO is primarily for infants that are > 34 wks gestation and > 2kg with <u>reversible</u> lung disease of less than 10-14 days duration, <u>with failure of other methods</u>.

In addition, the infant cannot have any systemic or intracranial bleeding or congenital heart disease.

---

[2] Extracorporeal membrane oxygenation; essentially temporary heart lung bypass.

BPD Graduates from RDS

BPD[3] is a **chronic lung disease** (CLD) previously believed to be due to prolonged mechanical ventilation and oxygen exposure. With therapeutic advances, it is now believed that it is due to the **arrest of normal lung development in premature infants**.

CLD is present in infants who still have an **oxygen requirement 28 days after birth** and/or continued **oxygen requirement at 36 weeks corrected gestation**.

BPD is treated with **diuretics**. Infants with BPD are at risk for **hypocalcemia** as a side effect of diuretic use.

The typical chest x-ray description in an infant with BPD is **diffuse opacities** as well as **cystic areas with streaky infiltrates**, and **ground glass appearance**.

Assessing Lethargic Infants while You are Lethargic

The most common causes of coma and lethargy in infants are **sepsis, metabolic disturbances,** and **asphyxia**. You can distinguish these on the exam by looking for signs in the history they present to you.

Make sure you go over the classic presentations of infectious and metabolic conditions in the Genetics, Metabolism, Infectious Disease, and Endocrine chapters in this book.

Neonatal hypoxic-ischemic encephalopathy (HIE)

Neonatal hypoxic-ischemic encephalopathy (HIE) would have to include a history of a **complicated delivery**. Added features could include metabolic disturbances such as **elevated serum ammonia, lactic acidosis, hypoglycemia, hypocalcemia, and hyponatremia**.

If you are presented with lab findings by all means calculate the anion gap. **If it is normal then HIE is a likely cause**

Sepsis

Remember all that is lethargic and floppy with "out of whack" labs is not sepsis. **Remember to consider:**

❑ Congenital Adrenal Hyperplasia
❑ Inborn Errors of Metabolism

---

[3] For psychiatrists, BPD is borderline personality disorder.

TREATMENT

The empirical treatment of suspected neonatal sepsis, like the long lines at DMV, have not changed in over 55 years.

PERIL

That treatment is still **ampicillin and gentamicin**. Don't be fooled into choosing ampicillin and cefotaxime. The latter is responsible for outbreaks of drug resistant *Enterobacter* and *serratia*.

Listeria monocytogenes

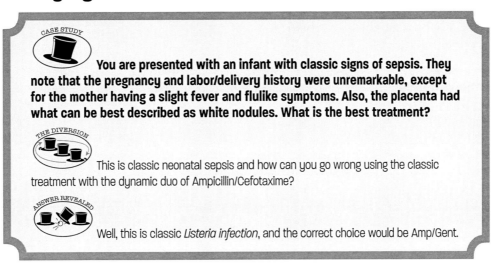

CASE STUDY

You are presented with an infant with classic signs of sepsis. They note that the pregnancy and labor/delivery history were unremarkable, except for the mother having a slight fever and flulike symptoms. Also, the placenta had what can be best described as white nodules. What is the best treatment?

THE DIVERSION

This is classic neonatal sepsis and how can you go wrong using the classic treatment with the dynamic duo of Ampicillin/Cefotaxime?

ANSWER REVEALED

Well, this is classic *Listeria infection*, and the correct choice would be Amp/Gent.

Group B Strep *(Strep agalactiae)*

BUZZWORDS

GBS can present with anything from asymptomatic bacteremia to septic shock. Respiratory symptoms, including **tachypnea, grunting, flaring, apnea and cyanosis** are the initial clinical findings in 80% of newborns regardless of the site of infection.

Onset Facts

HOT TIP

Group B strep (GBS) **early-onset infection** presents in the **first 7 days after birth**. It usually presents as sepsis or pneumonia. Meningitis occurs in <10 % of early onset GBS disease.

Indications for Intrapartum Antibiotics
- maternal colonization on screening or GBS bacteriuria during pregnancy
- preterm birth < 37 weeks
- ROM > 18 hours before delivery
- intrapartum fever > 38'C
- previous infant with invasive GBS disease

Late-onset disease presents generally in the first month of life, but may present **up to 90 days after birth**. It is usually not associated with obstetric or birth complications. It most commonly bacteremia without a focus or meningitis. It less commonly presents as skin/soft tissue disease.

Late-late-onset disease usually presents in preterm infants and may appear **at up to 6 months of age**.

Antenatal screening for GBS has now been changed to 36 0/7 weeks to 37 6/7 weeks of gestation.

Women who are positive for GBS, or have not been tested but have sepsis risk factors, require intrapartum antibiotic prophylaxis (IAP), **unless a C-section is performed before the onset of labor or rupture of membranes**.

Infants of mothers with suspected chorioamnionitis should have a **CBC and blood culture obtained** and **antibiotic therapy begun** pending culture results.

Even well-appearing infants should be monitored for **48 hours prior to discharge** if the mothers had inadequate treatment of GBS.

The drug of choice for treatment of definitive GBS disease is **penicillin G**. Ampicillin is an acceptable alternative. All other antibiotic choices or ANY antibiotic given <4 hours before delivery is not considered adequate intrapartum antibiotic prophylaxis (IAP) for GBS.

Flu Flip

If the **mother** was described as **asymptomatic** during pregnancy, **GBBS** is the more likely cause of the newborn's illness.

But if they describe the mother as having a **flu-like illness**, then consider **Listeria** infection instead.

Birth Trauma

Bleeding Caps

Caput Succedaneum crosses the suture lines and will be described as "soft, boggy pitting."

A **Cephalohematoma** is more localized and will be described as firm and tense since the blood is contained within the periosteum, and therefore can NOT cross suture lines.

And if all else fails, remember the phrase, "caput crosses."

Cephalohematoma has a pH in the word to help remember that it is "phirm" and an "L" to help remember that it is localized. Remember that it is unilateral and does not cross. It is also slower to heal.

A cephalohematoma is more likely to occur with prolonged labor or instrument-assisted delivery. 10-25% of cephalohematomas may be associated with underlying skull fractures. Cephalohematomas may calcify and remain as bony prominences for months.

Subgaleal hemorrhages are often associated with **vacuum-assisted deliveries** and involve bleeding between the epicranial aponeurosis and the skull periosteum. It presents as a mass that enlarged soon after birth and may lead to hemorrhagic shock and hyperbilirubinemia.

Clavicular Fracture

In most cases, watchful observation is all that is necessary, and you can expect the callus to recede within 2 years.

Watch for this if you are presented with a neonatal CXR. It is easy to miss the clavicular forest while focusing on the Lung and cardiac trees.

Erb's Palsy and Phrenic Nerve Palsy can occur with a clavicular fracture.

Brachial Plexus Injury

You will need to be familiar with the 2 classic types of brachial plexus injury and distinguish them based on their clinical presentations or their appearances in an image they might present to you. These occur in less than a **half a percent of deliveries**, but occur in a much *larger percentage of deliveries on the Boards*.

Erb's Palsy

Erb's Palsy occurs higher up (**C5-7**). It presents with the **classic Waiter's Tip** (adducted, internally rotated, with the wrist and fingers flexed). For those not familiar with this pose, picture a waiter with his hand to his side, wrist facing behind him expecting a tip. There is limited shoulder movement. Erb's Palsy is also associated with clavicular fractures. It occurs after a delivery where there was excessive lateral neck flexion.

Picture a **waiter** getting a big "**Herb Plant**" instead of a tip.

Phrenic Nerve paralysis leading to respiratory distress can occur with Erb's Palsy as well. Watch for this in the history. The diagnosis is made with fluoroscopy that will show an elevated hemidiaphragm on the affected side.

Klumpke Palsy

Klumpke Palsy occurs much lower down (**C8, T1**). It affects the muscles of the hand, resulting in the **claw hand**. It occurs when an abducted arm is pulled away from the body.

Picture this: "Klumpke the monkey" hanging onto a tree branch with one hand. This will help you remember the mechanism of injury and the way the hand will look.

They may also lose **the ability to grasp** with Klumpke Palsy, despite this initial presentation.

> ### Grasp the Difference!
>
> Erb's Palsy is more common than Klumpke palsy. With Erb's Palsy the nerve is stretched, not broken, and **the ability to grasp is preserved.**

It can be associated with **Horner syndrome**, so keep this in mind if this is noted in the history.

Think of Hand paralysis, Horner syndrome in a Hairy monkey (see above mnemonic) to help differentiate this from Erb's palsy.

Cord Issues

Clingy Cord

The umbilical cord should **fall off by the 2-week visit**. Keep this in mind if they present you with an anxious grandmother who is concerned that the cord has not fallen off within 48 hours!

If it stays attached **beyond one month**, think LAD (Leukocyte Adhesion Deficiency) or low WBC count.

It is important to note that, for the purpose of the boards, all that is needed for umbilical stump care is washing with soap and water and pat dry. There is no decreased infection risk by applying alcohol to the stump. Cultural remedies are okay, provided they do no harm.

Single Umbilical Artery

In the real world, most incidences of a single umbilical artery are **not** associated with renal disease. However, it must be considered, especially on the exam!

When presented with a newborn with a single umbilical artery, you are expected to know that a thorough physical exam is indicated since 25% have associated anomalies.

Renal US is no longer routinely recommended due to the low incidence of actionable findings.

Bloody Cord

Yes, the baby should be kept below the cord before clamping, for around 30 seconds, to prevent decreased red cell volume.

However, the obstetrician should not "milk" the cord toward the baby. This could lead to polycythemia.

Witch's Milk

Breast hypertrophy in a newborn is usually a benign finding. This is the case even if milk is produced. Historically this has been called witch's milk.

The correct answer is to leave it alone. Expressing the milk by squeezing it out will be the wrong answer. In fact, this will make it worse, since this stimulates prolactin and oxytocin secretion and will prolong it. It also increases the risk for mastitis.

Assessing Baby's Growth

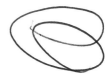

Definitions

Strict definitions of terms are important because they might describe something, or imply a disorder or problem, that does not meet the criterion for the "definition." If you fall into the trap you will get the question wrong.

LGA/SGA

The Boards can present you with a small baby an imply it is SGA. Unless you know the definition, you will be fooled. **An SGA baby is in the lower 10th percentile, and an LGA baby is above the 90th percentile, for weight for gestational age.**

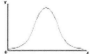

In addition, LGA is greater than 3900g and SGA less than 2500g. SGA babies have a **higher morbidity and mortality risk** than AGA babies. In the short term, they are at higher risk for **temperature instability**, **polycythemia**, and **hypoglycemia**.

SGA and IUGR

An **SGA** baby is small for its gestational age. SGA infants are born with Intrauterine growth retardation (IUGR). Preemies are not necessarily SGA if their weight is <u>appropriate</u> for their gestational age. **IUGR** means that a fetus did not reach its genetically determined growth potential for some reason (so not all SGA babies are IUGR). IUGR babies tend to have more difficulty tolerating labor, and therefore IUGR is often associated with perinatal asphyxia.

Infants of mothers with chronic illness are at higher risk for being SGA. Teenage mothers are at higher risk for delivering SGA babies.

SGA babies' growth may catch up nicely once they are removed from the restrictive uterine environment. If the growth failure is due to an inherent infant condition, like a congenital infection, growth will likely not catch up. This will often be your clue to a congenital problem.

Full Term

This is defined as 40 weeks plus or minus 2 weeks. Any baby born in the range of 38-42 weeks is considered to be full term; thus, a 42 week baby is actually considered term.

Post Term (Prolonged pregnancy)

Sometimes too much is too much. Babies born **post term**, i.e., more than 2 weeks post dates, also present with a whole host of problems.

> ## Tiny Tots
>
> **Symmetrical** IUGR: a fetus's head & body are proportionately small. Typically, it occurs early in a pregnancy so think of early infections, genetic abnormalities, chronic alcohol or tobacco use.
>
> **Asymmetrical** IUGR: a fetus's head growth is spared while its body is smaller than expected. Typically occurs later in pregnancy so consider placental issues, hypertension and/or preeclampsia.

Post term newborns may be described as having **dry skin that is peeling, long fingernails,** and **decreased lanugo on the back.** The **ears will have strong recoil.**

Fetal Deaths/Causes

The most **common causes of fetal demise are chromosomal abnormalities and congenital malformations.**

The normal arterial blood gas values for a newborn infant is a pO_2 60 – 90 mmHg and a pCO_2 35-45 mmHg.

Special Delivery

Newborns are at risk for heat loss because of the high surface-area-to-body-mass ratio. Heat loss is reduced by the use of a *radiant warmer* and drying with warm blankets.

Ultimately, the best source of warmth is skin to skin contact with the mother (which has emotional benefits as well). **Cold stress should be avoided because it can lead to depletion of fat and glycogen stores.**

The one exception to the radiant heat warmer answer is extreme premies, or ELGANs[4] as they are now known, who weigh less than 1 kg. Placing these tiny babies in an open air radiant heat warmer can result in too much evaporative fluid loss.

Therefore, a closed humidified environment is required for usually at least the first 24-72 hours of life. Basically, an isolette is better than open air radiant heat, even though access for procedures is less convenient.

> ### Clonus Bonus
>
> Remember that **bilateral ankle clonus** can be a normal finding in an infant, so don't let them trick you into thinking it's some sort of neurologic sign or seizure.

Apgar

Although Virginia Apgar was an anesthesiologist, her work is the domain of the pediatric boards. Know that **the 1-minute Apgar does not reflect long term problems if the 5-minute Apgar is fine.**

This is because the 1 minute Apgar reflects life in the uterus and his/her endurance of the delivery process to the harsh life outside the uterus.

The 5 minute Apgar reflects transition and adjustment to the new world. A 5 minute Apgar of 7 or less is reflective of difficult adjustment. We are assuming that anyone reading this is familiar with the Apgar measurement, having attended scores of deliveries by the time this book has reached your eyes.

No Time to Wait

You do not use Apgar results to make decisions regarding administration of CPR, since you would never "wait one minute" before making a decision.

---

[4] Extremely low gestational age newborn.

Preemie Dreamy

Some important points about preemies can, and will, be held against you. If you know the basics, you should be able to answer these questions with ease.

Very Low Birth Weight Infants (VLBW)

What exactly is a very low birth weight infant? **Any infant weighing less than 1500 grams should be considered to be VLBW.**

VLBW infants require D10 in order to provide sufficient glucose without fluid overload.

Factors which impact **prognosis** include the following:

- Gestational age (the most important factor)
- Morbidity while in the NICU
- Intracranial hemorrhage

Very Low Birthweight (VLBW) Infants and Apgars

Due to neurological immaturity, including poor tone, an Apgar greater than 6 cannot be expected in these tiny infants.

VLBW and Sepsis

In the absence of another explanation such as pre-eclampsia or placenta previa, infection must be considered as a trigger for premature delivery. Sepsis has to be ruled out in the VLBW infant unless an alternative cause of the preterm birth seems clear.

Coverage for common bacteria would be accomplished with the old standbys, ampicillin and gentamicin.

If the infant presents with vesicular lesions, neonatal herpes is likely, and treatment with **acyclovir** would be a correct choice. Thrombocytopenia, or even a bloody spinal tap, could be another sign of neonatal herpes.

Do NOT let the fact that the mom has no history of herpes throw you off the herpes diagnostic trail.

Meconium Aspiration

Meconium aspiration occurs almost exclusively in **term and postterm infants.** Passage of meconium in utero may represent **fetal hypoxemia**.

Premie Pressure

While there are no set norms for blood pressure in preemies, use the following if a question on this pops up on the exam.

The preterm baby's mean arterial blood pressure should not be less than the corrected gestational age in weeks.

Mec Delivery

BREAKING NEWS Babies born through meconium and meconium aspiration babies are now treated the same as any other baby in the delivery room.

CXR in cases of meconium aspiration usually shows **patchy areas of atelectasis alternating with areas of hyperinflation**. Pneumothorax is seen in 10-20% of infants who have meconium aspiration.

Infants with meconium aspiration are likely to present with respiratory distress and a **"barrel chest"** with **rales and rhonchi on auscultation**.

In the event they present you with a case of bona fide meconium aspiration syndrome, **persistent pulmonary hypertension** is the most likely complication they will be describing.

Counting Fingers, Counting Toes: The Routine Newborn Exam

Anuric Infants

If they ask you to evaluate an anuric[5] infant, the following stepwise approach would be in order

1) Recheck the plumbing by evaluating the abdomen and genitalia
2) Make sure fluid intake has been adequate
3) Obtain a cath urine specimen for analysis
4) Check the BUN and Creatinine
5) Order a renal ultrasound
6) If you do all this and the results are normal and then the baby starts to pee, you can stop now.
7) If anything comes up positive and/or the baby still hasn't been convinced to pee, then you can call in the urologist, even on the boards, but only if you are provided with the lab results that would be part of the initial workup.

The Passing of Meconium

If meconium has not been passed **in the first 48 hours**, this should be looked into.

The possible causes of **delayed passing of meconium** in an infant are:

• Meconium plug syndrome
• Hirschsprung's disease
• Imperforate anus

Too Cool for Stool

Step-wise evaluation of an infant who has not stooled in 48 hours involves:

• Repeat examination of abdomen and rectum
• Assess for adequacy of feeding
• Check barium enema to R/O Hirschsprung's disease
• Order surgical consultation for rectal biopsy
• Watch for signs of intestinal obstruction, hydration
• Hydration and feeding until a diagnosis is established

[5] No urine output for 24 hours.

Necrotizing Enterocolitis (NEC)

The following are some important points to remember about Necrotizing Enterocolitis (NEC).

NEC is associated with:

- **Hypoxic Injury** – RDS, birth asphyxia, and/or prolonged apnea
- **Bacterial Infection**

Blood cultures are often positive, and **pneumatosis intestinalis** is a common finding on x-ray.

 Some of the typical findings associated with NEC are general, such as **lethargy, apnea,** and **poor feeding,** while others are more specific, such as **bloody stools, erythema of the abdominal wall,** and **thrombocytopenia.**

Pneumatosis intestinalis, gas in the bowel wall, in and of itself, is not diagnostic, because it can occur with other disorders. However, on the Boards it should be present, and they will probably show you a film that also shows **air in the biliary tree** or **pneumoperitoneum**. The combination of these two findings would be sufficient for an assumption of a diagnosis of NEC and a slam-dunk for you.

The long term complication of NEC that you need to be aware of is **intestinal strictures**.

Management of NEC should include NPO status, replogle (double lumen tube) to low intermittent suction, broad spectrum antibiotics with anaerobic coverage, CBC, lytes, coags and serial abdominal films as indicated.

Surgical intervention is required up to half the time.

Neonatal Jaundice

Questions on this are certainly fair game. In addition to the basic garden-variety presentations like breast-fed and physiological jaundice, they will throw in some Yellow Zebras as well.

- A bilirubin up to 12.4 within the first 24 hours can be normal in a full term newborn.
- Visual diagnosis is generally unreliable, even more so in darker skinned infants.
- Near term infants 35-38 weeks are at higher risk for jaundice.
- Infants of Asian descent are at higher risk for hyperbilirubinemia.

What are the Causes of Indirect Hyperbilirubinemia? YELLOW

You Never Know: Gilbert Disease, Gilbert Goes Yellow

Endocrine: (Hypothyroid - Hypopituitarism); **E**nterohepatic Circulation Increased (Obstruction, Pyloric Stenosis, Meconium Ileus, Ileus, Hirschsprung's Disease)

Lucy Driscoll Syndrome: You never know, they could ask.

Lysed Blood Cells: Hemolytic Disease, Defects of Red Cell Metabolism, Isoimmunization

Overdrive: Some are both Direct and Indirect. Galactosemia, Tyrosinosis, Hypermethionemia (Cystic Fibrosis)

Wasted Blood: Petechiae, Hematomas, Hemorrhages anywhere, Cephalohematomas, Swallowed maternal blood

---

Physiologic Jaundice

Physiologic jaundice is an unconjugated hyperbilirubinemia that occurs on Day 2 through Day 5, usually peaks on Day 3, and may last 1 week, in an otherwise healthy infant with no other pathological explanation. It is a diagnosis of exclusion, but very common.

An elevated bilirubin that occurs during the first 24 hours is abnormal. It cannot by definition be called "physiologic jaundice." Likewise, a bilirubin level of 17 after 120 hours of life can no longer be considered physiologic.

If they ask what would be the "first step," it would be to check **a total and direct bili** (checking direct bilirubin is important before starting phototherapy).

Phototherapy is **contraindicated in infants** with an elevated **direct (conjugated) bilirubin** or a **family history of light sensitive porphyria**. They might describe the **"Bronze Baby Syndrome"** in a child started on phototherapy that did not first have a direct level checked. Phototherapy would be what caused the Bronze Baby Syndrome.

The incidence of neonatal jaundice is reduced with maternal heroin use.[6] It is also reduced with smoking, alcohol, and the double P's: Phenobarb/Phenytoin.

Breastfeeding vs. Human Milk Jaundice

Believe it or not, there is a difference between the terms. If you are confronted with the two in a multiple-choice situation, don't be fooled.

Breastfeeding jaundice occurs during the first days of life. It is the most common cause of unconjugated hyperbilirubinemia, and is due to decreased caloric intake leading to an **increase in enterohepatic circulation**. Mild dehydration and delayed passage of meconium also contribute to the appearance of breastfeeding jaundice.

Think of it is breast(NOT)feeding to help remember it is from lack of sufficient breastmilk intake.

Treatment of breastfeeding jaundice involves **increased breastfeeding**: 8-12 times a day in the first few days along with formula suplementation if the infant has lost more than 10% of birth weight.

Human milk jaundice, formerly known as **breast milk jaundice**, occurs from the 6th to the 14th day after birth and **may persist for 1-3 months**. It is due to inherent human milk factors too complicated and boring to get into here.

---

[6] However, this does not mean one should encourage heroin use!

The most important factors are

      1. the baby is growing well

      2. the hyperbilirubinemia is unconjugated

Treatment is the same as for physiologic jaundice.

Hemolytic Disease of the Newborn

Maternal antibodies to incompatible fetal RBC antigens, such as Rhesus (Rh) D, A, or B, can cause hemolysis *in utero*. Onset of jaundice **in the first day of life** or **prolonged or severe hyperbilirubinemia** should prompt investigation for hemolytic disease, which is usually **Direct Antiglobulin Test (DAT) positive**.

So what happens when the ABO and the Rh in-laws don't get along? ABO incompatibility may cause hemolysis in a **first-born child**. However, Rh incompatibility does not usually cause problems in a first born child, unless they were to mention a previous miscarriage/abortion.

Even with an ABO "setup,"[7] only **a small percentage will actually result in significant hemolysis**.

ABO incompatibility usually presents with jaundice; significant anemia is more typical of Rh disease.

Intensive phototherapy is usually sufficient to resolve ABO-associated hemolytic disease, but late-onset anemia may occur 1-3 weeks after birth.

Metabolic Issues of the Newborn

Sugar Babies

Hypoglycemia

Hypoglycemia is serum glucose less than 25 in a preemie and less than 35 in a full term newborn. In practice, it's less than 40. The Boards won't split such sweet hairs.

The very low birth weight infant is at risk for hypoglycemia due to small muscle mass and low glycogen stores. Maintaining adequate glucose levels and maintaining good body temperature are the most important steps for initial management and board questions.

> **Dextro Strip Deceptions**
>
> Blood samples contaminated with IV solution containing glucose can result in a falsely elevated result on the Dextrostix. In addition, shortened **time** on the strip will result in a **lower level**.
>
> Remember the "d" sticks are not totally accurate and, therefore, if that is the only value provided in the question, the "next" step is to **verify the result with serum glucose**.

Hypoglycemia can present in any number of ways such as the **classic jitteriness, lethargy** and **apnea**, as well as **cyanosis** and **seizures**.

Hypoglycemia is managed with a **2 -3 mL/kg D10 bolus and increasing enteral feeds or dextrose fluids**.

---

[7] E.g., mother with blood type O and baby with A or B.

BREAKING NEWS Diazoxide is a medication that can be used to treat persistent hypoglycemia due to hyperinsulinemism (i.e. in IDM babies).

BUZZWORDS "**A mother who has had tocolytics to arrest labor**" could be the tip-off; these agents can stimulate fetal insulin, resulting in hypoglycemia.

HOT TIP Remember: **tachypnea can be a sign of hypoglycemia**, and in fact it can be the only sign of hypoglycemia that they give you on the exam.

Infants of Diabetic Mothers

Fetuses of uncontrolled diabetic mothers are exposed to high glucose levels resulting in the fetus producing high levels of insulin in utero AND after birth, despite being cut off from their sugar source. Therefore, these infants often develop **hypoglycemia for several hours after delivery**. The increased insulin also promotes growth, which explains why they are typically **LGA**.

'Betes babies

Insulin dependent diabetic moms are at increased risk for congenital anomalies because the elevated glucose levels occur during organogenesis. **C**ommon problems include:

- **C**ardiac: **c**onotruncal, **c**ardiomyopathy
- **C**olon: small left colon
- **C**audal regression syndrome

HOT TIP Like all questions, they are not likely to test your knowledge of the obvious, in this case LGA babies and hypoglycemia. Another manifestation of infants of diabetic mothers is **polycythemia**, possibly due to increased erythropoietin. IDM babies commonly have RDS because the high glucose levels interfere with surfactant production.

MNEMONIC Remember **L**arge Body, **L**ots of red blood cells, and **L**ung problems.

Heme Dreams/Neonatal Hematology Issues

Anemia

DEFINITION At birth, 50% Hgb is Fetal HgbF. For a full term infant, Hgb less than 13 at birth is considered anemia.

The **Kleihauer Betke Test** detects for the presence of fetal cells in the mother's blood. It is used to evaluate neonatal anemia in the setting of fetometarnal hemorrhage.

Anemia in Preemies vs. Full Term Infants

In FT infants, the Hgb can fall to as low as 11 or even 9.

Pre-term infants often go as low as 7 to 8.

FT infants reach their "nadir" at 2 - 3 months; preemies can reach it in 1 - 2 months.

TAKE HOME MESSAGE The main point to remember is that in preemies the initial Hct is lower, and they bottom out earlier.

Polycythemia Arena

DEFINITION

Polycythemia is a **central venous HCT** of 65 or higher.

PERIL

The key phrase is **central venous**. If they give you a capillary measurement, and they are only trying to deceive you into working it up inappropriately. This is especially true if the infant is also acidotic and hypotensive.

TREATMENT

Treatment is indicated when the hematocrit is **greater than 70**. Polycythemia will often lead to **hypoglycemia, hyperbilirubinemia**, and/or **thrombocytopenia**. Treatment for symptomatic polycythemia is a partial exchange transfusion.

Hyperviscosity Syndrome

BUZZWORDS

Hyperviscosity syndrome results from polycythemia. This syndrome can result in **lethargy, hypotonia**, and **irritability**.

HOT TIP

Consider hyperviscosity syndrome in any infant with history of **twin to twin transfusion, delayed clamping of the cord, Down syndrome,** or an **infant of a diabetic mother**.

PERIL

They might list complications that could occur with hyperviscosity syndrome, and include hyperglycemia among the choices. Remember it is hypoglycemia that occurs with polycythemia.

MNEMONIC

To help remember hypoglycemia occurring with polycythemia, think of it as RBCs eating up all the glucose.

> ### Apt Test
>
> *HOT TIP*
>
> The Apt Test tests blood in the neonate's gastric aspirate to determine if it is actually maternal blood. For example, if they ask you what test you would order for a neonate that is being gavage fed, and there is blood in the residuals, "Apt Test" would be the correct answer.

Abdominal Defects

Omphalocele

DEFINITION

An omphalocele is a protrusion of the bowel and other organs (ie. liver) **through the base of the umbilical cord**.

COIN FLIP

With an **omphalocele**, the bowel contents will be **covered with a membrane**. The presence of the membranous cover is the key to distinguishing an omphalocele from gastroschisis.

Another clue is that omphaloceles tend to happen in big babies, (OOMPH!!), and gastroschisis in little babies.

Picture the O in Omphalocele as the membrane cover. Picture the membrane being made out of DNA strands to remind you that this can be **associated with chromosomal defects**.

Omphalocele is also associated with syndromes like **Beckwith Wiedemann**. An **echocardiogram** should be performed in all omphalocele infants.

Gastroschisis

Gastroschisis is the herniation of bowel through **a defect in the abdominal musculature to the right of the umbilicus**. This is usually seen in **small (IUGR) infants**. It is thought to be related to a vascular accident or vasoactive medications/drugs.

Whereas omphaloceles can involve intestines and other organs (e.g., liver), gastroschisis is usually **limited to intestinal contents,** and is **not covered with a membrane**.

You can choose to remember "O" for Organs and "G" for Gut.

> ### Special Delivery Packaging
>
> The most important initial management for both omphalocele and gastroschisis in the delivery room is to keep the abdominal contents warm and moist by covering them with saline-soaked sterile dressings.
>
> The newborn is also placed in a bowel bag up to the axilla to minimize fluid and heat losses. Special packaging for Special Delivery.

Diaphragmatic Hernia

If you hear the terms **"scaphoid abdomen"** with **"decreased breath sounds on the left side,"** and maybe even **"heart sounds on the right,"** look no further; you have been given a gift.

Initial management involves **intubation and ventilation, placement of an NG tube** to maintain the stomach decompressed, and **parenteral nutrition** to stabilize the infant until **surgical repair**.

Seizing the moment / Neonatal Seizures

If a neonatal seizure occurs **within 24 hours of birth**, it is likely secondary to **birth asphyxia**. Often there will be a hint of this in the history.

Most neonatal seizures are subtle.

Typical neonatal seizures include **staring spells, decreased motor activity, lip smacking,** and/or other **abnormal facial movements.**

Most full-term newborn infants who have neonatal seizures secondary to asphyxia **will not have any long-term neurodevelopmental sequelae.**

Neonatal encephalopathy and hypoxic-ischemic encephalopathy (HIE) are the most frequent causes of neonatal seizures in the full term infant.[8] When these infants develop seizures, there is more concern for impaired neurodevelopmental outcome. Nearly half of these infants may have abnormal outcomes, manifested by cognitive problems, motor problems, and/or epilepsy.

Phenobarbital will be the correct treatment.

Intraventricular Hemorrhage

Intraventricular hemorrhage (IVH), as with any intracerebral hemorrhage, should be managed like any other potentially unstable situation. Begin with the **ABCs** before anything else.

If imaging is needed in an unstable newborn, it should be done by **cranial ultrasound** at the bedside.

If the patient is stable and a subarachnoid or subdural hemorrhage is suspected, then a **head CT** would be indicated.

Many times IVH will be asymptomatic, but, if present, clinical signs may include **anemia, hyperglycemia, thrombocytopenia, hyponatremia,** and/or **acidemia.**

Grading IVH

Should they ask about grading:

> **Grade 1** is Germinal Matrix
> **Grade 2** is IVH without Dilation
> **Grade 3** is IVH with Dilation
> **Grade 4** is all this plus parenchymal involvement

Maternal Medication Machinations

Beta Adrenergics

Beta adrenergics such as *terbutaline* can be used for short-term tocolysis. Watch for these agents stimulating fetal insulin resulting in hypoglycemia in the neonate.

> ### Phenobarb is not Yellow
>
> Infants exposed to phenobarbital in-utero are often *jittery* and *irritable*. However, they are at lower risk for hyperbilirubinemia.

---

[8] However, metabolic causes have to be ruled out first.

General anaesthesia

General anaesthesia in the mother is considered to carry little long term risk to the newborn, but may cause a hypotonic, apneic newborn requiring resuscitation.

Corticosteroids

A single one-time use of corticosteroids imparts a **reduced risk of intraventricular hemorrhage, necrotizing enterocolitis,** and RDS.

Naloxone / Narcan®

These are opioid antagonists used to reverse the respiratory depression that can be seen when the mother received narcotic-based analgesics during delivery.

Naloxone/Narcan® will produce withdrawal symptoms in patients with chronic dependence. Since it has a short duration of action, multiple doses may be required.

Neonatal Abstinence syndrome

Neonatal abstinence syndrome refers to the **postnatal withdrawal effects in an infant after drug exposure in-utero**. This used to just refer to opioid withdrawal, but it has been expanded.

You are expected to distinguish between drug effects and withdrawal effects. The withdrawal effects vary from drug to drug.

Early discharge is not an option for an infant who has been exposed to drug use in utero. An infant at risk for NAS should be carefully monitored in the hospital for signs of withdrawal. The length of hospital observation depends on the drug of maternal use. Urine and meconium drug screens from the infant should be obtained within 24 hours of delivery.

The table below outlines several drugs and their withdrawal profile.

Drug	Withdrawal profile and Association
Alcohol	Hyperactivity, irritability Hypoglycemia can be seen in alcohol withdrawal as well
Cocaine	**No official withdrawal or abstinence syndrome exists.** However, while there is no known official withdrawal syndrome or teratogenic effects, these children are at increased risk for anomalies due to impaired uteroplacental circulation. This includes cerebral infarctions, limb anomalies, and urogenital defects. There is also an increased risk for placental abruption. Aggression has been described in boys exposed to cocaine in utero.

Drug	Withdrawal profile and Association
Marijuana	Maternal marijuana use has <u>not</u> been definitively shown to be associated with any specific infant features or developmental issues at this time. A few studies have low fetal growth concerns, but this is unconfirmed. There has been suggestion of abnormal vision response to light and/or infant tremulousness, but this probably won't be tested on the exam.
Amphetamine	Although there is no established withdrawal syndrome, children exposed to amphetamines in-utero are irritable and easily agitated with routine environmental stimulation. They often experience IUGR, and are prone to developmental and cognitive impairment.
Barbiturates	Hyperactivity, hyperphagia, irritability, crying and poor suck swallow coordination.
Opioid	Hyperirritability, tremors, jitteriness, hypertonia, loose stools, emesis and feeding difficulties. Seizure activity would also be consistent with opioid withdrawal. Methadone and/or oral morphine may be needed to manage withdrawal.
SSRIs	Obviously, this is not a drug of abuse, but recent studies have shown some withdrawal symptoms. Exposure later in pregnancy has increased risk of developing Neonatal Behavior Syndrome (excessive crying, irritability, jittery, vomiting, feeding / sleeping issues), LBW and even persistent pulmonary hypertension. Supportive care for Neonatal Behavioral Syndrome and appropriate indicated care for Persistent pulmonary hypertension of the newborn (PPHN) Usually resolves within 14 days.

Initial treatment of infants with signs of withdrawal includes minimizing environmental stimulation (both light and sound), swaddling the infant to limit autostimulation as well as responding quickly to the infant's signals (hungry, wet) and comforting the infant as able by rocking and swaying. Feedings should be small and frequent with hypercaloric formula or human milk to minimize hunger while providing for optimal growth.

Honorable Discharge

Most newborns are stable enough to be discharged within 24-48 hours after a vaginal delivery, or 48-72 hours after a C-section.

To be ready for discharge, a newborn must be feeding well, and have urinated and stooled. In addition, they need to be assessed for jaundice prior to discharge, and of course the family has to be deemed reliable to follow up.

Watch for signs in the question that would make the infant ineligible for discharge.

Chapter 16

Fluids and Lytes, and Everything Nice

Most Board candidates would rather be featured on *Tiger King* than study Fluids and Lytes. In fact, we dreaded editing this chapter.

This is a chapter that really doesn't lend itself to rote memory; it requires a clear understanding of the underlying principles. Some time invested in learning the logic can result in a clean sweep of this material, which comprises a large section of the exam.

You need to know a lot of the normal values, the abnormal ones, and the tricks they play to fool you. This can be a recurring dream or nightmare.[1] Follow the bouncing jokes and you will recognize the tricks and answer the questions correctly.

Once you understand the predictable patterns this can actually be an easy section to score points. There aren't really any tricks. The questions tend to be pretty straightforward.

Acid Base Metabolism

In determining the cause of an acid base disturbance, the following systematic approach should be helpful (technically, it is not acidemia until the pH is <7.36 or alkalemia until the pH is >7.44, but these are general guidelines):

Step 1: **Look at the pH**
- If the pH is > 7.40, you are dealing with alkalosis
- If the pH is <7.40, you are dealing with acidosis

Step 2: **Look at the Bicarb**
- If the bicarb is >25, you are dealing with a metabolic alkalosis
- If the bicarb is < 25, you are dealing with a metabolic acidosis

Step 3: **Look at the pCO_2**
- If the pCO_2 is > 40, you are dealing with a respiratory acidosis
- If the pCO_2 is < 40, you are dealing with a respiratory alkalosis

Calculating Osmolality

WARNING! You will be expected to be able to calculate serum osmolality using the following equation, which you should commit to memory.

Make a habit of calculating this each time you are presented with the electrolytes in the question.

2*Na (mEq/L)
+[BUN (mg/dL)/2.8]
+ [Glucose (mg/dL)/18]

 Normal serum osm is 265-285.

Higher than this and you are hyperosmolar or hypertonic. Lower and you are hypoosmolar or hypotonic.

How Much Bicarb?

DEFINITION The formula to correct metabolic acidosis is mEq Bicarbonate = Weight x 0.3 x the Base Deficit.

---

[1] Like the ones you still have about forgetting to study for a final scheduled in one hour.

These are general rules, since infants have lower bicarb levels than adults. The renal threshold for bicarb in term neonates is 21 mEq/L. Remember that their kidneys are not yet fully developed.

Whenever you are presented with an arterial blood gas, circle the components and write down whether each value would result in alkalosis or acidosis. This will go a long way toward understanding the clinical acid-base scenario you are facing.

Respiratory Acidosis

In this case, **hypoventilation is the primary cause of the acidosis,** so you would expect to see an elevated pCO_2; for example, **pH 7.15** and a **pCO_2 75.**

CNS dysfunction would be an example where respiratory drive is blunted, resulting in hypoventilation.

Respiratory Alkalosis

In this case, **hyperventilation is the primary cause of the alkalosis** so you would expect to see a low pCO_2 and an elevated pH; for example, **pH 7.55** and a **pCO_2 25.**

This would occur if a child moved to **Colorado** and was breathing rapidly because of the thin air. In this case, **hypoxia** would trigger **hyperventilation**, leading to respiratory alkalosis.

Metabolic Acidosis

This would result from increased acids or decreased bicarbonate. As a result, **pH would be <7.40** and **bicarb is depleted (<25).**

Diarrhea is the leading cause of metabolic acidosis in children.

Metabolic Alkalosis

In metabolic alkalosis, you are dealing with a **bicarb >25** and a **pH greater than 7.40.**

Vomiting, prolonged NG suction, pyloric stenosis and **cystic fibrosis** are common causes of metabolic alkalosis. This must be corrected preoperatively so it does not lead to postoperative apnea.

Compensatory Mechanisms

The body will try to buffer to minimize any changes in the pH. If the lungs caused the problem, the kidneys will try to fix the pH, and vice versa. However, **compensatory mechanisms are incomplete.**

Compensating for Metabolic Acidosis

Metabolic acidosis has too much acid (acidosis) and it's the kidneys' fault (metabolic), so the lungs would step in and blow off the acid it can (CO_2).

Compensated metabolic acidosis will still have a low pH but also a lowered pCO_2 in an attempt to compensate; for example, **pH 7.20** and **pCO_2 25.**

Septic shock (for example, secondary to meningococcemia) would be a clinical scenario where this may be seen.

Compensating for Metabolic Alkalosis

Metabolic alkalosis has too much bicarb "alkalosis" and it's usually the GI's fault "metabolic". Therefore, the kidneys will have to excrete more bicarb to increase the pH. If the kidney was the problem in the first place, you have a real problem!

A classic example of metabolic alkalosis is an infant with **pyloric stenosis** or an NG tube. The steps leading to **hypochloremic metabolic alkalosis** are as follows:

- Loss of stomach juices → Loss of hydrogen ions → Alkalosis
  → Loss of chloride ions → Hypochloremia

- Contraction of extracellular fluid → Increased bicarb reabsorption in the kidneys → worsening alkalosis
  → Kidneys retain chloride, so urine chloride is <10

Remember, the respiratory response to this metabolic alkalosis would be "hypoventilation" to retain CO_2. But this is also known as "not breathing," so hypoventilation can never adequately compensate for metabolic alkalosis.

CASE STUDY You are presented with a patient with pyloric stenosis, given a bunch of labs, and then you have to pick the one that is *inconsistent with the diagnosis.*

THE DIVERSION While this type of question may seem straightforward, it is not always so simple.

- First, it is crucial to write down in the margins the adjective description of the lab values, since this is how you have been studying. For example, a bicarb of 35 should be written down as "alkalosis."

- Second, when picking a lab which is *inconsistent with a diagnosis*, it is best to step back and *first cross off the ones which <u>are</u> consistent with the diagnosis*. Remember this, because on more than one occasion they have given a bunch of lab values and you had to choose the *one* that was inconsistent with pyloric stenosis.

ANSWER REVEALED Just remember that pyloric stenosis is associated with a **hypochloremic hypokalemic metabolic alkalosis.** Therefore, you would expect:

- High pH
- Low serum chloride
- Low serum sodium
- Low serum potassium
- **Hyperbilirubinemia may also be present**

PERIL High serum potassium would be inconsistent with a diagnosis of pyloric stenosis. Of course, a heel stick sample could have a high potassium level, but it would be due to hemolysis, not underlying pathology. It is highly doubtful that they would get that petty on the exam. Bottom line: understand the classic lab findings consistent with pyloric stenosis.

Compensating for Respiratory Acidosis

DEFINITION Since the lungs "respiratory" did not breathe enough and held on to too much CO_2 "acidosis", the kidneys need to step in and hold on to bicarb. What you see is **pH 7.30, pCO_2 50, and bicarb 32**.

Compensating for Respiratory Alkalosis

DEFINITION Since the lungs "respiratory" blew off too much acid CO_2 "alkalosis", the kidneys need to get rid of bicarb to decrease the alkalosis. What you would see is a **pH 7.48 and a pCO_2 of 20 with a bicarb of 15**.

Sorting Out Metabolic Acidosis

Fall into the Gap

Some folks shop at the *Gap®*, some folks visit the Delaware Water Gap, and others look at David Letterman's grin and obsessively focus on the distracting gap in his teeth. All of this is for later; right now we have to focus on the Anion Gap.

The first thing you should do when you have a patient **with acidosis** and you are given the patient's **serum sodium, chloride, and bicarbonate** is to **calculate the anion gap** as reflexively as an accountant calculating deductions on April 14th.

$$\text{Anion Gap} = \text{Serum Sodium} - (\text{Chloride} + \text{Bicarbonate})$$

A normal anion gap is between 8-12 mEq/L. The anion gap measures ions that are not accounted for in routine labs, including such delicacies as protein, organic acids, phosphate, sulfate, and lactic acid.

Normal Anion Gap

With **a normal anion gap,** the **serum chloride will be elevated.**

Acidosis with a normal anion gap is caused by either:

- Loss of bicarbonate
- Kidney dysfunction
- Diarrhea
- Addition of hydrochloric acid
- Renal tubular dysfunction

Diarrhea is the most common cause of a non-gap metabolic acidosis in children.

If you are presented with a child with a **normal anion gap metabolic acidosis but no diarrhea**, then you know he likely has **RTA**.

Pay attention if you are presented with a premie or former premie with chronic lung disease. If they note that they are taking a carbonic anhydrase inhibitor such as acetazolamide and / or potassium sparing Aldactone®/spironolactone. They are likely pointing you to normal anion gap metabolic acidosis.

> ### Normal Anion Gap Acidosis/Buying a Used Carp
>
> These causes can be referred to by the mnemonic device **USEDCARP**, which represents the following:
>
> - **U**reterostomy
> - **S**mall bowel fistula
> - **E**xtra chloride[2]
> - **D**iarrhea
> - **C**hronic diuretic use
> - **A**drenal insufficiency
> - **R**enal tubular acidosis
> - **P**ancreatic fistula

---

[2] Like from a large NS bolus

Renal Tubular Acidosis

HOT TIP

You will consider the diagnosis of RTA in a child with **a triad of failure to thrive, polyuria and constipation** who has a **metabolic acidosis** (pH <7.4, HCO3 <22) with an **elevated chloride** and a **normal anion gap**.

Both diarrhea and RTA result in a normal anion gap metabolic acidosis. They can be differentiated by the urine anion gap. For example with distal RTA (type 1) there is a positive urine anion gape and low ammonia excretion. This information would be included in the history.

Type 1 (Distal) Renal Tubular Acidosis

In **distal tubular acidosis,** also known as **classic RTA**, the proximal tubule is fine and it keeps all the bicarb it needs to. However, if the distal tubule is not doing its job, and H+ is not allowed into the urine compartment inside the distal tubule, so the **urine will have a high pH and cannot be acidified.** The urine pH **will always be greater than 5.5**.

Type 2 (Proximal) Renal Tubular Acidosis

HOT TIP

Proximal tubular acidosis is caused by the inability of the proximal tubule to take back its bicarb, resulting in excessive bicarb in the urine.

However the distal tubule can still do its job and show the H+ to the door (urine), so the **urine pH is less than 5.5**.

Type 3 Renal Tubular Acidosis

Type 3 is rarely used as a classification today because it is now thought to be a combination of type 1 and type 2.

Type 4 Renal Tubular Acidosis

Type 4 RTA is due to resistance to aldosterone (or to aldosterone deficiency); therefore, you can expect to see **hyperkalemia**.

Widening the Gap / Elevated Anion Gap

Acidosis with an elevated anion gap is usually due either to:

- Overproduction of organic acids
- Ingestion
- Inability to excrete acid, as in renal failure

Boxing Bicarb and Arranging Acid / All Else Falls into Place

Remember that the kidney is the key to acid-base metabolism, more than breathing is.

The **Proximal** Tubule **B**oxes and takes Bicarb **B**ack in.

The **Distal** Tubule **A**rranges for H/**A**cid to leave the building.

Any breakdown in one of these sites has obvious consequences.

RTA Imitators

RTA (Distal) Type I may be mimicked by use of potassium-sparing drugs like spironolactone.

RTA (Proximal) Type II is mimicked by use of carbonic anhydrase inhibitors like acetazolamide.

MUD PILES

The classic mnemonic for conditions that are associated with an **elevated anion gap** is **MUDPILES**:

- **M**ethanol
- **U**remia
- **D**iabetic ketoacidosis
- **P**araldehyde
- **I**soniazid (INH)
- **L**actic acid from organic acidemias, etc)
- **E**thanol / Ethylene glycol
- **S**alicylates

With an **elevated anion gap,** the **serum chloride will be normal.**

Sold on Sodium

Sodium is important because it is the big name in town that maintains osmolality, and if it shifts, it impacts the brain, resulting in a big ego for everyone (brain swelling) or injured ego (brain contraction).

 The daily requirement for sodium = 3 mEq/kg/day.

Preterm infants may require 2-3 times this amount due to their renal immaturity and their rapid growth.

Hypernatremia

 Hypernatremia is serum sodium **greater than 145 mEq/L.**

 When will you see hypernatremia? In two situations:

1. **Sodium Excess:**
   a. Improper mixing of formula (not enough water)
   b. Ingestion of sea saltwater
   c. Excessive sodium bicarb after resuscitation
   d. Breast milk with excessive sodium
   e. Iatrogenic[3]

2. **Water deficit**
   a. Diabetes insipidus
   b. Diarrhea (both sodium and water are lost, but water more than sodium in this case)

> ### Body Water
>
> Total Body Water (TBW) as a percentage of body weight changes with age. Almost 90% of the fetus's body weight is water. **As we age, this percentage decreases** so that ultimately in adolescents and adults, TBW represents only 60% of body weight.
>
> TBW is broken down into TWO main compartments: **intracellular** and **extracellular** fluids. Equilibrium is maintained between these two compartments by diffusion across cell membranes based on serum osmolality between the two compartments.

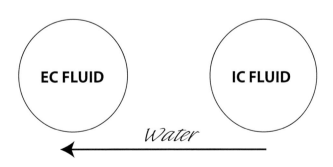

---

[3] Greek for "whoops!"

Extracellular fluid is maintained in hypernatremia. Remember, water chases sodium like a long lost lover. Wherever sodium excess is, water wants to go. Therefore, if there is hypernatremia, water is drawn out of the intracellular compartment. **This results in increased extracellular volume,** which can result in **pulmonary edema.**

Diabetes Insipidus (D.I.)

Kids with diabetes insipidus are urinating a lot, either because of a **lack of ADH (central D.I.)** or **resistance to it (nephrogenic D.I.)**

Diabetes "I am Sipping and Sipping this" – because you would sip and sip if you were peeing all the time.

Look for "**a child that is urinating profusely but has no sugar in the urine.**"

Labs will **show a high serum osmolality with inappropriately dilute urine**.

To differentiate D.I. from hypernatremic dehydration, **check the urine**. D.I. kids have continued urination with dilute urine, and dehydrated kids will have decreased urination with concentrated urine.

DI presents with polyuria, nocturia, polydipsi. Lab findings include low urine spec grav on 1st void in the morning, normal-high Na level. Watch for a history of neurosurgery, neurotrauma, or neuro-oncology.

Nephrogenic Diabetes Insipidus

This is an **X-linked** disorder, and is therefore **only found in males**. The kidney does not respond to the vasopressin (ADH), resulting in **dilute urine.**

Nephrogenic DI will fail to respond to **exogenous vasopressin,** and central DI will respond. Beware: if they describe a **familial pattern among males, nephrogenic DI is your answer.**

Hyponatremia

Hyponatremia is serum sodium **less than 130 mEq/L**. There are 3 categories of hyponatremia:

1. Hypovolemic
2. Euvolemic
3. Hypervolemic

The best study to order to determine the type of hyponatremia you are dealing with is **urinary fractional excretion of sodium (FENa).**

With a sodium < **120,** the patient may present with **lethargy** and **seizures**.

Hyponatremia is the result of one of two mechanisms:

    1) Loss of sodium

    2) Increased water (dilutional)

        ❑ Too much taken on board: **Polydipsia**

        ❑ Too little let out: **SIADH**

Sometimes, while sodium and water are both lost, more sodium is lost than water. The result, however, is still hyponatremia (3rd space losses post op, for example).

GI Losses

With hyponatremia secondary to GI losses, the kidneys will hold on to sodium, resulting in **low urine sodium** **(< 10).**

SIADH

No matter how well you know something, it is very easy to get confused in the heat of the battle, especially when a question asks, "are all true *except.*" Intelligent folks have missed questions like this by not being careful.

Remember, SIADH results in *diminished urine output.*

You can remember this logically as "ANTI - Diuretic" – the opposite of a Diuretic. Or think of it as "**S**yndrome of **I A**m **D**efinitely **H**ydrated (cause I ain't peeing)."

"Appropriate ADH"

Before we go on and on about inappropriate ADH, we should know when it is appropriate. Whenever there is **high serum osmolality,** you will want to retain fluid, and this results in concentrated urine secondary to "appropriate ADH."

> ## Post Op Fluid Management
>
> Postoperatively, there is a risk for increased ADH secretion: therefore, it is important to monitor for hyponatremia and restrict fluids appropriately.

Causes of SIADH

First, translate the labs into English. They might describe some **cerebral injury or insult** (trauma, tumor, etc.) Since the pituitary produces ADH, trauma or infection involving the brain can result in SIADH. In addition, certain **pulmonary or endocrine disorders can trigger SIADH**.

Chemotherapeutic drugs like vincristine and cyclophosphamide and the antiepileptic drug **carbamazepine** also may lead to SIADH.

Remember **SIADH**:

Surgery
Infection
Axon (neurological such as Guillain Barré, Brain Tumor)
D (Day After, Post Op, of any kind)
H (Head and Hemorrhage)

SIADH presents with hyponatremia; however, the underlying problem is **fluid retention, not excretion of sodium.** SIADH also presents with **normal serum potassium, elevated urine sodium.** Plasma volume is increased in SIADH.

The lab values expected in SIADH are as follows:

- **Low serum sodium** < 124 mEq/L
- **Elevated BP**
- **Decreased urine output - < 1cc/kg/day**
- **Renal function (BUN and Cr) will be normal**
- **Elevated urine Na concentration > 25 mEq/ L**

The **urine** in patients with SIADH will have **high osmolality** and **high sodium concentration.**

You will need to know how to **differentiate SIADH from hyponatremic dehydration**. Remember that: SIADH is **overhydrated**, so the serum osmolality will be low. Hyponatremic dehydration will have either normal or elevated serum osmolality.

Also, urine sodium is low in hyponatremic dehydration but high in SIADH.

BUN would be elevated in dehydration, but decreased in SIADH. Body weight would also increase with SIADH but decrease with dehydration.

The preferred **treatment for SIADH** is **fluid restriction.**

This may be difficult in infants and — no matter what — correction will be slow. SIADH is a diagnosis of exclusion, so you may need to rule out other disorders leading to hyponatremia before choosing fluid restriction.

If fluid restriction alone does not work, the use of **furosemide** and **hypertonic saline** is an option. **Demeclocycline** blocks the effects of ADH on the kidney. However, since it is a derivative of doxycycline, it is only indicated in children 8 years of age or older. **Lithium** also blocks the effects of ADH, but it is not usually recommended due to its side effect profile. However, it is still important to know in case it comes up on the exam.

3% sodium chloride would be indicated if the serum sodium is less than 120 mEq/L.

Thiazide diuretics would be incorrect in the treatment of SIADH, since they can lower sodium further.

CASE STUDY
You could be presented with a patient with a head injury or meningitis. They will either imply or come right out and tell you the patient has SIADH. You will then be asked to decide on a treatment. They will have to note that there are no neurological symptoms.

THE DIVERSION
Among the choices will be obvious ones that are incorrect, including maintenance, twice maintenance, and 1.5 times maintenance. Even if you realize that the correct answer is 2/3 maintenance and that 0.66 maintenance is the same thing (without pulling out a calculator), answering the question correctly may not be that easy. You will be expected to know when to use demeclocycline.

ANSWER REVEALED
Demeclocycline would be indicated if there is no clinical improvement with appropriate fluid restriction.

Renal Failure

BUZZWORDS
A patient with diminished urine output who is taking in fluid in excess of urine volume will develop hyponatremia. They will also have to present you with a clue that renal disease is present, i.e., **elevated creatinine.** The patient will likely also present with **edema** and **urine sodium > 20 mEq/L.**

PERIL
If you are presented with a patient who is **oliguric** and **hemodynamically unstable**, the correct initial treatment is with 20 mL/ kg of isotonic solution (e.g., normal saline, LR, packed RBC, or albumin). **This is true even in patients with renal failure.**

Once hemodynamically stable, adjustments would be based on the urine output, weight, and other symptoms included in the question, including the presence of pulmonary edema or other conditions.

PERIL
Chronic diuretic therapy may result in **hyponatremia.**

Medications that cause hyponatremia

The table below outlines medications that can cause hyponatremia.

Agent	Mechanism
Vincristine	SIADH
Cyclophosphamide	Diminishes water excretion
Chlorpropamide (oral hypoglycemic)	Stimulates vasopressin release
Thiazide diuretics	Blocks renal sodium and chloride reabsorption, decreasing the kidney's ability to produce dilute urine

Dilutional hyponatremia

- Dilutional hyponatremia is due to **water intoxication**
- **Total body sodium is normal**
- There are no signs of intravascular volume depletion
- Seizures occur due to cerebral swelling
- **Urine sodium concentration is increased >100 mEg/L**

Water intoxication is one of the most common causes of hyponatremia in infants. Mostly, this is due to **excessive dilution of formula** with water. Many of these infants present with **afebrile seizures, respiratory insufficiency,** and **hypothermia.**

Remember, **hyponatremic dehydration** causes pontine damage. That is easy to remember because hyponatremic dehydration and pontine both have an "**o**" in them.

Seizures in a patient with no history of seizures, no history of trauma, and no fever should make you think of metabolic causes, like hypoglycemia or hyponatremia. They might also mention that the child has spent a lot of time **swimming**, especially if it is a young child, because they **swallow a lot of water.** Other situations they may mention include **malnutrition, hypotonic IV fluids, glucocorticoid deficiency,** and **hypothyroidism.**

It is important to note that **the total body sodium is normal** in dilutional hyponatremia. Remembering this is worth at least one point on the exam.

You may need to distinguish dilutional hyponatremia from other similar clinical scenarios.

- **Third spacing of fluid** may occur after extensive surgery, due to either **1) endothelial damage and/or leakage** or **2) hypoalbuminemia** and **low oncotic pressure.**

- It also occurs in **nephrotic syndrome.** In this case, urine sodium concentration is low (less than 10 mEq/L). **Edema** is an important feature.

- **Cerebral and renal salt wasting** would also present as hyponatremia, but hypovolemia would also be a feature.

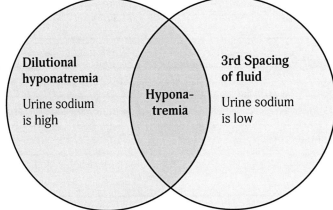

CASE STUDY You are presented with a patient who is post op for resection of a craniopharyngioma. The patient is noted to have hyponatremia and an elevated serum creatinine. Urine output is increased, and urine sodium is greater than 100 mEq/L with a urine osmolality of 350.

What is the diagnosis and what is the treatment?

THE DIVERSION This is a very tricky question. When presented with a patient with a cranial lesion, especially a craniopharyngioma, it is easy to immediately assume a diagnosis of SIADH. Those who write board questions know this.

If you picked SIADH and fluid restriction as the treatment of choice, you will be suffering from SIAQI or "Syndrome of Inappropriately Answering the Question Incorrectly."

ANSWER REVEALED Read the question carefully and you won't go wrong. With SIADH or "Syndrome of I Am Definitely Hydrated," urine output will be low and urine sodium concentration will be elevated. Hypervolemia is the result, and fluid restriction is the correct management.

The patient in this vignette, however, has elevated urine output and elevated urine sodium. Therefore, the correct diagnosis is **cerebral salt wasting,** and the correct treatment is replacement of fluid and sodium losses.

Pseudohyponatremia

This is one of the favorite tricky Board questions. They give you a **low sodium value** and then ask you if the **total body sodium** is normal, low, or elevated. Of course, the answer is not the obvious. Follow the logic arc here and you will slam-dunk this trick at least once and maybe twice on the same exam day.

Step 1

They will describe a situation where there are **elevated triglycerides** and/or **plasma proteins**. A typical example would be **nephrotic syndrome**.

Step 2

TGs take up a lot of room, so there is **less "water," but the "volume" is the same.**

Labs report sodium per volume, not sodium per water. The sodium level will be reported low, since water is the only part that actually contains sodium. Therefore, the **sodium level in circulation really is normal.**

Step 3

There is lots of water outside circulation in conditions of **edem**a. In fact, there is more water than usual and all this water **does contain sodium**. Therefore, **the Total Body Sodium is elevated.**

HOT TIP Remember: with edema secondary to decreased oncotic pressure, the measured sodium is low.

Potassium

 The daily requirement for potassium = 2 mEq/kg/day

Hypokalemia

 Hypokalemia is serum potassium **less than 3.5 mEq/L.**

 A typical scenario would be a child with a **history of diarrhea** presenting with **muscle pain** and **weakness, paralysis, constipation and ileus,** or **polyuria.**

Hypokalemia can be *caused by* diarrhea and *result in* constipation.

> Furosemide (Lasix®) is the classic diuretic that leads to hypokalemic alkalosis due to renal loss of potassium.
>
> If you want a potassium sparing diuretic, try spironolactone (Aldactone®).

Causes of Hypokalemia

❑ Poor Intake (Anorexia Nervosa)

❑ Loss

    • **GI**/Vomiting /Diarrhea

    • **Renal**/(i.e. diuretics, renal tubular disorders, or excess aldosterone)

EKG Changes

The EKG changes one would expect with hypokalemia are:

• **Flattening of T waves**

• **ST depression**

• **Premature ventricular beats**

In extreme cases, there may also be a **U wave** that appears just after the T wave.

CASE STUDY

    You are presented with a boy who has a 2-3 day history of vomiting and diarrhea. He has taken water and juice, but has become progressively weaker and has difficulty sitting or standing without support. You are then asked for the explanation for his weakness.

THE DIVERSION

    You will be presented with several diversionary electrolyte-based explanations for the child's weakness. Dehydration will be tempting, as will be hyponatremia. However, the question will specifically ask for the explanation for his weakness.

ANSWER REVEALED

    In any question asking for a specific explanation for weakness in the face of vomiting and dehydration, the answer will be hypokalemia.

Emergency Treatment of Hypokalemia

In **emergency situations**, potassium is replaced using **KCl 0.5 -1.0 mEq/L per kg over an hour**. The maximum would be 40 mEq/L.

However, this is only in emergency/urgent situations.

You must remember the following caveats:

- In mild cases, oral replacement of potassium is appropriate.
- If the hypokalemia is due to dehydration, then fluid replacement with added potassium is all that is needed.
- If **acidosis** is a factor, potassium **acetate** is used. That should be easy to remember phonetically.
- If hypophosphatemia is an issue, then potassium phosphate is used.

EKG monitoring is required during IV infusion of KCl.

There are other electrolyte abnormalities that can present with **weakness and EKG changes**:

- **Hypocalcemia** can present with **muscle weakness and prolonged QT interval**.
- **Hypomagnesemia** can occur in patients with **diarrhea**, as well as a **prolonged PR or QT interval**.

Hypoglycemia and **hyponatremia** will present with **muscle weakness but no EKG changes**.

Hyperkalemia

Hyperkalemia is serum potassium **greater than 5.0 mEq/ L**.

Causes of hyperkalemia

- ❏ Excess intake
- ❏ Not enough out (renal failure, HypO aldosteronism)
- ❏ *Redistribution* - Acidosis (H goes into the cell, K goes out of the cell)
- ❏ Cell breakdown (pseudohyperkalemia)

The initial EKG findings seen with hyperkalemia include **peaked T waves.** However, at substantially higher potassium levels, i.e. 10 or greater, you are likely to see the **absence of P waves, widened QRS complex, prolonged PR interval, ventricular fibrillation and asystole.** This is associated with **electromechanical dissociation (EMD).**

The widened QRS complex can be misinterpreted as **idiopathic bundle branch block (IBBB) or ventricular tachycardia.** However, they would not describe muffled heart sounds or absence of pulses in

IBBB. A pulseless state is possible with ventricular tachycardia at rates 200 or greater, but you would not have muffled heart sounds. Bottom line: read the question carefully.

Emergency Treatment of Hyperkalemia

 C BIG K DROP

      C - calcium gluconate

      B - bicarbonate and beta-agonist (albuterol)

      IG - insulin/glucose

      K - kayexelate (sodium polystyrene sulfonate - though acts super sllow)

      D - diuretic (Lasix), dialysis

If you are presented with a patient with potassium greater than 10 who has EKG changes, then the correct treatment is **IV calcium chloride or gluconate primarily to stabilize cardiac membrane**. Dialysis is also an option.

CASE STUDY

You are presented with an infant with an abdominal mass who becomes hypotensive. The physical exam is noteworthy for non-palpable pulses and distant heart sounds. The EKG shows a wide QRS complex. What is the appropriate *immediate* treatment?

THE DIVERSION

You might be tempted to pick a diversion, like a normal saline bolus to treat shock. Or perhaps you guessed correctly that the patient's abdominal mass is due to an adrenal tumor and the patient is experiencing hypovolemic shock; based on this, you might pick hydrocortisone IV, or maybe a pressor like dobutamine. But if you did, you might become pulseless yourself when you realize the correct answer.

ANSWER REVEALED

In this case, it is adrenal failure that has resulted in hyperkalemia. This has resulted in **electromechanical dissociation (EMD)**. The most appropriate *immediate* treatment* would be IV **calcium chloride**.

Potassium Acid/Base Montage

Few things strike more fear in mice and hens than this. However, it is also one of the most logical to keep straight. Here goes:

Alkalosis and Potassium

      Step 1: Alkalosis ➜ High pH ➜ Very little H in the EC Fluid

      Step 2: The Hs in the cells move out to help out their Cation brethren ➜H Moves from IC to EC ➜

Step 3: To replace the "H Cats" leaving the cell, the K Cats move from the ECF into the ICF ➜

Step 4: Therefore, **during alkalosis**, K heads in the house, resulting in ➜ **lower measured potassium levels.**

During alkalosis, K moves to the IC fluid and H moves out, resulting in lower measured serum potassium, but total body potassium is unchanged, it's just hiding.

Acidosis and Potassium

The opposite occurs:

Step 1: Acidosis ➜ Low pH ➜ Lots of H floating around the EC Fluid.

Step 2: There are just too many Hs running around the EC with too much time on their hands.

Step 3: They begin to "squat" where they don't belong by moving into the IC.

Step 4: And because there is only room for one positive ion for each seat, the weaker K gets kicked out of the ICF, and now there is increased K in the EC fluid.

Acidosis ➜ H moves in and K moves out, resulting in high measured serum potassium.

K increases 0.6 mmol/L for each 0.1 pH drop and vice versa.

Tonic for your Dehydration

Degree of Dehydration

At some point on the exam, you will be called upon to calculate fluids and to assess degree of dehydration. This really is a simple calculation with simple answers. The amount of rehydration will depend on the level of dehydration.

5% Dehydration

Tachycardia with **decreased tear production** may be descriptions you'll see. **Decreased urinary output** and **increased urine concentration** would be other signs of 5% dehydration.

Taking care of business:

> ❑ **5%** means the child is "short" **50 mL/kg** [50mL/ 1000mL].

> ❑ This can usually be done with oral rehydration, but if you need to do it IV for some reason, you simply add this to the maintenance fluid to come up with the total fluid the child should receive over 24 hours.

Calculating Fluid Maintenance

Okay, we all know the 100 mL/kg/day, 50 mL/kg/day, and 20 mL/kg/day calculation; well, the quick version to calculate the maintenance fluid hourly rate is:

4 mL/kg/hr (for the first 10 kg) PLUS

2 mL/kg/hr (for the next 10 kg) PLUS

1 mL/kg/hr (for each additional kg)

❑ **Half of this total is given over the first 8 hours.**

❑ **Half is given over the next 16 hours.** Hopefully, you and the child can then both go home.

10% Dehydration

Look for **tachycardia** plus **sunken eyes, poor skin turgor, and sunken fontanelle.**

> ### Signs of Dehydration
> **Tachycardia** is an **earlier sign.**
>
> **Hypotension, decreased skin turgor** and **bounding pulses** are **later signs** of dehydration.

Taking care of business once again:

❑ **10%** means the child is "short" **100 mL/kg** [100mL/ 1000mL].

❑ Over 24 hours, this would be **maintenance plus 100 mL/kg.**

❑ **Emergency phase** – This will be approximately **20 mL/kg over an hour.**

❑ Take whatever is left over and **give half over the next 7 hours** and the **other half over the remaining 16 hours.**

15% Dehydration

The same clinical signs you see with 10%, plus signs of **shock**, including **delayed cap refill time.**

Really taking care of business:

❑ Here the child is short a good **150 mL/kg** [150mL/ 1000mL].

❑ Over 24 hours, you need to give **maintenance plus the 150 mL/kg.**

❑ In this case, you keep giving **20 mL/kg boluses until you see some clinical improvement.**

❑ Then you can give **half of what is left over during the next 7 hours and the remaining half over the next 16 hours.**

Of course, now with the availability of PDA applications that do the calculations for you, the ability and necessity of learning these formulas has gone to the dustbin of history (along with the ability to spell, write cursive, and sit still for long periods of time).[4]

If you are presented with a patient in **septic shock**, they may require up to 3 boluses of 20 mL/kg normal saline which adds up to... hmm... let's see here... oh yes, a total of 60 mL/kg total.

If one of the choices is "the total amount is based on findings on frequent reassessment," this would be the correct answer.

Best Oral Replacement Fluid

All oral rehydration fluids must **contain glucose.** In order to cross the microvillus membrane of the GI tract, sodium molecules must be accompanied by a glucose molecule. Sodium is not permitted entry unless accompanied by a paid club member in the form of glucose.

When you are treating a patient with moderate to severe dehydration, i.e., a patient with **tachycardia** and **delayed cap refill**, you need to use **oral rehydration fluid**, which contains **75 mEq/L of sodium.** The rate should be 50 mL/kg over 1-4 hours, even if administered with a dropper.

---

[4] If you don't know what a dustbin is, I rest my case.

In cases of **mild dehydration**, you can use standard **maintenance hydration fluids**, which contain **50 mEq/L**. This solution can also be used once cap refill is normalized in cases of severe dehydration.

PERIL

Standard formula is the wrong answer if you are presented with an infant with moderate to severe dehydration.

The BRAT diet is **not part of AAP recommendations**, and therefore is **not the correct answer** on the exam for managing acute gastroenteritis.

CASE STUDY

You are evaluating a 5-year-old boy with a 3-day history of diarrhea and vomiting. He is now tolerating a small amount of fluids, although his vomiting is still intermittent. On physical examination, his mouth is pasty and he has good bounding pulses and a heart rate of 156 beats per minute.

What would be the most appropriate management in this patient?

THE DIVERSION

You could be given several choices that will take advantage of clinical urban myths, including IV fluids in the ER, admission and bowel rest, and discharge on a bland "BRAT" diet especially since the child is experiencing "intermittent vomiting."

ANSWER REVEALED

The correct answer would be oral rehydration and discharge home with a regular diet as soon as it is tolerated. The BRAT diet lacks adequate nutrition. Diluting formula is also incorrect. Complex carbohydrates, fruits and vegetables should be encouraged and fruit juices discouraged.

Isotonic Dehydration

DEFINITION

Isotonic dehydration would be dehydration with **serum sodium between 135-145**.

While sodium and water are lost proportionately, **more ECF than ICF fluid is lost**, resulting in a symptomatic patient.

Hyponatremic Dehydration

DEFINITION

Hyponatremic dehydration would be dehydration and serum sodium **less than 135**.

BUZZWORDS

This is usually due to GI losses, such as from **diarrhea**. But it may have an element of water intoxication. If the question mentions or hints at a dehydrated child that was **fed tea or water by a grandmother, think hyponatremic dehydration**.

Because fluid moves from the ECF to the ICF, it is this form of dehydration that causes the greatest circulatory disturbances, and the **patients are more symptomatic on presentation.** They might mention **poor skin turgor.**

CNS Effects

Free water moves into CNS cells with a **serum Na of 125**, and these patients may actually present with **seizures.**

Rehydration Time

Initial treatment is with **normal saline boluses.** If that doesn't work, then **hypertonic 3% saline in the** ICU would be correct. **Hypertonic saline is not indicated as the initial treatment.**

In addition to correcting the fluid part of dehydration (see below), you need to replace some of the sodium.

(Desired sodium - measured sodium) X weight X 0.6 = **A**

Maintenance sodium = 3 mEq/kg/day

Add maintenance to the A, and you have the amount of sodium you need to replace over 24 hours.

Sodium levels should not be raised by more than 12mEq/L in 24 hours. Rapid correction of hyponatremia can cause central pontine myelinolysis.

> ### Cystic Fibrosis
> Because cystic fibrosis is associated with an increased loss of sodium and chloride in sweat, it can lead to **hypo-chloremic hyponatremic metabolic alkalosis with dehydration.**

Hypernatremic Dehydration

Hypernatremic dehydration is dehydration with a serum sodium **greater than 145.**

It is due to either **water loss** or **sodium gain.** The **end result is a lot of sodium in the ECF.**

Infants with hypernatremic dehydration will often have a history of being fed **improperly mixed formula** (at least on the boards this will be the case). In the "olden days" before the rotavirus vaccine, **severe rotavirus diarrhea** was frequent cause as well. These infants are often **irritable, lethargic,** with **doughy skin** and a **high-pitched cry.** Eventually **seizures** can result.

Altered Mental Status

Remember: one of the ways the body deals with this is "extreme thirst." An **unconscious patient, infant,** or somebody who is **psychotic** will not act on the thirst mechanism and, therefore, **will likely have hypernatremic dehydration** (keep this is in mind in case you see one of those types of patients mentioned in the question).

Looks Aren't Everything!

With **hypernatremic dehydration**, water tends to go into the ECF, and this diminishes the clinical signs of dehydration; therefore, **assume 10% dehydration** regardless of clinical presentation.

Because of the **intracellular dehydration** that results from the mass water exodus heading out to the sodium, the shrinkage of brain cells can result in **tearing of bridging blood vessels** and **intracranial hemorrhage.**

Occasionally, however, the brain cells get smart, and with the water chasing its sodium mate, the brain cells take on a new lover, **idiogenic osmoles,** to lure the water back.

Idiogenic osmoles develop over 1-2 days, and do not go away so quickly either. Therefore the dehydration should be **corrected slowly over 2-3 days** in order to avoid cerebral edema as the water rushes in like an anxious lover to meet the new and improved mate-the idiogenic osmole.

The sodium should be **decreased no more than 10-12 mEq/L per day** in order to avoid this mad rush of water into the brain cells.

Rehydration Time

The treatment goal for hypernatremic dehydration is to correct the sodium concentration as well as circulating volume.

If the dehydration is chronic, sodium is reduced slowly at the rate of 0.5 mEq/L per hour.

Severe hypernatremia (170 or greater) should be corrected over 48-72 hours using 0.5 or 0.25 normal saline.

If there are signs of overcorrection, hypertonic solution should be used as a brake to slow the train down.

Potassium should be held until urine output is established.

Sodium Babbling Tower of Tables

It is very likely that you will get a table of lab values (on this and many other subjects) from which you will have to pick the correct diagnosis. This may include 6-10 questions that can be the difference between passing and failing. No pressure!

However, if you keep a cool head, this can be an easy 6-10 points for you to pick up on the exam.

The potassium will be normal in each of these.

Diagnosis	Sodium	Chloride	BUN	Glucose	Urine Specific Gravity	Abnormal Labs
Hyponatremic Dehydration	125	**85**	25	90	1.025	Decreased sodium and chloride Increased BUN and specific gravity
Hypernatremic Dehydration	152	120	25	90	1.025	Increased sodium, chloride, BUN and spec. gravity
Pseudohypo-natremia	120	108	15	**650**	1.015	Decreased sodium Markedly elevated glucose
SIADH	120	**85**	**5**	90	1.025	Decreased sodium, chloride and BUN Increased spec. gravity
Diabetes Insipidus	152	120	25	90	**1.002**	Increased sodium, chloride, BUN Decreased spec. gravity
Lab Error	120	108	15	90	1.010	Sodium is decreased and chloride is normal

Chapter 17

Genetics:
Everyone Into the (Gene) Pool

Prenatal Screening

In Utero Testing

- **Chorionic villus sampling** can be done at **12 weeks.**
- **Amniocentesis** can be done at **16 weeks.**

Fetal Ultrasound

Fetal ultrasound is used to track intrauterine growth over time. Structural anomalies (such as myelomeningocele) are best detected on ultrasound between 12 and 24 weeks gestation.

PERIL

Maternal obesity, if stated outright in the question, can be a complicating factor that blunts the accuracy of ultrasound findings.

Chromosomes and Genetics

Patterns of Inheritance

Understanding the inheritance patterns will enable you to eliminate 2-3 choices immediately. Knowing how to navigate the information in the question will allow you to instantly eliminate the incorrect choices deceptively left there for you.

HOT TIP

Genetic disorders may be caused by a mutation in one gene (**monogenic inheritance**), by mutations in multiple genes (**multifactorial inheritance**), or by a combination of gene mutations and environmental factors (**epigenetics**).

X-Linked Recessive

Males are affected and females are carriers. If they describe **ANY female relatives with the disorder**, then it is **not X-linked recessive.** There is **no male-to-male transmission.**

HOT TIP

If they "casually" mention in the question that "he had two uncles who had a similar problem," you know that **only males are affected** and they are pointing you towards an X-linked recessive disorder.

Recessive disorders in general, especially **X-linked** frequently involve an **enzyme deficiency**. The following disorders are x-linked recessive:

❑ **Androgen Insensitivity (formerly known as testicular feminization)** – Again the enzyme is defective. The patient will be phenotypically female but genetically male, so don't be fooled, it is still an X-linked recessive disorder.

❑ **Chronic Granulomatous Disease** – Here the enzyme to break down bacterial cells in the neutrophil is defective, so again it is an enzyme deficiency. Also remember it as CX GD.

❑ **Duchenne Muscular Dystrophy** – Remember it as DuXchenne.

❑ **Glucose-6-phosphate** dehydrogenase **(G6PD) Deficiency** – An enzyme deficiency, and remember it as GXPD deficiency.

❑ **Hunter Syndrome** –Also an enzyme deficiency.

❑ **Hemophilia A/B** – These are Factor 8 and 9 **enzyme deficiencies**

❑ **Nephrogenic Diabetes Insipidus** – Again, this is an enzyme deficiency. Think of it as NeXrogenic.

❑ **Retinitis Pigmentosa** – Also an enzyme deficiency, and you can remember it as retinitis pigmenXosa.

❑ **Wiskott Aldrich Syndrome** –To remember this change the name to "Whiskey All Rich" syndrome, so picture a bunch of "guys" sitting around drinking to help remember that it is X-linked recessive and affects males mostly.

CASE STUDY

Make sure you read the question carefully. They can present you with a scenario where the mother is a known carrier of an X-linked recessive disorder, and can then ask you one of two questions:

1. What are the chances of having an *affected male* **child**

2. What are the chances of having an *affected child*

THE DIVERSION

This question can be a slam dunk, but if you do not pay attention in the moment, you can easily miss the question. Highlight the word *male* or *child* and you won't be tricked with X-linked recessive disorders.

ANSWER REVEALED

The table that follows provides the logical conclusion to any question dealing with the chances of having a child with an x-linked recessive disorder when the mother is a carrier.

MALES	FEMALES	CHILDREN
50% will be affected 50% will not be affected	50% will be carriers 50% will not be carriers	25% will be carriers 25% will have disease 50% will be normal

X-Linked Dominant Conditions

There aren't that many X-linked dominant disorders. Just in case, here's how it works.

If **dad** has the gene on his X chromosome, and he only has that one X to give all his daughters, then clearly ALL his daughters will have the disorder. For the same reason, **none of his sons will have the disorder**.

If **mom** has the gene on one of her two X chromosomes, then 50% of her children will have it and 50% won't. **There are no carriers of a dominant trait. This is the same pattern for autosomal dominant**, making it difficult to distinguish and therefore a very unlikely question.

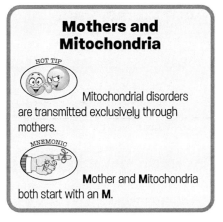

Mothers and Mitochondria

HOT TIP

Mitochondrial disorders are transmitted exclusively through mothers.

MNEMONIC

Mother and **M**itochondria both start with an **M**.

Remember, in X-linked disorders, whether recessive or dominant, there is **no male to male transmission**.

Once again, there aren't too many of these out there, and **they will most likely not ask you to pick this up from the question**. But in case they do, the disorders to consider are:

❑ Aicardi syndrome
❑ Alport syndrome
❑ Fragile X (a trinucleotide CGG repeat)
❑ Incontinentia Pigmenti
❑ Pseudohyperparathyroidism
❑ Rett Syndrome
❑ X-linked hypophosphatemic rickets[1]

These conditions affect females more often than males but they usually have a milder phenotype.

Autosomal Dominant

BUZZWORDS

Autosomal dominant inheritance is the only way a disease can be transmitted from father to son.

In addition, autosomal dominant disorders have the following characteristics:

- Variable expressivity
- Possible reduced penetrance
- High risk for spontaneous mutation with no prior family history.

Variability

Autosomal dominant disorders are associated with variable penetrance and variable expressivity.

Penetrance means there are people with the gene who exhibit it and people who do not.

Expressivity refers to the range of signs and symptoms that can occur in different people with the same genetic condition.

Examples include:

- Achondroplasia
- Apert syndrome
- Alagille Syndrome
- CHARGE syndrome
- FAP[3]/ ie Gardner syndrome
- Hereditary spherocytosis
- Marfan syndrome
- Neurofibromatosis[2]
- Noonan syndrome
- Osteogenesis imperfecta type 1, 2, 3
- Pseudohypoparathyroidism
- Pseudopseudohypoparathyroidism
- Retinoblastoma
- Tuberous Sclerosis

---

[1] See Endocrinology chapter for ongoing revised and often confusing changed nomenclature for this disorder.
[2] Neurofibromatosis can have variable expressivity with a high spontaneous mutation rate.
[3] Familial Adenomatous Polyposis.

Autosomal Recessive

Vertical transmission through 3 generations **rules out an autosomal recessive** disorder. Remember, recessive disorders usually involve enzyme deficiencies.

Examples include:

- Adrenogenital Syndrome
  (and Alpers Syndrome)
- Alpha-1 Antitrypsin Deficiency
- Ataxia Telangiectasia
- Chediak-Higashi syndrome
- Cystic Fibrosis
- Galactosemia
- Homocystinuria
- Hurler Syndrome
- Kartagener Syndrome
- Pickax = PKU
- Sickle Cell and Thalassemia
- Tay Sachs Disease
- Vitamin D dependent rickets, Vit D resistant rickets
- Wilson Disease

Mitochondrial Inheritance

In these conditions, both males and females are affected, but only females transmit the disease because mitochondria are inherited almost exclusively from the mother. The phenotype depends on the load of genetically abnormal mitochondria.

These family pedigrees will show all affected males and females being born to affected mothers, none to fathers. The history will likely include many deaths.

One example would be Leber hereditary optic neuropathy.

Mitochondrial inheritance is not the same as mitochondrial diseases. Many mitochondrial diseases are inherited in traditional Mendelian inheritance fashion, especially autosomal recessive fashion.

Genetic Anticipation... it's keeping me waiting!

In certain genetic conditions like myotonic dystrophy, the altered gene is passed down from one generation to the next.

The disorder may begin earlier in life and signs and symptoms become more severe in subsequent generations.

It typically presents in the neonaal period with respiratory issues and decreased tone.

This is referred to as genetic anticipation. In some cases, this happens because there is an increase in the length of the unstable region in gene.

add to the bottom

 In case it comes up Myotonic dystrophy type 1 is an autosomal dominant disorder caused by CTG trinucleotide repeat expansion of the gene DMPK.

Math Quiz

In an autosomal recessive condition, what portion of unaffected offspring are carriers? Answer is 2/3.

Genetic Testing

Karyotype

A microscopic evaluation of all the chromosomes which detects defects in number (ie. monosomies and trisomies), large rearrangements, and inversions.

You would request this to look for Down syndrome, Turner syndrome, etc. but nothing more subtle.

Fluorescent *in situ* hybridization (FISH)

Fishing is actually a good name for this because you have to know what you are fishing for to find it. You tell thelab what you are looking for and this has a single chromosome locus resolution to find it for you.

You would request this for Contiguous gene deletions or duplications(copy number variants).

Chromosomal Microarray Analysis (CMA)

This is like a karyotype and FISHing together. A detailed look at the entire genome.

You would order this for most children with abnormal phenotype or abnormal development if you do not know what's wrong with them (because if you suspect what's wrong with them you can order one of the two specific tests above since they are cheaper).

CMA does NOT detect point mutations, tiny deletions/ duplications (Fragile X), balanced chromosome rearrangements (translocations/ inversions).

It is important to counsel parents that CMA often finds variants of unknown significance or may find consanguinity, so might ant to ask before testing.

Molecular testing

This is also known as Sanger sequencing or whole genome sequencing and involves sequencis specific genes (usually left to geneticists).

Biochemical testing

Tests for metabolites (amino acids, organic acids, ammonium, acylcarnitine profile, etc) associated with metabolic diseases.

Methylation test

A test to check for a methylation pattern to see which of the parental copies of the gene got deleted.

This test is only necessary for imprinting disorders like Prader-Willi, Angelman, Beckwith-Wiedemann and Russell-Silver syndromes.

Counseling

When performing genetic testing, pretest and post test counseling are extremely important.

Pretest counseling includes why the test is being performed, as well as possible results and cost.

Posttest counseling includes not only the results, but the implications of the results, appropriate referrals and supports for the family.

Frequently Tested Genetic Disorders

Turner Syndrome (Primary Gonadal Dysgenesis)

Turner syndrome is associated with **short short stature, broad webbed neck**, and **left-sided congenital heart defects such as bicuspid aortic valve** or **coarctation of the aorta**.

Infants may present with **lymphedema of the hands and feet**.

Other characteristics include short 4th and 5th metacarpal ones, broad chest with widely-spaced nipples, occasional hypothyroidism, renal anomalies like horseshoe kidney, and primary ovarian failure presenting as delayed sexual maturation. They also have a higher likelihood of autoimmune diseases like celiac, IBD, Hashimoto, and diabetes.

In addition to the phenotypical features outlined above, there must be **a full or partial X chromosome deletion**. Turner syndrome can only be diagnosed in a female.

If you are presented with a male, turn left at the corner; Turner syndrome will be incorrect.

Know how to screen for the most common co-morbidities with Turner:

- Cardiac ECHO / 4 extremity blood pressures
- Renal US
- TSH
- Growth velocity

Don't Blame Mom Here

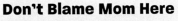 Since it is not a Trisomy, **Turner syndrome is NOT associated with advanced maternal age.**

Turner Delays

IQ is normal, but girls with Turner syndrome may have cognitive impairment including delayed speech, learning disabilities, and visual spatial problems.

They are not growth hormone deficient but their short stature is managed with growth hormone.

Turner syndrome is the most common chromosomal defect discovered in spontaneous abortions. 45XO is the most common form.

Buccal smear is woefully inaccurate for diagnosing Turner syndrome. A **karyotype** is necessary for definitive diagnosis.

Some girls who have Turner syndrome may have mosaicism. If you are "fishing" for Turner and initial chromosome analysis is normal, then turn to a **FISH study to look for mosaicism**. If you wish to carry this "fish story" further, then remember that elevated FSH can also be a feature of Turner syndrome.

Noonan Syndrome (Moon Man Syndrome)

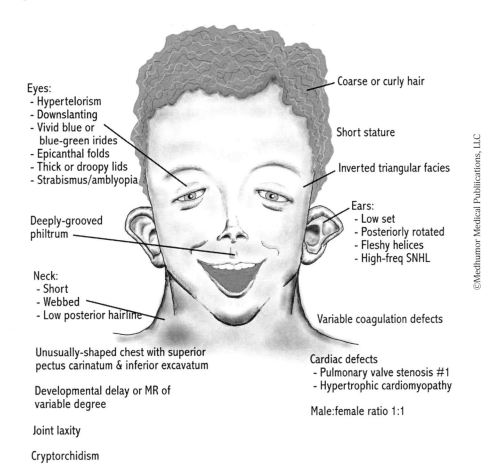

Eyes:
- Hypertelorism
- Downslanting
- Vivid blue or blue-green irides
- Epicanthal folds
- Thick or droopy lids
- Strabismus/amblyopia

Coarse or curly hair

Short stature

Inverted triangular facies

Ears:
- Low set
- Posteriorly rotated
- Fleshy helices
- High-freq SNHL

Deeply-grooved philtrum

Neck:
- Short
- Webbed
- Low posterior hairline

Variable coagulation defects

Unusually-shaped chest with superior pectus carinatum & inferior excavatum

Developmental delay or MR of variable degree

Joint laxity

Cryptorchidism

Cardiac defects
- Pulmonary valve stenosis #1
- Hypertrophic cardiomyopathy

Male:female ratio 1:1

©Medhumor Medical Publications, LLC

PERIL

Noonan Syndrome used to be known as "Male Turner syndrome," but it is not a male version of Turner. It **can** occur in **females,** so don't be fooled if they present the classic features in a female patient. These features include **pectus excavatum**, **webbed neck**, **low set ears**, and **pulmonic stenosis**.

The karyotype is normal.[4]

Marfan Syndrome

DEFINITION

Marfan syndrome is usually an **autosomal dominant**[5] connective tissue disorder associated with **skeletal, cardiac,** and **ophthalmologic** ramifications. The mutation is on **chromosome 15 in the fibrillin gene**. There can be great variation of the morphology among affected family members.

Skeletal abnormalities

Skeletal abnormalities associated with Marfan include:

- Tall stature
- High arched palate
- Dental crowding
- Hyperextensible joints
- Pectus abnormalities
- Arachnodactyly
- Disproportionately long extremities compared to the trunk

HOT TIP

An asymmetric pectus carinatum is almost pathognomonic for Marfan syndrome.

PERIL

Mitral valve prolapse is **not** one of the major criteria.

Cardiac Abnormalities

BUZZWORDS

Watch for murmurs associated with **aortic or mitral valve regurgitation**. They could give you a tall teenager presenting with a **spontaneous pneumothorax**.

HOT TIP

Patients with Marfan syndrome are at risk for **sudden death associated with aortic rupture** so they require a cardiac ECHO prior to

---

Turning on Noonan

Differentiating Turner from **Noonan** can be difficult. They are similar in many ways physically including a webbed neck, abnormal chest (wide nipples, pectus excavatum), cubitus valgus, and short stature. Pay attention to the following helpful clues to tell them apart in question stems:

COIN FLIP

- **Turner**: only females, **left**-sided heart lesions, typically have ovarian failure, normal IQ, abnormal karyotype

- **Noonan**: Males & females, **right**-sided heart lesion, females can have normal menses, coagulation defect, normal karyotype

---

The Major Criteria for Marfan

You need more than 2 criteria fto diagnose Marfan syndrome

1. Progressive dilatation or dissection of the ascending aorta
2. Lumbosacral dural ectasia
3. Ectopia lentis
4. Four skeletal manifestions
5. Family or genetic history

Marfan and Homocystinuria

COIN FLIP

Homocystinuria presents with a body type similar to Marfan's but the lens is usually **displaced downwards** instead of the upwards displacement seen with Marfan's.

Homocystinuria is also associated with **mental retardation** and **thrombosis**.

MNEMONIC

Marfan has a higher IQ so the lens goes **up / anterior** while homocystinuria has a lower IQ so the lens goes **down / posterior**.

---

[4] Technically speaking, genetics does play a role in Noonan syndrome; however, unlike in Turner syndrome, there are no identifiable genetic patterns on karyotyping.

[5] 25% of cases represent a new mutation.

sports participation. Close cardiac followup is important. Referral of other family members for genetic testing would be appropriate.

Pulmonary Abnormalities

Pneumothorax and apical blebs are minor criteria for diagnosis.

Ophthalmologic Manifestations

The ophthalmologic manifestation of Marfan syndrome to keep in mind is **ectopia lentis**, or upward and temporal displacement of the *lens of the eye*.

Serial slit lamp evaluation is important.

Smith-Lemli-Opitz Syndrome (SLOS)

Smith-Lemli-Opitz Syndrome (SLOS) is a rare autosomal recessive disorder where there is a problem with cholesterol synthesis.

Symptoms vary but some of the most common features are SGA with poor postnatal growth, microcephaly, intellectual disability and hypotonia.

Treatment is with cholesterol supplementation. Sadly, even with treatment, the prognosis is poor with most dying in early childhood.

If they mention syndactyly of the 2nd and 3rd toes, then SLOS is the most likely answer.

Trisomies

The incidence of all trisomies increases with advancing maternal age. **Trisomies are the only genetic disorders that increase with advancing maternal age.**

Trisomy 21 (Down syndrome)

Trisomy 21 can arise either from **nondisjunction** or from **translocation**.

There are no phenotypic differences between the two, but **the genetic implications are quite different**.

Translocation

If the infant has a translocation as the cause of the Trisomy 21, **chromosomal studies of the parents** are crucial.

If you find a carrier parent with a ***full*** translocation, there is a 100% chance of Down syndrome recurring. However, this is extremely rare.

With a ***partial*** translocation, the risk is closer to 15%. If the partial translocation is from the mother, the chances of recurrence are higher than if it is from the father.

Nondisjunction

The risk for recurrence here **equals the overall risk for the general population** (1%) plus the mother's age- related risk. At age 40, the age-related risk is 1/90. At age 22, it is 1/1,500.

> **Any question dealing with the risk of giving birth to a child with Down syndrome requires you to pause, take a breath, and read the question carefully.**
>
> **They could ask you which age group gives birth to more infants with Down syndrome.**
>
> Or
>
> **They could ask you which age group is at greater risk for having a child with Down syndrome.**
>
> These are very different questions.
>
> More children with Down syndrome are born to mothers in their twenties, since more women in their twenties have children, period.
>
> However, women in their 40s are at greater risk for having babies with Down syndrome.

The most **common** abnormality seen in Down syndrome is **hypotonia**, which is seen in 80% of cases. This may play a role in the **feeding difficulties** and **constipation** commonly seen in Down syndrome.

Balancing Translocations

Individuals with **balanced translocations** appear normal but will often have offspring with a genetic condition.

Individuals with **unbalanced translocations** have a genetic condition and will always have offspring with the same genetic condition.

Genetic counseling

Increased maternal age only increases the risk of Trisomy 21 due to nondisjunction (a.k.a. sporadic trisomy 21).

Inherited translocations can be a gift from either parent at any age. Thanks mom and dad!

The recurrence rate is higher is the mother is a carrier of a balanced translocation This would be described as 45,XX,t(14;21) in the mother.[6]

The recurrence rate is lower if the child has a freestanding chromosome 21.

This would be described as 47,XY, +21.

If the father is the carrier of the balanced translocation there is increased risk but much lower than with maternal balanced translocation risk. This would be described as 45XY,t(14;21).

Features of Down syndrome

- small head with brachycephaly
- small low set ears
- epicanthal folds
- upslanted palpebral fissures
- Brushfield spots
- single transverse palmar creases
- wide-space "sandal toe"
- fifth-finger clinodactyly
- short stature
- mild to moderate cognitive disability
- hearing problems
- cataracts

---

[6] One of the mother's number 21 chromosome is on the number 14 chromosome)

Physical features of Trisomy 21 include the following, most of which can be identified in the newborn period.

Clinical Associations

Children with Down syndrome are at increased risk for **leukemia, duodenal atresia,** and **cardiac disease**, especially **AV canal (endocardial cushion defect)** which throws off the axis in the EKG reading. Boards questions might refer to it a "**NW axis**".

Children with suspected Trisomy 21 need to have an echo performed and read by a pediatric cardiologist before they leave the hospital.

Children with Down syndrome are at particular risk for **atlantoaxial instability**. If you are asked what you should be concerned about when doing a sports physical on a patient with Down syndrome who wants to participate in Special Olympics, **atlantoaxial instability is your answer**.

Diagnosis of trisomy 21 is best made by fluorescence in situ hybridization (FISH) analysis to quickly confirm the diagnosis plus a high resolution chromosome analysis to figure out the cause of the extra 21.

Trisomy 18

Be prepared to see this in an infant in the picture section. Remember the following features and you will recognize it easily.

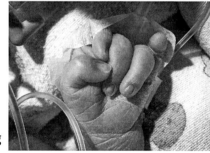

Clenched Fist

I remember the features as follows:

- ❏ I picture an **18** year old at a rock concert.
- ❏ He's dancing like he's having **seizures**.
- ❏ I then picture a **clenched fist**[7] and the **rocker bottom feet**.
- ❏ The fist has been clenched for days, resulting in **overlapping fingers** which is almost pathognomonic on Boards and **hypoplastic nails.**
- ❏ Such a person would be drinking a lot and too busy rocking back and forth to notice he is banging his head on the wall. This results in a **prominent occiput, microcephaly, microophthalmia** and **low set malformed ears.**
- ❏ He also would be too busy to go to the bathroom, resulting in the kidneys getting bent out of shape turning into **horseshoes** = Horseshoe Kidneys.

> **Second identity**
>
> You may also see Trisomy 18 called Edwards Syndrome (think **e**dward and **e**ighteen).

Not as light-hearted as the image above, these kids have heart malformations as well as severe growth and developmental delays and 95% die in the first year.

---

[7] They can also describe an overlapping of the index finger over the 3rd, 4th, or 5th digits.

Trisomy 13

It is the least common of the trisomies but is typically the most severe. Just focus on a few classic features and you will recognize this on the exam. They will likely show **punched-out scalp lesions.**

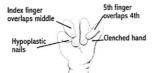

Trisomy 18
(Edward syndrome)

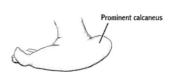

Trisomy 13 and 18

Since the #13 is considered bad luck, you can remember the features of trisomy 13 with the word "BAD LUCK".

Brain (Holoprosencephaly and Microcephaly and Mid Scalp Lesions)
Airs (Low Set Ears)
Digits (Extra Digits = Polydactyly)

Leukocytes (unique nuclear projections in the neutrophils)
Uterus (Bicornuate Uterus and Hypoplastic Ovaries)
Cleft Lip and Palate (Bilateral)
Kidneys (Cystic)

> **Trisomic Genetics**
>
> Remember that **birth of any trisomy increases the risk of having another child with other anomalies.**
>
> Therefore, genetic testing is indicated after the birth of any child with a trisomy.

> **Viable Trisomies**
>
> Trisomy 13, 18, and 21 are the only trisomies that make it to term.

Cutis aplasia is almost pathognomonic, especially on Boards.

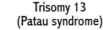

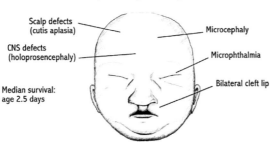

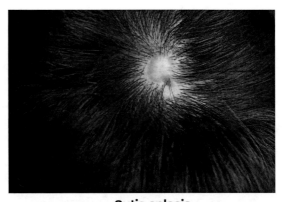

Cutis aplasia

Trisomy 13 can also present with rocker bottom feet.

Klinefelter syndrome (47 XXY)[8]

This is typically described as a teen that is **tall** with **small testes**[9] with **normal intelligence,** but 50% may have **delayed speech** and **mild learning disabilities.**

They may be described as **socially awkward**; 30% may have delayed emotional development and adults may have behavior problems.

They may also have **gynecomastia** with increased risk of breast cancer and mediastinal tumors.

You are presented with a patient who is noted to have delayed motor and language development. On physical examination, he is quite tall, with legs and arms longer than expected for his height. You also note 4 café-au-lait spots measuring between 4 and 5 mm each. His parents state that in school he is a bit of a loner. You note that he has a very calm demeanor. What would be the next most appropriate diagnostic step?

Here you are being diverted into suspecting neurofibromatosis because of the café-au-lait spots. In addition, the long arms and legs will divert you into believing this is Marfan syndrome.

The history is most consistent with Klinefelter syndrome, and the next most appropriate diagnostic step would be chromosome analysis. The café au lait spots are a true diversion, both in size and number. Six or more café-au-lait spots measuring at least 5 mm would be consistent with neurofibromatosis.

The word in German for small is *Klein.* That is a good way to remember the small testicles in "Kleinfelter" syndrome.

It can be difficult to differentiate between **Klinefelter** from **Kallman** syndrome, which is a central hypogonadotropic hypogonadism with anosmia. They are both tall, thin, and have small testes/cryptorchidism. The clue toward Klinefelter is gynecomastia. The clue toward Kallman would be normal social skills or anosmia.[10]

Treatment may include **testosterone supplementation.**

Contiguous Gene Conditions

Happens when chromosomal regions with similar (95-99%) sequences cause misalignment of homologous chromosomes, leading to either **deletions or duplications of those similar regions.** You probably have to read this twice and take a nap in between readings.

---

[8] 80% are 47, XXY. The other 20% are mosaic or variable (XXYY, XXXY, XXXYY, etc). The more extra X chromosomes, the more severe the symptoms.
[9] There is often a history of cryptorchidism.
[10] Also, females can have kallman syndrome whereas no female can have klinefelter.

Prader-Willi Syndrome

Guess which celebrity? Hint: **Slick Willy Syndrome**.

Neonatal hypotonia, failure to thrive as infant with **voracious appetite** starting at about age 2-3 and leading to **obesity, intellectual disability**, and **small hands and feet**. Additional physical features include almond-shaped eyes, thin upper lip and downturned mouth, short stature, hypogonadism. They can also have cognitive impairment and behavioral problems. A buzzword is OCD.

Much of the morbidity and mortality in kids with Prader-Willi syndrome comes as a result of complications of obesity (diabetes, sleep apnea, slipped capital femoral epiphysis).

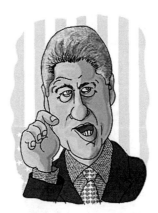

"I did not have dinner with that man ...Dr. Silverstein."

If the baby is **hypotonic and not Down's**, then order a methylation test for Prader-Willi.

First you "Pray They Will Eat" (Prader- Willi) and then you Pray They Will stop Eating.

Early diagnosis is key. Growth hormone and nutritional management is key during the first year of life.

Angelman Syndrome

Kids with Angelman syndrome are usually diagnosed between 3 and 7 years of age. All kids with this disorder will have **a distinctive facial appearance (big mouth always smiling showing off their widely spaced teeth and protruding tongue) and intellectual disability, early and profound speech impairment, ataxia and other movement disorders, and behavioral anomalies** such as frequent laughter, easy excitability, or short attention span. Many kids have **acquired microcephaly and seizures as well as spasticity and feeding problems**.

This combination of laughing and abnormal jerky movements led to Dr. Angelman calling these kids **"happy puppet children."**

Neurofibromatosis 1

Also a contiguous gene malformation and is discussed in the Dermatology chapter.

Beckwith Wiedemann Syndrome (BWS)

This is an overgrowth syndrome due to an alteration in Chromosome 11 p15.5.

2 From Dad ? or 2 From Mom?

It's extremely important to recognize, especially on Boards, that **Prader-Willi and Angelman syndromes both represent the same gene deletion: 15q11-13.**

If the dad's section is absent, you get Prader-Willi.

If the mom's section is absent, you get Angelman Syndrome.

Early in life, both present with feedings problems and developmental delays and are hard to distinguish from each other.

This is an example of **genomic imprinting**: the ability of a gene to be expressed depends upon the sex of the parent who passed on the gene.

Diagnosis is made by the **methylation test**.

Important features of Beckwith Wiedemann syndrome include:

- Hypospadias
- Omphalocele
- Macroglossia
- Macrosomia
- Hypoglycemia (Due to islet cell hyperplasia)
- Hemihypertrophy
- Renal anomalies

> **BWS children** are at risk for embryonal tumors including:
> - rhabdomyosarcoma
> - Wilm's (nephroblastoma)
> - hepatoblastoma
> - neuroblastoma

To help remember some of the features associated with Beckwith Wiedemann syndrome, think Big Width Wiedemann syndrome: picture a big man **eating M and M's** (**M**acroglossia and **M**acrosomia) with his "big tongue" and "big body," getting so large that he ends up with an eviscerated bowel covered with a membrane. Hypoglycemia is the driving force behind this ferocious appetite.

Since this is an imprinting disorder (the most common one!), diagnosis is made by methylation analysis.

Due to the increased predisposition to malignancy, these children need routine screening with AFP every 6-12 weeks from birth until 4yo and abdominal US every 3 months from birth until 8yo.

Williams Syndrome

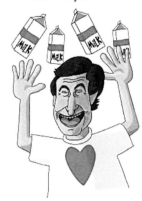

Think of the late Robin Williams as a zany character: **elfin facies** with **a prominent philtrum, big lips and mouth,** and an **upturned nose**. Kids with Williams syndrome usually have **mild intellectual disability**. They are also known to have a **"cocktail party personality"** because they are typically very friendly.

Hypercalcemia: Picture Robin Williams throwing milk containers around the room, eventually **winning the hearts** of everyone. You can think of the calcium as causing **supravalvular aortic stenosis.**[11]

Bye Bye DiGeorge Syndrome (22q11 Deletion Syndrome)[12]

DiGeorge Syndrome is no longer used in polite company. It has been switched to the descriptive **22q11 Deletion Syndrome** and **Velocardiofacial Syndrome.**

This is a contiguous gene syndrome that involves a **microdeletion** and an **autosomal dominant** inheritance pattern. It results in the spectrum of hypoplasia to asplasia of the hypothalamus and parathyroid glands.

> ## The Heart Hints
>
> Remember the buzz words between the following for easy points.
> - **Marfan:** dilation of the aortic root
> - **Noonan:** pulmonary stenosis, hypertrophic
> - **Turner:** bicuspid aortic valve > coarctation (think B before C to remember BAV is more common)
> - **Williams:** supravalvular aortic stenosis.

---

[11] It is not physiologically accurate, but it is one way of looking at it.
[12] DiGeorge syndrome is covered in greater detail in Chapter 15 Allergy and Immunology.

Conotruncal defects like Tetralogy of Fallot
Abnormal facies
Thymic aplasia and immunodeficiency
Cleft palate and Cryptorchidism
Hypoparathyroidism
22

The "eyes" have it

- **Trisomy 21**: brushfield spots
- **CHARGE** syn: coloboma
- **Williams** syn: stellate irises
- **Neurofibromatosis** Type 1: lisch nodules

In case you are asked for the most appropriate next step, the diagnosis is made by **Chromosomal Microarray (CMA).**

CHARGE Syndrome (CS)

The **CHARGE Syndrome** (previously CHARGE association but has been promoted) stands for the following:

Coloboma/cognitive deficits
Heart defects
Atresia or stenosis (choanal)
Retarded growth and development
GU abnormalities (genital hypoplasia)
Ear anomalies (hearing loss)

Double Jeopardy

Charge Syndrome is one of the most common causes of combined deafness and blindness.

You will need to recognize this on the exam.

It has been found to be an Autosomal Dominant (most are *de novo* mutations) in the CHD7 gene.

Intelligence is below normal. Think of it as since they are mentally challenged, someone else has to be in CHARGE of them.

Rubinstein-Taybi (Thumby) Syndrome

The key phrase or picture they will show is a **"broad thumb."** This is easy to remember by changing the name of the syndrome to **"Rubinstein Thumby"** syndrome. They also have **cryptorchidism.**

It is difficult to bring down an **undescended testicle** with a **broad-based thumb.**

Digit detangling

Pfeiffer syndrome: bilateral coronal craniosynostosis with significant proptosis and widely spaced eyes and wide thumbs.

Crouzon syndrome: similar head and facies to Pfeiffer, but no hand issues to differentiate it from these similar syndromes.

Apert syndrome: craniosynostosis of multiple sutures and mitten hands +/- feet.

In **Pfeiffer syndrome**, the thumbs and great toes are also short and broad; however, the eyes are prominent and widely spaced, just as they are in Crouzon syndrome. Therefore, a child who looks like a cross between Crouzon and Rubinstein-Taybi would likely have Pfeiffer syndrome.

Celebrity Dysmorphology

It is quite a challenge to remember the details of clinical syndromes and know the fine differences between them. For example, you will be expected to distinguish which syndromes are "autosomal dominant," which ones are associated with "sensorineural hearing loss," and which ones are associated with both.

When you have actually taken care of a patient with a given syndrome, it is easier to know this information cold. However, during the course of training and practice it is virtually impossible to "see" every syndrome. By associating them with well-known, popular and historical figures, you have essentially "seen the case" (See Prader-Willi above).

Fragile X Syndrome

Face elongated
Repeat CGG
Autism, ADHD
Giant genitals (macroorchidism)
IQ lower
Large hands and feet
Ears are big
X- linked dominant

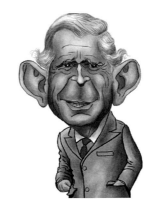

Prince Charles

> ### Disclaimer and Explanation
>
> We are not in any way trying to disparage children who suffer from any syndrome or their families, or even the celebrities. We are merely providing a memory aide for pediatricians to remember the syndromes.

Clues include: **male, mild to severe intellectual disability**, and a **positive family history of uncles** and other males who are weird.

Long narrow face, with a **prominent forehead, portruding ears, prominent jaw, difficulty with change, avoidance of touch, hyperactivity, hand biting and gaze aversion** as well as **macroorchidism**[13]—think of **Prince Charles.**

Sometimes they can go esoteric and mention the specific problem on the X chromosome that makes it "Fragile." This would be a **triplet CGG explansion**.

They might mention expansion of the CGG repeats in the FMR1 gene.

While Fragile X syndrome typically presents in boys, it *can* manifest in females. Females would not have physical features, but would be mildly intellectually affected, and may have attention or anxiety problems.

If you are asked how to evaluate a child for Fragile X, **choose DNA testing**. Technically, you are looking for the **FMR 1 gene.**

It is NOT detectable by Chromosomal microarray (CMA).

> ### Fragile X Distinctions
>
> • The most common *inherited* intellectual disability.
>
> • Overall the second most common *genetic* intellectual disability, after Down syndrome.[13]
>
> • The most common known single-gene cause of autism spectrum disorder.
>
> • The most common cause of X-linked intellectual disability.

---

[13] These classic dysmorphic features (long facies, prominent jaw, macroorchidism) become evident at the time of puberty.
[14] Remember that Down syndrome is genetic, but rarely inherited.

Not for Men only

BOTH male and female premutation carriers can have associated tremors or ataxias.

Therefore watch for a history where they note tremors in both male and female relatives.

Rett Syndrome

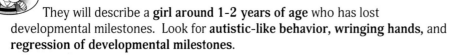

They will describe a **girl around 1-2 years of age** who has lost developmental milestones. Look for **autistic-like behavior, wringing hands,** and **regression of developmental milestones.**

These girls have **normal development at first**, but around 4 months of age their **head growth decelerates**. They then enter a period where they do not continue their development (**stagnation** - usually from age 6-18 months), followed by a loss of their milestones (**regression** - usually from 1-4 years of age). After this, there is usually no further decline. These children usually survive into adulthood (most only into their 20s), although they may not gain/regain purposeful hand use or functional speech.

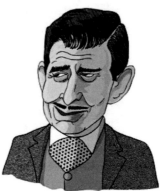

Most develop a seizure disorder. Other prime tidbits ripe for the test is that it is X-linked dominant inheritance but almost all diagnoses are de novo. **It is only seen in females because males with the diagnosis will not survive the pregnancy.**

Think of **Rhett Butler** (Clark Gable) from *Gone with the Wind*. Picture him **walking backwards**, wringing his hands, saying: "Frankly my dear, I don't give a damn, which is why I am **backing out** of the deal."

Teratogens

Fetal Alcohol Syndrome (FAS)

FAS may be diagnosed **with or without confirmed maternal alcohol exposure** if 3 criteria are present: 1. **characteristic facies** 2. **deficient brain growth** and 3. **prenatal and/ or postnatal growth retardation.**

- Facies
- Abnormal brain
- Small

Dysmorphology clues include: **flat philtrum** (that thing between your nose and your upper lip), **thin vermilion border of the upper lip, midface hypoplasia, and short palpebral fissures.**

Picture a **child drinking alcohol:**

❏ From having the bottle in his mouth so often, it forms a mark on the middle of his face (**midface hypoplasia**) and **thins out his upper lip and philtrum**.

Fetal alcohol syndrome (FAS) is the most common *preventable* cause of intellectual disability. In addition to intellectual disability, children with FAS can also have behavioral and psychiatric disorders (even in the absence of intellectual disability).

Fragile X syndrome and **Down syndrome** are the other most common *identifiable* genetic causes of intellectual disability.

But just to clarify, these two are **NOT preventable**.

Tobacco Exposure

Maternal smoking results in **low birth weight infants, higher miscarriage rates, placental abruption, placenta previa, IUGR, and prematurity**.

In addition, maternal smoking has been associated with **cleft lip/palate**.

Smoking during pregnancy is associated with **asthma, otitis media, wheezing and other sinopulmonary ailments**, independent of maternal smoking after delivery.

Maternal smoking increases the risk of **SIDS** as well.

In addition, there is some evidence that these infants also have **abnormal neurobehavior** extending into childhood that includes **deficits in mental development, language deficits, ADHD and lower IQ**.

Anticonvulsants

You will need to know the general and specific teratogenic effects of anticonvulsants, primarily valproic acid, phenytoin, and carbamazepine. Exposure to these meds is associated with an increased risk for **microcephaly, intrauterine growth retardation**, and other major malformations, such as the "**anticonvulsant face**" (**broad bridge of the nose, small anteverted nostrils, and a long upper lip**) and **fingernail hypoplasia**.

In addition, **cardiac defects, cleft lip, hypospadias** with **cryptorchidism**, and **clubfoot deformity** are associated with anticonvulsant use during pregnancy.

Valproic acid and carbamazepine both may result in neural tube defects. Change "carbamazepine" to "**Car-Bam**" and picture an auto accident resulting in "**spinal**" problems and "**facial deformities.**"

Valproic acid is mostly known for the facial deformities.

> ## Take THAT Neural Tube!
>
> Folic acid supplementation prior to conception can decrease the incidence of neural tube defects by **more than 50%**.

Phenytoin exposure can result in a pattern of defects in up to 10-15% of babies called Fetal Hydantoin Syndrome. To help remember the most distinguishing features remember **PHEN**:

- cleft **P**alate, **P**ostnatal bleeding
- microcep**H**aly,
- **AED**
- hypoplastic **N**ails

Malformations and Deformations

It is important to define the following to avoid confusion and getting a question wrong due to a technicality:

A **malformation** started out bad. A **deformation** started out well but met a roadblock and now is bad.

VACTER-L

This association has gone through a variety of incarnations. You will be asked to recognize it.

Vertebral Defects/ tethered cord
Anal Atresia
Cardiac Defects
TE Fistula
Renal Abnormalities

Limb abnormalities

At least 3 are required for diagnosis with no other explanation for the abnormalities.

It often presents with a "single umbilical artery," and growth deficiency is common. **Intelligence is normal.**

An **association** is the clustering of anomalies that cannot be explained by chance. An example would be VACTER-L association.

A **sequence** is the result of a localized abnormality early in fetal development. An example would be **Potter syndrome** (Oligohydramnios Sequence), whose effects all stem from oligohydramnios. **Pierre Robin sequence** is another example.

VACTER-L may be part of 22q11 deletion syndrome.

Craniosynostosis

Craniosynostosis is the **deformation** of the skull due to **premature fusion of one or more of the sutures**.

Craniosynostosis can be easily corrected, **but it must be recognized before five months of age,** since treatment is more successful when done prior to the period of greatest head growth. Neurological complications, such as **hydrocephalus** and **increased intracranial pressure**, are more likely to occur when two or more sutures close prematurely.

Positional plagiocephaly may be confused with craniosynostosis on exam, but head CT will reveal normal sutures. Positional plagiocephaly may look abnormal, but is **harmless** and **will improve over time** once babies do not spend so much time laying flat on their backs.

Molding helmets may be considered for moderate to severe cases not responding to more conservative therapy or at an advanced age (over 8 months) but they will probably not be the right answer for treating positional plagiocephaly on Boards.

You may be expected to distinguish between the closure of cranial sutures secondary to slow brain growth (which would result in a small, symmetrical head) and premature closure of a single cranial suture (which would present with an asymmetrically-shaped head). [15]

Cause	Resultant Head Shape
Positional plagiocephaly	Parallelogram head shape
Unilateral lamdoid synostosis	Trapezoidal head shape
Saggital synostosis	Dolichocephaly/ Scaphocephaly (long skinny egg-shaped head) #1 most common
Bilateral coronal synostosis[14]	Brachycephaly (short wide head) (Associated with syndromes like Crouzin, Pfeiffer syndrome)
Metopic synostosis	Trigonocephaly (triangle head) #3 most common
Multiple suture synostosis	Cloverleaf skull (think Apert syndrome)

Positional plagiocephaly can be difficult to differentiate from **unilateral lamboid synostosis**.

- **Lamboid synostosis** is rare and there will be ipsilateral posterior displacement of the ear and contralateral frontal bossing.
- **Positional plagiocephaly** is very common and there will be ipsilateral anterior displacement of the ear and ipsilateral frontal bossing.

These make sense when you think about the mechanics of what is happening. Look up some pics to cement it!

Sequences

Pierre Robin Sequence

These patients have **small chins** relative to their tongues, and **cleft palate** with **micrognathia**. They look like Margaret Thatcher.

Children with Pierre Robin sequence might also be described as having **posterior positioning of their tongues**.

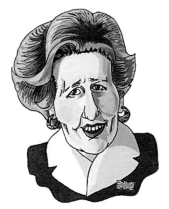

Therefore, picture **Margaret Thatcher singing like a robin**, and you will have this linked to long-term memory.

---

[15] Unilateral coronal synostosis II Anterior plagiocephaly (ipsilateral wind swept look) #2 most common.

Kids with Pierre Robin sequence have **glossoptosis** (tongue sticks out) – not because they have big tongues, but because their tongue is relatively large compared to their small chin. This is an important distinction, and not knowing it could cost you on the exam.

In addition, **extremity anomalies** are quite common, including **syndactyly, clinodactyly, hip and knee anomalies,** and spinal deformities like **kyphosis and scoliosis.** About half the kids have some sort of CNS involvement, including **language delay, seizures, and developmental delay.**

Upper airway obstruction caused by glossoptosis can lead to **cor pulmonale.**

Oligohydramnios sequence (Potter syndrome)

The "cause" here is **renal agenesis.** But the appearance of the infant is all due to **consequences of oligohydramnios.**

The 4 primary features are:

    1- Typical facies described as "pugilistic"

    2- Hypoplastic lungs

    3- Limb malformations like club feet and flattened hands

    4- Renal agenesis

They may also describe **"glove-like"** excess skin on the hands, and that the **fetal membranes are covered** by **yellowish nodules** which are collections of vernix (or the word **amnion nodosum**).

Genitourinary anomalies are an important part of the workup. Kids with Potter syndrome **ultimately die of pulmonary complications.**

Russell Silver Syndrome (Wrestle Silver Syndrome)

Features include **triangle face** (small chin) and **growth retardation.** These children are very small.

Picture a **small (growth retarded) wrestler** with a **triangle face made of silver.**

Prune Belly Syndrome

This will be obvious; **lack of abdominal muscle development** leads to the prune belly appearance. What else do you need to know? Let's go to the chalkboard.

It all starts with **bladder outlet obstruction,** which leads to **oligohydramnios.** The oligohydramnios results in **pulmonary hypoplasia** — and while we are down there, the **testes are undescended** (well, picture it as a pit of the prune that never came down).

Treacher Collins (Teacher Calling)

HOT TIP

The picture is very distinctive. One good look in the atlas and you will see it clearly. **Conductive hearing loss, a small jaw, ear abnormalities, and lower eyelid abnormalities** are part of the picture; **intellectual disability** is **not**. These structural abnormalities can be so severe that a G-tube or a tracheostomy may be required.

MNEMONIC

You can't be a teacher, or a Treacher, with abnormal intelligence.

HOT TIP

Since it is a **dominant trait**, picture a "dominating" teacher in control of a class. It occurs in several family members. They could show a family portrait in which several members have the same dysmorphic features. **One or more family members with a hearing aid could be the tip-off.**

> **DEFINITION**
>
> **Syndactyly** refers to the union of two or more fingers or toes. This typically only involves a skin connection between the two; however, it can also include fusion of bones.
>
> **DEFINITION**
>
> **Clinodactyly** is permanent deviation of one or more fingers, usually the 5th finger (pinky).

Achondroplasia

BUZZWORDS

Children (and adults) who have achondroplasia have the classic look of the "Munchkins" in the *Wizard of Oz* movie. They have **large heads** and **very short extremities**, which made for the "cute look" that the casting directors were after.

This is why it is also known as **"short-limbed dwarfism,"** especially of the proximal portion of the limb. This is called **rhizomelic shortening. They have short fingers and "trident hands".**

They also have **relative macrocephaly** and **frontal bossing.** Folks with achondroplasia have **genu varum** ("bowlegs"). Midface " retrusion" either described or illustrated would be another clue.

> ## Brand New Genes !
>
> **HOT TIP**
>
> Achondroplasia is **an autosomal dominant condition** with complete penetrance. And like all autosomal dominant conditions, it has a high rate of spontaneous mutation. This means a child can have it, even when the parents do not, which is what is seen in over 80% of cases of achondroplasia.
>
> New mutations are seen more often with advanced **paternal** age.

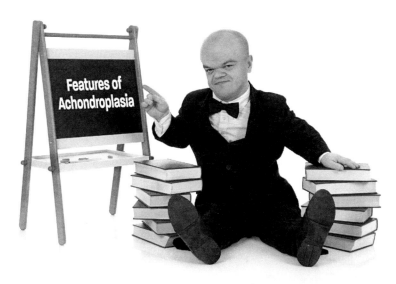

Achondroplasia

Lumbar lordosis gives them that puffed out chest appearance, and they also have small foramen magna, which can result in **nerve root compression.**

There are frequent respiratory problems – over 3/4 of kids with achondroplasia have **significant sleep apnea.** They also have increased incidence of otitis and hearing loss.

There is an increased risk of sudden death in infancy and early childhood.

Intelligence is normal.

CASE STUDY

You are presented with an infant who has the following physical findings: macrocephaly, frontal bossing, midface hypoplasia, and proximal shortening of the limbs. You astutely and correctly identify this as a child with achondroplasia. You now must either answer "What is the inheritance pattern" and/or "The most likely cause of sudden death in this infant..."

THE DIVERSION

The first diversion might be your inability to write the answer with your arm pinned behind you as you pat yourself on the back congratulating yourself for making the correct diagnosis. The inheritance pattern you will simply have to know, and the most likely cause of death can be deduced if you forget. You might be tricked into believing respiratory or cardiac failure, assuming these are associations and therefore most likely to cause sudden death. This would violate the "if-your-shoemaker-could-pick-a-choice-it-is-probably-wrong rule."

ANSWER REVEALED

The most common cause of sudden death in children with achondroplasia is cervicomedullary junction compression. The inheritance pattern is autosomal dominant.

Chapter 18

Inborn Errors of Metabolism

Inborn errors of metabolism involve the 3 substrates used for energy: protein, carbohydrates and lipids. The disorders include amino acid disorders, organic acidemias, urea cycle defects, fatty acid metabolism defects, and storage disorders. Basically, in anything metabolic you can think of, something can go wrong. Don't worry, we'll break it down for you so you don't have a breakdown.

Inborn errors of metabolism should come to mind when a previously healthy infant develops **poor feeding, hypoglycemia, lethargy, vomiting, tachypnea, irritability,** or **seizures**. In some cases, they will describe **coma, seizure,** and **apnea**.

Pay particular attention to any events they describe, no matter how inconsequential they may seem, i.e., feeding. This is often the crucial clue to getting the correct answer.

This can be presented to you on the exam in several forms. The more challenging form will be the "Best Answer" format where you need to diagnose a **classic "septic" infant that is not septic, or perhaps a repeat case of "Reye Syndrome."**

Many of these disorders are quite similar. This is another example where focusing on the "specific differences" between disorders will pay handsome dividends. **However, a logical approach to the question is something you cannot memorize.** If you use the step-by-step approach outlined below, the questions themselves will help you make the right diagnosis and get a series of questions correct.

> ## Wide Eyed Response to Infants in a Coma
>
> If you are presented with a **lethargic or comatose infant**, you need to keep the following principles in mind when answering the question.
>
> You will likely be presented with a **CBC, electrolytes, serum ammonia level, and urine organic acids**.
>
> You should **measure the anion gap** if you are presented with the corresponding lab values. Remember this is Serum Sodium - [Chloride + Bicarbonate]. Normal is 8-12 mEq/L.
>
> An **elevated anion gap** in this scenario should make you think immediately of **elevated ammonia**.

Approaching Inborn Errors of Metabolism

Given that so many **metabolic disorders present with vomiting and lethargy, distinguishing the fine differences between them can be a challenge.** Key phrases and wording are what distinguish one disorder from another. In fact, paying close attention to the fine differences between various disorders can help you score points on enough questions to push you over the top.

The Screen Door

The trend is to screen for most metabolic disorders so future generations of pediatricians will have no first-hand knowledge of or experience with them. You will still need to know them for the Boards.

Screening test are highly sensitive, rapid and inexpensive and followed up with specific testing.

The disorder must be associated with severe morbidity and mortality when untreated and early treatment must have the potential to improve outcomes.

PERIL

A positive screen must be followed up with a more specific confirmation test. That will be the correct answer.

Step 1: Afebrile

If they emphasize that the infant is afebrile, that is an indication that they are letting you know the **ID tree is the wrong tree**. Look for other clues in the question that this is not an infection such as a normal WBC and platelet count.

Step 2: Serum NH$_4$ (Ammonia)/ABG

> When approaching a question that seems to be an inborn error of metabolism, watch for the following clues in the question that will indicate which broad category is being tested.
>
> 1. **Glycogen storage disease** – will present in infancy, with recurrent hypoglycemia, ketosis, growth failure, and hepatomegaly.
>
> 2. **Organic/amino acid disorders** – These typically present in the neonatal period with lethargy, vomiting, seizures, strokes, hyperammonemia, metabolic acidosis. The clinical description might include signs of stroke and/or coma.
>
> 3. **Disorders of fatty acid metabolism** – These often present with hypoglycemia without **ketosis**.

ABG	Elevated Serum NH$_4$	Normal Serum NH$_4$[1]
Metabolic Acidosis	Propionic Acidemia Methylmalonic Acidemia Fatty acid oxidation defects	MSUD, some organic acidemias
Normal pH	Urea Cycle Defect Transient hyperammonemia	Aminoacidopathy Galactosemia[2] Non-ketotic hyperglycemia

Protein Metabolism Gone Astray

Organic Acidemias

Examples of organic acidemias include:

- Methylmalonic acidemia
- Propionic acidemia
- Isovaleric acidemia: "odor of sweaty feet"

BUZZWORDS

Organic acidemias typically present in the first 2 days after the **introduction of protein in the diet** with a "drunk-like" intoxicated picture, but the disease is life threatening. Important lab findings include **elevated serum ammonia levels (in many, but not all organic acidemias) acidosis (duh!), high anion gap,** and **ketonuria.**

---

[1] Normal serum ammonia value in a newborn is below 110mcmol/ L
[2] And just to make it more confusing — there may be an acidosis from sepsis.

In general, when they present you with an infant with a septic appearance with sepsis ruled out, a metabolic cause is likely; obtaining a **serum ammonia level** will often be the correct answer they are seeking.

Additional correct choices might include a serum **lactic acid level, serum pyruvate, total and free carnitine, and/or acetylcarnitine.**

The most important **initial step** after diagnosing one of these disorders is **hydration,** to maintain good urine output. After that **appropriate diet** is indicated.

The most important laboratory study will be measurement of **urine organic acid levels.**

Since metabolic acidosis can suppress bone marrow, **granulo-cytopenia** and **thrombocytopenia** may occur with organic acidemias. Therefore, do not dismiss the possibility of a metabolic disorder if you are given a history consistent with organic acidemia **and** a low platelet and WBC count.

Organic Acidemias

Think of organic acids as **very powerful alcoholic drinks**, because a child with this disorder will present as someone who is drunk.

Decreased appetite, falling down frequently, delayed developmental milestones, with no overt physical abnormalities or **dysmorphology** are all clues.

Of course, a **brain tumor** could present with balance problems and vomiting, but somewhere in the question will be the hint that the **symptoms have been progressively worse if it is a brain tumor.** They might also mention morning headaches and abnormal neuro exam to indicate a brain tumor.

Lipid Metabolism Gone Astray

Fatty acid oxidation defects are inherited in an **autosomal recessive** pattern.

Fatty acid oxidation is necessary to fuel hepatic ketogenesis when the intake of glucose decreases and the body needs an alternate source of fuel. Examples are Medium, Long, and Very Long Chain Acyl-CoA Dehydrogenase Deficiencies (MCAD, LCAD, VLCAD) and glutaric aciduria. **MCAD Deficiency is the most common.**

This will present in the first two years of life with **hypoglycemia** and possibly **hepatomegaly** and seizures. Watch for signs of a preceding benign illness, during which **oral intake was decreased** like viral gastroenteritis. **In between episodes, the child is fine.**

Note the **absence of reducing substances** and **ketones** in the urine as well as **normal serum amino acids** with **elevated ammonia** and **liver function tests.**

Chain Gang Tips

MCAD and VLCAD present mostly in neonates with congestive heart failure, multi system organ failure, dilated cardiomyopathy and arrhythmias Additional findings might include pericardial effusion, hypotonia and hepatomegaly.

Lab abnormalities that should tip you off to a lipid metabolism abnormality would include, hypoketotic hypoglycemia, elevated LFTs, elevated creatinine kinase, abnormal acylcarnitine profile, and increased dicarboxylic acid on urine organic acid analysis.

Definitive diagnosis is via the **plasma acylcarnitine profile** which is now included in the newborn screen.

Emergent IV 10% glucose and oral L-carnitine. Recommend future avoidance of fasting and dehydration. Low fat diet, medium chain triglyceride supplementation, frequent and regular feeding helps.

Carbohydrate Metabolism Gone Astray

Galactosemia

Infants with galactosemia will **appear normal at birth** until they are given their first meal containing **lactose**, which would include both items on the expected first menu: **formula** and/or **breast milk**. They then will present with non-specific findings, including **poor feeding** and **failure to thrive**.

ALL states test for galactosemia, but infants may develop symptoms before newborn screen (NBS) results are received. A newborn with appropriate symptoms or a positive screen should be **changed immediately to a soy-based formula** and the NBS should be repeated.

More specific findings would include:

- Abdominal distension with hepatomegaly
- Hypoglycemia
- Non-glucose reducing substances in the urine
- Lethargy and hypotonia

Watch for a history of **prolonged jaundice** and/ or infection with **gram negative organisms including** *E. coli.*

The disease is due to the deficiency of galactose-1-phosphate uridyltransferase (friends call him *GALT*). The definitive diagnosis is made **by measuring GALT in RBCs.**

Treatment is with a galactose-free diet ie. **soy formula.** Failure to treat may result in **cataracts, intellectual disability** and/or **liver disease.**

Cataracts are reversible with diet change.

Differential Diagnosis

Several glycogen storage diseases also present with hepatosplenomegaly. However, the mere mentioning of **positive reducing substances** in the urine should point you toward galactosemia.

- **Lactose Intolerance** – presents later in childhood and is much more benign
- **Maple Syrup Urine Disease** – presents with **hypoglycemia**, but also presents with **acidosis, increased tone, seizures** and as the name implies, the odor of maple syrup in the urine — yum!
- **Urea Cycle Defects** – in addition to **lethargy** and **poor feeding**, urea cycle defects present with **coma** and **hyperammonemia**.

You are presented with an icteric 4 day old newborn with lethargy and hepatomegaly. As a part of the septic workup, a lumbar puncture is done and is positive for gram negative organisms. What is the BEST additional study to obtain?

Well, well, well, what do you know — you have a newborn with a classic picture of sepsis confirmed with a positive gram stain of the CSF? Slam Dunk! The next study to perform is a culture of the CSF. You scratch your head, and say "What can be more straightforward than that?" You can continue scratching your head wondering why you got this one wrong.

While you don't want to over think every question on the exam, if something seems so obvious that even the members of the domestic engineering staff who have listened to morning report would know the answer, it cannot be that simple.

They note that the patient has hepatomegaly, and that is for a reason. You would need to realize that hepatomegaly and risk for gram-negative sepsis is the hallmark of galactosemia. However, even knowing this would not be enough — you would also need to know how galactosemia is diagnosed. It is diagnosed by measuring galactose-1-phosphate activity in RBCs, or as they can be alternatively described on the exam, erythrocytes.

When you are presented with an infant with a sepsis-like picture, with hepatomegaly and positive culture for gram-negative organisms, think of galactosemia lurking in the erythrocyte.

This must be coupled with knowing **all the associated findings of galactosemia**.

If they ask for the correct treatment, in addition to antibiotics, diet restriction would also be required.

If they ask for an associated finding, the answer might be **reducing substances in the urine**.

CASE STUDY You are presented with an infant with hypoglycemia and a variety of other symptoms such as seizures, hepatomegaly, or failure to thrive. What is the MOST helpful measurement to determine the etiology?

THE DIVERSION There may be choices there specific to the additional findings, in addition to hypoglycemia. For example, cortisol and growth hormone (if the infant is macrosomic), or they may include insulin level measurement. These are all diversionary choices.

ANSWER REVEALED The most important measurement to determine the etiology of hypoglycemia in infants would be **urine measurement of ketones and reducing substances.**

Hyperinsulinism

BUZZWORDS A typical presentation would include an **afebrile infant** presenting with **generalized seizures.** An important part of the presentation will be **persistent hypoglycemia**, remedied with an **injection of glucagon.** Additional findings could include, low beta hydroxybutyrate, low free fatty acids, and detectable insulin levels.

PERIL **Height, weight and head circumference** will all be in the upper limits of normal, typically in the 95th percentile for all parameters.

COIN FLIP Keep in mind the differential diagnosis in order to avoid picking the wrong answer on a technicality.

- **Beckwith-Wiedemann syndrome** – while this too presents with **macrosomia, watch for microcephaly rather than macrocephaly**. Additional findings include macroglossia, visceromegaly, and omphalocele
- **Adrenal Insufficiency** – also presents with **hypoglycemia**. However, in this case they will need to let you know about **ketonuria.** If they note the absence of ketones in the urine, they are ruling adrenal insufficiency out for you.
- **Galactosemia** – While this presents with hypoglycemia, it also presents with vomiting, failure to thrive, hepatomegaly, and, most importantly, non-glucose reducing substances in the urine.

HOT TIP In **Beckwith-Wiedemann syndrome,** the hypoglycemia is due to **islet cell hyperplasia.**

Glycogen Storage Diseases

Glycogen Storage Disease Type I (Von Gierke Disease)

In addition to non–specific findings such as **hypoglycemia** and a **distended abdomen,** watch for the description of a **doll–like** or **cherubic face. Consanguinity** is also a common feature in the history.

Additional features to remember are **poor growth, a large liver, seizures secondary to hypoglycemia,** and **elevated triglycerides and cholesterol.** Hypoglycemia and **lactic acidosis with fasting** is classic.

In case it comes up, this is due to a **deficiency of hepatic glucose-6-phosphatase.** This is the final step in the liver to produce glucose. Glycogen storage diseases often present **when an infant begins sleeping through the night,** which results in "**prolonged fasting.**"

Treatment is with **frequent snacks and meals, and sometimes continuous tube feedings.**

After the age of 2, **cornstarch** is often used, since it releases glucose slowly.

It is only the **continuous feeding of glucose** that is helpful. Choices that include the feeding of formula high in fructose or galactose will not be useful. Glucagon injections are not useful. They might present you with liver transplant, which might be appropriate down the road in the event of liver failure, but it will not be the appropriate initial treatment of course.

Glycogen Storage Disease Type II (Pompe Disease)

For those with the scorecard, this is a **deficiency in lysosomal breakdown of glycogen.**

They will describe this in an infant who was normal at birth by one month of age becomes **floppy, fails to thrive,** and develops **cardiomegaly and hepatomegaly** with **macroglossia.** Eventually death is due to **respiratory failure.** They also present with the odd combination of **hypotonia** and **muscles that are "hard"** on examination.

To remember this, change it to "**Pope**" disease. One of the features is "**cardiomegaly**"—and the Pope has a "big heart". He is also not afraid to speak out when necessary, so he has a large tongue = **macroglossia.**

Hypoglycemia and acidosis are not part of Pompe disease.

Protein Gone Astray

Urea Cycle Defects

Urea cycle defects present with **hyperammonemia** in the **absence of acidosis and ketosis.** In addition, look for a **symptom-free period,** followed by **hypotonia** and **coma.**

Respiratory alkalosis may be present, as well as **lactic acidosis.**

Hyperammonemia will result in symptoms consistent with **encephalopathy** (vomiting, lethargy and ultimately coma).

An example is OTC deficiency.

Treatment is to reduce the serum NH_4 by **reducing protein intake and increasing glucose intake by IV.** Dialysis might be needed on a PRN, usually acute, basis.

> ### Neonatal Hyperammonemia
>
> Neonates with **hyperammonemia, acidosis and ketosis** have **organic aciduria.** Those **without acidosis** and **ketosis** have **urea cycle defects.**

Amino Acid Metabolism Disorders

Maple Syrup Urine Disease

Besides the dead giveaway of "**maple syrup-smelling urine,**" they will describe an infant with **tachypnea,** with a **shallow breathing pattern** and **profound lethargy** (encephalopathy). They also can present with **irritability, poor feeding, hypertonicity** and **ketonuria.** The classic onset is during the **first week of life.**

To help remember which branched chain amino acids have elevated plasma levels[3] in Maple Syrup Urine Disease, think of the word **VIAL** (picture **maple syrup in a vial**):

>   Valine
>   Isoleucine
>   Alloisoleucine (never found in normal infants)
>   Leucine

The levels will be **elevated by the end of the first day of life.**

> ### Lesch-Nyhan Syndrome
>
> Lesch-Nyhan Syndrome is a disorder of uric acid metabolism and is characterized by motor dysfunction similar to cerebral palsy. Additional findings could include behavioral disturbances, cognitive impairment, and hyperuricemia.
>
>
>
> Self inflicted injuries is a hallmark of this disease.
>
>
>
> Urate: creatinine ratio > 2 (for a child < 10 years) (diagnostic).
>
> Hyperuricosuria and hyperuricemia are neither sensitive nor specific. Therefore you will need the additional signs outlined above to know you are dealing with Lesch-Nyhan syndrome.

---

[3] It is the inability to break down these amino acids that causes the disorder. More details can be found in the 30-pound biochemistry text of your choice.

Homocystinuria

Homocystinuria is actually an **error in methionine metabolism** where a cystathionine synthase deficiency results in **elevated blood homocystine and methionine levels** and **elevated urine homocystine levels**.

These patients present with **dislocated lens(es), skeletal abnormalities**, and often **cognitive deficits**. They could describe an **unpleasant odor**. They will very likely describe the patient as having **lighter-colored skin, hair, and eyes than other family members**. Thromboembolism can lead to early death. Additional features include a marfanoid habitus including, pectus excavatum, tall stature, long limbs and scoliosis.

Homocystinuria is diagnosed by confirming **homocysteine in the urine**.

Treatment involves a **diet low in methionine and protein as well as betaine, folate, Vitamin B12 supplementation**.

Both Marfan syndome and homocystinuria patients may present as tall and thin with pectus excavatum.

Marfan syndrome presents with **anterior lens displacement** and **no cognitive deficits**.

Homocystinuria presents with **posterior lens displacement** and **possible cognitive deficits**.

Nonketotic Hyperglycinemia

Yes this is spelled correctly, **hyperglycinemia**.

This will typically be described in a newborn presenting after being fed protein-containing formula for the first time.

They then become **lethargic** and eventually **comatose**. If they survive it, they often will have **spastic cerebral palsy**.

Phenylketonuria (PKU)

This is due to the deficiency of the enzyme that converts phenylalanine to tyrosine, thus **the accumulation of phenylalanine**.

Even though symptomatic PKU is not typically seen in the real world due to mandatory newborn screening, it can present on the boards. You need to be familiar with some of the important features.

PKU and Pregnancy

Any mother with PKU who is contemplating pregnancy should be treated **before conception**.

Otherwise, there is an increased risk for **miscarriage, SGA, microcephaly, cardiac defects**, and **intellectual disability**.

These patients will be **asymptomatic** for a few months (with **blond hair** and **blue eyes**). If they are not treated, they will ultimately present with **severe vomiting, irritability, eczema**, or a **musty** or **mousy odor**[4] of the urine.

It ultimately leads to **profound intellectual disability** and other neurological impairments.

Screening for PKU

It is important to note that most infants with a positive PKU screen do not necessarily have PKU. The positive screen only indicates elevated phenylalanine levels.

---

[4] I am not sure I know what exactly a mouse smells like, but if you see it described then consider PKU.

This can represent delayed enzyme maturation, hyperphenylalaninemia, or biopterin deficiency, rather than PKU.

PERIL

PKU screening is only valid after a **protein feeding**, which is why newborn screening must be done at 48-72 hours.

Treating PKU

TREATMENT

It is treated with a **low phenylalanine formula (Lofenalac®)**.

PERIL

Over-treatment is a potential problem. A child diagnosed with PKU who presents with increased **lethargy, rash, and perhaps diarrhea** is being over-treated, resulting in low phenylalanine levels.

Because phenylalanine is not synthesized in the body, overzealous treatment, especially in rapidly growing infants, can result in phenylalanine deficiency.

HOT TIP

In addition, it is important to note that **tyrosine becomes an essential amino acid in this disorder**, and its adequate intake must be ensured.

Lysosomal Storage Disorders

These involve disorders in which undigested or partially digested macromolecules accumulate in various organs. They are classified by the substance accumulated: mucopolysaccharidoses, sphingolipidoses, mucolipidoses, oligosaccharidoses, etc.

Mucopolysaccharidoses

With these, you must know the slight differences between similar disorders: **all of them present with coarse facies** (or faces for those unfamiliar with Latin). The differences start with the presence or absence of **corneal clouding** and **intellectual disability**. Modes of inheritance differ as well. Here goes:

Hurler syndrome (MPS Type I)

BUZZWORDS

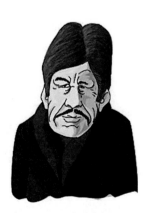

Hurler syndrome presents before age 2. In addition to **progressive facial coarsening**, they will likely note **hirsutism, hepatosplenomegaly, thick skulls, corneal clouding** and **severe intellectual disability** along with other neurologic deficits. I think of *Death Wish* star Charles Bronson.

They could also note lab findings significant for reduced **alpha-L-iduronidase** activity in WBCs.

Hunter syndrome (MPS Type II)

Coarse facial features are just the start. Watch for additional characteristics, including **organomegaly, joint contractures, and skin that appears "pebbly," especially over the upper back**.

They could also describe reduced **iduronate sulfatase enzyme** activity in WBCs.

Hunter syndrome does **NOT have corneal clouding** and it is **X-linked recessive**. Other differences from Hurler are that kids with Hunter's syndrome **are short and have skeletal abnormalities**. BOTH syndromes have **hepatosplenomegaly** and **progressive deafness**.

To remember that it is X-linked, picture a hunter with a bow and arrow. The tips of the arrows have giant X's. Their short stature and skeletal abnormalities help them get around while hunting without being seen. You can also remember that Hunter syndrome is not associated with corneal clouding because you need to "see in order to hunt."

In addition, focus on the following **H** pattern. Hunter and Hurler syndromes are associated with Hepatosplenomegaly and Hearing deficits.

Sphingolipidoses

Gaucher Disease

Gaucher disease is a lipid storage disorder that should be considered in any child presenting with **hepatosplenomegaly, bone pain, and easy bruisability**. **Short stature** is another important feature.

These symptoms are due in large part to **thrombocytopenia**. **Osteosclerosis** and **lytic lesions** on x-ray may also be present.

Picture a "Gaucho Cowboy" falling off his horse resulting in **bone pain, nose bleeds,** and lots of **bruises** to lock this association into long term memory.

Tay Sachs Disease

Tay Sachs disease is a result of a deficiency of activity in the **hexosaminidase A enzyme**, which is a lysosomal enzyme. It is inherited in an **autosomal recessive** pattern.

Lysosomal Disorders

These involve disorders in which undigested or partially digested macromolecules accumulate in various organs. They are classified by the types of substance accumulated as in: mucopolysaccharidoses, sphingolipidoses, mucolipidoses, oligosaccharidoses, etc.

Gaucher Disease

This comes in two flavors: "infantile" or "chronic juvenile."

Infantile Gaucher Disease

It is due to decreased beta glucosidase activity. This presents in a child in the first or second year of life with progressive hepatosplenomegaly and CNS deterioration.

Chronic Juvenile Gaucher Disease

This form isn't as severe and, usually, there isn't any CNS involvement. However, there is *splenomegaly* with chronic problems, including *thrombocytopenia* or *pancytopenia*.

The typical presentation of Tay Sachs is **normal development throug**[h] non-specific signs appear, including **lethargy** and **hypotonia**. Important signs specific to Tay Sachs include **exaggerated startle reflex, cherry red spot on the retina,** and **macrocephaly.**

This leads to progressive neurologic deterioration, including **blindness and seizures**, with death occurring by the age of 5.

While it is widely known to occur in **Ashkenazi Jews**, it can occur in other groups, including French Canadians. Screening is recommended even when only one parent is at risk based on ethnicity.

Niemann-Pick Disease

Like Tay-Sachs, Niemann-Pick Disease also presents with a **cherry red spot** and **CNS deterioration**, but there IS also **hepatosplenomegaly**.

Envision a "Pick Axe" attacking the liver and spleen, causing inflammation.

Mitochondrial Disorders

These are a group of disorders caused by functional abnormalities in oxidative phosphorylation, also known as the mitochondrial respiratory chain, which is the final common pathway in aerobic metabolism. I know, you're having flashbacks to biochem and had to read this sentence three times, using up 6.02×10^{23} ATP molecules in the process.

The point is aerobic means oxygen, and oxygen is very important to tissues, kind of like water to fish, and certain tissues get rapidly annoyed when deprived of oxygen. The tissues we're most concerned with here are the heart, the muscles, and the nervous system.

Accordingly, these children can present at any age and may initially affect a single organ or multiple organs; however, the main features tend to be **neurologic** and exhibit **myopathy** in most individuals. Other symptoms may include **short stature, sensorineural deafness, seizures, dementia, ophthalmoplegia, developmental delays,** and **stroke**.

Some additional general signs that could be included in this history are recurrent headache, vomiting, and evidence of stroke-like symptoms.

Prenatal screening for Specific non-NBS Conditions

Prenatal screening for many conditions is available through amniocentesis or CVS sampling.

The parents' carrier status does not need to be known. This may seem obvious, but they can present several choices that are based on the parents' carrier status. This would be nothing more than a diversion.

A family history of deaths due to metabolic disorders, ethnic background, and geographical origin are all important factors for screening disorders that are not screened routinely at birth. In this case, ethnic and racial profiling would be appropriate and helpful.

Cherry-red Spots

Besides Tay Sachs, cherry-red spots can be seen in infantile Gaucher disease, GM1 gangliosidosis, galactosalidosis, Niemann-Pick, and Sandhoff disease.

Hepatosplenomegaly is how we distinguish Tay Sachs from Niemann-Pick.

Gaucher - has more hematological and skeletal manifestations such as anemia and thrombocytopenia. In addition to hepatosplenomegaly, osteolytic lesions, fractures and short stature are additional clues you may be given for the diagnosis of Gaucher disease.

Sandhoff – Some of the important clues to know the question is about Sandhoff syndrome would include, cerebral degeneration, cortical blindness, macrocephaly and hyperacusis. Of course, hyperacusis would not be used, instead they would describe a child who is sensitive to sound. You should get in the habit of writing down a one word medical description of what is being described to jog your memory.

Diabetes mellitus can also develop in children with mitochondrial disorders. Watch for lab findings that suggest lactic acidosis in the blood as well as the CSF.

MELAS - **M**itochondrial **E**ncephalopathy with **L**actic **a**cidosis and **s**troke-like episodes.

Mitochondrial Genetics

Mitochondrial disorders can result from gene mutations or deletions in the nuclear DNA or in the mitochondrial DNA so they can be inherited in autosomal, X-linked, or maternal inheritance patterns since mitochondrial DNA is transmitted exclusively from the mother.

IEM: Putting It All Together

"But How Do I Put This All Together?" Easy, we've already done it for you. Here you go!

Class of Disorders	Age, Characteristics, Lab Findings
Glycogen Storage Disease	When **meals are more spread out**, i.e., the infant is sleeping more
Fatty Acid Oxidation Disorders	When meals are more spread out, i.e., the infant is sleeping more **Illness or stress** increase metabolic demands, leading to hypoglycemia, metabolic acidosis, and hyperammonemia **Nonketotic**
Organic Acidemias	Metabolic acidosis, increased anion gap, **hyperammonemia, hypoglycemia** Neutropenia and thrombocytopenia can be a part of the picture with organic acidemias
Urea Cycle Defects	Hyperammonemia **without acidosis, Respiratory Alkalosis**
Amino Acid Disorder	Acidosis and **hypoglycemia**
Galactosemia	Acute encephalopathy, **no metabolic acidosis, no hyperammonemia**
Non-ketotic Hyperglycinemia	Poor feeding, prolonged jaundice, and FTT when fed lactose; cataracts; positive reducing substances in urine
Mucopolysaccharidoses	Coarse facies, hepatosplenomegaly, progressive deafness. Hunter's s X-linked. Hurler's has corneal clouding and intellectual disability.
Sphingolipidoses	Late infancy or early childhood, with **slowly progressive** symptoms
Mitochondrial	Classically maternal inheritance; progressive neurologic symptoms and myopathy.

Allergy and Immunology

All In The Family

Atopic conditions present in a specific order referred to as "the atopic march":

1. **Atopic dermatitis** in infants
2. **Allergic rhinitis** in children
3. **Asthma** in children and adolescents

The most important component is a **parental history of atopy.**

However, genetics is not the only contributing factor. There are **environmental influences/exposures** (including indoor pets, cigarette smoke, respiratory infections, particularly RSV, and diet) that may increase or decrease risk.

The first step to controlling atopic dermatitis, rhinitis, and asthma is avoidance of allergens.

> **RSV wheezing**
>
> Infants with symptomatic bronchiolitis from RSV are at increased risk of wheezing in the first few years of life.

Asthma

❑ **The mortality of asthma is on the increase**, which is something that they might want you to know.

❑ Asthma is more common in boys, African American, and Hispanic children.

❑ HFAs used with spacers are just as effective as nebulizers, even in infants.

❑ **Routine pulmonary function testing** is indicated for the initial diagnosis of asthma and for ongoing management.

Vitamin D deficiency and obesity are risk factors for the development of asthma and its persistence into adulthood.

> **Spying on Spirometry**
>
> Some important points regarding spirometry that you should be aware of:
>
> Spirometry measures inspiratory and expiratory flow rate. It requires expiration for more than 6 seconds. Good luck getting a child younger than age 6 to do this.
>
> PERIL
>
> Spirometry does not measure total lung capacity or residual volume.
>
> MNEMONIC
>
> So remember, spirometry does not provide TLC or a ride home with an RV, you're on your own for that.

Asthma[1] will typically be described as a **chronic nighttime cough** which is not alleviated by over-the-counter medications. The special thing about asthma is it is characterized by airway hyperresponsiveness that is reversible with beta agonists.

A **nighttime cough** could also be associated with **sinusitis** and **gastroesophageal reflux**. However, if this is the diagnosis they are looking for, they will be obligated to provide you with additional signs and symptoms.

Classification of asthma

Classification	Clinical manifestations	Treatment and management
Intermittent	Exacerbations occur at most once a year	Short acting beta agonists when necessary only Asthma action plan
Respiratory tract infection (RTI) triggered	Infants and young children with episodic wheezing induced by respiratory tract infections Symptoms do not occur in the absence of RTI	Inhaled corticosteroids (ICS) at the start of illness Short acting beta agonist as needed
Persistent	Symptoms twice or more per week	Depends on severity as noted below
Mild	Symptoms occur twice a week	Depends on severity as noted below
Moderate	Daily symptoms	Same as mild plus Long-acting beta agonists
Severe	Daily symptoms occurring multiple times throughout the day. Extreme limitations in daily activities	Daily high dose ICS with long-acting beta agonists plus Leukotriene receptor antagonist with short acting beta agonists when necessary

Physicians tend to prescribe antibiotics for children who have a history of asthma and develop fever and cough. **Viral infections** are implicated much more commonly than are bacterial infections as triggers in children who have asthma. Bacterial infection will be incorrect on the exam.

A **typical chest XR** in asthma will show **peribronchial cuffing and hyperexpansion**. DO NOT confuse this finding or atelectasis as a sign of pneumonia.

Side effects of beta adrenergic agonists include **tremors, tachycardia, hypokalemia,** and in some cases **hyperglycemia** and **hypomagnesemia**.

---

[1] Also known as Reactive Airways Disease or hyperresponsive airway disease, which is how it is described at pulmonary wine and cheese parties to justify 3 years of fellowship training.

Levalbuterol has no hard data to support its therapeutic superiority over albuterol.

It would only be indicated in patients who have demonstrated excessive side effects such as **tachycardia, tremor,** and/or **irritability** with albuterol.

There is no role for inhaled mucolytics or chest physical therapy as part of routine care for asthma exacerbations.

> ## Controlling Persistent Asthma
>
> An **inhaled corticosteroid** is the best method because it not only **decreases bronchial inflammation,** but also **reduces bronchial hyperresponsiveness**.
>
> Patients should be instructed to rinse their mouth after use of ICS to prevent oropharyngeal candidiasis (thrush).

Regardless of the baseline asthma severity, patients can experience severe exacerbations. In general, if you are presented with a patient who is having an **acute exacerbation of asthma** which is not responding to beta adrenergic agonists, **systemic steroids** are the next step.

Steroids only inhibit the **late phase reaction of asthma**, not the early phase. On the other hand, **leukotriene inhibitors** primarily block the early phase inflammatory pathways, and are useful not only in asthma, but also in allergic rhinitis, young children with recurrent viral-URI exacerbations, and children with exercise-induced symptoms..

Hypercapnia and Asthma

A **low pCO$_2$** in the setting of acute asthma would reflect **tachypnea**.

However, an **increasing pCO$_2$** would reflect **CO$_2$ retention and fatigue and signals impending respiratory failure**.

Signs of **hypercapnia** would include **agitation, flushing, mental status change** (including **disorientation**), **headache,** or **tachycardia**.

Know that in an acute exacerbation, the child may **not be moving enough air to elicit a wheeze**. In this case, giving an albuterol nebulizer will actually make the **wheezing worse**, but it is a good sign!

Asthma Triggers

The following triggers will often be noted in the history to tip you off to a correct diagnosis of asthma:

- Weather changes
- Aspirin
- Beta Blockers
- Viral URI
- Preparing for and taking the boards (i.e. stress)
- Exercise
- Allergies
- Tobacco or other smoke

> ## Foreign Body vs. Asthma
>
> **Respiratory infection that is not clearing,** a **wheeze that is localized and fixed,** reduced breath sounds over one lung, a mediastinal shift that is seen on CXR, or a very sudden onset suggests foreign body as the cause of wheezing.
>
> If the foreign body is not removed, recurrent pneumonia, atelectasis, or bronchiectasis could result.

- Air pollution and smog
- Cold or hot air
- Strong perfumes or other irritants
- Mold

Allergies

80% of asthmatic children have positive immediate-type allergy skin tests.

Therefore, any description of allergic signs and symptoms should make you think of asthma.

Exercise Induced Asthma (EIA)

EIA is coughing and wheezing within a few minutes of initiation of vigorous **exercising**, with gradual improvement with 20-30 minutes of rest, although they can last up to 90 minutes when left untreated.

Cold, dry air is the worst; warm, moist air is the best. Therefore, figure skating on a rink in Lake Placid is the worst exercise for children at risk for EIA.

It is important to keep in mind that children with asthma should be encouraged to remain active. EIA exacerbations may be a result of poor asthma control.

If the asthma problems occur ONLY with exercise, treatment would involve the use of a short acting beta agonist (SABA) **30 minutes before exercise**.

Bad bad Asthma

Signs and symptoms of poorly controlled asthma include:

- asthma symptoms 2 or more days/ week
- nighttime awakenings > 1-2/ month
- interference with activity
- albuterol use > 2 days/ week (except for exercise induced asthma)
- FEV1 <80% of predicted
- oral steroids 2 or more times per year

Rule of 2's

- Symptoms **2** or more days a week
- Waking up at night **2** times a month
- Albuterol more than **2** times a week
- Oral Steroids more than **2** times a year

And if we stretch a bit here --> FEV1 is less than (100-80= **20**% of predicted)

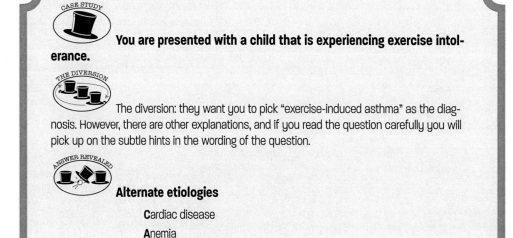

You are presented with a child that is experiencing exercise intolerance.

The diversion: they want you to pick "exercise-induced asthma" as the diagnosis. However, there are other explanations, and if you read the question carefully you will pick up on the subtle hints in the wording of the question.

Alternate etiologies

Cardiac disease

Anemia

Muscle weakness

Poor conditioning

And sometimes due to **D**epression or **D**istraction

Increased Asthma Risk

The following are important risk factors for asthma-related morbidity and mortality.

- Severe asthma
- Frequent use of beta agonists
- Previous loss of consciousness or hospitalizations
- Previous life threatening episode
- Reliance on Emergency Room for asthma care
- Poor adherence to medication
- Lack of perception of asthma symptoms
- Steroid dependence

Asthma Prognosis

Risk factors for asthma persisting into adulthood:

- ❏ Onset before age 3
- ❏ IgE Elevation
- ❏ Parental history of asthma
- ❏ A confirmed diagnosis of atopic dermatitis

The Agony of Beta Agonist risks

Patients needing repeated treatments with beta-agonists for bronchodilation are at risk for their side effects which include:

- agitation
- irritability
- tremors
- insomnia
- tachycardia
- arrhythmia
- agitation
- hypokalemia

HOT TIP

Patients with diabetes mellitus are at risk for hyperglycemia due to stimulation of hepatic glycogenolysis.

PERIL

Excessive daily use of beta agonists has been associated with increased mortality and with diminished symptom control.

Allergic Reactions

The Mt. Rushmore of Allergic Reactions: Types 1-4

The following will help you remember the four types, or just remember 1,2,3,4 and A,B,C,D:

Type 1	IgE Mediated = Anaphylactic Reaction	MNEMONIC Anaphylactic
Type 2	Mediated by Antibodies	MNEMONIC antiBody
Type 3	Immune Complex/Arthus	MNEMONIC Complex
Type 4	Delayed Hypersensitivity = Poison Ivy	MNEMONIC Delayed hypersensitivity (poison IV)

Allergy Testing

Allergy testing would be indicated any time symptoms are significant and/or require specific treatment, such as in the case of:

- Severe atopic dermatitis
- Allergic rhinitis unresponsive to routine treatment
- Food allergy
- Persistent asthma
- Insect sting allergy
- Vaccine or drug allergy
- Latex allergy

Antibiotic Allergies

The only antibiotic reaction that can be "skin/IgE tested" is **penicillin allergy**. Should they get specific, the IgE mediated reaction is one that **begins within 24 hours of exposure**. If the reaction occurs later, then it is not IgE mediated and not verifiable by skin testing.

About 10 percent of the population reports a penicillin allergy, And only 10-20% of those are true IgE-mediated allergies. The chances of a child who had a previous skin reaction to penicillin having a similar reaction to a cephalosporin are less than 10%.

Allergic Rhinitis

Allergic rhinitis presents with symptoms of **runny nose, sneezing, and itchy, swollen, or watery eyes. Eosinophils** will be present in nasal secretions.

Non-allergic rhinitis with eosinophilia syndrome (NARES), presents with allergy symptoms and eosinophils on nasal smear BUT skin tests are negative and serum IgE levels would not be elevated.

Perennial allergic rhinitis is due to exposure to indoor allergens such as dust mites, animal dander and annoying older brothers.

Treatment of allergic rhinitis

The first step in treating allergic rhinitis is to **identify and eliminate the offending allergen**, followed by medication if necessary.

Skin Testing/ False Negatives

Look in the question for any hint of anti-histamine use. This WILL interfere with the results of skin testing, but not IgE testing.)

Sometime they can be tricky, e.g., antidepressants or other medications that have antihistaminic effects will interfere with some testing. Here is another example of the importance of noting something seemingly irrelevant in the question.

What is Allergy really?

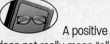
A positive "allergy test" does not really mean "allergy", it really means "sensitization".

Now, if there is an actual reaction on exposure, so you have Mast Cell Activation to go along with the Sensitization, then you actually have an Allergy.

In Vitro Allergy Testing[2]

In general, in vitro allergy testing correlates well with skin prick testing.

It is particularly helpful with children on chronic antihistamines because there is no need to stop these medications.

It is also preferred in children with extensive eczema or skin infections limiting testing area.

It would seem too obvious to mention, but it's also extremely handy in testing children who have had life-threatening allergic reactions to the suspected trigger.

Limitations of IgE testing include **higher cost** and **higher false positive rate**.

---

[2] The test formerly known as RAST testing.

Nasal steroids are the first line treatment for allergic rhinitis. However, **oral antihistamines or antihistamine-containing eye drops** may be used when indicated.

Not all noses that run are allergic rhinitis. You will be expected to distinguish conditions with similar presentations as follows:

- **Infectious rhinitis** presents in **younger children** with nasal congestion that is **worse in the winter**

- **Vasomotor rhinitis** presents with **congestion, rhinorrhea,** and **post-nasal drainage, unrelated to any specific triggering or infectious agent.** It can, however, be triggered by **emotions, pollution, cold drafts, rapid temperature changes, or changes in humidity.** This is probably where the old wives' tale regarding wearing a hat to avoid "catching cold" came from.

- **Rhinitis medicamentosa** is a rebound reaction to **adrenergic nose drops,** resulting in severe nasal congestion.

It can occasionally occur with **recreational cocaine use.** However, when due to cocaine abuse **nasal septum perforation** should also be mentioned.

Beware of the history if you are being led to believe that a child is allergic to pollen, especially if they throw in the word "hay fever" in quotes. **Seasonal (outdoor) allergic rhinitis requires repeated exposure over years, and is usually not seen before age 3.** The most likely diagnosis is **recurrent upper respiratory tract infection** in a child younger than 3 presenting with recurrent rhinorrhea.

Food Allergies

Food allergies are **most common in early childhood** and diminish with age.

The prevalence of food allergy is much higher in **children with atopic diseases** like allergic rhinitis, eczema, and asthma.

Infants with **severe eczema** and children with **persistent asthma** should be sent for food allergy testing.

Pets and Allergies

PERIL **Getting rid of a pet may not always be the answer.**

When it is the clear cause of an exacerbation of symptoms, taking steps to reduce the exposure is usually the answer. This is because of the emotional attachment children have to their pets.

At the very least, the pet should be **kept out of the child's bedroom** at all times.

Aspirin Asthma and Allergies

Aspirin may exacerbate asthma and lead to AERD (Aspirin-Exacerbated Respiratory Disease). This is usually a diagnosis for young adults.

The Aspirin triad presents as chronic nasal congestion and anosmia and consists of

1. nasal polyps
2. aspirin intolerance
3. asthma

Signs of Sinusitis

Children with allergic rhinitis are at risk for sinusitis, which is often underdiagnosed.

Watch for signs of sinusitis if you are presented with a patient with chronic allergic rhinitis. These patients are also at increased risk for otitis media.

Oral Allergy Syndrome

Oral allergy syndrome is caused when certain allergens come in contact with the oral mucosa.

BUZZWORDS This will typically be presented in a child with allergic rhinitis who complains of a tingling sensation in or around the mouth when eating a specific food, typically a **raw fruit or vegetable**.

The **most common food allergens** in the pediatric population are:

- cow milk
- eggs
- peanuts
- tree nuts
- soybeans
- wheat
- fish

Latex Fruit Syndrome

You could be asked to choose which fruits somebody with latex allergy should avoid.

The following fruits are examples of those that should be avoided:

Avocado, banana, chestnut, fig, kiwi, peach, and tomato. The typical reaction to consumption of these would be oral allergy syndrome.

Milk, egg, and **soy** allergies are often **outgrown** by 5 years of age.

Allergies to peanuts, tree nuts, and seafood typically are not outgrown.

When a 5 year old makes a **MES** it can be cleaned up: **M**ilk **E**ggs **S**oy.

IgE-mediated reactions are usually rapid in onset and **occur within minutes of ingestion** and up to two hours afterward. Food poisoning usually presents 6 or more hours after ingestion.

Peanut allergy

Peanut is the most common food cause of anaphylactic reactions. Previous recommendations were to avoid peanut introduction in the diet until childhood in an effort to avoid triggering this allergy, but recent research shows we need to do the exact opposite (i.e. early introduction).

Infants with NO history of atopic disease, should have peanuts introduced into their diet by 4-6 months.

Infants with history of SEVERE eczema or egg allergy should have skin or blood IgE testing for peanut allergy, and if the test is negative (less than 0.35 kU/L means low risk of reaction), may proceed with introduction as above. Those with IgE testing >0.35 kU/L to peanut should be advised NOT to introduce peanuts until evaluated by an allergist.

Infants with history of mild to moderate eczema should be introduced to peanuts around 6 months of age and do not require testing.

Managing Food Allergies

Positive skin prick and IgE testing have **low positive predictive value** for food allergy, ie. up to 60% of positive tests do not reflect actual symptoms on ingestion. On the other hand, negative tests virtually rule out food allergy. As a review, allergy tests are good scree**N**s, which are se**N**sitive to rule out conditions, but not s**P**ecific to diagnose them!

TREATMENT

After food allergy has been identified, the only proven therapy is **strict elimination** of the specific food. Children with anaphylactic reactions should be prescribed **autoinjectable epinephrine**.

CASE STUDY

You are presented with a toddler with moderate to severe atopic dermatitis and are asked to determine which foods could be triggering it.

THE DIVERSION

You will be tempted to go for several choices. Since you already know that milk, eggs, soy, wheat, and peanuts represent 90% of the foods that can cause atopic dermatis, eliminating these from the diet would seem to be the most logical answer. Logically illogical that is!

ANSWER REVEALED

Randomly eliminating multiple foods without evidence of a correlation will be the wrong answer. Allergy shots will be incorrect. The correct answer will be referral to an allergist, in order to specify any food allergies contributing to the atopic dermatitis.

Urgent and Emergent Allergic Reactions

Anaphylaxis

BUZZWORDS

A typical anaphylactic reaction will be categorized as **respiratory distress, urticaria,** and **general discomfort**. Children will often describe a **sense of doom**. Additional signs could include **angioedema of the lips and eyelids** and, of course, **wheezing, respiratory distress,** and/ or **cough**. Children may even vomit or have diarrhea. Anaphylaxis involves more than one organ system such as dermatologic, respiratory, cardiovascular (hypotension), GI.

PERIL

By far, the #1 cause of anaphylaxis in children is **foods**. Other causes include **insect stings, and medications**.

TREATMENT

All patients in anaphylactic shock are considered unstable. Airway is the first concern, followed by the administration of **0.01 mg/kg of epinephrine 1:1,000** (the strong stuff, NOT 1:10,000). IM (max 0.5 mg) every 15 minutes as needed. Fluids are secondary.

HOT TIP

The sooner epinephrine is given, the lower the mortality. All of the symptoms may not develop until 2 hours after ingestion. In cases where readily injectable epinephrine is available, the dosing is **0.30 mg for patients weighing 30 kg or more**, and **0.15 mg for those weighing less than 30 kg**.

HOT TIP

On the test they will likely present a patient having symptoms of anaphylaxis/shock then ask what is the best next step.

1. Airway
2. Epi
3. Oxygen as needed
4. Fluid bolus for hypoperfusion
5. Albuterol
6. Adjunctive therapies (antihistamines)

The dosing of epinephrine is easy to remember. A child weighing **30 kg** or greater gets a **0.30 mg** dose.

A second dose of injectable epinephrine may be necessary 10-20 minutes after the first injection if symptoms return. It is for this reason that patients must ALWAYS have 2 epinephrine injectors available.

Antihistamines may diminish symptoms when given to a child experiencing an anaphylactic reaction. However, this would only serve to give a false sense of security, and it will always be the wrong choice in a question on treatment of anaphylaxis. Steroids also have no role in anaphylaxis.

> ### Eosinophilia
> In addition to being associated with allergic disorders, this can be a tip-off to parasitic diseases.
>
> Envision a giant E becoming a worm (with legs if you prefer).

Acute Urticaria

This lasts less than 6 weeks and is often seen in atopic in children and young adults.

Chronic Urticaria

Urticaria, defined as hives with or without angioedema, is considered chronic if it lasts **longer than 6 weeks**.

Watch for clues in the history including new drugs, evidence of infection, history of recent travel, and any chronic medical conditions. They could describe signs of underlying conditions. Laboratory tests could include a CBC with differential, markers for inflammation (ESR or CRP), and a thyroid-stimulating hormone level.

> ### The Bigger Itchy Picture
> Chronic urticaria is most often seen in individuals over 20 years of age. No external trigger can be found in 80-90% of cases and foods are a rare cause.
>
> It can be associated with various auto-immune conditions, most specifically thyroid disease.

The most appropriate **long-term** treatment of chronic urticaria is 2nd or 3rd generation **antihistamines** such as fexofenadine (Allegra®), loratadine (Claritin®), and cetirizine (Zyrtec®).

First generation antihistamines, such as diphenhydramine and hydroxyzine, can be used for break-through exacerbations.

Steroids only necessary for severe exacerbations in the treatment of chronic urticaria. **Allergy testing has no role** in identifying a trigger for chronic urticaria.

A positive skin test for an allergen in a patient with chronic urticaria does not necessarily mean that allergen is the cause of the chronic urticaria. Remember, these are good screens, with low positive predictive value.

Mast cell mediated Reactions

Contrast Media

Contrast reactions are not IgE-mediated. They are an osmolality- hypertonicity reaction that triggers degranulation of mast cells and basophils with release of mediators, which then cause the reactions.

CASE STUDY

A 5 year old boy who has experienced a severe allergic reaction to shrimp in the past needs a CT scan with IV and oral contrast. What precautions should you take?

THE DIVERSION

You will be given several choices including pre-treatment with antihistamines and prednisone. This will be a tempting choice, since you have been given the red herring allergy to shrimp.

ANSWER REVEALED

The correct answer will be reassurance, since the risk of a reaction is negligible. The association of shellfish allergy to radiocontrast material (presumably because of the iodine content) is a myth.

MYTH

The only time **pretreatment with prednisone and diphenhydramine** would be indicated is with a documented history of an **adverse reaction to radiocontrast media**.

Red Man Syndrome: Vancomycin

With IV infusions of vancomycin, patients may develop flushing of their face/neck. Vancomycin directly stimulates mast cell degranulation releasing histamine. This can be improved by slowing the infusion rate and administering an antihistamine.

Hymenoptera Stings

The Sting of Age

BUZZWORDS

These involve stings/bites from bees, wasps, yellow jackets, hornets, and ants. Yes, we said ants! One presentation of a local reaction would be a child sustaining a sting, and the following morning local erythema has spread dramatically. However, to distinguish this reaction from cellulitis they will note that the child is **afebrile** and the swelling is **non-tender**.

Most reactions are local. If a child experiences a **localized nonsystemic reaction, even hives**, they are not at increased risk for future systemic reactions and **do not require allergy testing or desensitization**.

PERIL Hymenoptera stings may cause a **triad of systemic reactions**:

- hypotension
- wheezing
- laryngeal edema

TREATMENT Removal of the stinger as quickly as possible (within 10-20 seconds) minimizes the amount of venom delivered. It must be scraped with a credit card or fingernail and not squeezed with tweezers because that may release more venom.

HOT TIP Any child with a systemic reaction to a bee sting requires a **referral to an allergist** and needs to be prescribed **injectable epinephrine to carry at all times**.

Any child with a life threatening reaction to a bee sting requires **venom immunotherapy,**[3] which is **98% effective** in preventing future reactions.

Allergic or Not?

HOT TIP Regarding insect sting allergy, there is a 25% false negative rate for both skin testing and in vitro testing, which renders false test results marginally reliable. Therefore, if in vitro is negative, skin testing is done and vice versa. The testing must be done 4-6 weeks after the reaction to be reliable.

Allergy testing with insect bites is limited to those experiencing reactions beyond simple local inflammation. When testing is done, it should be general, not for a specific insect.

Immunodeficiencies

The Significance of Efficiency in the Deficiencies

There are a variety of immunodeficiencies you need to know for the exam. It is a well-represented topic on the exam and is worth taking the time to learn. The core information to focus on is as follows.

PERIL You will almost certainly be presented with a patient whose parents are concerned over the number of infections their child has. It is important to note that the typical child can have one "infection" a month with "reassurance" being the correct answer. This is especially the case if all they have are self-limited GI and respiratory ailments.

Most immunodeficiencies are inherited in a recessive pattern, X-linked or autosomal recessive.

HOT TIP Infants and children **not growing or gaining weight as expected** and who suffer from **recurrent severe or atypical infections**, would be a clue that they are presenting a child with a potential immunodeficiency.

Innate Immune Defects

Chronic Granulomatous Disease (CGD)

DEFINITION Chronic Granulomatous Disease is **a disorder of phagocytic function**. The defective phagocytes cannot undergo the **respiratory burst** needed to kill ingested bacteria and fungi, leading to life-threatening

---

[3] Immunotherapy is allergy shots.

infections with these pathogens. About two-thirds of CGD is X-linked, and the remainder are autosomal recessive.

Most kids present within the **first 5 years of life**. To remember which organs are most commonly involved, think of which ones are barriers to infection: skin, GI tract, lungs, liver, lymph nodes, and spleen. In addition to infection, patients often have granulomas of the skin, GI tract, and GU tract which may lead to urinary retention and bowel obstruction.

The most common infections are **deep abscesses, pneumonia, lymphadenitis, osteomyelitis,** and **systemic infections** usually with *S. aureus, B. cepacia, Serratia species* and fungi.

The diagnostic test is the **nitroblue tetrazolium (NBT) test**, which assays the phagocytic oxidase activity. Believe it or not, you may be expected to know this.

Prophylaxis is with **trimethoprim/ sulfamethoxazole** and **itraconazole.**

CGD Buzzwords:

NADPH oxidase defec.t

Diagnosed via Nitroblue tetrazolium reduction [NBT] or dihydrorhodamine [DHR].

Organisms: **B-SPACES**

Burkholderia
Staph aureus
Aspergillus
Candida
Enterobacter
Serratia

To give or not to give?

Children with Innate Immune Deficiencies MAY receive live viral vaccines, but they should NOT receive live bacterial vaccines such as oral typhoid or BCG.

Leukocyte Adhesion Deficiency (LAD)

LAD is a **defect in chemotaxis**, which is essentially a problem with the white blood cells getting where they have to go and in adhering to the endothelium.

These kids may have a **high white blood count** (20,000) and infections such as a **perirectal abscess, indolent skin infections,** and **omphalitis**. The infected areas have **no pus** and **minimal inflammation** (because of the poor chemotaxis). **Wound healing is delayed.**

LAD typically results in **recurrent infections in the skin, mucosa, and respiratory tract.**

Although not usually the presentation in real life, on the Boards, LAD may have a history of **delayed umbilical separation.**

Diagnosis is through flow cytometry.

Bone marrow and **hematopoietic stem cell transplantation** can be curative.

Chediak-Higashi Syndrome (CHS)

This should be a slam-dunk if memorized properly. Inherited in an autosomal recessive pattern. Abnormal LYST (gene).

The WBCs contain **giant inclusion bodies (lysosomal granules)** and have **abnormal chemotaxis.**

Apart from **frequent infections**, the other symptoms to keep in mind are **easy bruisability** and **oculocutaneous albinism.**

Remember: Infections in CHS mostly occur in the **lungs** and **skin**, and the most common pathogens are *Staph aureus, Strep pyogenes,* **and pneumococcus.** They may ask you this in one form or another.

"**Cadillac Hibachi:**" If you sat on a hibachi (grill) instead of a Cadillac and tried to drive, you wouldn't go far (**poor chemotaxis**) and your butt would have some serious granules (**lysosomal granules**). A Cadillac is a receding "auto," which should help you remember that CHS is **AUTOsomal recessive.** The Hibachi would burn your skin and the smoke would make you cough (infections of the skin and respiratory tract).

Think of a very fair-skinned, blonde, blue-eyed kid with frequent bad skin infections and you won't forget Chediak-Higashi.

The diagnosis is made on blood smear with **giant granules in the neutrophils.** Without bone marrow transplant, most kids die before age 10.

Humoral Immune Deficiencies

The antibody deficiencies are **the most common** immunodeficiencies.

The typical presentation is **recurrent sinopulmonary infections** with **encapsulated bacteria.** Symptoms do not appear until **4-6 months of age** due to initial protection by **maternal antibodies.**

Except for isolated IgA deficiency, these children should also **NOT receive live vaccines** because they are unlikely to be immunogenic due to the passive receipt of IvIg used for their treatment.

IgA Deficiency

Selective IgA deficiency is **the most common primary immunodeficiency.** Over 80% are asymptomatic. **Recurrent sinopulmonary infections** are the most frequent manifestations.

IgA deficiency is **NOT an indication for IVIg replacement** because commercial replacement immunoglobulins contain very little IgA.

Bruton's X-linked Agammaglobulinemia (XLA)

X-linked agammaglobulinemia (XLA) **primarily affects B cells. The T cell count is often elevated.**

The absence of B cells means that serum levels of **IgG, IgA, IgM, and IgE are very low** and that lymphoid tissue such as tonsils, adenoids, Peyer's patches, peripheral lymph nodes, as well as the spleen are **reduced in size**. The most common presentation is that of a **baby boy with recurrent infections** with **encapsulated pyogenic bacteria** such as *Strep pneumo* and *H. flu.*

Pretty simple to follow: **B** as in Bruton's. Remember it as **"BruXon's"** disease to recall that it is X-linked.

Diagnosis is made by first measuring **immunoglobulin levels**. When they are all found to be low, confirmation is made by **measuring B and T cell subsets**.

Children with XLA **require IVIG** to protect them from recurrent bacterial infections.

They are at risk for **bronchiectasis** and **chronic pulmonary insufficiency**.

> Credit to the classic mnemonic such as this for encapsulated organisms.
>
> **SHNE SKS**
>
> **S**trep pneumoniae
> **H**aemophilus **i**nfluenzae B
> **N**eisseria meningitidis
> **E** coli
>
> **S**almonella
> **K**lebsiella
> **S**trep agalactiae (group B strep)

Common Variable Immunodeficiency (CVID)

CVID is **the most common *clinically significant*[4] antibody deficiency** and is characterized by a defective antibody response. The B-lymphocytes do not differentiate into plasma cells, so there is a **deficiency of the immunoglobulin subtypes**. In addition, most patients have a **T cell defect as well**.

Patients with CVIC present with **normal CBCs**. Watch for that in the history.

Kids are susceptible to **recurrent infections** of the upper and lower **respiratory** tract and frequent **gastrointestinal** symptoms, including malabsorption and chronic diarrhea. In addition, recurrent herpes and zoster infections are common.

There is a frequent association with **autoimmune diseases** such as rheumatoid arthritis, cytopenias, or thyroid abnormalities. There is also a greatly increased risk of **lymphoma**, usually EBV-associated.

Like children with XLA, these kids **require IVIG** to protect them from recurrent bacterial infections.

X-Linked Hyper IgM Syndrome

X-linked immunodeficiency with Hyperimmunoglobulin M is caused by a **disruption of B cell differentiation**.

---

[4] IgA deficiency is actually the most common primary immunodeficiency but it is usually not clinically significant.

B cells usually produce IgM. Normally CD40 Ligand on activated helper T cells is required to signal class B cells and signals them to differentiate into other immunoglobulin [IgA, IgE, IgD, IgG] production. Hyper IgM is due to a defect in this CD40.

Classic presentation in childhood is a **male** infant 6-12 months of age with frequent **otitis** and **sinopulmonary infections**, as well as **diarrhea** although most cases are diagnosed in adults. There is also a high incidence of **opportunistic infections**.

Lab studies show **low levels of IgG, IgA, and IgE**, with **high levels of IgM**.

The hallmark of Hyper IgM Syndrome is marked **lymphoid hypertrophy** despite antibody deficiency.

Treatment is with IVIg.

Hyper IgM Syndrome would explain the **presence of *Pneumocystis carinii* in the absence of HIV infection**. It is a **T cell abnormality that prevents conversion of IgM to IgG**.

Job Syndrome = Hyper IgE

Hyper E can easily be remembered as 3 Es: Eosinophilia, Eczema, (don't forget recurrent skin infections), and elevated IgE (picture a giant E on the nose, and you will remember **recurrent sinopulmonary infections** as well).

Infections are usually with **Staph aureus**. Kids also get **chronic thrush** and **abnormal facies** as well as **multiple fractures** and other **skeletal abnormalities**.

Hyper IgE is **often mistaken for atopic dermatitis**, but in the latter there will be no skeletal abnormalities or abnormal facies like in Hyper IgE.

Boys with Wiskott-Aldrich typically have a milder rash than Hyper IgE, and have bleeding problems from the thrombocytopenia — a problem not seen in Hyper IgE.

Treatment is with **antibiotics** and **steroids**.

Transient Hypogammaglobulinemia of Infancy

Unlike XLA and CVID, there is no intrinsic B cell deficiency. Instead, decreased T-helper function leads to lower than normal amounts of IgG and IgA.

The disease usually begins to **manifest itself by age 6 months or so** (as the infant breaks down more and more of the mother's immunoglobulins). Kids tend to **outgrow it by 3-6 years of age**.

Laboratory exam shows a **severely low IgG level**. IgA may also be low, but IgM is usually normal.

Cellular Immune Deficiencies

Defects in T-lymphocyte function present with infections due to **opportunistic organisms**, such as Candida, CMV, and *Pneumocystis jiroveci*.

A **low lymphocyte count** would correlate with T cell dysfunction, since the majority of circulating lymphocytes are T Cells. In general, **live vaccines should be avoided** in this scenario.

Ataxia Telangiectasia (AT)

If they describe the following combination - **ataxia** with **discoloration of the conjunctivae**, as well as **frequent sinus infections** and **developmental regression** - unwrap your gift.

This is an **autosomal recessive** condition.

AT is discussed in more detail in the Neurology chapter.

22q11 Deletion Syndrome (previously known as DiGeorge syndrome)

This is a group of disorders caused by deletions on the long arm of chromosome 22. It is also known as "velocardiofacial syndrome".

Known by the mnemonic **CATCH-22**:

       Conotruncal cardiac anomalies and VSD

       Abnormal facies

       Thymic aplasia and hypoplasia

       Cleft palate

       Hypoparathyroidism

       22 (Chromosome)

This is now known to be a contiguous gene sequence microdeletion (usually a *de novo* mutation) inherited in an autosomal dominant pattern. It is diagnosed by chromosomal microarray (CMA).

The syndrome may be characterized by **neonatal tetany, congenital heart disease**, and **abnormal T cell function**. In the history, they may describe **dysmorphic facies** (low set ears), **loud murmur**, and **tetany** (secondary to hypocalcemia).

Innate and Adaptive Immunity

These are the two components of the immune system:

The **innate system** responds without requiring previous exposure to the trigger. This includes leukocytes, phagocytes, and the complement system.

The **adaptive system** responds to a previous exposure to produce antigen-specific antibodies. The adaptive system is composed of the **cellular and humoral immune systems**.

There is **no parathyroid** and a **small or absent thymus** (due to poor development of the pharyngeal pouches).

Infection may be the major presenting problem - these kids can **present like SCID**, depending on the degree of thymic hypoplasia. In addition, parathyroid deficiency can lead to **diarrhea** and **hypocalcemia**, which leads to tetany.

20% have intellectual disability. Learning disabilities and psychiatric conditions such as schizophrenia are also seen more frequently.

Treatment is aimed at the underlying problems (hypocalcemia, infection, cardiac defects). In general, the prognosis is poor, and children may die from sepsis. The **best therapeutic approach (for the complete syndrome)** would be **thymic transplantation**.

Severe Combined Immunodeficiency (SCID)[5]

SCID is caused by a **complete absence of lymphocyte (both B and T cell) function**.

Infants usually present in the **first 3 months of life** with a history of **failure to thrive, chronic diarrhea**, and **recurrent opportunistic infections including thrush**. Other than these findings, the physical exam may be normal.

Most kids have a **low white count**, so a **CBC is the best screening test**. But a normal lymphocyte count does not rule out SCID.

No matter what the white count is, there will be a **complete absence of T cell function**.

Treatment is **initially supportive**, with care aimed at the underlying infections. **Bone marrow transplant** is essential and curative. Left untreated, children with SCID will die within two years of birth.

The **Bubble Boy** had a form of this – **ADA deficiency** (adenosine deaminase, if you must know), which results in dysfunctional B and T Cells.[6]

For fans of *Seinfeld*, the Bubble Boy made an appearance, and a catch phrase from the show was "yada, yada, yada" = easy to remember **ADA**. Just don't get carried away and yada yada yada the whole exam.

Wiskott–Aldrich Syndrome (WAS)

WAS is an **X-linked** immunodeficiency featuring a triad of **eczema, thrombocytopenia**, and **cellular immunodeficiency**.

The typical presentation is a **male** infant with **eczema, recurrent sinopulmonary infections**, and **unusual bleeding** (bloody diarrhea, bruising, and/or bleeding from circumcision).

---

[5] All US states now test for SCID via newborn screen.
[6] It can also be associated with abnormality of HLA antigen expression, and abnormal assembly of the cytokine receptors. However, this is way too boring for the main text of this book and even for those who write Board questions, so stop reading this stuff and get back to the material that actually matters.

- WBC problems
- Atopic problems
- Small and few platelets

Workup will show **a low platelet count** with **small platelets**[7] as opposed to idiopathic thrombocytopenic purpura which has a low platelet count with large platelets.

The initial infections usually are **sinopulmonary** involving **encapsulated bacteria**. Eventually, infections are with **opportunistic infections** including herperviruses and *P jirovenci*.

Treatment involves management of bleeding and infections. Bone marrow or stem cell transplantation can be curative.

These boys also have an extremely high rate on **lymphoma**, and this is actually the **most common cause of death**.

Complement Deficiency

All of the described components of the complement pathway are associated with clinically significant deficiencies.

Deficiencies affecting **C1-C4** present with **recurrent sinopulmonary infections** due to **encapsulated bacteria**.

Deficiencies affecting the **terminal components C5-C9** of the complement cascade are associated with **recurrent *Neisseria* infections** and an **increased risk of meningitis**.

Most complement deficiencies are inherited as **autosomal recessive**.

Complement conditions are **screened by checking a CH50 assay**. There is **no therapy** for complement disorders.

These children may receive ALL vaccines.

---

[7] The only time looking at the MPV is of use- to see small platelets in Wiskott-Aldrich.

Testing the Immune System

The following table summarizes which lab tests are used to measure the efficacy of a given component of the immune system.

Test	Component of Immune System
NBT (Nitroblue Tetrazolium)	Tests neutrophil activity (not number). Normal turns blue, abnormal stays colorless. **Chronic granulomatous disease** reflects this deficiency.
CH50	Tests the **complement system.** You order this if they describe **repeated serious bacterial infections.**
TB/Candida Skin Test	Tests for cell-mediated immunity associated with T-cell defects such as AIDS.
Immunoglobulin Levels	Tests the "**humoral system**," whose defects usually manifest as recurrent "less serious" infections (therefore, more "humorous," humoral, get it?) It is rarely seen before 6 months of age (because of the presence of Mom's antibodies). BUZZWORDS Look for the words "healthy until 6 months" in the question.
Flow cytometry	Test to diagnose Leukocyte Adhesion Deficiency.
Blood Smear	Giant granules are seen in the neutrophils of Chediak-Higashi.
Specific Antibody Tests	IgG levels may be normal. If a humoral defect is still suspected, check for subclasses from vaccination (e.g., tetanus, rubella, pneumococcus, etc.)
Complete Blood Count	Checks lymphocyte count in cellular deficiencies associated with opportunistic infections. LAD may have WBC over 20,000.

Chapter 20

You Give Me Fever: Infectious Diseases

Bacterial Infections

Bug Preview

Many bacterial infections reveal themselves by their choice of patient. These should automatically jump into your "Aha!" brain on the Boards.

Age	Etiology of Septicemia
Neonates (<1 month)	Group B strep, *E. coli, Streptococcus pneumoniae* (pneumococcus), and *Staph aureus*
Infants (1-12 months)	Group B strep, *E. coli, Streptococcus pneumoniae* (pneumococcus), *Staph aureus*, and *salmonella*
Immunocompromised patients	Gram-negative bacilli *(Pseudomonas, E. coli*, and *Klebsiella)* and *Staph*
Asplenic patients[1]	All encapsulated organisms (*H. flu, N. meningitidis*, and *Streptococcus pneumoniae*)

Meningitis

You need to be aware of causes of meningitis according to age as follows:

Age	Cause
Neonatal	-Usually **bacterial** -Sometimes **enteroviral** infection, especially in the spring or summer -Most common bacteria are **Group B strep**, ***Listeria monocytogenes,*** and ***E. coli.***
Young Children	*Streptococcus pneumoniae, Neisseria meningitidis, enteroviruses, Borrelia burgdorferi, Rickettsia rickettsii*

---

[1] They will simply note a condition where functional asplenia is common, ie. sickle cell disease, without coming right out and telling you that asplenia is a factor.

Complications of meningitis

Neurological sequelae include **seizures** as well as **focal deficits** (including aphasia, visual field deficits, and hemiparesis).

Because of the risk of SIADH, urine output and serum electrolytes and osmolality need to be monitored closely.

If there are **focal signs**, a **CT** must be obtained **before** doing an LP.

Chlamydophilia and Chlamydia (Clam Eyelid-a)

There are 3 species of *Chlamydia* that are pathological to humans: *Chlamydia trachomatis*, *Chlamydophilia pneumoniae*, and *Chlamydophilia psittaci*.

Gynecological and Peripartum Disease

Chlamydia trachomatis is the most common reportable STD in the US. Besides sexual transmission, transmission occurs from mothers to infants, mostly via vaginal birth.

It can also be transmitted with C-section delivery even with intact membranes.

If they describe a newborn (first 2 months of life) with an **afebrile "staccato cough"** and **tachypnea** with or without eye discharge, think of chlamydia trachomatis. **"Intracytoplasmic inclusion bodies"** in the scrapings is another phrase to look out for.

Definitive diagnosis of *Chlamydia trachomatis* is by **PCR**.

Chlamydia conjunctivitis is treated with **oral erythromycin,** azithromycin or sulfonamides if erythromycin is not tolerated. **Topical treatment will be the wrong choice.**

Picture "clams" instead of eyes with discharge, coughing. **Cold clams have no fever.** If you put the eye drops in there, **they gobble it up and the rest of the body gets none** (therefore, systemic antibiotics are needed). Lab findings could also include Eosinophilia. Treatment is with Erythromycin. Both begin with an **E.**

Developing Nations

With any child from a developing country, look for either something that **U.S. kids are immunized against**, a **chronic condition** that was not diagnosed previously, or **infectious diseases that are more common in the "developing world."**

TB, HIV, typhoid fever, invasive *H. flu*, and *sickle cell disease* would be examples of diseases they might describe in children from developing countries.

Macrolides in newborns

Most macrolides have been linked to infantile hypertrophic pyloric stenosis in newborns; the greatest risk is associated with erythromycin use in infants in their first 6 weeks of life.

Azithromycin is thought to have less association with infantile hypertrophic pyloric stenosis, and with once daily dosing, is becoming the preferred drug for Chlamydial infections.

The Eyes Have It

Although silver nitrate prophylaxis is effective at preventing GC conjunctivitis, it does not protect against Chlamydia conjunctivitis.

Therefore, 0.5% erythromycin ointment is the preferred prophylaxis immediately after birth.

Erythromycin → Eye ppx for GC

Pneumonia in Adolescents Too

They could very well throw you an adolescent with a **low-grade fever and infiltrates**. Mycoplasma won't be one of the choices. In that case, *C. pneumoniae* will be the answer.

It is diagnosed with **immunofluorescent antibodies**. Picture "glow-in-the-dark clams".

Chlamydophilia pneumonia is either treated with **azithromycin** for 5 days or **erythromycin** for 14 days.

Rickettsial Diseases

Rocky Mountain Spotted Fever

Rocky Mountain Spotted Fever (RMSF) is **the most common fatal tick-borne disease** in the US.

Rickettsia rickettsii is the bacteria which causes RMSF. The peak times for infection are **spring and summer**. The incubation period is 3-12 days.

If they present symptoms during the winter, it is unlikely to be RMSF. Despite its name, the disease only rarely occurs in the Rocky Mountain states (less than 2% of all cases).

The trick with ticks... and rashes

The question can include clues about the direction that rashes develop which is often a dead giveaway regarding the diagnosis and answer

- **RMSF** rash on wRists then spreads centrally
- **Parvo** begins with slapped cheeks then lacy rash on trunk and extremities
- **Varicella** rash begins on trunk then spreads peripherally

---

Rocky Mountain Spotted Fever

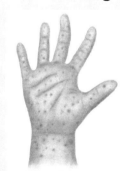

The illustration would be consistent with the physical findings of early rocky mountain spotted fever.

The rash is an erythematous papulrar rash on the palms. It can also start on the soles of the feet and the wrists. The rash typically spreads to the trunk within hours.

Rocky mountain spotted fever can present without the typical rash. However this is unlikely to occur on the boards.

If You Delay You Pay

Paired serologic testing (via indirect immunofluorescent antibody assay) is done on presentation and 2-4 weeks later. The diagnosis is based on a 4-fold increase in titers.

Treatment is indicated even if the initial titers are negative. In fact, on the exam, we can almost guarentee the initial titers will be negative without mention of the repeat titers. That would be too easy a question !

The rash is **"mac pap"** or a **"purpuric macular rash,"** which becomes **petechial**. The rash **starts on the wrists and ankles, palms and soles**, 2-4 days after the onset of fever and spreads centrally. They will always describe a **headache**. They may also describe **myalgias**.

Around one quarter of affected individuals will have CNS symptoms, mainly **confusion** and **lethargy**.

Think of a **Rocky Mountain climber** who develops a rash on his **hands and feet** from climbing the Rocky Mountains. His hands come in contact with tiny microscopic stones, which form tiny **red dots (petechiae)**.

In about 20% of cases, RMSF will present without a rash. In this case, watch for **hyponatremia** along with **depression of one or all three cells lines of the CBC** as your clues to the diagnosis. Can also have elevation of AST and ALT.

CASE STUDY

You may be presented with a patient with the classic signs of Rocky Mountain Spotted Fever (RMSF), with a trip to Long Island thrown in to throw off those expecting to see a trip to the Rocky Mountains mentioned.[2] Sometimes you will read through the entire one page vignette written in 0.5 Helvetica font and the last sentence tells you the diagnosis. You may then be asked several questions:

- **What is the most important immediate step?**
- **What is the treatment?**

THE DIVERSION

Among the choices will be *direct immunofluorescence* of a skin biopsy. After all, isn't documentation of a diagnosis important before treatment? Among the choices of treatment will be *doxycycline*, which everyone knows can't be used in a child younger than 8, so you go ahead and cross out this diversionary answer.

ANSWER REVEALED

Well this is a disease that has 2 exceptions to these rules. During the acute phase, the only reliable test is direct immunofluorescence of a skin biopsy. This test is not very sensitive, and patients should receive treatment whenever the disease is suspected. In other words, "treat first and ask questions later." ***Waiting for test result is never going to be the correct answer when Rocky Mountain Spotted Fever is suspected***. Despite treatment, the mortality rate is still around 4%. Quick diagnosis based on acute clinical assessment is key.

Chloramphenicol used to be the treatment of choice; however, the current preferred treatment is **doxycycline**, even in a child younger than 8, as the risk of teeth staining from a single course is actually quite low.

Treatment should be continued until there is clinical improvement and for at least 3 days after fever resolution.

Ehrlichiosis

Human ehrlichiosis can be clinically indistinguishable from Rocky Mountain Spotted Fever. Symptoms may include **fever, headache,** and **myalgias**.

---

[2] A trip to the Rocky Mountains would never be included.

While both Rocky Mountain Spotted Fever and erlichiosis can present with **thrombocytopenia** and **hyponatremia**, human ehrlichiosis is more likely to present with **leukopenia** and **elevated liver function tests**.

Haemophilus Influenzae Type B (Hib)

The advent of the Hib vaccine has dramatically decreased the amount of *H. flu*, type B meningitis and invasive disease.

Therefore, *Haemophilus influenzae (H. flu)* is another example of a disease that is seen less and less frequently in clinical practice, but remains a popular Boards topic. It is also another blow against the theory that "just reviewing the cases you have seen in residency will mean that you pass the Boards."

H. Flu type B causes **neonatal sepsis, childhood meningitis, periorbital cellulitis, pyogenic arthritis,** and **epiglottitis**. The mortality and morbidity rates from these infections are high.

A typical presentation is in a child coming from *(fill in the developing country) or in a child whose parents are against immunizations.* They may describe a **gram-negative pleomorphic organism, or gram-negative cocci in pairs,** on gram stain.

Remember the other gram-negative cocci in pairs would likely be *N. meningitidis*.

Watching and waiting are **not** appropriate, because it is an aggressive organism. **Ceftriaxone or cefotaxime** are the treatments of choice. Alternatives include meropenem or chloramphenicol.

STEROIDS, when given concurrently for *H. flu* meningitis can decrease the risk of hearing loss. Steroids may also be considered for pneumococcal meningitis.

The vaccine does **not** provide protection from **non-typeable** *H. flu*, which is a cause of otitis media (and conjunctivitis-otitis) and pneumonia.

> **Beware the Eye and Ear**
>
> The conjunctivitis-otitis combination is typically caused by *H. influenzae* and it requires oral amoxicillin-clavulanic acid.
>
> Amoxicillin or topical ophthalmic antibiotic alone or in combination would be the incorrect answer.

Along with *Strep pneumo* and *Neisseria meningitidis, H. flu* is an **encapsulated organism**. Remember these three when thinking about **splenectomized patients**.

Chemoprophylaxis following *Hib* exposure

Household Contacts

In households with a contact **younger than 12 months of age** who has **not received the primary series of Hib vaccine**, all household members should receive **rifampin prophylaxis**.

If there is at least 1 household contact **younger than 4 who is incompletely immunized**, then **rifampin prophylaxis** would be indicated for all household contacts, regardless of age.

If there is one **immunocompromised child** in the household, even if the child is older than 4 and fully immunized, then all members of the household need to be given **rifampin prophylaxis** because of the possibility that immunization may not have been effective.

Chemoprophylaxis is **not recommended** for occupants of households where all members are immunocompetent and have been fully immunized.

If the index case has non-typeable *H. flu,* then it is a trick and nobody needs rifampin.

Childcare and Preschool exposure

If there are **2 or more cases** of invasive *Hib* infection occurring **within 60 days** and **unimmunized** or **incompletely immunized** children attend the child care facility or preschool, then **rifampin prophylaxis** is indicated for ALL attendees and child care providers.

Prophylaxis for nursery school or childcare children older than 2 who have only been exposed to one index case is to be decided on a case-by-case basis.

> **Post-exposure immunization**
>
> Besides chemoprophylaxis, unimmunized or incompletely immunized children should receive the **Hib vaccine** and proceed the with **regular vaccine series**.

Bordetella Pertussis

Pertussis has three phases:

Catarrhal	Paroxysmal	Convalescent
1-2 weeks	4 weeks	1-2 *months* or "100 day cough"
Typical cold-like symptoms	Paroxysms of coughing, sometimes inspiratory whooping, post-tussive emesis, cyanosis, or apnea (in infants)	Waning symptoms over several weeks
Antibiotics given here may improve symptoms	Antibiotics at this stage will decrease communicability but will be unlikely to improve symptoms	

One week prior to the catarrhal stage is an asymptomatic incubation period.

Pertussis presents as indistinguishable from the common cold in the catarrhal stage, but progresses to **paroxysms of coughing**, sometimes with **inspiratory whooping, perioral cyanosis,** and possibly **posttussive emesis.** Typically the patient is **afebrile.**

If you see a **WBC count of 20-40K** with increased **lymphocytes,** think of pertussis. Again, they will imply **lack of immunization**; for example, parents who are against immunization, recent immigrants, etc.

In **infants**, the presentation can be atypical, with a very short catarrhal stage. Watch for a description of an infant who is having trouble sleeping with resultant fatigue, and having trouble feeding from the persistent cough, yet well appearing between the paroxysms or cough. Infants younger than 6 months of age are at the greatest risk for complications including apnea and respiratory failure.

The typical duration of pertussis can last **up to 10 weeks**.

It might help if you remember that pertussis in the olden days was known as "the 100 day cough".

Neither infection nor immunization provides lifelong immunity. Many **adults with protracted "colds" with cough** may actually have pertussis, and pass it on to an unimmunized neonate. Look for this in the history. In fact, pertussis vaccine booster is now recommended for all pregnant women, all teenagers and all adult household contacts of newborn infants.

> ## Immunize Anyway
>
> In the past, if an infant had bona-fide documented pertussis, he or she did not need to be immunized. However, this is not the case anymore. The duration of immunity following clinical disease is unknown. The correct answer now is that such children should go through the full series.

Pertussis is transmitted **via close contact or via aerosolized droplets**. Therefore droplet precautions are indicated for all hospitalized patients with pertussis until 5 days after treatment started or 21 days of cough onset.

PCR testing is now the new gold standard for diagnosis, because it is faster and more sensitive than culture.

Treatment

Erythromycin estolate, clarithromycin, and **azithromycin** during the *catarrhal stage* would improve the cough (of course at that point the cough is mild).

Supportive care is the mainstay of treatment since the diagnosis is usually made during the paroxysmal stage.

If given **during the paroxysmal stage** (the actual whoop and cough stage), **antibiotic decreases the period of communicability, but does NOT shorten the coughing stage.**

Post-Exposure Prophylaxis

Asymptomatic close contacts (face-to-face contact within 3 feet for over one hour), regardless of immunization status, need to be **treated prophylactically with erythromycin, azithromycin, or clarithromycin** in order to **prevent the spread.**

Salmonella

Chickens and humans are the carriers. *Salmonella* can be contracted from foods such as **chicken** or **eggs**, **red meat**, **unpasteurized milk and ice cream**, contaminated unwashed **raw fruits and vegetables**, contaminated **medical instruments**, or pets such as **turtles**, **snakes** and **hedgehogs**.

BUZZWORDS

If they describe a group on a **picnic** in the **summer**,[3] and then **1-2 days later** several attendees present with **watery loose stools** with **vomiting, abdominal cramps,** and **fever**, think of *Salmonella*. Diagnosis is made from **stool culture**.

Treating Salmonella

CASE STUDY

You are presented with an otherwise healthy patient with a classic history for *Salmonella* diarrhea, including the picnic and undercooked chicken salad made with mayonnaise that sat out in the sun for 8 hours. What is the oorrcot treatment?

THE DIVERSION

You will be provided with a smorgasbord of antibiotic delights, all there for your culinary and diversionary pleasure.

ANSWER REVEALED

Pick any of these other than supportive care and you have taken a step to studying for the boards in the hot sun next summer right next to the baking mayonnaise.

HOT TIP

Remember, treatment for *uncomplicated (non-invasive) Salmonella* gastroenteritis is not necessary. In fact, it may lead to the carrier state.

TREATMENT

Treatment is indicated in **infants younger than 3 months** of age and anyone else at risk for invasive disease. This list would include those with **hemoglobinopathies malignancies, severe colitis,** or anyone who is **immunocompromised** (asplenia, HIV).

Ceftriaxone, azithromycin and the quinolones are appropriate initial treatment choices pending culture and sensitivity confirmation.

Typhoid Fever

BUZZWORDS

You could be presented with a patient infected with the Typhi serotype of *Salmonella* who has general **systemic signs**, including **headache, abdominal pain, malaise, and high fever**.

Additional signs would include **hepatospleno-megaly**, as well as **"red" or "rose" spots**, and **"fever pulse dissociation"** where pulse does not increase with fever as expected.

HOT TIP

A classic history is a patient who has just emmigrated or returned from a visit to another country such as India.

TREATMENT

Treatment is the same as above: cefotaxime and cefriaxone.

---

[3] Likely eaten: chicken salad, egg salad, fruit and veggies that sat in the sun too long.

Shigella (Shake-ella)

The initial presentation is of **watery diarrhea** and **fever**. The characteristic **bloody diarrhea appears after the fever subsides**. There is also an increased number of **bands on the CBC**, regardless of the actual white blood cell count.

If they describe a child with **bloody diarrhea who is also having a seizure**, then the diagnosis is *Shigella*. They might describe the seizure without mentioning the diarrhea, but they will provide some "hint" somewhere that it is Shigella. That hint might be WBCs or RBCs in the stool with a left shift on CBC.

"**Shake – ella**". Get it? "Shake" as in tonic clonic seizure.

Oral rehydration is the primary treatment.

In the US, most Shigella are NOT toxin-producing, so treatment is not indicated, but on the Boards, toxin-producing Shigella are still quite common. Treating Shiga-toxin producing infections can make things worse by releasing toxin upon death of bacteria. Therefore treatment is recommended only for those with **severe disease, dysentery,** or those who are **immunosuppressed**.

Drug of choice depends on regional susceptibility and include **ceftriaxone**, and **azithromycin** in children, and ciprofloxacin if the question involves a non-pregnant patient over 18.

Campylobacter can present with a picture similar to *Shigella*. It can cause "pseudoappendicitis" and may be linked to Guillain-Barre syndrome.

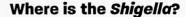

Where is the *Shigella*?

Watch for a history of water exposure, as in pools, hot tubs, lakes and oceans, as even swallowing a small amount of water with fewer than 10 organisms can cause illness.

These hearty bacteria can survive 6 months in water and one month in food! The onset of illness is just a few days after ingestion.

Shigella sonnei is a common cause of gastroenteritis in daycare centers and spread through fecal-oral contact.

Pseudomonas

Pseudomonas may cause **osteomyelitis/osteochondritis** as a result of **puncture wounds**. Often, they will describe it **after a nail goes through a shoe**.[4]

Pseudomonas is also the cause of **otitis externa** (swimmer's ear) and infections from **mechanical ventilators**. Water is the common denominator.

Pseudomonas aeruginosa is a major cause of **sepsis** and **pneumonia** and has a very high mortality rate. *Burkholderia cepacia* (formerly *Pseudomonas*) is a major cause of pneumonia and death in kids with **cystic fibrosis**.

Cancer patients, especially those experiencing **neutropenia**, are at risk for *pseudomonas* infections.

---

[4] The most likely skin infections at all times are caused by *Staph* and *Strep*. However, when the lesion involves soil and water, also consider *Pseudomonas*.

Piperacillin/tazobactam and **gentamicin** are effective against *pseudomonas* infection.

Carbapenems (**imipenem** and **meropenem**) and **ceftazidime** can be used for pulmonary infection.

Ciprofloxacin and **levofloxacin** are the only quinolones that are effective against *pseudomonas*.

Remember ertapenem does not work against *pseudomonas*.

Ceftaz is the "Tazmanian Devil" of cephalosporins and can treat *pseudomonas*.

> ## Pseudomonas/ Leukemia and Cystic Fibrosis
>
> Here is another example where you need to know two diseases that have something in common. **CF** and **malignancy** patients are both at risk for **Pseudomonas** infection.

Brucellosis

This is often transmitted via **unpasteurized milk** and **dairy products such as cheese**. While the history and physical findings are generally nonspecific, i.e., patients have **fever and malaise**, they will always note **exposure to cattle, sheep or goats** within the preceding 2 months. This is because Brucellosis is really **a zoonotic disease**. Humans are accidental hosts.

Picture a COW going BRUUUUUCE instead of MOOOOO.

Treatment is with **T**etracycline or **T**rimethoprim/sulfamethoxazole (depending upon age).

> ## FUUUUUUUUO
>
> Remember to consider Brucellosis in children with fever of unknown origin (FUO).

Think of a cow being milked. Milk is delivered through the cow's **teat** (yes that's how it is spelled by farmers). Cow Teat ➜ T = Teat ➜ T = Treatment ➜ T = Tetracycline[5] ➜ T = Trimethoprim/ sulfamethoxazole.

Clostridioides (formerly *Clostridium*) *difficile*

C. difficile most commonly presents as **pseudomembranous colitis**.

This is a severe form of diarrhea that develops after a course of **clindamycin OR ANY antibiotic including penicillins or cephalosporins**.

In the clinical description they will describe **bloody mucous diarrhea** and they might mention **a recent antibiotic course**.

> ## *C. diff* Diagnosis
>
> Isolation of *C. diff* from stool is not useful because colonization does not necessarily indicate causation.
>
> This is particularly true in infants who approach 30% *C. diff* colonization.
>
> To diagnose *C. diff* disease, you must find *C. diff* toxin using enzyme immunoassay.

---

[5] More specifically, doxycycline.

The diarrhea does not have to be grossly bloody – they may mention that the stool was "heme positive" or "guaiac positive."

Infection control measures include meticulous hand washing, especially with diaper changes, disinfecting fomites (things that are contaminated with the pathogen that can transmit the disease), and limiting use of antimicrobials in general.

In this case, using plain old **soap-and-water is much better** than alcohol-based hand sanitizers, because **alcohol does not kill** *C. diff* **spores from contaminated hands!**

Children with *C. diff* **must be excluded from child care settings until the diarrhea is resolved.**

Treatment is **with oral metronidazole (Flagyl®).** Vancomycin PO (NOT IV) would be the alternative drug in patients who do not respond to metronidazole or have severe disease.

Streptococci

Streptococcus pneumoniae

Strep pneumoniae are part of the **normal upper respiratory flora** and are **spread person-to-person via large droplets.**

Penicillins and **cephalosporins** are generally effective against *Streptococcus pneumoniae.*

The exception would be **meningitis**, where a combination of **vancomycin and cefotaxime/ceftriaxone** would be necessary.[6] **Rifampin** would be an appropriate alternative in the case of cephalosporin allergy.

Strep pyogenes (Group A beta-hemolytic Strep, GAS, GABHS)

Group A Strep (GAS) is transmitted with close contact via **inhalation of organisms in large droplets** or by **direct contact with respiratory secretions.**

Strep Pharyngitis

Strep pharyngitis will present with **sore throat** as well as **fever,** and sometimes **headache** and **abdominal pain**. It could be described as **erythema and edema of the posterior pharynx** and always think Strep if **palatal petechiae** and **strawberry tongue** are mentioned. Cough is usually absent.

> ### Show me the Strep
>
> *Strep pneumoniae* is the leading bacterial cause of **respiratory tract infections** and the most important cause of **otitis media**.
>
> It was a leading cause of **bacteremia and meningitis** until the introduction of the vaccine, but it's still present ubiquitously on Boards, especially in kids who are **underimmunized** or from **developing countries**.
>
> The risk of colonization with antibiotic resistant strains correlates with **age younger than 2 years, child care attendance, and recent antibiotic administration**.
>
> A clue in the question might be **unresolving otitis media**.

---

[6] Vancomycin is added for possible cephalosporin-resistance until susceptibilities are known.

Scarlet fever could be described with an associated **rash** that **blanches** easily and s**pares the face, palms, and soles**. Watch for the description of **pastia lines**, which are red lines in the skin folds of the neck, axilla, groin, elbows, and knees. They could describe the typical **sunburn-like sandpapery** rash as well as **perioral pallor**.

A positive rapid strep test is sufficient for diagnosis. However, negative tests require specimens sent for additional culture or nucleic acid amplification test NAAT (PCR) for confirmation.[7]

Antibodies to streptolysin O (ASO antibodies) would be useful to **confirm a recent infection** but not a current infection.

The preferred treatment for strep throat is **penicillin**, although amoxicillin is an acceptable alternative for small children due to taste. Those allergic to penicillin should be treated with erythromycin, azithromycin, clindamycin, or a first generation cephalosporin.

Asymptomatic contacts do not have to be treated.

Treatment for strep throat is to **prevent acute rheumatic fever**. It does not prevent poststreptococcal glomerulonephritis.

Strep Cellulitis

Strep cellulitis could be described as rapidly growing inflammation with **red skin, fever** and **chills**.

Erysipelas refers to infection of the dermis with well-defined borders and develops quickly vs cellulitis which has ill-defined borders and develops more slowly. They could describe red streaks associated with **lymphangitis**.

Necrotizing fasciitis (NF)

Watch for the start of infection with a **relatively minor trauma**, which **rapidly evolves** to erythema, marked inflammation, and bullous formation.

Marked pain that seems **out of proportion** to the appearance of the lesion is classic.

Varicella is a well-known risk factor for invasive group A Strep/ Strep pyogenes (GAS) and necrotizing fasciitis (NF.)

Arcanobacterium (Previously called Corynebacterium) haemolyticum

This little catalase-negative, weakly acid-fast, facultative, hemolytic, anaerobic, gram-positive, slender, sometimes club shaped bacillus was formerly classified as Corynebacterium haemolyticum.

It causes an acute pharyngitis that mimics Group A Strep with fever, pharyngeal exudate, lymphadenopathy, rash, and pruritus but without palatal petechiae and strawberry tongue. Respiratory tract infections mimic diphtheria with membranous pharyngitis, sinusitis, and pneumonia.

Invasive infections, including septicemia, peritonsillar abscess, brain abscess, orbital cellulitis, meningitis, endocarditis, pyogenic arthritis, osteomyelitis, urinary tract infection, pneumonia, spontaneous bacterial peritonitis, and pyothorax have been reported. No nonsuppurative sequelae have been reported.

It is susceptible to erythromycin, azithromycin and clindamycin, but not penicillins.

---

7 Fancy way of saying "Don't trust a negative rapid Strep Test".

Toxic Shock Syndrome

It starts out as **fever, nausea, vomiting, diarrhea**, and **erythroderma**. This then evolves to **shock and organ failure**.

It may also be caused by strains of Staph, EB virus, coxsackievirus, and adenovirus.

For bacterial caused toxic shock syndrome, an antibiotic which targets toxin production is recommended (i.e. clindamycin).

Strep agalactiae (Group B beta-hemolytic strep or GBS)

GBS is mainly a pathogen or **newborns**, so it is discussed in the newborn chapter.

Staphylococci

Methicillin sensitive *Staph aureus* (MSSA) infection is treated with beta lactamase-resistant agents such as **oxacillin/nafcillin**, which may be more effective than cephalosporins or vancomycin (especially for certain infection sites).

For more invasive infections such as endocarditis, bacteremia, or meningitis, **gentamicin or rifampin** may be used as well.

MRSA in the USA

You can expect to be tested on **Methicillin resistant** *Staph aureus* **infection (MRSA)**. The following are specific points regarding hospital acquired MRSA and community acquired MRSA.

Hospital Acquired MRSA

Hospital acquired MRSA infections account for over 50% of hospital acquired *Staph aureus* infections.

Nasal and skin carriage is the primary source for *S. aureus,* and therefore this is the highest risk factor for developing hospital acquired infection. The nasal carrier state can persist for years.

Hospital acquired MRSA infection is usually **multidrug resistant**. If you are presented with a case of hospital acquired MRSA, you should assume that it is **susceptible only to vancomycin**.

Coagulase Negative Staph

Coagulase-negative infections with *S. epidermidis* typically occur as a result of **indwelling IVs** and **central venous catheters**.

It is important to be able to discern whether a positive culture for coagulase-negative staphylococci represents specimen contamination or infection. In general, if the patient does not have a **foreign body**, the culture will represent **contamination**.

Toxin- mediated Staph diseases

S. aureus causes 3 toxin-mediated syndromes: **toxic shock syndrome (TSS), scalded skin syndrome, and food poisoning**.

TSS is associated with acute onset of fever, generalized erythroderma, rapid-onset hypotension, and signs of multisystem organ involvement. TSS is usually related to **menstruation, childbirth** or **abortion**.

Community Acquired MRSA

Community acquired MRSA infection usually involves **skin and soft tissue**. However, more invasive disease such as **pneumonia** can also occur, especially after viral respiratory infections such as influenza.

Although community acquired MRSA is resistant to all beta-lactam antimicrobials, its resistance is not as widespread. Community acquired infection is often susceptible to several antibiotics including **trimethoprim-sulfamethoxazole** and **clindamycin**.

MRSA abscesses **smaller than 5 cm** only require **incision and drainage**, not antibiotics.

Botulism

There are three types of botulism:

(1) **Food-borne botulism** – from ingestion of improperly packaged or incorrectly stored food

(2) **Wound botulism** – from systemic spread of the organism from an infected wound

(3) **Infantile botulism** – from intestinal colonization in infants, as their intestinal flora is too underdeveloped to prevent infection

An infant, *younger than 6 months of age*, might present with poor sucking or feeding, progressive descending generalized weakness and hypotonia, loss of facial expressions, ocular palsies, loss of head control and ptosis. Additional findings could include **weak cry, poor gag reflex, and constipation**. Infants often have several days of constipation before other symptoms present.

For botulism, think **6 Ds** in a bottle:

Diplopia
Dysphagia
Dysarthria
Dying to pee and poop (urinary and stool retention)
Dysphonia
Descending symmetrical paralysis

You can also picture **6 Ds** as if they were 6 bees **buzzing around in a bottle of honey.**

Botulism is the reason **honey** should not be given to infants younger than 12 months.

Don't look for a history of honey intake because it won't be there. Still, botulism will be the correct answer.

Mechanism of Action

This may seem trivial, but it is precisely the kind of information they will test you on.

In the **food form** of botulism (from poorly canned goods), preformed **botulism toxin is ingested**. This makes sense; this is why your mother told you (or she should have) to never eat from a can that is expanded.

In the **infantile form, spores are ingested and they germinate after ingestion.** Then toxin is produced and absorbed in the GI tract. Picture an infant eating a jar of honey, which then expands in the GI tract.

In infant and wound botulism, the diagnosis is made by **demonstrating** *C botulinum* **toxin** or organisms in feces, wound exudate, or tissue specimens.

PCR is *not* used in the diagnosis of infantile botulism.

They DO expect you to know the pathophysiology of the botulism toxin. It will also come in handy when you are rounding with a toxicologist.

The toxin blocks the release of acetylcholine into the synapse. Picture a GIANT bottle of honey sitting in the way of "a little Colleen."

> ### Calling all Cars !
>
> Any case of suspected botulism is a **nationally notifiable disease** and is required by law to be reported immediately to local and state health departments.
>
> Immediate reporting of suspect cases is particularly important because of possible use of botulinum toxin as a **bioterrorism weapon**. Note in case this is included in the question.

> ### Spore the Rods !
>
> *Clostridium tetani, botulinum,* and *perfringens* are anaerobic, gram positive, spore-forming rods.

Treatment

> **You are presented with an infant with infantile botulism and are asked for the** *most* **appropriate treatment.**
>
> Of course, 4 out of the 5 choices are antibiotics and none of them will be correct, especially the aminoglycoside as explained below.
>
> *Supportive care* will be the correct answer. However, presented with antitoxin ("BabyBIG" for cases of infant botulism, standard antitoxin for the rest) as an option for treatment, it would probably be the correct choice.

Aminoglycosides can potentiate the paralytic effects of the toxin. Antimicrobial therapy is not indicated in infant botulism.

Most cases of infant botulism **progress to complete respiratory failure**, sometimes requiring 2-3 weeks of ventilation.

> ### Treating Wound Botulism
>
> In cases of wound botulism, **penicillin** or **metronidazole** should be given after antitoxin has been administered.

Treponema pallidum (syphilis)

The great imitator

Infection can be divided into 3 stages.

1° **The primary stage** appears as one or more **painless indurated ulcers (chancres)** of the skin or mucous membranes at the site of inoculation approximately 3 weeks after exposure and heal spontaneously in a few weeks.

2° **The secondary stage**, beginning 1 to 2 months® later, is characterized by **rash, mucocutaneous lesions,** and **lymphadenopathy.** The polymorphic maculopapular rash is generalized and typically **includes the palms and soles.** In moist areas around the vulva or anus, **condylomata lata** can occur. This stage also resolves spontaneously without treatment in approximately 3 to 12 weeks, leaving the infected person completely asymptomatic. A variable latent period follows.

3° **The tertiary stage** of infection occurs **15 to 30 years after the initial infection** and can include **gumma formation, cardiovascular involvement,** or **neurosyphilis.**

Acquired syphilis almost always is contracted through **direct sexual contact with** lesions of the primary or secondary stages.

RPR, VDRL, FTA-ABS, EIEIO, and BINGO was his Name - O

Presumptive diagnosis of syphilis is made using **serologic tests.**

The **nontreponemal tests (RPR and VDRL)** may be positive with other viruses such as EBV, varicella, and hepatitis, so they **may not be used for actual diagnosis,** but serve as good screens.

Any reactive nontreponemal test result must be **confirmed by one of the specific treponemal tests** to exclude a false-positive test result, but **treatment for syphilis should not be delayed** while awaiting the results of the treponemal test results if the patient is symptomatic or at high risk of infection.

The main treponemal test used is the **FTA-ABS.** People who have reactive treponemal test results usually **remain reactive for life, even after successful therapy.** Treponemal test antibody titers correlate poorly with disease activity and should not be used to assess response to therapy.

What's Up ?
What's Down ?

For **botulism** and **myasthenia gravis** think top-down (starts ocular and descends). **Guillain-Barre syndrome** however, is an **ascending** paralysis.

With myasthenia gravis, the Tensilon® (edrophonium) test will be positive and onset is more gradual. With botulism, Tensilon will be negative.

Call me Anytime

Manifestations of neurosyphilis can occur at any stage of infection, especially in people infected with human immunodeficiency virus (HIV) and neonates with congenital syphilis.

All patients who have syphilis should be tested for HIV infection.

Treponemal tests also are not 100% specific for syphilis; positive reactions occur variably in patients with other spirochetal diseases, including Lyme disease. Interestingly, nontreponemal tests can be used to differentiate **Lyme disease** from syphilis, because the VDRL test is nonreactive in Lyme disease and positive in syphilis.

FTA-ABS is **F**orever.

Definitive diagnosis is made when **spirochetes** are identified by **microscopic darkfield examination** or **direct fluorescent antibody (DFA)** tests of lesion exudate, nasal discharge, or tissue, such as placenta, umbilical cord, or autopsy specimens.

Parenteral penicillin G remains the preferred drug for treatment of syphilis at any stage.

Parenteral penicillin G is the only documented effective therapy for patients who have neurosyphilis, congenital syphilis, or syphilis during pregnancy and is recommended for HIV-infected patients. Such patients always should be treated with penicillin, even if desensitization for penicillin allergy is necessary.

Syphilis in Pregnancy

Congenital syphilis is contracted from an infected mother **via transplacental transmission at any time during pregnancy or possibly at birth from contact with maternal lesions**.

All women should be screened serologically for syphilis early in pregnancy with a nontreponemal test (eg, RPR or VDRL) and preferably again at delivery.

Remember that treating the mother with penicillin automatically treats the infant because **penicillin crosses the placenta**. Picture a paper-thin P (for Penicillin) passing through the placenta.

Do you Treat the Newborn?

If the mother was treated during the pregnancy, do you need to treat the infant?

- **No, if she was treated with penicillin more than a month before delivery**
- Yes, if she was treated within the last month of pregnancy
- Yes, if she was treated with anything other than penicillin
- Yes, if the baby's titers are higher than the mother's titers

CASE STUDY You may be presented with the infant of a mother who tested positive for syphilis and was treated with erythromycin 2 months prior to delivery. What treatment should the infant receive?

THE DIVERSION "Well," you say to yourself, as you embark on a long diversionary journey to the incorrect answer, "They are testing me to see if I know that if the mother was treated more than one month prior to delivery, then no treatment is necessary." And there sitting for you, all made up in attractive diversionary clothing is "no further treatment."

ANSWER REVEALED Well, they actually are assuming you know that no treatment is needed if the mother was treated more than one month prior to delivery. What they were testing you on is whether you knew that *erythromycin doesn't cross the placenta*, and therefore starting the infant on penicillin is the actual correct answer.

Congenital Syphilis

Congenital syphilis is often not recognized at birth.

BUZZWORDS In addition to non-specific signs, look for **snuffles** (copious, highly infectious nasal secretions), **bullous lesions, osteochondritis** and **pseudoparalysis** of the joints. They may also describe **poor feeding**.

Additional associations include include **lymphadenopathy, mucocutaneous lesions, pneumonia, edema, thrombocytopenia, hepatosplenomegaly, hemolytic anemia, jaundice,** and a **maculopapular rash** at birth or within the first 4 to 8 weeks of age.

Corynebacterium diphtheria

DEFINITION An irregularly staining, **gram-positive**, nonspore-forming, nonmotile, **pleomorphic bacillus.** Humans are the sole reservoir. Organisms are spread by **respiratory tract droplets** and by **contact with discharges from skin, nose, throat, and eye lesions.** Clinically significant disease is caused by toxin-producing strains.

BUZZWORDS In the respiratory tract, diphtheria causes **membranous nasopharyngitis** that is associated with a **bloody nasal discharge** and **low-grade fever.** Cutaneous diphtheria leads to **extensive neck swelling** with cervical lymphadenitis (**bull neck**).

Untreated Congenital Syphillis

One would hope you won't encounter this anywhere else but on the Boards. This is a description of what you can expect if you do.

Untreated infants may develop symptoms **after 2 years of age** that involve the CNS, bones and joints, teeth, eyes, and skin.

The **Hutchinson triad** of such consequences includes **interstitial keratitis, eighth cranial nerve deafness**, and **Hutchinson teeth** (peg-shaped, notched central incisors).

Diphtheria Dropline

We of course vaccinate against diphtheria (DTaP, Tdap) so the test question would likely drop a hint that suggests the child is not immunized

The history might include the fact that the patient was adopted from another country or the parents objected to immunizations.

Life-threatening complications of respiratory diphtheria include **upper airway obstruction** caused by extensive membrane formation, **myocarditis**, which often is associated with heart block, and **cranial and peripheral neuropathies**.

Treatment is with 14 days of erythromycin or penicillin and a single dose of **equine antitoxin** obtained through the CDC.

Enterococci

Enterococci are **gram positive cocci in chains** that are ubiquitous in the normal GI flora, and are generally of low virulence. They may cause **neonatal and catheter-associated bacteremia** and other infections in **patients with anatomic abnormalities** such as recent surgery and indwelling urinary catheters.

Enterococcal infections are more common after **recent antibiotic use**. Enterococci are **resistant to ALL cephalosporins**, and typically respond to **ampicillin** and **vancomycin**, but resistance to vancomycin is increasing (VREC).

Kingella kingae

Kingella organisms are fastidious, **gram-negative coccobacilli** previously classified as Moraxella. The human oropharynx is the usual habitat. The organism more frequently colonizes young children and can be transmitted among children in child care centers, generally without causing disease. Infection may be associated with **preceding or concomitant stomatitis or upper respiratory tract illness**.

The most common infections associated with Kingella kingae are **suppurative arthritis, osteomyelitis**, and **bacteremia**. Almost all skeletal infections occur in children younger than 5 years of age. In addition to **fever**, children with K kingae bacteremia frequently have **respiratory** or **gastrointestinal** symptoms.

Cephalosporins are the drugs of choice. Some beta-lactam resistance is seen in US strains so unless susceptibilities are given, administer a 1st, 2nd, or 3rd generation cephalosporin or ampicillin-sulbactam would be the correct answer.

Listeria monocytogenes

Listeria is a **facultative anaerobic**, nonspore-forming, motile, **gram-positive bacillus** that multiplies intracellularly.

Listeriosis transmission predominantly is **foodborne** (think lunch meats, cheeses, ice cream, unwashed produce) and occurs most frequently among **pregnant women** and their **fetuses or newborn infants**, people of **advanced age**, and **immunocompromised patients**.

In pregnant women, infections can be asymptomatic or associated with an **influenza-like illness with fever, malaise, headache, gastrointestinal tract symptoms, and back pain**.

Neonatal illnesses have early-onset and late-onset syndromes similar to those of group B streptococcal infections.

Although **ampicillin alone** is sufficient to treat mild infection in immuncompetent individuals, initial therapy is traditionally with intravenous ampicillin and an aminoglycoside, usually gentamicin. Individuals with penicillin allergy should undergo desensitization. **Cephalosporins are not active against *L monocytogenes*.**

Neisseria meningitidis

Meningococcemia is an important etiology to keep in mind for septic shock.

Neisseria meningitidis presents with mild non-specific symptoms, including **runny nose, headache, lethargy, myalgias, and/or joint pain**. This quickly evolves to a **petechial/purpuric rash**. Patients may also present with signs of **meningeal irritation**.

Invasive infection usually results in meningococcemia, meningitis, or both. Infection may progress to limb ischemia, coagulopathy, pulmonary edema, shock, coma, and death in a few hours despite appropriate therapy.

N. meningitidis is an aerobic, nonmotile gram-negative catalase- and oxidase-positive diplococci that grows best in chocolate or blood agar. **Humans are the only known reservoir.**

Diagnosis is made by culturing the organism from blood, CSF, skin or another normally sterile site. PCR may help in pretreated patients.

Initial therapy includes **cefotaxime** or **ceftriaxone**.[9] Once the microbiologic diagnosis is established, treatment can often be completed with penicillin if the organism is susceptible. **Droplet precautions should be continued for 24 hours after antibiotics started.**

Spread of meningococcal disease

The organism colonizes the upper respiratory tract. Transmission occurs from person-to-person through droplets and requires close contact.

High risk populations include:

- college students who live in dormitories
- military recruits in boot camp
- those with terminal complement component deficiencies
- those with anatomic or functional asplenia[8]

Risk factors for epidemics include:

- overcrowding
- poverty
- malnutrition

---

[8] Remember: *N. meningitidis* is encapsulated!
[9] For septic shock of unknown cause, start with Vancomycin and Ceftriaxone.

Meningococcal prophylaxis

Regardless of immunization status, close contacts of all people with invasive meningococcal disease are at high risk and should receive chemoprophylaxis.

Chemoprophylaxis is recommended for

- **Household contacts**
- Child care or preschool contacts at any time during **7 days** before onset of illness
- Direct exposure to index patient's **secretions** through kissing or through sharing toothbrushes or eating utensils, at any time during **7 days** before onset of illness
- Anyone who frequently **slept in same dwelling** as index patient during **7 days** before onset of illness
- Anyone with prolonged contact (>8 hours) in close proximity (3 feet or less) during **7 days** before onset of illness
- Health care workers exposed directly to the index patent's secretions who did not wear a surgical mask in the first two days of therapy.

The drug of choice for prophylaxis for most children is **rifampin.**[10]

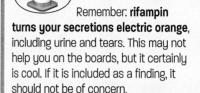

Electric Rifampin

Remember: **rifampin turns your secretions electric orange,** including urine and tears. This may not help you on the boards, but it certainly is cool. If it is included as a finding, it should not be of concern.

Shots against N. meningitidis

Vaccines against strains MenACWY-D (Menactra®) or MenACWY-CRM (Menveo®) are given as primary vaccines in infants/toddlers.

Vaccination against B strains can be given to those at increased risk (>16 yo/ college-aged, complement deficiencies, etc.)

Campylobacter jejuni

This is the most common cause of bacterial gastroenteritis in the developed world. The highest rates of infection occur in children younger than 4 years of age and transmission is common in **daycare centers**.

Many **farm animals** can harbor the organism. **Pets,** especially pet shop puppies, dogs, cats, hamsters, and birds, are potential sources of infection.

Improperly cooked poultry, untreated water, and unpasteurized milk have been the main vehicles of transmission. Transmission also occurs via direct contact with fecal material from infected animals or people.

Immunocompromised hosts can have **prolonged, relapsing, or extraintestinal infections**.

Infection can present as **fever, abdominal pain, intestinal cramping, and/or bloody diarrhea "dysentery"**.

Abdominal pain by *Campylobacter* may **mimic** that produced by **appendicitis** or **intussusception**.

Maintaining hydration status is the mainstay of treatment for all children with diarrhea. **Azithromycin** shortens the duration of illness and excretion of organisms.

---

[10] Alternative is ciprofloxacin.

Yersinia

Bubonic plague is caused by *Yersinia pestis* but *Y. enterocolitica* is a more commonly seen infection, although rarely in the United States. The principal reservoir is **swine**.

Enterocolitis due to *Yersinia enterocolitica* can be mistaken for acute appendicitis.

Watch for a history of ingestion of **unpasteurized milk** or **raw meat** including **chitterlings** (pork intestines), typically in a child younger than 5. History might also include contact with pets and/ or farm animals and exposure to dead animals and/ or rats.

It can present with **bloody diarrhea**, along with "pseudoappendicitis", including **RLQ pain** and **elevated WBC**.

Diagnosis is made by stool culture.

In otherwise uncomplicated cases, **no intervention is needed**.

Bacteremia most often occurs in children younger than 1 year of age and in older children with **predisposing conditions**, such as excessive iron storage (eg, sickle cell disease, and beta-thalassemia) and **immunosuppressive states**. In those cases, treatment would include trimethoprim-sulfa, cefotaxime, aminoglycosides, (and fluoroquinolones in patients older than 18).

First generation cephalosporins and penicillin would not be recommended due to resistance.

The Plague

Yes, bubonic plague still exists, and if you are not familiar with its manifestations and treatments it can become the plague of your existence if you have to take the exam again.

If you don't believe that the plague still exists, take a nice long trip to India. Be sure to drink tap water and eat all the street food you can get your hands on.

The physical findings include "**buboes.**" What's that, you ask? Buboes are **swollen painful lymph nodes**, usually inguinal. They can also involve the cervical and axillary nodes.

WHY ask Y ?

"Y" is key: App**Y** mimickers include **Y**ersinia and Camp**Y** infections.

Escherichia coli

The most important manifestations of E. coli are neonatal septicemia/ meningitis, urinary tract infections, and diarrhea, each covered in their respective chapters.

E coli is a gram-negative enteric rod. Invasive disease is broadly covered with a 3rd generation cephalosporin or with ampicillin.

Bartonella

Following a scratch or bite from a cat (or sometimes a dog) or inoculation with infected flea feces, the regional draining **lymph node** can become **swollen** and **tender** – this is cat scratch disease, a **self-limiting** illness that also causes **anorexia** and **malaise**. The disease can be **serious in AIDS and other immunocompromised patients**.

The diagnosis can be confirmed by **serologic testing** with **enzyme immunoassay (EIA)** or the **immunofluorescent antibody (IFA) test**.

The etiology is ***Bartonella henselae,*** and the treatment of localized disease is **supportive**.

CASE STUDY

You may be presented with a patient who has a draining lymph node that was preceded by a bite from a cat. The patient has no other underlying disorders. You will be asked to pick the most effective treatment.

THE DIVERSION

This is an excellent question that can easily divert you from the correct answer. After all, you have a draining lymph node following an episode where the skin integrity was breached. Must be a staph infection! What about trimethoprim-sulfamethoxazole (Bactrim®), cephalosporins, or doxycycline? What about penicillin, amoxicillin, or nafcillin? If you pick any of these diversions in an *otherwise healthy child* and if remaining on the hospital staff is pinned to your passing the boards, you took a step in the wrong direction.

ANSWER REVEALED

Despite the presence of malaise and anorexia, cat scratch disease is usually a self-limited disease that only requires supportive treatment.

HOT TIP

Now if it had been a cat BITE with acute infection, amoxicillin-clavulanate (Augmentin) would be the correct answer, to cover for Pasteurella.

Treatment would be indicated for **hepatosplenomegaly, large painful adenopathy,** and with **immunocompromised patients**.

The following antibiotics are appropriate when clinically indicated:

- Azithromycin
- Erythromycin
- Trimethoprim-sulfamethoxazole
- Rifampin
- Doxycycline.

HOT TIP

INEFFECTIVE antibiotic treatment for Cat Scratch Disease includes penicillin, amoxicillin, and nafcillin.

Painful suppurative nodes may be treated with needle aspiration for relief of symptoms. However **incision and drainage can lead to fistula formation and other complications**.

PERIL

Incision & drainage and surgical excision are to be avoided.

Tuberculosis (TB)

You will need to know the proper management of tuberculosis, whether infection or disease, and when it's TB or not TB.

Dealing with the Faces and Phases of TB

Children (and adults) infected with *Mycobacterium tuberculosis* are initially **asymptomatic** and the primary pulmonary focus (which is also known by its *nom de Guerre* "the Ghon Complex") is not always visible on CXR. Therefore, the PPD and its new BFFs the Quantiferon (QFN) and T-spot, are the "eyes and ears" in the field looking for this guerilla warrior, the Ghon Complex.

If a PPD, QFN or T-spot is positive, a chest X-ray is indicated.

If the X-ray is negative, the diagnosis is TB **infection**.[11]

If the X-ray is properly abnormal[12] (usually with perihilar adenopathy or cavitary lesions), then pulmonary TB **disease** is likely.

> ### Armed Armadillos?
>
> A cousin of TB is *Mycobacterium leprae*, the agent that causes leprosy.
>
> Yes, it's still possible to get leprosy. The organism's favorite resevoir is armadillos.

Treatment of Tuberculosis Infection

Isoniazid (INH) monotherapy would be indicated for a full gestational period = **9 months**.

You could be asked about side effects of INH and how to prevent them. ,

Peripheral neuritis or **seizures** can be prevented by administration of **B6 (pyridoxine)**.

Peripheral neuritis can be prevented by Pyridoxine.

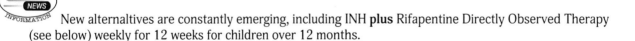

Rifampin is given for 6 to 9 months if it is an INH-resistant strain or if INH is not tolerated.

New alternaltives are constantly emerging, including INH **plus** Rifapentine Directly Observed Therapy (see below) weekly for 12 weeks for children over 12 months.

Treatment of Tubercolosis *Disease*

Classic symptoms of pulmonary TB are rare in children but may be present in their infectious contacts: **low-grade fever, weight loss and persistent cough, sometimes with hemoptysis.**

---

11 Formerly known as "latent" TB Infection (LTBI).
12 We say "properly" because sometimes it shows nonspecific findings and needs to be repeated.

Referral to ID is indicated to check for resistance and to decide on the treatment plan which usually includes 4 meds.

RIPE therapy for TB includes:

Rifampin
INH
Pyrazinamide*
Ethambutol

Extrapulmonary Tuberculosis

Pulmonary is a guerilla warrior, but extrapulmonary fights fair and is diagnosed after symptoms or signs have presented themselves. It's all out in the open; therefore, they are easily **MAPD**:

Meningitis
Adenitis
Pleuritis
Disseminated (Miliary disease)

Other Mycobacteria (Non-TB)

These are found in the environment, water, etc.

M. marinum can cause skin and soft tissue infections.

M. avium complex (MAC) can cause indolent lymphadenitis, pulmonary infections, or disseminated disease (in immunocompromised).

Opportunistic Infections

Pneumocystis jiroveci (carinii) Pneumonia (PCP)

PCP and HIV go hand in hand. It occurs **early** and is often **fatal**.

Trimethoprim/ sulfamethoxazole TMP-SMX (Bactrim® and **Septra®)** is used prophylactically as soon as the diagnosis of HIV is made and starting at 4 weeks of age for infants born to HIV positive mothers.

The mode of transmission of PCP is unknown.

Watch for respiratory distress but they will not mention HIV. Look for the buzzword **ground-glass appearance** if they describe an x-ray. They could also describe **general perihilar infiltrates** that can evolve to **interstitial infiltrates**. Patients will invariably have significant hypoxemia so pay attention if the description includes low oxygen saturation.

PCP pneumonia is also common in **cancer/bone marrow transplant patients**, which is why they receive **TMP-SMX prophylaxis** for 3 consecutive days each week.

Cryptosporidium

Extensive Crypto outbreaks may result from **contamination of municipal water and swimming pools**. Transmission to humans may also occur from **farm livestock** and especially **petting zoos**. Person-to-person transmission is common **in child care centers** due to poor hygiene after diaper changes.

Cryptosporidium diarrhea typically presents as severe, *non-bloody, watery diarrhea* similar to viral gastroenteritis, except it lasts a lot longer. Consider this diagnosis if they mention **chronic diarrhea in an immunocompromised patient**.

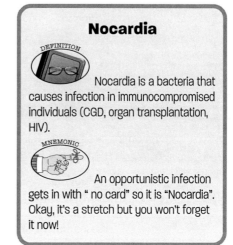

Nocardia

Nocardia is a bacteria that causes infection in immunocompromised individuals (CGD, organ transplantation, HIV).

An opportunistic infection gets in with " no card" so it is "Nocardia". Okay, it's a stretch but you won't forget it now!

Antibiotic Antics

Aminoglycosides

GNATS (**g**entamicin, **n**eomycin, **a**mikacin, **t**obramycin, **s**treptomycin)

Unlike other antibiotics, **effectiveness** is dependent on **high peak levels**. **Toxicity** (such as **ototoxicity**) is associated with **high trough levels**.

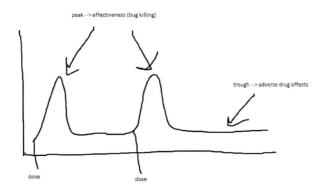

peak --> effectiveness (bug killing)

trough --> adverse drug effects

dose   dose

AminOglycOsides
Adverse effects include OtOtoxicity and nephrOtoxicity.

Peak levels are measured 30 minutes after the dose is given. Trough levels are measured 30 minutes before the next dose.

Penicillin

Penicillins are ß-lactam antibiotics that bind to bacteria's PBP (penicillin-binding-proteins) in order to inhibit bacterial cell wall formation. "High dose Amox" attempts to overcome PBP resistance.

Beta lactamase producing bacteria produce penicillinases, which cleave penicillin. Penicillinase-resistant antibiotics (oxacillin, nafcillin, dicloxacicillin, etc) are required for these organisms, including *Staph* organisms. "High dose Amox" would not overcome ß-lactamase production.

Penicillin is the treatment of choice for Strep throat, syphilis infections, as well as susceptible meningococcal infections.

High dose amoxicillin 80-90 mg/kg/day is indicated for routine otitis media, sinusitis, pneumonia, and initial treatment of UTIs.

 Ampicillin with or without gentamicin would be the treatment of choice for *Listeria monocytogenes* infection.

Cephalosporins

Like Star Wars® and its prequels and sequels, we have several generations to track and contend with.

Cephalosporins work by time-dependent killing. Their effectiveness is related to time spent above MIC (minimum inhibitory concentration).

The first generation drugs cover move gram positive bacteria. Gram negative increases as you move to subsequent generations.

First generation	First generation cephalosporins are effective against **gram positive** bacteria and are useful to treat skin infections, including methicillin **sensitive** *Staph aureus*. They are not effective against methicillin resistant *Staph aureus*. Read the question carefully, at first blush these can be confused with each other. First generation does not penetrate CSF well and should **not be used to treat meningitis**. They are also not effective against *Listeria* or enterococcus.
Second generation	2nd generation cephalosporins are the struggling underappreciated middle child of the cephalosporin family. Second generations are best **against beta lactamase producing gram negatives**, including *Enterobacteriaceae*, *H. influenzae*, and *Moraxella catarrhalis* (however, they are generally not as good at this as the 3rd generation). They have some effectiveness against gram positives, but not as good as first generation.
Third generation	Third generation cephalosporins have **excellent CSF penetration** and cover a broad spectrum. They are, therefore, **a good choice for meningitis**. Cefpodoxime and cefdinir are effective oral medications for otitis media and sinusitis, as well as group A beta hemolytic strep. Ceftibuten and cefixime are effective against urinary tract infections or respiratory infections. Warning: Extensive use of cephalosporins has lead to resistant strains of *Klebsiella*, *E. coli*, *Proteus mirabilis*, and *Pseudomonas aeruginosa*.

Fourth generation	**Cefepime** is a fourth generation cephalosporin. It is a broad-spectrum agent that may be used for **gram negatives** such as *pseudomonas*. It also has good activity against **gram positives** such as *S. aureus* MSSA (not MRSA).

Clindamycin

Clindamycin is **bacteriostatic**, not bactericidal, so it is usually used with another antibiotic.

This antibiotic binds to the 50S subunit of bacterial ribosomes and inhibits protein synthesis so it's often used in toxin-mediated processes (toxic shock syndrome, staph scalded skin, etc.)

Clindamycin is active against the following

- **Aerobic gram positive cocci:** streptococcus, staphylococcus, and *Corynebacterium diphtheriae*
- **Anaerobic gram positive cocci:** *Peptostreptococcus* sp, gram-positive non spore-forming bacilli (*Actinomyces* sp, *Propionibacterium* sp), clostridia except for *C. difficile*, and *C. perfringens*.
- **Anaerobic gram negative cocci:** *Bacteroides, Prevotella, Fusobacterium* sp
- **Chlamydia:** *Chlamydia trachomatis*
- **Protozoa:** *Plasmodium sp, Pneumocystis jiroveci (carinii), Toxoplasma gondii,* and *Babesia* sp.

Macrolides

Macrolides would be indicated for *Mycoplasma, Moraxella catarrhalis, H. flu, S. pyogenes, Strep viridans, Chlamydia,* pertussis, *Bartonella,* and *Legionella pneumophila*, as well as nontuberculous mycobacteria.

Azithromycin and clarithromycin are as effective as erythromycin, with fewer GI side effects. Therefore, erythromycin is rarely a first line medication.

There is high azithromycin resistance in *Moraxella* and *H. flu*.

> **Azithromycin for Atypicals**
>
> Macrolides work well for the following causes of respiratory infections: Mycoplasma, Chlamydia, and Legionella.

Rifampin

Rifampin would be appropriate **prophylaxis** when indicated for **meningococcal** or **Hib exposure**.

Rifampin is also indicated for **invasive and/or resistant *Staph* infection**, including osteomyelitis and endocarditis. It also has a role in the treatment of **latent and active tuberculosis**.

If presented with a pregnant patient, rifampin is **absolutely contraindicated**, because of its potential for teratogenicity.

Tetracyclines/Doxycycline

Tetracyclines are usually not recommended in children younger than 8 due to risk of teeth staining, except for the use of **doxycycline** in **Rocky Mountain Spotted Fever**, in which it is indicated regardless of the age.[13]

 If it's Rocky, give Doxy.

 Doxy has recently been approved for treament for Lyme disease in younger children as well.

Trimethoprim with sulfamethoxazole (TMP-SMX)

Trimethoprim with sulfamethoxazole can be used to treat acute UTI, inflammatory bowel disease, burns, umbilical cord care, and *Chlamydia* urethritis. TMP-SMX is also very useful against minor MRSA infections.

It would be indicated for GI infection due to *Salmonella* or *Shigella* in immunocompromised patients or those with severe disease.

TMP-SMX is also indicated for PCP prophylaxis in HIV and cancer/ bone marrow transplant patients.

Side effects include Stevens Johnson Syndrome, as well as rash, neutropenia, anemia, and thrombocytopenia.

Vancomycin

Vancomycin would be indicated for **MRSA** infection in patients who do not tolerate other medications. It is also used to treat **endocarditis**.

Vancomycin would be treatment of choice for **resistant corynebacteria** and **resistant pneumococcus**.

An important side effect is **Red Man Syndrome**. This is a **rate-dependent infusion reaction** caused by histamine release causing redness and itching, usually of the head and neck. It is treated by **slowing the infusion rate and giving diphenhydramine**.

Protozoal Infections

Entamoeba histolytica

 E. histolytica causes amoebic dysentery.

---

[13] Newer studies have shown that up to 21 days of a tetracycline can be used in patients of any age with minimal adverse effects.

Groups at increased risk of infection include **immigrants** from, or travelers to, areas with endemic infection (developing countries such as Latin America, Africa and Asia), **institutionalized people**, and **men who have sex with men**. *E. histolytica* is transmitted by the **fecal-oral route** via **contaminated food or water**.

Amebic dysentery (acute amebic colitis) starts with 1-2 weeks of **crampy abdominal pain, diarrhea, fever** and **tenesmus** (painful but ineffectual urge to defecate). Stools are liquid, consisting mainly of **water, blood,** and **mucus**.[14]

Clinical course can range from asymptomatic (90%) to invasive disease (amebiasis) with **liver and brain abscesses** and **lung disease**.

Stool exam may identify hematophagous trophozoites or cysts. Stool cultures are usually positive.

Definitive diagnosis is by **enzyme immunoassay in stool (EIA)**.

Enter amoeba "hysterical:" picture a crazy, hysterical amoeba playing tennis (tenesmus) in your bowels causing bloody mucous diarrhea.

Don't forget! Amebiasis can cause a liver abscess. Abdominal ultrasound is a minimally invasive and cost-effective diagnostic tool.

Symptomatic patients should be treated with **metronidazole** or **tinidazole**, followed by a therapeutic course of **iodoquinol** to clear the cysts from the intestines.

Asymptomatic patients with positive screening only need the iodoquinol.

Follow up stool studies and **screening of household members** is recommended.

Corticosteroids and antimotility drugs administered to people with **amebiasis** can worsen symptoms and the disease process. In general anti-motility drugs should be avoided in ALL patients with infectious diarrhea.

Malaria: *Plasmodium* species

P. falciparum **is the most deadly parasite in the world.**

Malaria is endemic throughout the **tropical areas of the world** and is acquired from the bite of the **female** nocturnal-feeding **Anopheles genus of mosquito**.

> ## Vector-borne infection prevention
>
> In general to prevent against mosquito and tick-borne diseases the following are recommended:
>
> 1. insect repellent,
> 2. long clothing
> 3. mosquito netting when in malaria endemic areas.

---

[14] Apologies from the editors if you were studying while eating your lunch.

The classic symptoms of malaria are **high fever** with **chills**, **rigor**, **sweats**, and **headache**. Anemia and musculoskeletal pain are common. Without treatment, fever occurs **every 2-3 days**.

Treatment is with **quinidine**.

Toxoplasmosis *(Toxoplasma Gondii)*

With toxoplasmosis occurring **early in pregnancy**, there is a **lower chance of fetal infection**, but when infection does occur, the **consequences are more severe**. The opposite is true later in pregnancy—**there is a greater chance of infection, but the sequelae are less severe**.

Most affected pregnant women show no clinical signs, and when they do, **lymphadenopathy** may be the sole symptom.

Congenital Toxo

The majority of newborn infants with congenital toxoplasmosis are asymptomatic in the neonatal period. When symptoms are present at birth, common findings include **microcephaly, hydrocephaly, chorioretinitis, cerebral calcifications, jaundice, thrombocytopenia,** and **hepatosplenomegaly**.

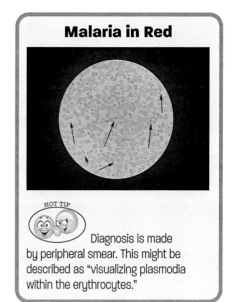

Malaria in Red

Diagnosis is made by peripheral smear. This might be described as "visualizing plasmodia within the erythrocytes."

Later Signs include

- ❏ Deafness
- ❏ Impaired vision
- ❏ Seizures
- ❏ Mental retardation
- ❏ Learning disabilities
- ❏ Cognitive deficits

CMV vs. Toxo: Cerebral calcifications in CM**V** are peri**v**entricular.

Think of the **V** in CM**V** and peri**V**entricular."

With toxoplasmosis, they are diffuse cerebral calcifications.

Acquired Toxo

Toxoplasmosis is why we tell pregnant women that they can get out of **changing the kitty litter** while they are pregnant – this is a mode of transmission for toxoplasmosis.

Toxoplasmosis may also be acquired by consumption of **contaminated water and food**, such as **unwashed garden vegetables, inadequately cooked meat**, and **unpasteurized goat milk**.

Because most cases acquired (not congenital) toxo infection are self-limiting, specific drug therapy is not required.

Acquired toxoplasmosis **would** require treatment in **symptomatic**, especially **immunocompromised**, patients, such as those with **HIV and receiving chemotherapy.**

Viral Infections
The Herpes Viruses (1, 2, 4, 5, 6)

Herpes Simplex Virus (HSV)

HSV in the Newborn Period

The typical presentation is an infant in the neonatal period (first 28 days) with signs of **sepsis, meningitis, and seizures.** In addition, they may tip you off by telling you the **gram stain on CSF is negative.**

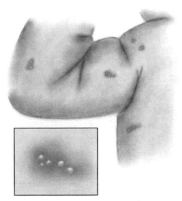

Herpes Simplex lesions

Any **seizure in the newborn period** should have you considering a herpes infection. This is especially the case if they describe a **temporal lobe seizure.** The **mother will be described as asymptomatic** because there is usually "no history" of herpes documented when an infant presents with systemic HSV, despite our best efforts at eliciting one. Most invasive neonatal herpes infections are caused by **Type 2 HSV.**

Rapid diagnosis of HSV meningitis can be made by CSF **PCR,** especially in CSF. CSF culture is not the method of choice because of false negatives.

Direct fluorescent antibody staining is a reliable method to identify HSV in **vesicle scrapings.**

Herpes can also be transmitted as an ascending infection through the infected birth canal **(even with intact membranes); therefore, delivery via c-section does not rule out transmission of perinatal infection.**

Neonatal infection can also be transmitted postnatally from an adult with a cutaneous, genitourinary, breast or oral lesion. **It is NOT transmitted through breast milk itself.**

Acyclovir

Acyclovir is used **for primary genital and mucocutaneous HSV infections** for **prophylaxis and treatment in immunocompetent patients.**

HSV in Childhood

Toddlers, with primary HSV will present with fever, tender adenopathy, and oral lesions (gingivostomatitis). Other presentations in older children may include cold sores, herpetic whitlow, aseptic meningitis, or eczema herpeticum.

HOT TIP

If you are presented with a prepubertal patient with a genital herpes simplex type 2 infection, **sexual abuse** should be suspected.

Presenting Neonatal Herpes !

There are 3 presentation of Neonatal HSV. All require IV acyclovir.

- **SEM** (skin eye mouth))- localized disease
- **Disseminated**- involving multiple organs especially liver and lungs
- **CNS**- Brain

IV acyclovir would also be indicated in **immunocompromised patients** with **varicella** or **disseminated zoster**, as well as to treat **HSV encephalitis in any patient**.

Neonates with skin or mucous membrane manifestations of herpes are initially treated with IV acyclovir, followed by extended PO treatment.

EBV (Epstein-Barr Virus)

Humans are the only known reservoir of EBV a.k.a. **human herpesvirus 4**, and primary infection results from exposure to oral secretions of infected individuals and by blood transfusions.

Infectious mono can present with **fever, tonsillitis, and enlarged lymph nodes**, as well **hepatosplenomegaly** and **atypical lymphocytosis**.

Watch for a description or suggestion of splenomegaly. You will need to be aware of the need for the patient's restriction from contact sports for *weeks* after diagnosis.

EBV Serology

The heterophile antibody test confirms the diagnosis but is not reliable in children under age 4. EBV serologic tests are especially useful for heterophile-negative patients.

The most commonly performed test is for antibody against the IgG **viral capsid antigen** (VCA) that appear early in infection and persist for life, so it is not helpful in differentiating acute from convalescent infection. **IgM is key to diagnosing acute infection**.

Antibodies to EBNA (Epstein Barr nuclear antigen) appear several weeks to months after onset of infection and persist for life so a positive test excludes an active primary infection. This makes sense of course, the immune system will see viral capsid antigen first and make corresponding antibodies in acute/ recent infection.

EBV Infection	VCA	EA	EBNA
Acute	POS	POS	NEG
Convalescent/Past	POS	LOW	POS
Reactivation	POS	HIGH	POS

EBV-Associated Disorders

 EBV infections can **evolve to lymphoma** in immunocompromised hosts.

EBV-associated lymphoproliferative disorders result in a number of complex syndromes in patients who are immunocompromised, such as **transplant recipients** or people infected with **human immunodeficiency virus (HIV)**.

> **HOT TIP**
> A **rash** can develop following **ampicillin** or **amoxicillin** treatment in patients who have infectious mono. This is not an allergic reaction.[15]

CMV (Cyto–Megalo–Virus)

CMV a.k.a. **human herpesvirus 5** transmission occurs **horizontally** (by direct person-to-person contact with virus-containing secretions including sexual transmission), **vertically** (from mother to infant before, during, or after birth), and **diagonally** via transfusions and transplantations.

Patients may **shed the virus in urine, saliva, or genital secretions. CMV may cause serious disease in immunocompromised patients.**

Young children are little disease vectors that transmit CMV to their parents, including mothers who may be pregnant, and other caregivers including child care staff.

Calcifications
M
peri**V**entricular

Congenital CMV

These babies can get thrombocytopenia with subsequent petechiae and purpura ("***blueberry muffin baby***").

Additional findings would include **hepatosplenomegaly, jaundice, SGA** and **microcephaly**. Neurological findings would include **seizures, hypotonia,** and **weak suck**.

HOT TIP
Although this is the classic presentation, **congenital CMV infection is usually clinically silent**. However, some infants with silent congenital infection, are later found to have **sensorineural hearing loss** or **learning disability**.

> **Hear Ye! Hear Ye!**
> **HOT TIP**
> Congenital CMV infection is the leading nongenetic cause of **sensorineural hearing loss** in children in the United States.
>
> This hearing loss may appear years after birth, so a normal newborn hearing screen is not enough. These kids need close audiologic follow up until at least age 6.

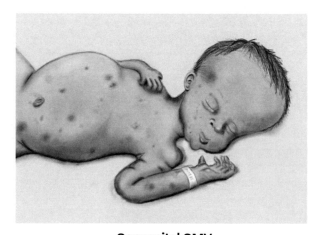

Congenital CMV

---

[15] This is often called "the poor man's mono test", and we're not recommending it. However this can be presented on the exam so please be aware of this.

A **urine culture or PCR for CMV in the urine or saliva within the first 3 weeks of life** is the definitive diagnostic study[16] for congenital CMV infection.

Serologic tests have absolutely no utility in the diagnosis or congenital CMV.

CMV, think **5 Cs**: **C**horioretinitis, **C**erebral **C**alcifications with diagnosis confirmed with urine **C**ulture and the potential for **C**ensorineural hearing loss (Sensorineural hearing loss).

Drug of choice is ganciclovir.

Acquired CMV

CMV can present with a clinical picture **much like mono** with **prolonged fever** and **mild hepatitis**. If mono is described and EBV is not an option, CMV is the answer.

Viral culture and PCR are the preferred methods to diagnose acquired CMV. Serologic assays have no role in diagnosis here either because IgM can persist for months after primary infection.

Roseola Infantum (Roses)

The formal name is **human herpesvirus type 6 (HHV-6).** It is also known as **exanthem subitum** (sudden, in latin).

Look for a well-appearing infant or toddler with "3-5 days of high fever." After the fever passes, a generalized "mac-pap rash" will appear.

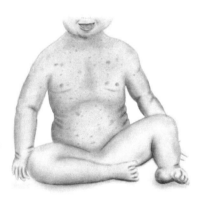

Think of the rash as a dozen roses being presented AFTER the fever's performance to say goodbye; thus, Roses = Roseola.

A **febrile seizure** is not an uncommon occurrence with roseola infection. They could present you with a classic clinical scenario of roseola followed by a seizure, and ask you for the most likely cause. Of course the correct answer will be human herpesvirus type 6.

And the work up? Just say NO to everything, like a typical 2 or 13 year old.

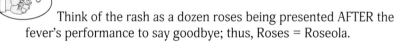

Meet the Human Herpes Virus (HHV) Family

HHV1 = a Herpes Simplex Virus 1 (HSV-1)

HHV2 = Herpes Simplex Virus 2 (HSV-2)

HHV3 = Human Herpesvirus 3, Varicella Zoster Virus

HHV4 = EBV

HHV5 = CMV

HHV6 = Roseola

HHV7 = Similar to Roseola

HHV8 = Kaposi sarcoma

---

[16] The "shell-vial assay" is an adaptation of tissue culture, which is more rapid than standard cultures.

Vaccine-Preventable Viral Infections

Rubella (German Measles)

Rubella really is only a mild viral illness. It only becomes important when an **expectant mother** is infected, leading to **congenital rubella syndrome**. 50% of infants infected during their first trimester are affected – most commonly with **cataracts and PDA**.

They will never use the terms "German Measles" or even "Measles." They will use the more formal terms. Therefore, it is important to keep **rubella** and **rubeola** straight, in a way that you won't forget in the heat of the battle.

For rubella think of **BELL** in the middle of the word.

Rubella is German measles: picture a "bell" ringing in Germany during Oktoberfest and the image is with you. The bell has a white eye on it (the cataract).

As with measles and mumps (MMR), pregnant women should NOT be vaccinated.

> **You are asked to evaluate a boy who was recently adopted with unknown immunization status. He presents with a low grade fever, generalized maculopapular rash and enlarged occipital and preauricular lymph nodes. He does not appear to be toxic. Which of the following is the most likely diagnosis?**
>
> You will be presented with several diversionary choices, including EBV infection, rubeola, HIV infection, and TB.
>
> The key to answering this question of course is the uncertain immunization status. The maculopapular rash, low grade fever, and subacute clinical picture are consistent with rubella. Rubeola, or measles, would also present with a maculopapular rash. However, the clinical description would include cough, coryza, and conjunctivitis. Likewise, EBV virus would present with higher fever and a more toxic clinical presentation.

RubeOLa (Measles)

The typical buzzwords for rubeola are **confluent macular papular rash**, **Koplik spots** (which are pathognomonic, at least on Boards), and **conjunctivitis** in a miserable or "measle-rable" kid.

Also look for **FCC: F**ever, **C**ough, **C**oryza (think of the FCC[17] in charge of airborne messages). This, along with the mac pap rash and conjunctivitis, will be the keys to recognizing this in the picture section. They can also have **photophobia**.

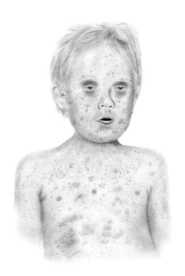

Rubeola / Measles

Measles is **transmitted by airborne droplets with an incubation period of 8-12 days**. Humans are the only natural hosts.

The sequence of signs and symptoms can be confusing. Here is the roadmap:

- The incubation is 8-12 days.
- The prodrome is on the first two days.
- Koplik spots appear shortly after.
- Then the rash comes around day 5.
- The rash is worst after about a week and begins to resolve around day 10.

They are most contagious from 4 days before to 4 days after the rash, so **airborne transmission precautions** are indicated for 4 days after the onset of rash in otherwise healthy children and for the duration of illness in immunocompromised patients.

Isolation isn't enough to protect immunocompromised patients. They would also require **immunization** and **immunoglobulin**.

If they describe a *preschool* age child from a developing country with FCC as the presentation, think measles (preschool because hand-washing practices are lacking in this group). Even with proper immunization there ARE measles outbreaks in the US. Therefore, arriving from another country is not a prerequisite for a child with measles.

If you are presented with a patient with coryza and cough, along with vomiting and diarrhea, the most likely diagnosis is influenza, not measles.

Post Exposure Management

If exposure has been **within 6 days, immune globulin** should be given, to **infants under 12 months, pregnant women, and immunocompromised individuals**.

Persons exposed to measles who are not completely immunized, including infants 6 to 12 months of age, should receive the **measles vaccine**.

Measles vaccine given **within 3 days of exposure** might help prevent the onset of disease.

M has 3 down strokes; therefore, remember 3 days for Measles vaccine.

---

[17] FCC= Federal Communications Commission.

HOT TIP

MMR doses given before the first birthday will not count towards completion of the series.

PERIL

Vaccination must wait **5 months after the IM immunoglobulin was given**, and until the child is at least 12 months of age.

CASE STUDY

If you are presented with a 7 month old infant who is exposed to measles, what should you do?

THE DIVERSION

You could be presented with all sorts of choices. If you pick one of the diversions, you won't even get one "measly point" toward passing the boards! Here is the correct way to answer a question which tests your knowledge of this protocol.

ANSWER REVEALED

If given within **72 hours**[13] **of exposure**, the measles vaccine will protect against infection. This rule applies to infants who are at least 6 months: therefore, a 7 month old infant falls into this category.

If the exposure is **greater than 72 hours but less than 6 days**, measles immunoglobulin should be given.

Rubella (German Measles)	Rubeola (Measles)
Low fever, rash	High fever
Prenatal infection is associated with congenital cataracts and PDA (patent ductus arteriosus)	Patients can develop SSPE (subacute sclerosing panencephalitis) years after measles infection
Sensory reminder: bell ringing in Germany during Oktoberfest	Sensory reminder: Sing to the tone of Head, Shoulders, Knees, and Toes: "Head, shoulders, measles, toes. Eyes, and ears, and mouth and nose. Head shoulders measles toes." This song will remind you of the direction which the rash appears (head down to toes) with the associated signs/symptoms (eyes- conjunctivitis, mouth- kolpik spots, nose- coryza)

Mumps

Mumps is another example of a disease that is rarely seen in clinical practice. Mumps virus is a **paramyxovirus.**

---

[18] Which to most of us is also known as 3 days, so put down the calculator, already!

General symptoms of mumps are **fever, headache, malaise,** and **muscle aches**. Swelling of the **parotid gland** can be described with **unilateral facial swelling anterior to the ear,** with **difficulty opening the mouth**. There will be no abnormalities noted in the oral cavity.

Complications may include **parotitis, meningitis/encephalitis, orchitis,** or **pancreatitis** (look for abdominal pain in the description).

So, besides the obvious parotid gland swelling, complications of **MUMPS:**

Meningitis/encephalitis (fever and headache)

Unable to open mouth

Muscle Aches/malaise

Pancreatitis

Swelling of testicles

Epididymoorchitis is the most common complication of mumps; and presents as abrupt onset of high fever and usually unilateral testicular pain with swelling and erythema of scrotum.

Impaired fertility is seen in only 15% of orchitis cases.

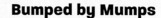

Bumped by Mumps

Even though many of you have never had or treated mumps, you may be expected to manage a mumps outbreak at a school located on the boards.

What to do?

- Children who are fully immunized can remain in school
- Children who are due for the booster vaccine need to get the booster vaccine
- Children who never received the vaccine need to receive it before returning
- Children whose parents refuse to immunize must wait 26 days after the last person in the class developed symptoms
- The child who has mumps can return to school 9 days after the onset of symptoms

Differentiating Mumps from Viral Parotitis and other Imitators

CASE STUDY

You are presented with a child with a *high fever* **who is** *toxic appearing* **and is** *fully immunized*. **Physical exam is noteworthy for unilateral preauricular and submandibular swelling. What is the diagnosis?**

THE DIVERSION

The diversionary choice sitting right there will be mumps. However, if you are specifically being told that the patient is fully immunized, then mumps will not be the correct answer.

ANSWER REVEALED

The combination of high fever and toxic appearance makes for a diagnosis of bacterial parotitis. Mumps is associated with low-grade fever and a non-toxic appearance.

A **stone in the salivary gland** will likely cause "**intermittent swelling.**"

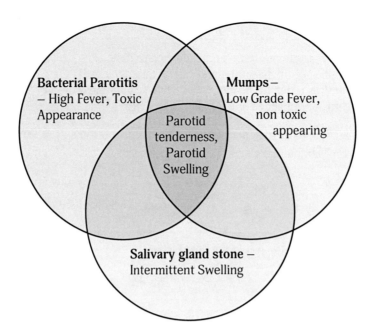

Bacterial Parotitis – High Fever, Toxic Appearance

Mumps – Low Grade Fever, non toxic appearing

Parotid tenderness, Parotid Swelling

Salivary gland stone – Intermittent Swelling

CASE STUDY

You may be presented with a teenage boy with a typical clinical presentation of mumps, parotitis. You are then asked for the most likely additional manifestation.

THE DIVERSION

Of course, you will be dazzled by choices like deafness, thyroiditis, arthritis, nephritis, pancreatitis and encephalitis.

ANSWER REVEALED

Although all of the above can occur, they are rare. Orchitis however, is a relatively common manifestation although infertility is rare.

TREATMENT

Treatment of mumps is **supportive**.

Erythema Infectiosum (Fifth Disease)

MNEMONIC

This is caused by **parvovirus B19** (single-stranded DNA virus) and spread by respiratory droplets (if in doubt, choose this for any question of what causes **hydrops fetalis**[19] in pregnancy, **aplastic crisis in sickle cell disease**, and, I believe, the controversy over the 2020 US Presidential election ballots.

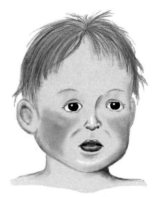

Slapped Cheek Rash in Fifth Disease

---

[19] There is no congenital infection or birth defect associated with parvovirus. Either the pregnancy is lost or it is fine.

The prodrome is non-specific, with fevers, sore throat, runny nose, headache, and malaise. This is followed by the classic **"slapped-cheek" rash**. Over the next few days, a **"lacey" rash on the extremities may develop**. **Polyarthropathy** may also develop.

There is a lesser known entity of parvo called **Purpuric Glove and Socks Syndrome** which has painful, purpuric papules, petechiae, and purpura on hands and feet with associated fever.

Parvo has 5 letters... Fifth Disease

It presents as malaise and fever then followed by rash

P- Pregnancy-associated hydrops fetalis

A- Anemia, Aplastic crisis

R- Rash (slapped cheeks then lacy rash)

V- Roman numeral V

O- pOlyarthralgia

Varicella Zoster Virus (VZV)

Varicella infections are becoming as rare as toilet paper at the start of the COVID-19 pandemic. However, both are fair game on the Boards. It is also known as human herpes virus #3.

Varicella zoster is a highly contagious virus and humans are the only source. Infection results when the virus comes in contact with the **mucosa of the upper respiratory tract or the conjunctiva**.

Person-to-person transmission occurs by the **aerosolized route** or by **direct contact with the lesions or respiratory secretions**.

In addition to standard precautions, **airborne and contact precautions** are recommended for patients with varicella **for a minimum of 5 days after onset of rash and until all lesions are crusted**, which, in immunocompromised patients, can be a week or longer.

Airborne and contact precautions are recommended for neonates born to mothers with varicella and, if still hospitalized, should be continued **until 21 or 28 days of age** if they received Varicella-Zoster Immune Globulin or IGIV.

Remember that kids are **contagious** from **several days before they have their rash** until all the lesions are crusted over. Anyone around a child during this period should be considered "exposed." **An immunocompromised child exposed during this period would need to receive varicella zoster immune globulin (VZIG) to help prevent infection.**

Most children who contract varicella do fine. **Varicella tends to be more severe in infants, adolescents, and adults than in young children.**

The most common complication is **superinfection** with *Staph aureus* involving skin. In more severe cases, invasive infections may lead to **pneumonia** and **osteomyelitis**.

However, **immunocompromised kids** (chemotherapy, AIDS) are much more susceptible to disseminated varicella, and can develop **viremia, pneumonia, encephalitis**, or other complications.

Bad Varicella

Patients on chemo have a lot to fear regarding varicella. You are expected to know that varicella-zoster immunoglobulin is indicated for any patient on chemo who is exposed to varicella.

Follow the Zoster

Zoster (shingles) is the secondary infection of varicella, caused by reactivation of VZV from latency.

Children with zoster can return to school if the lesions can be covered or once they are crusted.

These patients should receive Varicella Zoster Immune Globulin or IVIg as soon as possible.

Newborns

VZIG is the treatment of choice for a newborn exposed to chickenpox. What constitutes exposure? If the mother develops chickenpox between **5 days before delivery through 2 days after delivery**, then the infant is at risk.

Now how do you keep that straight? In the heat of the battle, you could find yourself asking (put on your best Clint Eastwood voice) **"Did he say 5 days before and 2 days after or is it the other way around? Huh, Punk!?"**

Well, there is no need to be concerned. Just remember the following and it will be impossible to forget. The Roman numeral for 5 is **V**. V is in the beginning of the word **V**aricella so it is 5 days **before** delivery. There are 2 **L**s at the end of the word, so it is 2 days **after** delivery. Therefore, normal infants older the 2 days who were exposed to varicella after 2 days of age do **not** need to receive VZIG.

VARICELLA

Fi**V**e days before	2 days after (**LL**)

> ### Acyclovir use in Varicella
>
> Oral acyclovir or valacyclovir are **not recommended** for routine use in otherwise healthy children with varicella.
>
> Oral acyclovir or valacyclovir should be considered for otherwise healthy people **at increased risk of moderate to severe varicella**, such as unvaccinated people older than 12 years of age, people with chronic cutaneous or pulmonary disorders, people receiving long-term salicylate therapy, and children receiving short, intermittent, or aerosolized courses of corticosteroids.
>
> Intravenous acyclovir therapy is recommended for immunocompromised patients, including patients being treated with chronic corticosteroids.

VZIG is considered to be a preventive measure rather than treatment, and it needs to be administered within 96 hours of exposure.

Respiratory Syncytial Virus (RSV)

The most common manifestation of RSV is bronchiolitis. The clinical description will likely be an **infant** with **expiratory wheeze, crackles, nasal flaring, retractions, tachypnea,** and the nonspecific description of **fever** and **URI symptoms**.

The CXR will have **diffuse infiltrates** and **hyperinflation.**

Humans are the only source of infection. Transmission usually is by **direct or close contact with contaminated secretions,** which may occur from **exposure to large-particle droplets at short distances or fomites.** RSV can persist on environmental surfaces for several hours and for a half-hour or more on hands.

Confirmation is **not necessary** for management.

Diagnosis: Immunofluorescence is how it is confirmed. Picture a "Really Shiny Virus" because it lights up.

If they ask how healthcare providers can **BEST** prevent the spread of RSV, the answer is "**good hand washing**."

Pure RSV bronchiolitis does not respond to albuterol or corticosteroid therapy and on the Boards, choosing either treatment will always be the wrong answer. **Management is largely supportive.**

Monthly injections of **Palivizumab** (Synagis®) given during RSV season in a particular region do NOT reduce the risk of acquiring RSV disease but reduce the severity of the disease if acquired. Pavalizumab is recommended for infants with **chronic lung disease (CLD), preterm birth** and **congenital heart disease.**

Palivizumab is not effective in treatment of RSV disease and is not approved or recommended for routine RSV bronchiolitis.

Influenza

Influenza typically begins with **sudden onset of high fever**, often accompanied by **chills** or **rigors, headache, malaise, diffuse myalgia,** and **nonproductive cough.** Upper respiratory symptoms like sore throat, nasal congestion, and rhinitis.

Complications and rates of hospitalization are greater in **newborns** and children with **high-risk conditions** such as hemoglobinopathies, bronchopulmonary dysplasia, asthma, cystic fibrosis, malignancy, diabetes mellitus, chronic renal disease, and congenital heart disease.

Rapid antigen screen is the quickest and most useful method to identify influenza.

Supportive therapy is indicated for most uncomplicated cases.

Antiviral medications would be indicated for severe disease or those patients at risk for complications or who have close family contacts at risk.

In the United States, 2 classes of antiviral medications are available for treatment or prophylaxis of influenza infections: neuraminidase inhibitors (**oseltamivir and zanamivir**) and adamantanes (amantadine and rimantadine). **Due to resistance, only the neuramindase inhibitors are currently recommended.**

Parainfluenza

Parainfluenza viruses are the major cause of **laryngotracheobronchitis (croup),** but they also commonly cause upper respiratory tract infection, pneumonia, and/or bronchiolitis

Rotavirus

The words to look for are: **1-2 day history of fever**, **watery stools**, and **intermittent vomiting**. Evidence of **dehydration** will also be described.

Diagnosis is done by **antigen testing of the stool** (of course). There is a 1 to 3 day incubation period.

There is no specific treatment for rotavirus, but small infants may need to be hospitalized because of dehydration.

HIV: For Life

Human Immunodeficiency Virus (HIV) is a **lentivirus** in the **retrovirus family**. It has an affinity for the **CD4 T-lymphocytes**. In the pediatric age group, it has two major forms of transmission: **mother to child** and **behavioral**.

Chronic non-specific symptoms in a child or neonate should make you consider HIV infection. These include **weight loss, fevers, or night sweats**. A history of **recurrent or persistent thrush** may be a clue. The main laboratory finding is **a decreased CD4 count**.

Perinatal

Vertical transmission of HIV during delivery is the most common mode of transmission in kids. **Breast feeding** is another important mode of transmission.

Since mother-to-child transmission is almost always preventable with a combination of maternal antiretroviral therapy, intrapartum maternal zidovudine (AZT), neonatal zidovudine,[20] and not breastfeeding, **routine prenatal HIV screening is now recommended for all women**. C/S reduces risk of transmission by 50% in mothers with active viremia.

HIV Testing

Because maternal antibody to HIV is an IgG (free ride across the placenta), serologic testing in infants under 18 months is unreliable. Therefore in the United States, **the HIV DNA polymerase chain reaction (PCR) is the gold standard for HIV testing under 18 months of age.**

For those 18 months and over, **enzyme immunoassays (EIAs) are used as the initial test for serum HIV antibody**. Positive EIAs are verified by Western blot analysis. Rapid tests for HIV antibodies also require confirmatory testing.

Breast is Best

Breastfeeding is almost always best, but there are a few Infectious contra-indications to breastfeeding...

- **Maternal HIV** (in resource rich countries),
- **Active TB** (until treatment has been given for 2 weeks, then breastfeeding is safe.

Active HSV lesion on nipple.

It is okay for a mother to breastfeed if she has Hepatitis B. Assuming the infant has received HepB Immunoglobulin, and hep B vaccine, the theoretical risk of hep B transmission through breastmilk is eliminated.

Maternal HIV in developing countries is not always a contradiction to breastfeeding.

---

[20] If a mother's HIV viral load is greater than 50 copies/mL near delivery, then the infant will receive three drug antiretroviral treatment and serial testing. The regimen always includes AZT.

HIV Manifestations

One presentation is a clinical description consistent with **Pneumocystis *jiroveci* (formerly known as *Pneumocystis carinii*[21] pneumonia (PCP))**. Remember that your buzzwords for PCP are **"ground glass appearance"** on chest x-ray and hypoxia.

Other manifestations of pediatric HIV infection include **unexplained fevers, generalized lymphadenopathy, hepatosplenomegaly, failure to thrive, persistent or recurrent oral and diaper candidiasis, recurrent diarrhea, parotitis, hepatitis, central nervous system (CNS) disease** (eg, hyperreflexia, hypertonia, floppiness, developmental delay), **lymphoid interstitial pneumonia (LIP), recurrent invasive bacterial infections**, and other **opportunistic infections** eg, viral and fungal.

The **recurrent bacterial infections** during the first year of life are due to an **increased** production of **nonfunctional antibodies**. The developmental delay is likely due to **encephalitis**.

> ## TMP-SMX
>
> Kids with HIV need to receive **trimethoprim-sulfamethoxazole prophylaxis** against PCP as soon as the diagnosis is made, and starting at 4 weeks of age for infants born to HIV-positive mothers. It may be stopped when their CD4 counts are stable.

Exposure

If somebody is going to **seroconvert**, it will occur during the **first 6 months of exposure. Testing** and **tracking** should be done **at time of exposure, 6 weeks, 12 weeks, and 6 months.** This would apply to any form of exposure, including child abuse.

The use of antiretroviral (ARV) agents is limited to needle sticks where there is a strong **likelihoood of HIV transmission**, but testing is always done.

Arbovirus

Arboviruses can cause encephalitis in the **late spring** and **early summer** months. The viruses are transmitted by **ticks** and **mosquitos**. Disease is best prevented by tick and mosquito control.

Arboviruses include:

- St. Louis encephalitis
- La Crosse encephalitis
- Western and Eastern equine encephalitis
- California encephalitis
- West Nile encephalitis
- Colorado tick fever
- Dengue fever

> ## Remember bug prevention
>
> Long pants, long sleeves, insect repellent, and mosquito netting.

---

[21] Somehow PJP doesn't have the same ring to it as PCP.

Typical presentation includes **fever, irritability, change in mental status**, and **headache**.

Enteroviruses (echo, coxsackie)

 High fever, rash, and perhaps signs of **viral meningitis in the summer**.

You will most likely be presented a patient younger than 5. They typically present with **vague symptoms** inducing **malaise, fever**, and **vomiting**. Additional findings would include **pharyngitis** and/or **conjunctivitis**.

 Neonates can develop severe disseminated infection if exposed at birth. This may be indistinguishable from sepsis due to a bacteria.

Enteroviruses can be identified **via PCR** within 24 hours.

Contact precautions are indicated.

Coxsackie B

Coxsackie B can result in myocarditis.

Myo "Coxsarditis"

Adenovirus

You are presented with a patient who has a combination of conjunctivitis, pharyngitis, and otitis media. They casually mention that this is during the summer, so your patient has likely been swimming.

The diversion is the expectation that you are to treat with antibiotics.

However, the correct answer will be supportive measures only. Remember that the combination of conjunctivitis and pharyngitis is often the way adenovirus is presented on the exam, especially if the patient presents during the summer.

 Adenovirus can cause **conjunctivitis, pharyngitis, adenopathy**, and even **intussusception**. Pay special attention if they mention **summer** in the question.

Enteric adenovirus and norovirus can cause **diarrhea**.

Adding Adeno!

Adenovirus can also cause severe pneumonia, hepatitis, and hemorrhagic cystitis but these are rare.

Rabies Virus

If you are bitten by a rabid board question about rabies, here are your guidelines.

Think of rabies if the animal is bat, raccoon, skunk, fox, coyote, or bobcat or any carnivore in a rabies-endemic area.

Rabies in small rodents (squirrels, hamsters, guinea pigs, gerbils, chipmunks, rats, and mice) and lagomorphs (rabbits, pikas, and hares) is rare.

Perhaps it is easier to remember the animals that can carry rabies in groups, to the tune of **"Frère Jacques"**.

> Foxy foxes
> 'coons and skunks
> 'possums and BATS!

A dog, cat, or ferret that appears healthy and has bitten a human should be **confined** and observed by a veterinarian for **10 days**. Human prophylaxis is given only if the animal develops signs of rabies.

Rabies prophylaxis (4-dose rabies vaccine and HRIG infiltrating the wound) should be started for a bite from an animal suspected of being rabid. It is important to consult with your local health department to assess the risk of rabies in the area, especially if the animal is unknown or cannot be contained and observed.

Bats can transmit rabies to humans even without known bites. Therefore, if you are presented with a patient who wakes up in a room with a bat, treatment for rabies would be indicated, even in the absence of a known bite taking place.

> **IG and vaccine**
>
> For hepatitis B and rabies, their respective vaccines should be given *at a body site other* than where the immunoglobulin was administered.

Once symptoms have developed, neither rabies vaccine nor Rabies Immune Globulin (RIG) improves the prognosis.

Helminthic Infections

Ascaris Lumbricoides (A Scary Lumbar-Coilee)

A. *lumbricoides* is **the most prevalent of all human intestinal nematodes (roundworms)**, with more than 1 billion people infected worldwide.[22]

Adult worms live in the lumen of the small intestine. Female worms produce approximately 200,000 eggs per day, which are excreted

> **Tricky Trichinella**
>
> *Trichinella spiralis* is another roundworm known as the "pork worm" because it is often found in undercooked pork. Besides pigs, it can be found in horses and bears (so it can be acquired through eating undercooked bear meat as well). Fill in your own Bulls get rich, Bears get rich, and pigs get slaughtered one liner here.
>
>
>
> Interestingly, it can cause severe eye pain.

---

[22] Don't worry, there's no way you're one of them.

in stool and must incubate in soil for 2 to 3 weeks for an embryo to become infectious. Infection follows **ingestion of eggs**, usually from **contaminated soil**.

Most infections with *Ascaris lumbricoides* are actually **asymptomatic**, although moderate to heavy infections may lead to **malnutrition** and **nonspecific gastrointestinal tract symptoms**. But on Boards, they will describe someone visiting or returning from a faraway place where ascaris is endemic, presenting with symptoms consistent with **obstruction or abdominal pain**.

Ascaris might also be found in a toddler with **pica** or is otherwise fond of **ingesting dirt**.

CASE STUDY

You might be presented with a child with signs of acute abdominal obstruction, with the implication of appendicitis or other surgical cause. Buried in the question will be a history of immigration from or travel to a tropical region.

THE DIVERSION

The diversion will be the signs of obstruction, which will be emphasized in the question, with the risk for parasitic infection barely mentioned or certainly not emphasized.

ANSWER REVEALED

If you read the question carefully, you will realize that the obstruction is due to *ascaris lumbricoides* infestation, and pick the correct diagnosis and treatment if there is a second followup question.

MNEMONIC

"A Scary Lumbar Coilee:" picture a scary coil tangled up in the lumbar spine causing abdominal pain and obstruction.

It can also cause a cough and transient pneumonitis as the larva move through the lungs (**Loeffler syndrome**).

TREATMENT

The following would be appropriate treatment for asymptomatic[23] or symptomatic *Ascaris lumbricoides*.

- **Albendazole**
- **Ivermectin**
- **Pyrantel pamoate**

---

[23] I know, you're saying "If it's asymptomatic, how would I know they have it? Refugees are screened for stool O&P prior to arrival and again on arrival to US. Therefore keep this in mind regarding questions in this clinical setting.

Necator americanus (hookworm)

BUZZWORDS

Infection is often **asymptomatic**, but chronic infection is associated with **hypochromic microcytic anemia, physical growth delay, deficits in cognition**, and **developmental delay**.

After walking barefoot on contaminated soil, initial skin penetration of larvae, can cause a **stinging or burning sensation** followed by **pruritus** and a **papulovesicular** rash that may persist for 1 to 2 weeks.

HOT TIP

Watch for questions that describe or show pictures of a serpigenous, red, itchy rash on the lower extremities.[24]

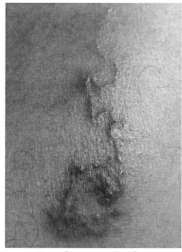

Serpigenous Lesion

Tapeworms (*Taeniasis* and *Cysticercosis*)

BUZZWORDS

Taeniasis caused via ingestion of larvae is often asymptomatic, but **nausea, diarrhea**, and **pain**, can occur. Tapeworm segments may sometimes be seen migrating from the anus or in feces.

Cysticercosis in humans is acquired by **ingesting eggs of the pork tapeworm (*T. solium*)**, through **fecal-oral contact** with a person harboring the adult tapeworm, or by **autoinfection**. The eggs hatch within their human host. The organisms travel throughout the body by way of blood vessels and lymphastics and cause cysts within tissues (even brain! eek!). So wash your hands and cook your meat. Eggs are found **only in human feces** because **humans are the obligate definitive host**.

Toxocariasis

BUZZWORDS

Toxocariasis is due to a roundworm that goes by the name of *Toxocara canis*, a Board classic. It can present with **GI symptoms** (hepatomegaly and abdominal pain) and **respiratory symptoms** (wheezing). This is because it **migrates everywhere**.

Exposure to dogs and cats is the risk factor and they might tip you off with **eosinophilia**. Look for the **preschooler who has been eating dirt**.

There are 3 clinical manifestations of toxocariasis:

1) **Visceral larval migrans** – these patients present with fever, hepatomegaly, and wheezing.

2) **Ocular larval migrans** – as you can guess, these patients present with visual disturbances.

3) **Covert toxocariasis** – patients with covert toxocariasis may present with GI symptoms as well as pruritus and a rash.

---

[24] Ulcerations with irregular margins that literally look like a serpent in the skin as seen in the photo.

CASE STUDY You could be presented with a patient with abdominal pain and wheezing, with the casual mention of exposure to cats and dogs thrown in to further throw you off. They casually note eosinophilia and bury hepatomegaly in the cascade of physical findings. They might note that the child was seen eating dirt while playing. You will be asked to make the diagnosis.

THE DIVERSION This is an excellent method to throw you off on several diversionary paths. The combination of abdominal pain and wheezing suggest pneumonia. The exposure to cats suggests asthma and allergies. The presence of eosinophilia further substantiates this diversionary path. Treatment and steps to address each of these issues will be there for your diversionary pleasure.

ANSWER REVEALED The key to separating the correct answer from the diversions will be the hepatomegaly, which again will be buried in the physical findings, but not to those who tease it out by noting on the scratch paper provided for you at the test center. If they mention the child eating dirt, it should also help pull you away from the diversionary choices and help you identify the correct answer: visceral larva migrans. If the question asks for the most appropriate test to make the diagnosis and the correct treatment, we have this information below.

HOT TIP **ELISA** is the test to diagnose VLM. In order to rule out other parasitic infections, **stool cultures** should still be done.

TREATMENT Treatment is with **albendazole** or **mebendazole**.

PERIL You can remember this with the "L" links. Longhaired cats and Licking dogs cause Larval disease in the Lungs and the Liver.

Enterobius vermicularis (pinworms)

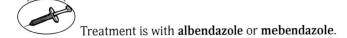

BUZZWORDS These children will present with **perianal** or **perivulvar itching**.

Egg transmission occurs by the **fecal-oral route** either directly or indirectly via **contaminated hands or fomites** such as shared toys, bedding, clothing, toilet seats, and baths. Reinfection is very common.

Diagnosis is made when **adult worms** are visualized in the perianal region, which is **best examined 2 to 3 hours after the child is asleep** or by the "scotch tape test".

TREATMENT Treatment is with **pyrantel pamoate** or **albendazole** at diagnosis and again 2 weeks later.

Fungal Infections

Candidiasis

The most likely cause of **a *mild* Candidal** infection is **antibiotic use**. With **chronic or systemic candidiasis, immunosuppression** is the most likely cause, e.g., bone marrow/organ transplant, malignancy, or corticosteroids.

To remember the most likely causes of **systemic candidiasis**, try the following (**YEAST**):

Y (Widespread immunosuppression) - Malignancy/ HIV
Extensive Burns
Antibiotics
Steroid use
Transplant recipients

Oral candidiasis in immunocompetent hosts is treated with oral nystatin suspension. **Fluconazole** or **itraconazole** can be used for immunocompromised patients. **IV amphotericin** is the treatment of choice for neonates with invasive disease.

Cryptococcosis

Cryptococcus neoformans is an encapsulated yeast. It causes both **pulmonary disease** as well as CNS disease **meningitis/meningoencephalitis**. The meningitis is often indolent. **It is most commonly associated with AIDS infection.**

Even though in the real world antigen testing is the rule, this is the boards' world. Therefore they could show you a picture of an organism with India ink stain. If they do, think cryptococcus.

Look for a history of exposure to **bird droppings (e.g., pigeons)**.

Picture someone **stuck with a bunch of pigeons** in a **giant CRYPT**. There is no air so he can't breathe and he is getting a **headache** so severe it feels like **meningitis**.

Amphotericin B, in combination with **oral flucytosine or fluconazole**, is effective.

Coccidioidomycosis

These patients present with **vague influenza-like symptoms including fever, night sweats, headaches, chest pains and muscle aches**. They often will tip you off by mentioning recent travel to **California, Arizona, or Texas**. Symptoms develop within a month of exposure.

CAT: California, Arizona, Texas. Change the disease name to **CAT CITY –oido-Mycosis** and you'll have this memorized.

Treatment is with **amphotericin B, fluconazole, or itraconazole**.

Aspergillosis

Think of **aspergillosis** when they present an **asthmatic with worsening symptoms despite treatment**. There are increased **eosinophils** and **infiltrates** noted on CXR. Invasive aspergillosis usually occurs in immunocompromised patients.

Diagnosis is made by **positive serum galactomannan**, which is an antigen in the Aspergillus cell wall.

Voriconazole is the drug of choice for invasive aspergillosis, except in neonates, for whom **amphotericin B** in high doses is recommended.

Histoplasmosis

Histoplasmosis is found throughout the Ohio, Missouri, and Mississippi river valleys. Most people infected remain asymptomatic, and those who get sick are usually immunocompromised.

They will describe general **influenza-like symptoms**. Hilar or mediastinal lymphadenopathy may be seen on chest x-ray. **Hepatosplenomegaly** in the clinical description is the key to choosing this as the correct answer.

Like crypto, histoplasmosis is also obtained from **bird droppings**. Histo patients may also have a history of cave exploring which is referred to as "spelunking".

Immunocompetent children with uncomplicated disease only **require supportive care**.

For **disseminated disease**, especially in immunocompromised patients, **amphotericin B** is recommended. If necessary, **fluconazole** would be the most appropriate azole. Yes! We agree the term "azole" does sound funny!

> ## Dropping like birds
>
> Both histoplasmosis and cryptococcosis are associated with bird droppings.
>
> **C**rypto hurts your **C**ranium (indolent meningitis).
>
> **H**isto gives you **H**epatosplenomegaly.

Modes of Transmission

You will be expected to be familiar with the mode of transmission of a variety of infectious agents, as well as the precautions necessary to prevent spread.

Droplet Transmission

Infections spread by droplet transmission, primarily by **sneezing** and **coughing**. These do not remain suspended for prolonged periods of time. Therefore, the only precautions are **covering your mouth** when sneezing or coughing, or in the hospital, wear a mask.[25] They do not require any special air ventilation systems to prevent spread.

Examples of organisms transmitted by droplet transmission include **mumps, rubella, plague, meningococcus, parvovirus, influenza,** and **pertussis**.

Airborne Transmission

These are organisms that can remain airborne for prolonged periods of time. Therefore they can spread through the hospital ventilation system. **Specialized masks (N95)** and **special air handling units** are needed to prevent spread.

Examples include **aspergillosis, tuberculosis, measles, varicella,** and **disseminated zoster.**

Picture an **ATM** as a hospital air conditioning system delivering **V**s and **Z**s as droplets to remember that the hospital ventilation system can spread varicella and zoster.

Legionella pneumophila, Candida parapsilosis, and *Pseudomonas aeruginosa* ironically do not spread through the hospital ventilation system and therefore only require standard precautions.

Contact Transmission

Contact precautions involve gown and glove with hand washing preceding and following gowning and gloving.

Infections transmitted via contact include *S. aureus, herpes*, RSV, metapneumovirus, poliovirus, Salmonella, Smallpox, Cholera, and Varicella.

Multidrug resistant organisms are also handled with contact precautions, as are wound drainage and diarrhea patients.

Universal Precautions

Universal precautions are routine practices that should be followed by all health care workers with all patients.

---

[25] At the time of this printing, everyone is wearing a mask everywhere due to COVID19. We are hoping that this will no longer be the case in very short order !

The cornerstone of Universal Precautions is **good handwashing**.

Coronavirus

2020: The year which shall not be named brought us the terms covid-19, MIS-C, and social distancing. If you are as tired as we are about it, you can skip this section. There are so many unknowns with coronavirus, its sequelae, and management. Therefore, it will hopefully not appear on the exam any time soon. We do, of course, feel compelled to include some information about it here, just in case .

Covid-19, SARS-CoV2, Corona, The Rona

The newest member of the SARS family, a single-stranded RNA virus, has been found to cause a wide array of disease. This has ranged from upper respiratory infection symptoms, diffuse pneumonia, anosmia, ageusia, diarrhea, and numerous others. We are learning more and more about this disease each day and the considerable variability in its management once again makes it an unlikely topic of the boards.

As of this printing the vaccine has not been approved for children younger than 12.

For your learning pleasure we will provide the following:

> **Diagnostics**: PCR testing for acute disease is the current gold standard.
> **Treatment** may include antivirals, steroids, and/or mono- or poly-clonal antibodies.

MIS-C: Multisystem Inflammatory Syndrome of Children

Not long after SARS-CoV2 became widespread, pediatric patients began presenting with a hyperinflammatory syndrome now referred to as MIS-C. This disease entity has a specific case definition provided by the CDC which includes several days of fever, known covid exposure or positivity, and two or more organ system involvement.

Some of these kids may have physical exam findings **similar to Kawasaki Disease** (conjunctivitis, rash, lymphadenopathy, strawberry tongue), while others may be in florid shock and require vasopressors.

Either way treatment involves IVIG. Severe/refractory cases may require additional immunomodulatory treatments.

For the most up-to-date recommendations on management of Covid-19 and MIS-C, see information from the CDC and IDSA. It is not likely to be tested but it is definitely possible.

Chapter 21

Is That an Orchidometer in Your Pocket?: Endocrinology

Sexual Differentiation

In order to better understand the breakdown in sexual differentiation, it is worthwhile to first review normal sexual development and differentiation, and point out potentially confusing concepts now rather than later.

This is important, as there are many questions on the exam covering this subject.

HOT TIP

Know that, **the default pattern** of differentiation of the genital system is **toward phenotypic "femaleness,"** unless the system is dominated by the influence of androgens and müllerian inhibiting factor, aka Anti-mullerian hormone.

- The **presence of androgens** is responsible for the formation of male external genitals
- The **presence of müllerian inhibiting factor** results in the regression of female internal duct structures

Male Pubertal Development

The sequence of male pubertal development is

Testicular growth → Pubarche → Penile growth → Peak height velocity

- The **first sign of pubertal development in males is testicular enlargement**, with testicular length greater than 2.5 cm (greater than 4 ml in volume) indicating the onset of puberty and the end of childhood as the boy once knew it.

Testicular enlargement before age 9 in boys is considered abnormal.

HOT TIP

Pubic hair development and penis enlargement **in the absence of testicular enlargement** suggests androgen stimulation **from outside the gonadal area.**

Gynecomastia

If they describe gynecomastia in a male in early puberty or asymmetric breasts in a female, the choice will usually be "normal; only **reassurance** is necessary." However, gynecomastia is also associated with **Klinefelter syndrome 47, XXY**, so watch for other features of Klinefelter in the history.

PERIL

Gynecomastia before puberty, or in late puberty, or after puberty should be investigated and may be due to to medications such as **ketoconazole. Galactorrhea** may be due to **marijuana use**. If this does not work as a deterrent for male teens not to smoke pot, I don't know what will.

Female Pubertal Development

The sequence of female pubertal development is

Breast Budding (thelarche) ➜ Pubarche ➜ Peak height velocity ➜ Menarche

- Puberty may begin as young as age 8 in females; prior to that is considered abnormal

Delayed Puberty

Puberty is defined as delayed if there are no pubertal signs **by age 14 in boys** or **by age 13 in girls**.

> **How late is too late?**
>
> In general, menarche is considered delayed if has not occurred by age 16, or 3 years after thelarche.

The most likely cause of delayed puberty in boys is constitutional delay of puberty. In constitutional delay of growth and puberty, the chronologic age is higher than the bone age.

Girls may also have constitutional delay of puberty, but **functional gonadotropin deficiency**, as in anorexia nervosa, is also common. It is also important to consider **primary ovarian failure**, as in Turner Syndrome 45, XO.

Delayed puberty has various **psychosocial effects on teens**, boys more than girls. Many feel inadequate and report that their lack of development has affected their success either at work, at school, or socially.

These children should be **evaluated by an endocrinologist**. Psychosocial difficulties in boys with constitutional delay of puberty are an indication for **IM testosterone**. Girls are treated with **estrogen** (oral or transdermal); higher doses are required for those girls with Turner Syndrome. This will initiate puberty and with it, the pubertal growth spurt.

Premature Adrenarche

The presence of **androgenic sexual characteristics** (axillary hair, pubic hair, acne, and/ or adult body odor) without estrogenic sexual characteristics (breast development and menarche) and without the growth spurt of puberty, is termed **premature adrenarche**.

> **Premature NON Puberty**
>
>
> Premature adrenarche and premature thelarche are by definition benign conditions that DO NOT represent true precocious (central) puberty. The bone age must NOT be advanced more than one year. If the bone age is advanced, you must consider other causes for the symptoms.

This would correlate with **elevated serum dehydroepiandrosterone (DHEA)** and **dehydroepiandrosterone-sulfate (DHEA-S) levels.**[1] It would also correlate with **low concentrations of testosterone.**

However, adrenarche can also be caused by **exogenous androgen** or an **endogenous androgen-secreting tumor**. It can also be caused by **late-onset congenital adrenal hyperplasia**.

Premature adrenarche could be an early sign of **polycystic ovary syndrome** in adolescent girls.

---

[1] DHEA-S is made by the adrenal gland and is a marker of adrenal androgen production.

Premature Thelarche

Premature thelarche is **breast development in girls younger than 8 in the absence of other sexual characteristics**.

Although usually benign and due to premature activation of the hypothalamic-pituitary axis, premature thelarche could also be due to exogenous estrogen.

Sources of **exogenous sex steroids** could be hinted at in the question, including **skin preparations, oral contraceptive medication exposure, weight lifting steroids,** and **plant-based phytoestrogens**. You must also consider estrogen-producing tumors.

Central "True" Precocious Puberty

When development of secondary sexual characteristics are accompanied by **acceleration in linear growth** (ie. crossing percentiles) or **advanced bone age**, this is indicative of true central puberty. When this true central puberty starts before age 9 in boys and before age 8 in girls, it is defined as precocious.

The only significant consequence of true precocious puberty is **short adult height**.

HCG Oh Boy !

HOT TIP

Tumors producing HCG can cause pubertal change in boys, but not in girls. Girls require LH and FSH to stimulate ovarian estrogen production.

Benign Premature Thelarche

DEFINITION

Benign premature thelarche, as the name implies, is a relatively benign finding, usually in infants/ toddlers but resolves by age 4.

In 10% of the cases, true central precocious puberty will develop later on. In girls there is an increased risk for developing **ovarian hyperandrogenism (PCOS)**.

Crazy CAL

In cases of precocious puberty, watch for cafe-au-lait spots with jagged borders suggestive of McCune Albright syndrome.

Search from Top to Bottom

It is always good to think anatomically from top to bottom when working up precocious puberty. This systematic approach can make this potentially complex topic a quick slam-dunk.

Top/Central

Terms like "optic fundus abnormal" and "visual field deficits" tip you off to a CNS lesion, possibly a pituitary mass.

Bottom/Abdominal

For **androgenic**, look for descriptions like "acne", "facial and axillary hair" and "muscle bulk" (in boys). For **estrogenic**, look for a change in vaginal color and more prominent labia minora.

The Friendly Radiologist

HOT TIP

Ultrasound can help in the investigation of adrenal or ovarian masses. If presented with androgenic symptoms - look at the adrenals. If presented with premature breast development - look at the ovaries.

Bone age x-rays are helpful in drawing a comparison between bone age and chronological age.

Brain MRI will find many causes of central precocious puberty (true precocious puberty) including:

- Hamartomas
- Hydrocephalus
- Arachnoid or ventricular cysts
- Meningitis
- Encephalitis
- Neoplasms
- CNS trauma

Central precocious puberty is often idiopathic in girls, but boys are significantly more likely to have CNS pathology, so they routinely need CNS imaging.

The Friendly Lab

LH, FSH, and adrenal steroids will help differentiate peripheral from central disorders.

If caught early enough, one possible treatment involves very expensive injections of the **GnRH agonist leuprolide** to arrest the progression. This is more often recommended in male patients, those younger than 6, those with very rapidly advancing symptoms, and those with psychosocial disturbances.

Ambiguous Genitalia (What's in an Organ?)

Androgen Insensitivity Syndrome[2]

Recall from earlier in this chapter, androgens are required for male genitalia development. In these individuals their end-organs do not recognize the hormones in question resulting in phenotypically female external genitalia. These are **genetic males** with **end organ insensitivity to androgens** resulting in

1) the inability to develop male external genitalia

2) a blind-ending vagina and no uterus.

On the outside, there is nothing ambiguous about the genitalia. They are **perfectly normal looking females** BUT they are **genetically male (XY)**.

Ironically, this is an X-linked disorder (transmitted from mother to son who looks like a daughter).

True Hermaphroditism

True hermaphroditism (both ovarian and testicular tissue) is extremely rare, even on the Boards, and thus it is unlikely to be the correct answer.

Panhypopituitarism

Panhypopituitarism is a deficit in all hormones produced by the pituitary gland.

It can present as **micro-penis**, and when it does, **hypoglycemia** will also be included in the description.

You will then want to check **ALL pituitary hormones**.

Panhypopit can be part of the following syndromes: **Prader-Willi** (slick Willy), **Kallmann** (poor sense of smell), or **septo-optic dysplasia**.

---

[2] Testicular Feminization Syndrome was the previous name of Androgen Insensitivity Syndrome, but not the current preferred term.

These girls may sometimes present with **inguinal masses**, which turn out to be testes.

These patients tend to present one of two ways:

1. a prenatal amnio says baby is XY but is born a girl or

2. a teenaged girl has primary amenorrhea and the workup reveals no uterus or ovaries and then of course, the karyoptype reveals the XY factor.

Müllerian inhibiting factor IS produced by the Y chromosome; therefore, no uterus or ovaries develop, which is the reason for the vagina ending in a blind pouch.

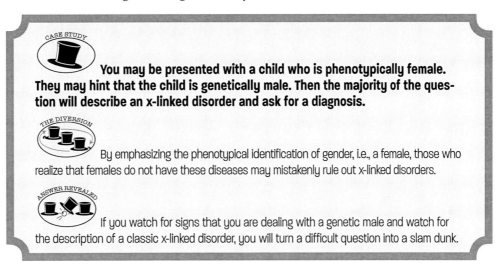

You may be presented with a child who is phenotypically female. They may hint that the child is genetically male. Then the majority of the question will describe an x-linked disorder and ask for a diagnosis.

By emphasizing the phenotypical identification of gender, i.e., a female, those who realize that females do not have these diseases may mistakenly rule out x-linked disorders.

If you watch for signs that you are dealing with a genetic male and watch for the description of a classic x-linked disorder, you will turn a difficult question into a slam dunk.

Adrenal Disorders

The adrenals can simply stop functioning on their own (primary), or shut down if they are not receiving the signal from the pituitary gland (secondary).[3]

The most common cause of adrenal insufficiency in infants is congenital adrenal hyperplasia, and the rest are usually autoimmune, which is the primary cause in adults.

Congenital Adrenal Hyperplasia (CAH)

It's hypERplasia. Think of this as a super active adrenal which will produce plenty of DHEA and testosterone (leading to virilization in females).

Congenital Adrenal Hyperplasia will often[4] present in the **newborn period** with a **shocky/septic picture**.

• With **males**, there will be **no ambiguous genitalia,** but there could be **excessive scrotal pigmentation**, so look for this in the question. Since there may be no physical signs, the newborn screen will be crucial in identifying the males, before they present in crisis.

---

[3] The signal coming from the pituitary is ACTH.
[4] But not always.

- With **females,** the increased androgens will probably lead to ambiguous genitalia, but a big clue will be no palpable testes. This is why bilateral undescended testes at birth always need an evaluation prior to discharge.

They will not come right out and hit you over the head with a hammer and say **ambiguous genitalia**. Instead they will note **posterior labial adhesions** and **clitoral hypertrophy**.

Not for Newborns Only

> **CASE STUDY** **You are presented with a patient with growth delay. They point out that the patient "has received no medical care to date." They casually point out a recent history of hirsutism and amenorrhea. They ask for the most likely underlying condition.**
>
> **THE DIVERSION** The diversion here is their noting that the child has received no medical care to date. This will set you away from what is usually seen as a congenital condition causing growth delay.
>
> **ANSWER REVEALED** The correct answer will be congenital adrenal hyperplasia. This is an autosomal recessive disease. Remember that congenital adrenal hyperplasia can present beyond the newborn period. Therefore, do not rule this out just because they note that the child has required no medical intervention to date. There is also a *late-onset form of congenital adrenal hyperplasia* that should be considered as a possible cause of growth delay.

And now you're having flash backs to the huge adrenal hormone production pathway from physiology and step 1. To simplify: aldosterone, cortisol, and DHEA (and testosterone) are the final products of this pathway. A missing enzyme at any junction causes shunting of the pathway into overproduction of the other hormones.

Another Traffic Report

Congenital adrenal hyperplasia (CAH) can be due to **cortisol production being blocked** along the endocrine highway. Like any highway with a bottleneck blockage, traffic builds up along the inroad that feeds it. The endocrine highway is no different.

21-Hydroxylase is needed to produce both **aldosterone** and **cortisol**. When blocked, production of steroids leading up to the block is increased, just like cars behind a traffic jam stack up.

HOT TIP This is the reason for the **increased levels of testosterone** resulting in virilization.

> ### Gel Should Ring a Bell!
>
> **PERIL** Watch for their mentioning a history of family members taking **prescribed testosterone gels** for hypogonadism. If precautions are not taken, this can be absorbed by close contacts, resulting in **virilization** in both males and females.

You are presented with labs that will imply other "salt-wasting disorders,"and the question may mention a family history of early death. Buried in the description will be the implication of ambiguous genitalia.

The implication and diversion is a diagnosis of cystic fibrosis, (CF) because CF has an increased amount of sodium present in sweat, resulting in decreased serum sodium, and therefore, in "salt wasting."

Yes, cystic fibrosis is another salt waster. However, CF does not have anything to do with ambiguous genitalia, which all but rules out CF for the purpose of the exam.

Labs

While there are different varieties and flavors, the most common cause of CAH is **21-hydroxylase deficiency**. There is also a "salt wasting" variety that will present with **hyperkalemia** and **hyponatremia**.

Remember, with 21-hydroxylase deficiency, **17-hydroxyprogesterone levels are elevated**[5] and this is the first-line diagnostic test for CAH.

Screening for CAH

Newborn screening for CAH is done in all 50 states via the **17-hydroxyprogesterone assay**.

This 17-HP steroid precursor builds up in the most common form of CAH (over 90% are due to 21 hydroxylase deficiency).

If elevated, **repeating the test** is the next step.

If the repeat is positive, then **measurement of serum electrolytes and urinary sodium/potassium excretion** would be the next step.

Treating CAH

Pharmacological treatment of congenital CAH consists of **dextrose containing isotonic fluids**, **mineralocorticoids** (like fludrocortisone) and high doses of **corticosteroids** (IV hydrocortisone).

---

[5] The precursor just before the deficient enzyme.

Adrenal Crisis

The two main hormones secreted by the adrenal glands are **aldosterone**, which helps control the amount of salt and fluid in the body, and **cortisol**, which helps control how the body uses sugar and how it responds to stress.

Excess glucocorticoid from any source (endogenous or exogenous) can lead to suppression of the hypothalamic-pituitary-adrenal axis and to adrenal crisis in times of stress.

An **adrenal crisis** is most likely to occur in **primary adrenal deficiency** because of the associated mineralocorticoid deficiency and salt loss. Adrenal crisis is a medical emergency that may lead to **shock and death** if not recognized and treated promptly.

Symptoms of adrenal crisis are sudden and vague, including **anorexia, vomiting, abdominal pain, weakness, fever, fatigue, weight loss, lethargy, hypotension, confusion, and coma.** Electrolyte abnormalities include **hypoglycemia, hyponatremia "salt-wasting", hypercalcemia, and hyperkalemia, and possibly elevated renal and hepatic tests.**

First, give **20 mL/kg of NS IV over one hour, followed by isotonic fluids at 2x maintenance. Then, add IV hydrocortisone.** Correct hypoglycemia as needed. Finally, after the crisis has been treated, add **glucocorticoid replacement.**

Primary Adrenal Deficiency

The adrenals stop working for a variety of reasons, ranging from **autoimmune disease** to **infection** to the always popular **idiopathic.**[6]

When the adrenals stop functioning, the message to the brain is "pour out ACTH by the bucketful."

The increased ACTH levels explain the **hyperpigmentation.**[7] And no matter how much ACTH you pour out, aldosterone isn't produced, and **salt wasting, hyperkalemia** and **hyponatremia** are seen. **Fatigue and weight loss** are other signs.

Patients with adrenal deficiency are usually **maintained on fludrocortisone** for the mineralocorticoid replacement, and **hydrocortisone** for the glucocorticoid replacement.

These patients will need stress (extra) doses of steroids during times of surgery, illness, strenuous exercise, or other significant stressors (like taking the Boards).

Addison disease is usually an **autoimmune disorder.** Patients with Addison disease are also at risk for other endocrine disorders, including diabetes, ovarian failure, and hypothyroidism.

Secondary Adrenal Deficiency

With secondary adrenal deficiency, there is **no problem with the adrenal gland itself.** The problem is with the organ it takes orders from, the pituitary, which is "asleep at the wheel."

---

[6] Latin for "we really don't know".
[7] The elevated ACTH stimulates melanin production.

COIN FLIP

The pituitary makes ACTH. As they say, "No squirt, no ACTH, no cortisol service," or something like that. **In this case, ACTH levels are low.** With primary adrenal deficiency, ACTH levels are high.

BUZZWORDS

Since there is normal aldosterone, there is **no hyperkalemia, hyponatremia, or salt wasting** here. There is also **no hyper-pigmentation** because there is no excess ACTH.

HOT TIP

Remember, CRH (corticotropin releasing hormone) stimulates the pituitary to release ACTH. CRH can be used to distinguish pituitary disorders from hypothalamic failure in secondary adrenal deficiency.

The **cosyntropin[8] stimulation test (ACTH stimulation test)** is used to test the adrenals, and results in no rise in cortisol levels in primary adrenal deficiency (since the adrenals are "broken" and can't respond). If you have secondary disease, then the adrenals usually have normal cortisol stores, and cortisol will be released during the test.

> ### Adrenal Deficiency due to Medication Withdrawal
>
> Patients who abruptly stop taking adrenocorticoid or glucocorticoid medications can present with signs of adrenal deficiency, including **muscle weakness**, as well as decreased cardiac function (with **increased pulse** and **decreased blood pressure**).
>
> **HOT TIP**
>
> *Electrolyte imbalance would not be seen in this case.*

BUZZWORDS

Look for clues in the question of **midline defects**, such as cleft lip and/or palate. This will be their way of telling you the problem is probably in the **pituitary** and, therefore, **secondary adrenal deficiency**.

> **CASE STUDY**
>
> **You are presented with a patient who is treated chronically for adrenal deficiency with oral mineralocorticoid and hydrocortisone. The patient will either be going for surgery or will have an acute febrile illness, including vomiting and you will be asked how to adjust the medications.**
>
> **THE DIVERSION**
>
> You will be presented with several diversionary choices including IV/ IM mineralocorticoid and a variety of oral medication variations including doubling or tripling the usual oral dose.
>
> **ANSWER REVEALED**
>
> Since there is no such thing as a parenteral mineralocorticoid, that choice will always be wrong. In the context of a patient who is vomiting or is going in for surgery, they should be given **parenteral hydrocortisone**, typically hydrocortisone hemisuccinate.

Cushing Syndrome (CS)

DEFINITION

Cushing syndrome refers to glucocorticoid excess of any origin. **Cushing disease** specifically refers to the excessive production of corticotropin by the pituitary gland, which leads to excess cortisol production by the adrenal gland.

---

[8] Synthetic corticotropin (ACTH 1-24).

Classic features of Cushing syndrome include **acne, purple striae, hirsutism, virilization,** and **buffalo hump**. In children, Cushing almost always leads to **increased BMI with growth arrest** (ie. gain in weight without gain in height).

The growth arrest is important if they present you with an obese child and ask you for the most likely diagnosis. Obesity due to increased caloric intake leads to both gain in weight and gain in height. In addition, children with Cushing will have **delayed bone age**, while children with non-Cushing obesity will have normal to advanced bone age.

The most common cause of Cushing syndrome, in both children and adults, is exogenous, specifically the **chronic use of topical, inhaled, or oral corticosteroids**. The treatment in this case would be cessation of the medication.

Laboratory tests to confirm excess cortisol production, either endogenous or exogenous:

- **24-hour urinary free cortisol excretion** is the gold standard for confirming hypercortisolism.
- **Midnight sleeping plasma cortisol level** has the greatest sensitivity of all tests for CS in children.
- **Dexamethasone suppresion tests** should lead to undetectable plasma cortisol levels after dexamethasone administration (as the test implies).

In cases of Cushing syndrome from adrenal tumors, levels of morning corticotropin would be undetectable. The next step would be adrenal CT or MRI to try to locate the tumor.

If morning corticotropin levels are elevated, pituitary MRI should be performed.

> **Steroid side effects**
>
> Side effects of chronic corticosteroid use include weight gain, growth arrest in children, sleep issues, mood disturbance, osteoporosis, myopathy, immunosuppression, hyperglycemia, acne, cataracts, hypertension, gastritis, and peptic ulcer disease.

> *HOT TIP*
>
> Excess glucocorticoids from any source (endogenous or exogenous) and lead to short stature.

> *HOT TIP*
>
> Cushing syndrome in infants is often caused by **McCune Albright syndrome.**

Langerhans Cell Histiocytosis (LCH)

This presents as a classic triad of:

1. Diabetes Insipidus
2. Exophthalmos
3. Lytic bone lesions
4. Recurrent otitis media

This is a posterior pituitary disease.

The posterior pituitary is only responsible for ADH and oxytocin. All the other hormones are the product of the anterior pituitary.

Stature

The key to getting all these right on the Boards will be know the difference in the growth curves due to different causes. We will walk you right through it.

 Height velocity, BMI, weight-for-length ratio, and bone age will be terms to become intimately familiar with to breeze through this section of the test. They will help identify the growth pattern presented.

Peak Growth

❏ **Prior to Puberty:** 5-6 cm/year and there is a slight but significant deceleration in height growth just before puberty.

❏ **During Puberty** There will be a gradual increase in growth rate. Peak growth velocity reaches its maximum **around SMR 3 in both boys and girls**. Peak growth in boys occurs roughly 2 years after girls, as all middle school boys well know.

In girls, peak growth velocity occurs ~1.5 years before menarche at SMR 3. Once girls have reached menarche, they are within 6-8 cm of their adult height.

Maturing earlier usually means a shorter adult height. For boys, that may mean being the bigger, tougher kid in class, only to be shorter than average later in life. For girls, it will mean being taller than even most of the boys at first.

Let's look at some of the specific causes of short stature.

Growth Hormone Deficiency (GHD)

Intuitively, growth hormone deficiency is the easiest cause to think of, but it is rarely the cause of short stature on the Boards.

When you are presented with short stature, look for clues for other causes (including hypothyroidism, syndromes,[9] chronic illness (like IBD or renal disease), familial short stature, or constitutional short stature).

There are two correct scenarios for GHD: One would be a child with **headaches** and **growth attenuation** due to a space-occupying lesion. The other would be **congenital GHD**.

Congenital growth hormone deficiency usually presents during infancy (typically around 6-12 months of age), with severe growth failure. The triad of GHD includes **micropenis, hypoglycemia,** and **short stature.** Other clues would include **septo-optic dysplasia, breech presentation, and prolonged jaundice.**

Bone age may be significantly delayed.

> ### Aging Your Bones
>
> You will not be required to actually recognize a bone age by looking at it. That is what they have radiologists in dark rooms with flashlights, dictaphones and disco balls for. However, on the exam, they will tell you what the bone age is, usually in comparison to height and chronological age.

> ### Cranial Irradiation and Growth Attenuation
>
> Cranial irradiation can impact pituitary hormone secretion, including growth hormone secretion.
>
> It is important to monitor for growth hormone deficiency in children receiving cranial irradiation therapy. This could be worth a point on the exam.

---

[9] Examples would be Hurlers, Hunters, and Turner syndrome.

CASE STUDY

You are presented with a 4 year old child who was at the 50th percentile for both height and weight at birth. She is now at the 25th percentile for weight, but her height is below the 5th percentile. There is no family history of short stature. Physical exam is otherwise non-contributory. What is the cause of the short stature?

THE DIVERSION

You will be given lots of diversionary choices such as **poor nutrition, constitutional growth delay, or neglect.**

ANSWER REVEALED

This time, the choice you might ignore (because it would be the obvious choice to even those who have no medical training) would be right. In this case, the masses would have picked **growth hormone deficiency** correctly and you, the well-trained pediatrician that you are, would have picked the wrong answer.

Constitutional growth delay would be ruled out by their telling you the parents have no significant history. The weight is at a reasonable 25th percentile, so Inadequate nutrition is not a factor. If she went from the 50th percentile for height down to less than the 5th percentile, then she has not tripled her height or grown 5 cm/year. As noted above, this would most likely be due to growth hormone deficiency. Hypothyroidism could also be correct if it were one of the choices.

HOT TIP

Children and adolescents with acquired GH deficiency should undergo CNS imaging and evaluation for other pituitary hormone deficiencies.

Nutrition Deficiency

TAKE HOME MESSAGE

These children would be underweight as well as underheight as evidence of chronic malnutrition. Bone age would be normal.

CASE STUDY

You are presented with a child with growth delay who is otherwise asymptomatic. You are then asked for the most likely cause or the next step to establish a diagnosis.

THE DIVERSION

Among the choices you will be presented with will be Crohn's disease. However, since you have been told that the child is asymptomatic, you may be diverted into crossing out Crohn's disease among the choices.

ANSWER REVEALED

Crohn's disease can result in growth delay, which can precede the GI symptoms. Therefore, *ordering an ESR* could be the correct answer. Similarly, an elevated ESR in the lab values could be your clue in the question, and the correct answer will be Crohn's disease.

Constitutional Delay (Late Bloomers)

This is the classic "late bloomer." It is **more common in males**.

Typically they will describe a family history of a similar growth pattern in other family members with late menarche in females and late age to start shaving in males.

- The **growth curve** may show a **decrease in growth rate**, usually in **early teen years. Delayed onset of puberty** and **bone age below chronological age** is the rule.
- There is a later onset of increased growth velocity. The growth rate may accelerate at around age 16 years.

If the bone age is Lagging, this Late Bloomer has consitutional growth delay.

Bone age is below (younger than) chronological age (think of the gap as the "bud" for the later bloomer to blossom in the spring). In addition to height, sexual development also lags behind.

If they ask for the best way to assess for growth delay, the answer is to compare **bone age** to chronological age. A look at family history is also important. Remember, the least invasive and less exotic the answer, the more likely it is to be correct.

Growth velocity may be blunted in early adolescence. However, when this is preceded by poor weight gain, it is abnormal and a workup may be warranted. Celiac disease is an example of a cause which may be distinguished from constitutional growth delay through lab studies.

> **CASE STUDY**
>
> You are presented with a 15-year-old boy who is short for his age, with a low SMR. His growth velocity is normal. The family notes that the father had the same "problem" and received "shots." You are asked to pick the most appropriate intervention at this time.
>
> **THE DIVERSION**
>
> The father receiving IM shots is the diversion.
>
> **ANSWER REVEALED**
>
> The correct answer would be to reassure and wait, since the correct diagnosis would be constitutional growth delay. The fact that the father received IM shots tells you nothing, especially if it's in quotes. If they note a history of maternal delayed onset of menarche, this too is associated with constitutional growth delay in both boys and girls.

Familial Short Stature
(Just Plain Short/Genetic Short Stature)

Sometimes short kids are just kids who are from "short stock," and will grow up to be short adults. They will start to decelerate at 6-18 months of age to around or below the 5th percentile for height, with a **bone age equal to chronological age.** Growth velocity will be normal. They may even mention that the parents are short as well.[10]

> ### Large Apples Fall from Large Trees
>
> For a rough estimate of mid-parental height (MPH), (ie. genetic potential"):
>
> - First add the parents heights in inches. If they present this data to you in centimeters, you will use 13 instead of 5 in the following equations.
> - Then "correct" by adding 5 in to mother's HT if your patient is a boy and subtracting 5 in from father's HT if your patient is a girl.
> - Divide by 2 (for the average).
> - "Target" height will be +/- 2 inches from this result.

CASE STUDY

You are presented with a patient whose parents want to know his potential height. They will present you with the parents' heights, but buried in the question will be an implication that one or both of the parents were malnourished growing up.

THE DIVERSION

The diversion here is their providing you with the parents' height. You will be diverted away from factoring in the parents' failure to reach their genetic potential due to malnourishment.

ANSWER REVEALED

The correct answer will be that the child will likely be taller than the parents, assuming the child is receiving adequate nutrition.

Coming Up Short

Turner syndrome (45, XO)

Turner syndrome is an example of a syndrome that might not become evident until puberty.

If they drop hints like **pedal edema, webbed neck, shield-like chest,** or **scant breast tissue,** consider a **karyotype** as part of the workup to rule out Turner syndrome.

HOT TIP

Consider Turner syndrome in **any short female** even if they do not mention any of the phenotypic hints above.

---

[10] More than likely, they will simply tell you the parents' height and let you figure out that they are short.

Turner syndrome patients are often **treated with growth hormone**.

Achondroplasia

Your clue is that the short stature is **not proportionate**.

Premature Puberty

The increased androgens result in **premature closure of the growth plates**.

Hypothyroidism

With hypothyroidism, they will be **short AND overweight**, but it won't be described that way.

Children will have **delayed bone age**, so they could describe an 11-year-old with height consistent with a 9-year-old, and a bone age of a 7-year-old.

They may even drop in some hidden clues consistent with hypothyroidism, such as **cold intolerance, constipation, dry skin, or myxedema**.[11]

Tall Stature

Tall stature is defined as above the 97th PCT for the reference population.

 If you are presented with a child who is "tall" for age, and are asked for the most important determinant for ultimate adult height, the answer will be **sexual maturity rating**. A **bone age** x-ray could be used to predict adult height. This will help determine how much additional growth is left.

Klinefelter Syndrome (47 XXY)

While these kids will appear **physically normal at birth**, eventually they will be tall. In addition to tall stature, they could have **learning disabilities** and **small testicles. Gynecomastia and delayed puberty** may be seen.

Marfan Syndrome

One of the main features is a **cardiac defect**, including **aortic aneurysm**. These individuals are at risk for **sudden death**.

---

[11] Relatively "hard edema" of the subcutaneous tissue.

Patients with Marfan syndrome have **disproportionately long arms** (arm span to height ratio >1.05) and significantly long tapering fingers described as **arachnodactyly**, or spider fingers.

Soto's Syndrome

Besides tall stature, they will likely also decribe **macrocephaly** as well as **cognitive deficits**. This would most likely be presented in the context of **parents who are not tall**.

High Caloric Intake

Here they will be **tall**, often **overweight** and have **normal to advanced bone age**.[12]

- Children with **exogenous obesity** tend to be **tall**.

- Children with **endogenous obesity** secondary to endocrine disorders, on the other hand, tend to be **short**.

Thyroid Disorders

Congenital Hypothyroidism

Neonatal screening thyroid tests are now performed routinely, making untreated hypothyroidism a rare disorder in real life, except on the Boards.

Thyroid dysgenesis is the most common cause of congenital hypothyroidism in the United States. It occurs sporadically. More than 95% of hypothyroid infants have **no clinical manifestations at birth**. Treatment should be initiated by 2 weeks of age, which is why newborn screening is so important. Symptoms develop over time.

When they are symptomatic, watch for non-specific findings like **poor feeding** and **prolonged jaundice**, as well as **constipation**, **hypotonia**, **hoarse cry**, **large tongue** (also known as macroglossia), **umbilical hernia**, and **large anterior fontanelle**.

85% of congenital hypothyroidism is **sporadic**, usually due to **thyroid dysgenesis** (aplasia, hypoplasia, ectopy).

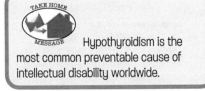

Hypothyroidism is the most common preventable cause of intellectual disability worldwide.

For **newborn screening**, most states use **initial total TSH** testing followed by T4 testing as needed. Infants who fail a thyroid newborn screen, need **immediate test of free T4 and TSH**.

---

[12] In other words they are big and fat.

Treatment is with oral levothyroxine (Synthroid®) 10-15 mcg/kg/day, once confirmation tests are back and by 2 weeks of age.

The oral levothyroxine (Synthroid®) tablets should be crushed and mixed in formula, human milk, or water, but **NOT with soy formulas** because it reduces the absorption.

Delayed treatment can have long-term consequences, including learning disabilities, cognitive deficits, as well as clumsiness and diminished fine motor skills. In general, the longer the diagnosis and treatment are delayed, the lower the IQ.

Thyroxine binding globulin (TBG) Deficiency

This can be a very confusing issue. Therefore, it is ripe for testing on the boards.

This would only be an issue in BOYS in the states that start their newborn screens **checking for serum total T4**. They would have to specifically mention this in the history.

- T4 and T3 are reversibly bound to **thyroid binding globulin (TBG)**.
- However, it is the **free unbound hormone which is metabolically active**.

So even though the total T4 is LOW, the key step you need to keep in mind is checking the **free** T4 and TSH. These will be normal confirming the diagnosis of X-linked TBG deficiency. You will be one question closer to being board certified.

This is X-linked, so of course you should only expect to see it in boys.

The diagnosis is confirmed by **measuring aTBG level**.

A key point to remember is that **thyroid replacement therapy isn't necessary**. Normal free T4 concentrations are maintained and the patients remain euthyroid.

Acquired Hypothyroidism

Hashimoto Thyroiditis

> **TSH #1**
>
> A TSH level (elevated) is the best way to diagnose primary hypothyroidism.

This is also known as **chronic autoimmune thyroiditis**. Hashimoto's disease is an **autoimmune disease** characterized by **antibodies to thyroid tissue** and **lymphocytic infiltration**. As with most autoimmune conditions, it is **more common in females**.

Patients are **clinically euthyroid or hypothyroid**. Most are **asymptomatic** and are discovered by the **presence of a goiter**. In such cases, **TSH should be checked regularly**.

Secondary Hypothyroidism

Hypothyroidism can be caused by **hypothalamic or pituitary disease**. In this case, TSH levels may be low or normal. Free (unbound) T4 is low in this case.

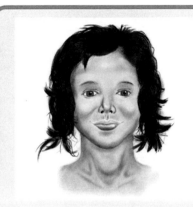

Goiter

The key features in the illustration include a diffuse, soft, symmetrical enlargement. This would be consistent with a thyroid goiter.

They might throw in that the mass moves when the patient swallows. Additional physical findings might include a bruit on auscultation.

Thyroid ultrasound is not routinely indicated in children with simple goiters or suspected autoimmune thyroiditis.

Think Hashimoto

Hashimoto thyroiditis is the most common cause of acquired hypothyroidism and of goiter in iodine-sufficient areas.

In some cases, however, patients can develop **thyrotoxicosis** known as **Hashitoxicosis**. Therefore, watch for clues for Hashimoto disease in a patient who is also **hyperthyroid**.[13]

Hashimoto can also be a part of polyendocrine autoimmune syndromes, and is the most common autoimmune condition seen with Type 1 diabetes.

It is also **common in those with chromosomal disorders**, such as Down syndrome, Turner syndrome and Klinefelter syndrome.

The Shake on TSH

In general, if you are presented with a teenager with lab results inconsistent with treatment, *poor compliance* will likely be the correct explanation.

If you are asked which lab results are important before changing the dose of thyroxine, the correct answer would be both free T4 (fT4) and TSH levels.

TSH levels are often mildly elevated in obese children and adolescents but free T4 is normal.

TSH is the key, since T4 can be normal in compensated hypothyroidism. In addition, look for the presence of **anti-thyroid peroxidase (TPO) antibodies**.

Hashimoto has two "O's" to remind you that hypothyroidism is the more typical presentation. It has an "I" to remind you that it can present with transiently high thyroid hormone.

Lifelong levothyroxine replacement is required.

---

[13] We included this under hypothyroidism since it is the more typical presentation.

Hyperthyroidism

Graves Disease

DEFINITION

Graves disease is the most common cause of hyperthyroidism in adolescents. Thyrotropin receptor antibodies are associated with Graves disease.

BUZZWORDS

With Graves disease, they may describe **bulging eyes** (infiltrative ophthalmopathy) which is pathognomonic. Since children with Graves disease tend to be "revved up," they could emphasize the **emotional lability** (trying to trick you into a psychiatric diagnosis), **weight loss, sleep disturbance,** and/or **heat intolerance**. They may even describe **lid lag**.

Some of the findings can be more subtle, especially in more mild disease. Subtle findings could include **increased appetite with weight loss** or **decreased muscle strength or endurance**.

Additional signs could include **itching, tremors, sweating,** or **increased urination at night**. Females might present with **decreased menstrual flow** and/or **decreased frequency of menses**.

There are other causes of hyperthyroidism, but Graves will almost certainly appear on the test, so this is one to know well.

TREATMENT

Methimazole is the first line agent. It blocks the organification of iodide and so decreases thyroid hormone synthesis.

PERIL

PTU is not preferred in children or adolescents because of the risk of severe hepatitis, neutropenia, and drug rashes.

Hyperthyroid in Graves and Hashimoto: Telling the Difference

COIN FLIP

Since Hashimoto and Graves can both present with hyperthyroid symptoms, how can you tell the difference? Glad you asked.

Do the "eyes" have it? No. The presence of bulging eyes may tip you off that it is Graves, but the absence doesn't rule it out, especially on the Boards.

Can you measure the human thyroid stimulating immunoglobulin? You can, but not everywhere. Both a nuclear medicine thyroid uptake and scan together can help resolve the question.

Antithyroid therapy would be appropriate with Graves disease, but would be inappropriate with Hashimoto (which is usually transitory and requires only monitoring).

ADHD or Attention Deficit thyroid disease?

Think hyperthyroidism, or even the hyperthyroid stage of Hashimoto (Hashitoxicosis), in children with new onset ADHD since they often develop decreased school performance and hyperactivity.

CASE STUDY

You may be presented with a patient with emotional lability and hyperactivity, with information hinting at a diagnosis of Graves Disease buried in the question.

THE DIVERSION

The diversion is to draw you away from a diagnosis of Graves and towards a diagnosis of bipolar disease or ADHD by emphasizing the emotional lability or disorganization.

ANSWER REVEALED

Remember to consider a diagnosis of Graves disease in emotionally labile and disorganized children, especially if they provide physical and other findings consistent with Graves disease.

Neonatal Thyrotoxicosis

Neonatal thyrotoxicosis is due to **maternal thyroid stimulating antibodies crossing the placenta**, which remember can happen even if mom's thyroid has been ablated since the antibodies remain.

Watch for these details in the history they present to you! Since mom is on Synthroid replacement, you may think she has hypothyroidism, but she actually has a history of hyperthyroidism.

The baby comes out with a super activated thyroid with: **irritability, tremors** and **tachycardia** in the immediate newborn period. This is precisely how this would be differentiated from any inborn errors of metabolism, which usually do not manifest in the immediate newborn period. **Symptoms in utero can include increased heart rate and a high output state.**

Failure to thrive, feeding problems, and hyperbilirubinemia are other associated findings.

Laboratory testing would reveal **low TSH** and **high free T4**.

Because of the risk of cardiac arrhythmias, an immediate post-birth thyroid level is indicated.

Treatment is again with **methimazole** until the maternal antibodies are cleared.

Thyroid Nodules

Palpable thyroid nodules in children are almost always benign BUT there **is a greater chance of a thyroid nodule being malignant in an adolescent than in an adult.** Therefore, watchful waiting is not an option in children, even though it is an accepted practice in adults.

Most children with thyroid carcinoma have an asymptomatic thyroid mass and normal thyroid function tests.

Thyroid US is usually the first test performed and is the only time a thyroid US will ever be indicated in children.

Fine needle aspiration (FNA) is the diagnostic test of choice. FNA can identify virtually all thyroid malignancies.

Past history of **exposure to "ionizing radiation"** is a risk factor for malignancy; exposure to "ultraviolet radiation" is not.

131-iodine thyroid scan, once in vogue to distinguish hot from cold nodules, is no longer felt to be useful and will now be the wrong answer on the exam.

> ### Midline neck masses
>
> A single midline firm solitary mass with normal thyroid function tests may actually represent a thyroglossal duct cyst because thyroid nodules are usually off center with abnormal thyroid function test results. A thyroglossal duct cyst will move upward with protrusion of the tongue.

Diabetes Mellitus

Since these are the Pediatric Boards and not the Endocrine Boards, a few good facts and concepts should set you up to be prepared.

The ADA defines a diagnosis of diabetes by **meeting 1 of 4 criteria** in the **presence of symptoms of hyperglycemia** OR **1 of 4 criteria on 2 separate occasions in the absence of symptoms**.

The 4 criteria are:

- HbA1c => 6.5%
- A random glucose value equal to or greater than 200 mg/ dL (11.1 mmol/ L)
- Fasting glucose equal to or greater than 126 mg/ dL (7.0 mmol/ L)
- 2 hour glucose tolerance test equal to or greater than 200 mg/ dL (11.1 mmol/ L).

Since diabetes is usually precipitated by acute illness, it is important to look for signs of diabetes when children present with routine illnesses, such as URI, influenza, and VGE.

Type 1 Diabetes (T1DM)

Type 1diabetes is due to **progressive islet cell destruction** resulting in the inability to produce insulin.

The progression begins with genetic predisposition, proceeds to antibody positivity, then altered glucose metabolism, and finally clinical symptoms and diagnosis when islet function is down to about 20%. This is also known as **insulin dependent diabetes**.

Type 1 diabetes presents with the classic **polyuria, polydipsia, increased appetite,** and **weight loss**.

Important tests at time of diagnosis include glucose and electrolyte panel, venous pH, UA for ketones, serum ketones, and baseline Hgb A1c.

Treatment would consist of **short and long acting SQ insulin**. Insulin pumps are also used with a baseline rate and manual override for bolus doses for meals. Health maintenance in children older than 10 would include an **eye exam. Lipid levels are monitored starting at age 12.**

Family education regarding disease management is a **crucial component of effective treatment**.

Patients with type 1 diabetes are at **increased risk for other autoimmune diseases**. Highest risk is for autoimmune thyroid disease and next highest is for celiac disease. Patients should be screened for both at diagnosis and periodically thereafter.

Honeymoon Phase

Soon after the diagnosis of type 1 diabetes mellitus (DM), there will be a gradual reduction in the amount of insulin needed.

This is because the last drops of insulin are being squeezed from the islet cells.

This does not mean the diagnosis is incorrect. Not remembering this on the exam can come back to haunt you.

This is the honeymoon phase but like any honeymoon, it is short-lived.

Diabetic Ketoacidosis (DKA)

DKA is present IF there is:

- a **blood glucose level** greater than 200 mg/dL
- a **venous pH** less than 7.30 or a **bicarb level** less than 15 mmol/L
- ketones are present in urine/serum.

DKA may be seen in type 1 or type 2 diabetes. Poor compliance and intercurrent illness are the two top triggers.

Symptoms of DKA above worsen until they develop **nausea, emesis** and **abdominal pain.** This leads to **metabolic acidosis.** To compensate for the acidosis, patients develop **hyperpnea (Kussmaul respirations).** This may progress to **drowsiness** and **coma.** Fruity breath is also a sign of DKA.

Fluid Replacement

In DKA, you should assume **5-10% dehydration**. The first step is **rapid volume expansion** with **10-20 cc/kg of normal saline (NS) or lactated ringers (LR) boluses over 1-2 hours**. The rest of the rehydration should be administered evenly over the next 48 hours.

Watch the Bouncing Na

The initial **measured** sodium level should be low due to a dilutional hyponatremia.[14]

If the initial sodium is high, it is a sign of **severe** dehydration.

The sodium level should gradually come up with rehydration.

If the measured sodium does not rise as the glucose falls during treatment, it can be attributed to overzealous fluid correction and this represents an increased risk for cerebral edema.

This is important if you are presented with a patient with mental status change during DKA corection.

Putting the K in DKA

In DKA, there is a **K deficit**, regardless of the initial value they give you. Up to 60 mEq/L of K can be given when the serum potassium is low at presentation, **provided urine output is established.**

Reality Compliance Check

The best way to check long term compliance in a diabetic is the **glycosylated hemoglobin test (Hemoglobin A1C)** which is a reflection of glucose levels over the **past 3 months**. This is fair game and and a concept that is likely to be tested.

Dilutional Delusional Hyponatremia

In DKA, the hyperglycemia draws water into the intravascular compartment through osmotic pressure.

This increased water, results in the dilutional hyponatremia seen in DKA.

The sodium levels do not go down and as the hyperglycemia is corrected the hyponatermia should resolve accordingly.

Where did the potassium go?

During the correction of DKA, *the K levels* will fall for a variety of reasons, mainly having to do with correction of acidosis. K goes back into the cells plus more K is lost in the urine with correction.

---

[14] If you must know how to calculate the corrected l sodium you use the following boring formula : Corrected (i.e. actual) Na = measured Na + 0.3 (glucose - 5.5) mmol/l.

Sugar and Spice

You begin to **add insulin** in the IV fluids **after the initial 1-2 hours of fluid rehydration.**

Dextrose should be added to the fluid **when the blood glucose drops below 300.**

Insulin should be **given IV** until the **acidosis has resolved** (pH > 7.3 and bicarb >15) and the patient is well enough to tolerate oral intake. The insulin is then **changed to SQ.**

Watch that Sign

When rehydration is too rapid, one thing to watch out for is cerebral edema. The treatment will be the same for any case of increased ICP, so this could be the last part of a series of questions.

Just say NO to Bicarb

Insulin and IV fluids are the only treatments needed to correct the acidosis. Bicarb should NOT be used in DKA because its use has been associated with cerebral edema.

Type 2 Diabetes (T2DM)

Type 2 diabetes is primarily **due to insulin resistance.**

The typical presentation is an **obese child.** Physical findings, in addition to obesity, could include **acanthosis nigricans,** which will be described as *dark, thickened, velvety patches of skin* usually in the back of the neck or in the axillae.

Screening criteria for T2DM include being overweight (ie. BMI >85th PCT) plus any 2 of the following risk factors:

1. Family history of T2DM in 1st or 2nd degree relative
2. High-risk race or ethnicity (ie. Native American, African American, Latino, Asian American/ Pacific Islander)
3. Signs of insulin resistance (ie. acanthosis nigricans, hypertension, dyslipidemia, or polycystic ovary syndrome).

Testing **should begin at age 10**, or sooner if **puberty** occurs sooner.

Preferred screening test: **fasting plasma glucose.**

Are you My Type?

Type 1 and Type 2 diabetes can be distinguished from each other by measuring **autoantibodies against pancreatic beta cells, which should only be present in type 1 diabetes**.

In addition, T1DM patients tend to be thin and T2DM patients tend to be overweight.

T1DM patients are more likely to present with classic diabetes symptoms. T2DM patients tend to present after puberty and are much more likely to have a first-degree relative with diabetes.

Initial treatment of Type 2 diabetes is non-pharmacological. This means **improved nutrition, less sitting, and more exercise**. If this does not work, then **metformin**, an oral hypoglycemic agent, is used.

Treatment of type 2 DM involves initiation of insulin at diagnosis if HbA1c >8.5 or glucose >=250. Screening for complications are done at the time of diagnosis for DM2 and annually. This includes an eye exam, microalbuminuria, blood pressure, serum lipids. These should occur at diagnosis and yearly.

Hyperosmolar Non-ketotic Coma

Type 2 diabetics who are insulin resistant with high glucose may present with hyperosmolar non-ketotic coma.

The presentation will include **elevated serum osmolality** and **serum glucose**.

The goal of treatment is the same as DKA, which is to make the patient euvolemic and euglycemic without throwing the patient into cerebral edema. Fluid replacement should take place over 36-48 hours (similar to managing hypernatremic dehydration, for those of you who like to make connections).

Metabolic Syndrome

Metabolic syndrome is a series of clinical and laboratory findings that are felt to be **the result of insulin resistance** and result in cardiovascular disease and Type 2 diabetes. The current definition of Metabolic Syndrome includes:

1. Obesity
2. Dyslipidemia
3. Hypertension
4. Glucose intolerance

Management includes primarily **weight loss** and adoption of **healthy lifestyle** including **regular exercise**.

Recommended screening for children and adolescents with BMI 85th percentile or higher include screening for

1. Hyperglycemia (fasting glucose, Hgb A1c, or glucose tolerance test)
2. Hyperlipidemia (fasting lipids)
3. Liver transaminases (primarily ALT)
4. PCOS in females
5. Obstructive sleep apnea
6. Psychiatric comorbidities.

There is **no current recommendation for the use of metformin** in treating metabolic syndrome.

Calcium Metabolism

I always found this a bit difficult to follow. It involves way too many organs and levels to measure and keep straight. However, it is well worth the time invested to study. So let's go to the blackboard.

Hypercalcemia

Hypercalcemia = serum calcium greater than 11 mg/dL.

Think elevated calcium if they present a patient with **prolonged immobilization.**[15] Symptoms of hypercalcemia range from **decreased appetite, weight loss, dehydration, polyuria, vomiting, constipation, fatigue** and **depression,** to **muscle weakness** and **changes in sensorium, including coma.**

HyperCalcemia can cause issues with:

Bones

Groans (abdominal pain), and

Psychiatric overtones

Calcium Shakedown

If you are presented with a patient who is immobilized, this can be associated with HYPERcalcemia dur to an imbalance between the breakdown and formation of new bone.

A wishbone is made of calcium, so think of the word **WISH** to remember the causes of hypercalcemia:

Williams Syndrome
Ingestion (Vitamin D and A Intoxication, Thiazide Diuretics)
Skeletal Disorders (Dysplasias and Immobilization/Body Casts)
Hyperparathyroidism

Treating Hypercalcemia

High volume fluid, furosemide (Lasix®), and EKG monitoring. In rare cases calcitonin is used.

Hyperparathyroidism

Parathyroid hormone (PTH) acts on kidney, skin and bone to increase serum calcium and decrease serum phosphate.

Primary hyperparathyroidism causes hypercalcemia.

---

[15] Hypercalcemia due to immobilization is caused by an imbalance between bone formation and resorbtion.

Secondary hyperparathyroidism is reactive and due to low serum calcium.

 Treatment is with Calcitriol or Vitamin D and calcium depending on the cause.

Hypocalcemia

Hypocalcemia = Ionized calcium lower than 4.5 mg/dL (1.0 mmol/L), and a total calcium lower than 8.5 mg/dL.

A classic presentation of hypocalcemia could include the following:

- **Painful muscle spasms (hypocalcemic tetany)**
- **Generalized seizures**
- **Vomiting**
- **Prolonged QT interval on EKG**

In particular, watch for a seizure that is resistant to diazepam. Also look for the classic **Chvostek** and **Trousseau signs. Watch out for hypomagnesemia as well.**

Chvostek sign is elicited by tapping just anterior to the ear lobe below the cheek bone. Contraction of the distal muscles is a positive finding.

Trousseau sign is much easier, it is elicited by inflating the blood pressure cuff above systolic pressure and leaving it there for 2 minutes (ouch! Don't forget to come back to the patient!) A positive finding would be carpal muscle spasm on that side.

> ### Heading: Ying and Yang and more Ying
>
> A combination of *hypocalcemia* and *hyper-phosphatemia* correlates with *hypoparathyroidism*.
>
> The reverse is also true: the combination of *hypercalcemia* and *hypophosphatemia* should make you consider *hyperparathyroidism*.
>
> *Hypocalcemia* and *hypo-phosphatemia* correlate with vitamin D deficiency.

Remember the causes of hypocalcemia by picturing somebody getting drained of all the calcium (which is colored white = milk). Well, if you were drained of all of your pigmentation, you would look quite **PINK**.

Pseudohypoparathyroidism[16]

Intake (nutritional deficiency), **I**mmune Deficiency (DiGeorge syndrome)

Nephrotic Syndrome *(with a lowered albumin level, there is a lower calcium level)*

Kidney *(renal insufficiency results in higher phosphate, lower calcium, and a secondary hyperparathyroidism)*

---

16 Peripheral tissue is resistant to the effects of the parathyroid hormone; they are just not listening so PTH levels are high.

CASE STUDY

An infant with hypocalcemia has been receiving calcium replacement and continues to show signs of hypocalcemia. What is the best next step?

THE DIVERSION

Among the choices will be to continue to administer calcium or get a repeat value of calcium. However, these would be incorrect.

ANSWER REVEALED

The correct next step would be to administer magnesium, because serum Mg and Ca levels are directly correlated. An elevated Mg will decrease PTH secretion. Hypomagnesemia can result in intractable hypocalcemia that won't respond to calcium replacement until you correct the magnesium.

Hypoparathyroidism

DEFINITION

Due to either low PTH or resistance to PTH action (pseudohypoparathyroidism).

If the PTH is low, the serum calcium with be low.

PTH tells the body to increase serum calcium levels by reabsorbing it from bone, decreasing urinary calcium excretion, and increasing calcium absorption from the intestines.

BUZZWORDS

Patients with hypoprathyroidism have short stature and truncal obesity. Almost all are due to genetic conditions and many have a family history of fetal and neonatal demise. There is often a family history of other endocrinopathies like GH deficiency, hypothyroidism, and hypogonadism.

HOT TIP

X-Ray of patients with longstanding hypoparathyroidism often show short 4th and 5th metacarpals and metatarsals and calcification of the basal ganglia.

Pseudohypoparathyroidism would present with high PTH *AND* **hypocalcemia,** because of end organ (kidney) resistance to the hormone.

Rickety Rickets

Navigating the bridge of Rickets can get quite "rickety" indeed. However, if you take our hand and don't look down, we can navigate this bridge together and get across unscathed.

Beware the March of IDM

HOT TIP

If you are presented with a neonate who is LGA and hypoglycemic with hypocalcemia, there is a strong probability that you are being presented with an infant of a diabetic mother, even if this is not stated outright.

Emergent Calcium

Calcium may be needed emergently in the case of:

- ❏ Hypocalcemia (duh!)
- ❏ Hyperkalemia
- ❏ Calcium Channel Blocker ingestion (hey, it could happen, especially on the Boards)
- ❏ Hypermagnesemia

First what is **Rickets**? **Rickets is the deficient mineralization of bone at the growth plate.** Therefore, rickets cannot occur after the growth plates are closed. If the deficient mineralization happens at the bone matrix instead, that is **osteomalacia**.

Normal mineralization **requires both calcium and phosphate.**

> If the problem is with calcium, you have **calcipenic rickets.**
>
> If the problem is the phosphate, you have **phosphopenic rickets.**
>
> *You will be expected to determine which one it is, based on the clinical presentation and the lab findings.*

Many, many, many, many disorders (and we mean many) can result in low calcium and/or low phosphate and subsequently, rickets. The boards may make you think you need a degree in metabolism, fluids, and lytes, but, rest assured that if you use the testing tips, and think through the question, you'll be A-OK.

Regardless of the type of rickets (which we'll jump into in a moment), there are classic characteristics in the history that should lead you to consider rickets as a diagnosis.

> ## Anticonvulsing into Rickets"
>
> Children on certain **anticonvulsant medications** are at risk for developing rickets. Watch for this in the history.

Children with rickets present with a combination of **bone pain, anorexia, decreased growth rate, widening of the wrist and knees, delayed eruption of teeth** and **bowed legs.** In particular, look for the enlarged costochondral junctions, known as the **"rachitic rosary,"** and softening of skull bones, called **craniotabes.** Expect to see an x-ray of either the rachitic rosary or long bones of rickets with fraying and cupping.

Serum alkaline phosphatase levels will be elevated in all forms of rickets.

Calcipenic Rickets

So you're probably thinking, "oh this is easy, calcium is low". Not so fast. "Calcipenic" means not enough calcium to meet the needs of growing bones. **The serum calcium may actually be normal or low!**

There are three types of calcipenic rickets:

> 1. Vitamin D deficient rickets
> 2. Vitamin D dependent rickets
> 3. Hereditary Vitamin D resistant rickets

Parathyroid hormone is always elevated in calcipenic rickets. Think of this as the bone phoning home for more calcium!

> ## Calcipenic Rickets
>
> Calcipenic rickets may also result from secondary defects in Vitamin D metabolism and from defects in Vitamin D or calcium absorption.
>
> Rickets may be seen in extremely severe liver disease or in intestinal disorders, such as celiac disease.

Vitamin D Deficient (Nutritional) Rickets

This is **the most common type of rickets** so know it well.

There are a number of risk factors to watch out for in the presenting history that should point you toward a diagnosis of nutritional rickets:

1. **Breast-feeding** without vitamin D supplementation
2. Poor exposure to natural sunlight (pay attention if they note the baby is **dark skinned**)
3. **Low birth weight**, prematurity, or both
4. Infants on **strict vegan diets** which exclude dairy products. If the mother was on a nondairy diet while she was pregnant, the infant may be born with congenital rickets.

African American babies are at particular risk, because of lower absorption of UV light. A typical presentation would be an African American infant, born in the fall or early winter, who is being breastfed without vitamin D supplementation.

Watch for children who are **lactose intolerant** since, by stating such in the history, they will expect you to realize that the patient (by avoiding dairy products) is vulnerable to Vitamin D deficient rickets.

Of all the calcipenic rickets, **Vitamin D deficient rickets is the only one where a 25-hydroxy vitamin D level will be low.** Seems kind of obvious when you think about it.

Treatment is with **vitamin D** and **calcium** supplementation.

The serum calcium and phosphorus levels may be normal in the face of rickets, so don't be tricked. However, serum alkaline phosphatase levels will always be elevated.

Liver Disease and Rickets

When rickets occurs with chronic liver disease, it is not due to the lack of hydroxylation. **It is usually a result of reduced availability of bile salts in the gut and subsequent decreased absorption of vitamin D.** Fat-soluble vitamins: D, A, K, E.

Newborns and Vitamin D

Infants needs 400 IU of vitamin D daily and Vitamin D is not very bioavailable in breast milk.

The current AAP recommendation is actually for ALL infants, regardless of feeding method, receive supplemental vitamin D_3 (cholecalciferol) in infancy.

D Levels

25-hydroxy-Vitamin D reflects the amount of Vitamin D stored in the body.

1,25-dihydroxy-Vitamin D is the active metabolite of Vitamin D.

The (25) is added by the liver. The (1) is added later by the kidney.

See the Nutrition chapter for the more formal names for the different forms of Vitamin D.

The Ticket to Rickets

Here is what they will describe and what you will see:

Head/ Craniotabes: Delayed suture and fontanel closure, skull thickening, "frontal bossing," and bad tooth enamel.

Extremities: Widened physes of wrists and ankles, femoral/tibial bowing.

Chest: "Pigeon chest," rachitic rosary (the costochondral joints are enlarged). They could show this as a picture.

 Rickets can occur with liver disease.

 To remember that Rachitic Rosary is associated with Rickets, change it to "RICKETIC Rosary."

Vitamin D Dependent Rickets

 This used to be known as Vitamin D dependent rickets Type 1. It is autosomal recessive and due (autosomal recessive) is due to **inadequate renal production of 1,25 dihydroxy vitamin D.**

Serum calcium is low as well, but the 25 hydroxy vitamin D is normal because the liver is still doing its job.

This topic is confusing enough as a stationary target. But it is even more difficult when the nomenclature is a moving target.

This is also known as pseudo-Vitamin D-resistant rickets. What can possibly be more frustrating than studying and not even knowing if you are reading about the same disorder with two different names?[17]

Clinically, the presentation is the same as vitamin D deficient rickets.

Treatment is with **Vitamin D$_2$ and 1,25-dihydroxy vitamin D.**

Hereditary Vitamin D Resistant Rickets

This used to be known as vitamin D dependent rickets Type 2. It is an autosomal recessive hereditary condition due to **end organ resistance to vitamin D.**

Phosphopenic Rickets

In phosphopenic rickets, it's the **phosphate that is low.** The calcium and the PTH may actually be normal. The most common form of phosphopenic rickets in children and adolescents is due to **renal phosphate wasting.**

X-Linked Hypophosphatemic Rickets

 Here, the problem is **excessive phosphate loss through the kidneys.**

It's one of those rare **X-linked dominant diseases,** and it's the most common cause of rickets in industrialized countries.

 Treatment is with **phosphate supplementation.** In addition, **1,25-dihydroxy vitamin D** is needed.

---

[17] Like Prince, later known as The Artist Formerly known as Prince, and even later as The Artist Formerly Known as The Artist Formerly Known as Prince. #RIPPrince

Crossing the Rickety Rickets Bridge

Knowing this information cold will be worth several points on the exam.

	Vitamin D deficient	Vitamin D Dependent	Vitamin D resistant	X-Linked hypo-phosphatemic	Renal Disease
THE UNDERLYING CAUSE	Nutritional Deficit OR Poor UV Light Exposure	1-alpha hydroxylase deficiency	End Organ resistance	Defect in tubular reabsorption of phosphate	Defect in phosphate excretion
Phosphate	Low or normal	Low or normal	Low or normal	Very Low	High
Calcium	Low or normal	Low	Low	Normal	Decreased
Alkaline Phosphatase	High	High	High	High	High
PTH	High	High	High	Normal	High
25-Vitamin D	Low	Normal	Normal	Normal	Low
1,25 Vitamin D	Normal	Low	Very High	Normal	Low

TAKE HOME MESSAGE   Ultimately, the easiest way to know this information is to know and understand how PTH and Vitamin D affect serum calcium and phosphate normally.

Chapter 22

GI:
Chew ! From Top to Bottom !

This is the section where you literally have to know everything from soups to nuts. Which soups, which nuts, and where can you find them floating around—that is the trick to passing.

Abdominal Pain

Acute Abdominal Pain

Acute abdominal pain isn't very cute at all, especially if you encounter it on the Boards. You need to take into account the age and gender of the child, as well as all the different bits of information they throw at you in the question. The following are common causes of abdominal pain and how they will be described.

> **CASE STUDY**
>
> **A 6 year old with periumbilical pain yesterday now presents with RLQ tenderness and guarding, but no rebound tenderness. What is the best diagnostic test to determine if surgery is necessary?**
>
> **THE DIVERSION**
>
> By noting that there is no rebound tenderness, they are hoping that you'll be fooled into believing that appendicitis is not in the differential, and therefore will choose a study that will rule out something else in the differential, i.e. *Yersinia* infection, mesenteric adenitis, or Crohn's disease.
>
> **THE DIVERSION**
>
> The correct answer is U/S because it has less radiation exposure than CT.

Appendicitis

Appendicitis should be considered in any child presenting with persistent severe abdominal pain. It is more common in children over 2, but may certainly present in infants so don't count them out. The diagnostic spot for pain is known as **McBurney's**[1] **point**.

DEFINITION The classic pain will be described as having started mid abdomen and moved to the right lower quadrant area, along with **nausea, vomiting, anorexia,** and **low-grade fever**. On physical examination, they might describe the **psoas sign** (pain on straightening out the leg).

---

[1] Apparently McBurney staked his flag about 1/3 of the way between the anterior-superior iliac crest and the umbilicus. Therefore, if you want a location on the abdomen with your name on it, you will have to move to another location.

X-ray findings include the **sentinel loop** and the **absence of air in the right lower quadrant**. A **fecalith**, which is a hardened mass (usually of stool), would be an important clinical sign that the patient has appendicitis. More often than not, the x-ray with appendicitis is **negative**. DO NOT let that dissuade you from considering this as a correct choice.

A child who wishes to eat is unlikely to have appendicitis. Do not look for severe vomiting to suspect appendicitis. The absence of an elevated white blood cell count does not rule out the diagnosis.

The Cute Players of Acute Pain

Remember some other causes of acute abdominal pain as follows:

If you attended a summer camp known as **"CAMP HITS"** your abdomen would hurt for sure. Remember the causes of acute abdominal pain as follows:

Constipation (Cyst-Ovarian)
Adenitis (Mesenteric)
Mono
Pancreatitis

Hepatitis
Infection (UTI)
Trauma
Surgical (Intussusception/Malrotation/Volvulus)

Recurrent or Chronic Abdominal Pain

Some of these children will have an etiology found for their pain (like celiac disease) while some of these children will continue with pain for which no cause can be found.

Before you succumb to recurrent abdominal pain as a result of this confusion, we offer you the following causes to chew on.

Functional Dyspepsia

All of the following must be present at least once per week for at least 2 months before diagnosis:

Recurrent pain in the **upper abdomen** above the umbilicus. The pain cannot be relieved with defecation. There must also be **no evidence of inflammatory, anatomic, metabolic, or neoplastic process**.

If they describe the above clinical scenario in a child with a **recent history of acute viral gastroenteritis**, this is not functional dyspepsia. It is post-viral **gastroparesis**. Remember, this will be described after the viral illness has resolved.

The slippery heels of Helicobacter pylori

Even if the test for *H. pylori* is positive in the context of recurrent abdominal pain, it does not mean there is a causal relationship.

So why order the test? Good question! That is why routine testing for *H. pylori* in a question involving a patient with functional dyspepsia will likely be the wrong choice.

Having said that, *H. pylori* is associated with low socioeconomic status, especially in those living in crowded housing. It is also more common in people immigrating from developing countries.

BREAKING NEWS The AAP and NASPGHN[2] recommend that only children with endoscopic or radiographic evidence of gastric or duodenal ulcers, or those with MALT lymphoma be tested for *H. pylori*.

---

2 North American Society for Pediatric Gastroenterology, Hepatology, and Nutrition.

If there are "red flags" described, such as **pain radiating to the back, bilious vomiting, bloody emesis, difficulty swallowing, or melena,** they are pointing you in another direction. Systemic findings, including **weight loss, fever, night sweats, or anemia** are also signs that point away from a diagnosis of functional dyspepsia.

If you are sure that functional dyspepsia is what they are describing, then it is treated by eliminating items that can exacerbate symptoms, including **NSAIDs, spicy foods,** and **soda** (especially sodas containing **caffeine**). Dyspepsia may improve with smaller, more frequent meals.

If you are presented with medications, **histamine-2 receptor antagonists** or **gastric proton pump inhibitors** would be correct treatment choices.

Although not proven in children, **low dose antidepressants** could be the correct answer, since they work in adults.

Irritable Bowel Syndrome (IBS)

If each of the following is present once a week for at least 2 months in the clinical history, they are describing irritable bowel syndrome.

Abdominal discomfort **improved with defecation, change in stool frequency, or change in stool consistency**. There also has to be **no organic explanation for the symptoms**.

Besides the stool changes, they could also describe **straining or bowel urgency**, with **feeling of incomplete evacuation**. Passage of **mucus, bloating, and abdominal distention** are also consistent with the diagnosis.

If the clinical description includes any of the following "red flags", you are **not** dealing with irritable bowel syndrome: **pain limited to the night time, unexplained weight loss, oral ulcers, rash, pallor, or bloody stools.**

Inflammatory bowel disease is the more likely diagnosis if they describe more systemic signs, such as anemia, fever, arthritis, delayed puberty, short stature, or a family history of inflammatory bowel disease.

High fiber diet, antispaspodics, peppermint, tricyclic antidepressants, probiotics, **addressing psychological issues** (cognitive behavioral therapy) are all appropriate answers if asked about management and treatment.

Anti-Anticholinergic Policy

Anticholinergic Meds

Watch out for a patient with recurrent abdominal pain presenting with

- Urinary retention
- Tachycardia
- Blurred vision
- Dry mouth

A patient presenting with these symptoms along with a history of recurrent pain may have been *inappropriately* prescribed anticholinergic medications to treat the recurrent abdominal pain.

Anticholinergics should not be administered to children who have either acute or chronic diarrhea.

Childhood Functional Abdominal Pain

 As always, they must describe the following as having been present at least once a week for the past 2 months.

Episodic or continuous abdominal pain that does not meet the diagnostic criteria for other GI disorders. In addition, there must be some evidence of **loss of daily activity** and presence of additional symptoms, including **headache, limb pain, or sleep disruption**.

Treatment is the same as for IBS.

Abdominal Migraines

 Acute, incapacitating, periumbilical abdominal pain that lasts for more than 1 hour and interferes with normal activities.

Must be associated with at least 2 of the following: **pallor, anorexia, nausea, vomiting, headache, or photophobia.**

There must be at least 2 episodes in the last 12 months. There must also be **symptom-free periods**, lasting weeks to months in between episodes. A family history of migraine headaches could be included. There must be no other cause for the symptoms.

Treatment includes triptans and other medications as for regular migraines.

If you are presented with a patient with signs of any of the above categories of functional abdominal pain, ordering lab and imaging studies would be incorrect choices. Watch for signs or indications of psychological stressors.

Vomiting

Vomiting occurs for different reasons in different age groups. Again, the presenting symptoms and facts included in the question, coupled with the age, should make these easy pickings.

Inborn Errors of Metabolism

These are common causes of vomiting in early infancy. The description is similar to that of a septic infant so how can you tell?

Look for metabolic acidosis (with an elevated anion gap), hypoglycemia, hyperammonemia, and no fever as your clues pointing to inborn errors instead of sepsis.

Duodenal Atresia

The key point to remember is that this presents as **bilious vomiting during the first few hours of life.**

Be ready to recognize the classic **double bubble sign** on x-ray.[3] Because of diminished enterohepatic circulation, these infants are frequently **icteric.** There will be **no air distal to the site of atresia.**[4]

Remember "duo" means "two" so in the Duodenal Atresia x-ray you see a double bubble.

What else is there?

If you see a baby with duodenal atresia, also check for:

- Down syndrome
- Malrotation
- Congenital Heart Disease

Malrotation

Abnormal intestinal rotation and fixation leading to small bowel obstruction.

It is caused by the **cecum's failure to descend while being handcuffed to the posterior right abdominal wall.** Therefore, it compresses the duodenum, causing duodenal obstruction.

Malrotation will typically present as **bilious vomiting** and **abdominal distention.** The patient could also have **crampy abdominal pain** and could be passing **blood via the rectum.**

This is a **surgical emergency** that requires immediate intervention and is almost always on the Boards.

Volvulus

Presents in infancy as **bilious vomiting** and **right-sided abdominal distention.** It is associated with **Ladd Bands,** which constrict the large and small bowel.

X-ray findings will be described as **gastric and duodenal dilatation,** as well as **decreased intestinal air** and **corkscrew appearance** of the **small bowel** — whatever that is. This is an example where knowing the association is the key.

Intussusception
(You Don't Want This on a Spelling Bee)

Classic presentation is a healthy child **3 months to 6 years**[5] who has sudden onset of **abdominal pain** with **drawing up his legs** and **vomiting,** then has a period of being perfectly fine, then pain recurs. They may have fever and anorexia. The pain may be relieved with the passing of a stool. However, the child **ultimately becomes lethargic.**

Camp Town Races

Recurrent crampy abdominal pain in a **febrile** child, that isn't quite as severe as the pain found in intussusception or appendicitis, could be *Campylobacter jejuni* or *Yersinia* infection.

---

[3] This represents the stomach and proximal duodenum.
[4] You will then of course remember to think of Down syndrome since there is a clear association.
[5] Highest incidence is in children younger than 2 years.

HOT TIP

They probably won't describe the typical **currant jelly stool**. They might mention **bloody stool** and palpation of a **sausage-like mass** in the right abdomen.[6]

MNEMONIC

In the later stages, intussusception might be described as **bilious vomiting** with **shock-like symptoms**, so don't miss the diagnosis if you see **green** (bile) and **no red** (currant jelly stools) in the question.

COIN FLIP

They sometimes portray this as a toddler who is **afebrile,** and toxic-appearing with lethargy and pallor **mimicking sepsis,** but with no GI symptoms.

TREATMENT

Treatment facts: "Air enema" resulting in hydrostatic reduction will **diagnose and "cure"** in most cases.

HOT TIP

Cause is usually idiopathic under age 3, but need to consider pathologic lead points (Meckel's, polyps, HSP vasculitis, lymphoma) in children over 3.

CASE STUDY

A 20 month old presents with colicky abdominal pain and a right lower quadrant mass. He is intermittently in severe pain and lethargic between episodes. What would be the BEST diagnostic study to order?

THE DIVERSION

If you are well prepared for the exam, there really isn't a diversion here. You should realize by now that they will not deliver a fast ball down the middle by noting that there are "currant jelly stools." There are sufficient code words, like *lethargic* and *severe pain,* here to let you know that this patient has intussusception. However, you could be thrown by their mentioning the abdominal mass, and think the correct diagnostic study is CT.

If they provide you with 2 correct choices, remember they want the best choice. Ultrasound may be correct, but it is not the best choice.

ANSWER REVEALED

The correct choice is *air contrast enema*, since this may be both diagnostic and therapeutic.

---

[6] I never knew what "currant jelly" was prior to medical school, but since training in pediatrics, I have never been tempted to try it, for obvious reasons.

GE Reflux in Infants

Gastroesophageal reflux (GER) can present with **severe emesis**, sometimes even out the nose.

It manifests as **effortless regurgitation** (or "spitting up" if you will), in infants who are perfectly well in every other way.

Many infants have daily episodes of spitting up at 4 months of age and it is normal, on the boards at least.

It is important to remember that regurgitation is a normal finding in infants. Reassurance is the correct answer. It can also be a sign of "overfeeding;" therefore, if they specifically mention the amount the baby is being fed along with signs of reflux, then reducing the amount in the feedings may be the correct answer.

GER disease (GERD) is defined as GER with abdominal pain, arching with feedings, apnea, or failure to thrive. This might require further workup and/or treatment.

GER and GERD are clinical diagnoses: no diagnostic tests are indicated. The tests below may be necessary to rule out other causes of vomiting or to quantify the severity of the disease if intervention is a consideration.

Upper GI Series	To assess for malrotation and hiatal hernia
pH probe study (or esophageal impedance)	Measures the extent and duration of reflux over a 24 hour period
Gastric emptying scan	Tests for gastroparesis
Esophageal motility evaluation	Measures peristalsis and esophageal sphincter pressure

Prognosis for Infants with GERD

Infants who simply have physiologic reflux will **outgrow it by 1 year of age** without any consequences.

However, if you are presented with the following in the history, they probably expect you to realize that there are higher risks for complications. These would include **prematurity, underlying neurological impairment**, or a **family history of severe GERD**.

Sandifer Syndrome

They will describe unusual **dystonic movements** of the head and neck along with **GER**.

Remember this by picturing a "sandpiper" blowing sand out of the pipe, as a reminder of reflux and the "twisted pipes" as a reminder of the twisting movements.

Anti serotonin antiemetic

Zofran®, which is also known as ondansetron, is an important antemetic. They might just ask you its mechanism of action; if they do, you will know that it is a serotonin receptor antagonist.

Rx for GERD

Medications including antacids (ranitidine), and proton-pump inhibitors (omeprazole and lansoprazole) are frequently used to treat GERD but they really just decrease the heartburn pain, they can't decrease the actual reflux. **They will rarely be the correct answer on the Boards.** On the Boards they usually want "reflux precautions" and "reassurance".

Surgery is only indicated if the infant is having severe consequences (like failure to grow or respiratory compromise) and medication has failed. Duh!

Hypertrophic Pyloric Stenosis (HPS)

Pyloric stenosis occurs more commonly in **white males**. Since it is rarer in females, it stands to reason that a **maternal history of PS increases the risk more than paternal history.**

Progressive non-bilious vomiting is the description. They will not mention **projectile vomiting**[7] with **palpable olive.**[8] It typically occurs during the second month of life.

Shine a Lyte: Pyloric stenosis presents with **hypochloremic hypokalemic metabolic alkalosis.** The alkalosis would make sense because they are vomiting acid. And they will be low on Cl as well because they are throwing up HCl.

> You may recall from the ID chapter:
>
> Macrolides (erythromycin, azithromycin) in infancy may be associated with development of hypertrophic pyloric stenosis

They could present you with a patient with HPS and then ask you to choose which value is not consistent. Therefore, know this well.

Elevated indirect Bili can occur in pyloric stenosis in up to 2.5% of cases, so don't let that throw you if it is included in the question of an otherwise classic description of PS. This is not a trick, just extra information.

Ultrasound Findings – Pyloric stenosis is diagnosed via ultrasound. In case they expect you to know the mind numbing ultrasound diagnostic criteria is:

A pyloric length **greater than 14 mm**
or
Pyloric muscle thickness **greater than 4 mm**

Surgical repair (pyloromyotomy) is indicated after IV rehydration and correction of electrolyte imbalances.

CASE STUDY

A 2 month old infant with Down syndrome presents with projectile non-bilious vomiting with hypochloremic metabolic alkalosis (or they might just present the lab findings themselves). What imaging study results are most likely?

THE DIVERSION

The diversion is their telling you that the infant has Down Syndrome. Among the choices will be the double bubble sign. This, however, is just a diversionary choice, and if you are not careful the double bubble will be double trouble for you.

ANSWER REVEALED

The correct answer will be "pyloric muscle measures over 6 mm in thickness" and the "pyloric channel 18 mm in length;" or, if they are actually fair and realize that this is not the pediatric radiology boards, "thickening and elongation of the pyloric muscle." They note that the infant is 2 months old, the time when a patient is likely to present with pyloric stenosis. Duodenal atresia will present in the first day of life, not at 2 months.

---

[7] Or if they do, you can be sure they're trying to trick you and go ahead and cross HPS off your list.
[8] With or without the pimento.

DKA

Don't forget this as a cause of vomiting. The lab findings would be suggestive of the diagnosis (see Endocrinology chapter).

Cyclical Vomiting Syndrome

This entity may have **emotional overtones** with a precipitating event. Children with cyclical vomiting are also at risk for **migraines and irritable bowel syndrome**. It is a diagnosis of exclusion, so they will also need to tell you what has been ruled out.

If the diagnosis is cyclical vomiting, they will present a patient with **intense periods of vomiting** that last **up to 48 hours**. The most common time for vomiting is early morning (like brain tumors) but will have an otherwise normal physical exam. The patient will be described as **feeling well between episodes**.

You also need to know that conditions other than migraine variant can present with severe episodic vomiting, including **pancreatitis** and **metabolic defects**. Therefore, a workup that includes metabolic studies and imaging might be the answer they are looking for, depending on the context.

> ### Another hot shower really?
>
> Depending on the age, it will be important to rule out **Cannabinoid Hyperemesis Syndrome (CHS)** in a patient with repeated vomiting. It is related to chronic marijuana use. Interestingly, these patients have found that hot showers alleviate the symptoms, so if the parents are suddenly so proud that their grungy teenaged son has developed a passion for the shower, this may be the other reason.

CASE STUDY

A 5 year old is experiencing vomiting episodes that typically last 48 hours, and end suddenly after a long nap followed by an episode of Sponge Bob Square Pants. The mother has a history of severe headaches, and his uncle Billy, who accompanied them, has gone to the bathroom twice during this office visit. What is the most appropriate treatment at this time?

THE DIVERSION

By noting the symptoms of the mother and Uncle Billy, they are letting you know that there is a family history of migraine headaches and irritable bowel syndrome. Both are associated with cyclic vomiting, which typically lasts 48 hours.

TREATMENT

Long-term pharmacological treatment is similar to migraine treatment, i.e. cypro-heptadine, propranolol, or tricyclic antidepressants.

ANSWER REVEALED

If they ask for the best treatment at this time, the answer would be IV hydration.

Rumination

Rumination is the frequent passive regurgitation of ingested food into the mouth that is then re-chewed and swallowed or spit out. They will appear calm during episodes.

Rumination may be seen in **infants** of **severely disturbed caregivers**, and in older kids who are themselves **disturbed or developmentally delayed.**

These children may **induce vomiting to seek attention** in environments where there is a failure in reciprocal interaction between the infant and caregiver.

Resolving the emotional trigger is the treatment of choice.

Going From Top to Bottom

Let's travel from the mouth to the other side of the GI tunnel.

Chew on This: The Mouth

If they describe a cyst on the floor of the mouth as a "mucocele," think **ranula**.

Take out your atlas and take a good look at what these both look like.

Treatment for a ranula is excision.

However, a "midline mass" could be **ectopic thyroid**, which should not be removed.

Too Few Teeth

Ectodermal Hypoplasia

This can present with underdeveloped or absent teeth.

Change ectodermal to **"empty dental,"** and the image is clear and linked to the diagnosis. It is **X-linked**: in place of teeth, picture small X's sitting on the gums.

It is diagnosed by skin biopsy, which shows lack of sweat pores.

Down the Tunnel: The Esophagus

Esophageal Varices

Liver disease leads to **portal hypertension** with **bright red, bloody, hematemesis,** and **tarry stools, esophageal varices.** Remember esophageal varices CAN cause tarry stools.

Tracheo-Esophageal Fistula

The TE fistula with a **blind upper esophageal pouch** is the most common type. It will often present as **coughing and vomiting with feeding in the newborn period.** They often show you a film with a feeding tube **coiled up** in the blind-ending esophagus.

It is managed by making the child **NPO** and **draining the blind-ending esophagus** prior to **surgical correction.**

Copious oral secretions, polyhydramnios, coughing and cyanosis with initial feeding, and **inability to pass a feeding tube** are all descriptions associated with TE fistula.

The other TE fistulas will present in older children as respiratory symptoms (namely cough) associated with eating and/ or drinking.

You could be asked for further studies and you should know that you should be ruling out other associated findings common with **VACTERL syndrome.**

Eosinophilic Esophagitis (EE)

This is a **chronic immune/ antigen-mediated condition** that presents as GERD and/ or dysphagia. Food impaction (dysphagia with certain solid foods).

Antigens are typically foods (milk, soy, wheat, eggs, nuts, and fish) but may be environmental triggers as well. 50 % of patients have an atopic history.

Diagnosis is made by history along with biopsy showing **eosinophil-predominant inflammation in the esophageal wall** (specifically >15 eosinophils/high powered field on microscopy).

Treatment is with PPIs, diet changes, and corticosteroid therapy.

Treatment of Peptic Ulcer Disease: How It Works!

There are 4 primary meds used to treat PUD in children: H2 blockers, sucralfate, prostaglandins, and PPIs.

1. The **H2 Blockers block** gastric acid secretion.

2. **Sucralfate** "coats" damaged gastric mucosa, protecting it from further damage.

3. The **prostaglandin analogues** enhance bicarb production, and to some extent decrease gastric acid production as well.

4. **Proton pump inhibitors (PPIs)** inhibit the gastric acid pump.

 Misoprostol is an example of a prostaglandin that is used but **shouldn't be used in pregnant teens**; you can remember this by telling patients not to kiss under the "mistletoe" – misoprostol.

On the Bubble: The Stomach

Peptic Ulcer Disease

This will be described in its classic form, which is vomiting after eating[9] and **epigastric pain severe enough to wake the child up at night**. They could throw in **guaiac positive stools**, which would be the clincher.

A **plain KUB** would be an important **first study** when evaluating the child with abdominal pain, **but is not helpful when PUD is suspected.**

The best diagnostic study is an **upper gastrointestinal endoscopy,** so that a biopsy can be done and esophagitis can also be ruled out.

NSAID SO Sad

NSAIDs cause GI symptoms by interfering with prostaglandin synthesis.

Uncomplicated dyspepsia due to NSAIDs can be managed with antacids and food.

Intestinal Fortitude to Learn Intestinal Disorders

Celiac Disease

Classic presentation includes **abdominal distention, anorexia, diarrhea, failure to thrive, weight loss, proximal muscle wasting and nonresolving iron-deficiency anemia.**

Gluten is found in foods that contain **wheat or rye,** and must be avoided. **Oatmeal is fine in some patients, and therefore, can be tested initially. Vitamin supplementations** are needed.

As long as they verify that the patient has **normal IgA levels,** the best way to screen for celiac disease would be to test for **elevated levels of IgA antibodies against tissue transglutaminase (anti-tTG) or IgA antibodies to endomysium.** However, **diagnosis is confirmed by biopsy.**

Besides iron deficiency, children with celiac disease are also at risk for deficiency of folate, Vitamin B12, the fat-soluble vitamins (D,E,A,K), and zinc.

You could be presented with a a patient with **dermatitis herpetiformis**, the characteristic rash associated with celiac disease, and ask you to order lab tests to aid in diagnosis. All of the follow would be correct: IgA level, tissue transglutaminase antibodies, and endomysial antibodies, but endoscopy with biopsy would be the **gold standard** for diagnosis.

---

[9] Postprandial emesis for those who prefer Latin terms.

Alone in the Colon

PTEN Hamartoma Syndrome

DEFINITION

Also known as Cowden syndrome and Multiple Hamartoma syndrome, it consists of macrocephaly, papillomatous papules, mucocutaneous lesions, acral keratosis. The skin hamartomas are usually present by the mid 20s. Also have increased risk of breast, endometrial and thyroid cancers.

Familial Adenomatous Polyposis (FAP)

BUZZWORDS

Begins with benign adenomatous polyps in colon in the teens and the polyps will become malignant over time. Sigmoidoscopy or colonoscopy should begin at age 10 to 12 in patients with FAP. Average age of colorectal cancer is 39 years if colectomy is not done before that.

PERIL

Turcot syndrome is FAP that has colonic polyps plus CNS tumors.

Gardner's Syndrome

DEFINITION

This is one of the FAP syndromes associated with **extra teeth** and **polyps (pre-malignant) in the large and small intestines. Osteomas and soft tissue tumors** are also part of the picture, and it is inherited in an **autosomal dominant** fashion.

TREATMENT

Treatment is surgical.

MNEMONIC

Picture a gardener working his garden, but instead of the usual leaves, he has a garden made out of **bones** and **colonic polyps** (that's right — we have another delightfully grim and morbid image for you here). The polyps are indeed **pre-malignant,** and eventually win out by dominating the bones (to remind you that it is an **autosomal dominant** trait). However, along comes a power lawnmower driven by a surgeon to remind you that surgery is the answer. The lawn mower is made of supernumerary (extra) teeth that will pull out the bones and polyps.

Peutz-Jeghers Syndrome

BUZZWORDS

Mucocutaneous pigmentation of lips and gums that starts in infancy around mouth, nostrils and buccal mucosa and associated with **hundreds of polyps** in the stomach and colon which may lead to intussusception and become malignant.

Rectal Prolapse

Cystic fibrosis is known to be associated with rectal prolapse. Other causes of rectal prolapse are anything that results in increased intra-abdominal pressure, such as **pertussis** and **tenesmus,** as well as **chronic constipation**.

Rare causes include **meningomyelocele** and **parasites** (especially if they tell you the child recently traveled or is a new immigrant from a place where parasites are endemic). This can even occur in some cases of pinworms.

HELLO POLYP

Intestinal polyps can present with rectal bleeding, abdominal pain, or intussusception. They may also be found incidentally.

Solitary juvenile polyps are the most common and should be removed even if found incidentally.

If <5 polyps are found and there is no family history of polyp syndromes, no further evaluation is needed.

There is risk of cancer in many organs including colon, pancreas, stomach, lung, testes, breast, uterus, ovary, and cervix. Overall, there is a 70% risk of cancer by age 70.

Treatment consists of routine colonoscopies removing any mean-looking polyps plus specific screening guidelines for each organ.

Inflammatory Bowel Disease

Ulcerative Colitis vs. Crohn's: There can be several questions on both of these and you will have to know the similarities and differences.

Ulcerative Colitis

Ulcerative colitis (UC) typically presents in a **teenager** with a history of **chronic crampy lower abdominal pain, with or without a history of bloody stools**.

Severe colitis can present with **fevers** and **hypoalbuminemia**, as well as **anemia**.

Ashkenazi (European) Jews are at particular risk for UC.

Severe cases require initial hospitalization for rehydration and/ or blood transfusion. When the disease is actually a medical emergency, **fluids, blood transfusions,** and **steroids** are required, and when infection is suspected, **metronidazole** is the treatment of choice.

The **first line of medical treatment is 5-ASA** (or 5-aminosalycylate, if they write the whole thing out); however, if this were not successful, the **second line of treatment would be:**

- Corticosteroids
- 6-mercaptopurine or azathioprine or methotrexate
- Cyclosporine or tacrolimus

Drug therapy does help prevent relapses.

A surgical consult is also needed because of the risk for perforation. **A barium enema is never the right answer with acute UC, because of the risk of perforation.** If possible, pain meds should be avoided, since the masking of pain makes it difficult to track the clinical status.

B27 Cousins

Both Crohn's and UC are associated with **HLA B27 antigen** just like ankylosing spondylitis.

Colectomy

Colectomy will eliminate the risk for cancer in children with ulcerative colitis. This is not a small consideration given that the cancer rate is 20% per decade after the first 10 years of disease.

The "extracolonic" manifestations of ulcerative colitis include arthritis, mucocutaneous lesions, and liver disease.

Colectomy does not stop the progression of ankylosing spondylitis.

IBD Clues

The picturesque IBD patient would have abdominal pain with occult + stools, short stature, elevated ESR, and anemia (usually microcytic), hypoalbuminemia, and elevated fecal calprotectin. You will only be given a few, not all, of these clues with which to make the diagnosis.

Crohn's Disease (Regional Enteritis)

HOT TIP

Crohn's can present as weight loss even before overt GI symptoms present. *The elevated ESR may be the only clue they give you.* Obtaining an **ESR** may be the correct answer in a child presenting with **short stature**.

BUZZWORDS

Skip lesions on x-ray, **cobblestone** appearance on endoscopy, and **transmural lesions**, as well as **noncaseating granulomas**, are all typical descriptors of Crohn's disease.

TAKE HOME MESSAGE

Tuberculosis can be mistaken for Crohn's disease, because it can result in nodularity and mucosal thickening of the terminal ileum.

TREATMENT

The medical management includes the use of **corticosteroids, aminosalicylates, immunomodulators,** and **antibiotics (metronidazole [Flagyl®])** in addition to nutritional support.

Just as in ulcerative colitis, **5-ASA** is now used instead of Azulfidine® (sulfapyridine).

COIN FLIP

> ### Extraintestinal Sightings and Crohn's Disease
>
> They can give you a case with no GI symptoms, and only the extraintestinal manifestations of Crohn's disease, such as:
>
> ❏ Pyoderma gangrenosum of the foot
> ❏ Erythema nodosum (red tender nodules over the shin)
> ❏ Ankylosing spondylitis/ sacroiliitis
> ❏ Arthritis
> ❏ (Eyes) Uveitis
> ❏ Liver Disease
> ❏ Renal Stones
>
> **MNEMONIC**
>
> Think of it as "Cone" disease, since cone sounds like Crohn. The cone affects where you **sit** (sacroiliitis), where your shoe **fits** (pyoderma gangrenosum), where you get **kicked** (erythema nodosum), and where you can see **IT** (eyes – uveitis), and turns your liver into a useless **mitt** (liver disease).

	Ulcerative Colitis	Crohn's Disease
Lesions are continuous – no skipped lesions	YES	NO
Surgical excision is curative	YES	NO
Toxic megacolon can occur	YES	YES
Growth retardation and pubertal delay	YES	YES more common than with UC

HOT TIP

Crohn's can present initially as an acute abdomen, mimicking appendicitis. Oral **aphthous** ulcers and **perianal fistulae** can also be presenting signs of Crohn's.

TREATMENT

Treatment: Meds do not change the long-term course of CD; they just decrease morbidity. Those with mild symptoms are treated as outpatients, and those with more severe symptoms (e.g., massive weight loss, significant systemic symptoms) are hospitalized.

Steroids induce remissions in 70% of patients with small bowel involvement. There is a **high relapse rate after steroids are weaned.**

Constipation

Fecal overflow incontinence /Encopresis

 This is constipation that disguises itself as diarrhea. Typical presentation is a previously stool-continent school aged child with **daily soiled pants** who does not have weight loss, fever or other systemic manifestations. Their rectum is so full that they are now having leaving leakage of stool.

Treatment is in 3 phases

1) **Education** – family must know that episodes are out of the child's control and not a purposeful behavior. Punishment and blame should be avoided.

2) **Emptying the colon** – Clean out with enema, and then mostly oral cathartics and stool softeners.

Enemas and suppositories may traumatize the child, and are not recommended unless there is encopresis.

3) **Maintenance program** – adjusting doses of medications until colon regains tone and one soft stool a day is obtained.

Hirschsprung's Disease

Hirschsprung's Disease (Congenital aganglionic megacolon) is due to the **absence of parasympathetic innervation of the internal anal sphincter.** The affected recto-sigmoid segment is contracted, the region proximal to the aganglionic segment then becomes distended with stool.

 No passage of meconium in the first 48 hours is the classic presentation. Think of Hirschsprung's disease for any significant defecation problem in a newborn, especially a male. In addition to constipation or failure to pass first stool in the hospital, infants with Hirschsprung's disease can also present with **bilious vomiting, poor PO intake,** and **abdominal distension alternating with periods of diarrhea.**

Hirschsprung's Disease is associated with **Down syndrome.**

Diagnosis is by **rectal biopsy.** Treatment consists of **surgical excision** of the aganglionic segment, followed by colostomy and ultimately end-to-end anastomosis.

You may be called upon to distinguish just plain old constipation from Hirschsprung's. Keep the following in mind:

	Functional Constipation	Hirschsprung's
Delayed passage of meconium in the newborn period	RARELY	YES
Signs of obstruction	RARELY	YES
Soiling	YES	RARELY
Failure to thrive	NO	YES
Present after age 2	YES	NO[10]
Difficulty with toilet training	YES	NO
Stool in the rectal ampulla on PE	YES	NO

Occasionally "squirt sign" is described in children with Hirschsprung's- this is when there is explosive passage of stool after digital rectal exam.

Differential Diagnosis

Anal Stenosis - infants strain to pass small liquid stools, and there is a tight band narrowing on the anus. This is self limited and remits by age 1.

Functional Constipation - typically presents in infants fed cereal at an early age. Delayed passing of meconium will not be described in the vignette.

Congenital Hypothyroidism – in addition to constipation, the patient will present with poor growth, a hoarse cry, umbilical hernia, and delayed closure of the anterior fontanelle.

> ## Cool Stool Facts
>
> Ninety-nine percent of healthy newborns will deliver their first stool within their first 24 hours and the other 1% will within 48 hours.
>
> **Hirschsprung's disease** and **cystic fibrosis** should be your first considerations when there is **no stool production in the first 48 hours**.

Gastrointestinal Bleeding

When you are presented with a GI bleed, the first consideration is appropriate **immediate fluid resuscitation** if there are signs of hypovolemia. Then Nasogastric lavage will help you distinguish upper GI from lower GI bleeding.

Upper GI Bleed (UGB)

Hemetemesis is the vomiting of blood and reflects bleeding **proximal to the Ligament of Treitz**. Bright red blood signifies active bleeding. Coffee ground material signifies cessation of active bleeding.

> ## Upper GI Bleeding for All
>
> The most common cause of upper GI bleeding in all age groups is gastritis due to **peptic or acid irritation**.

---

[10] It is usually treated before age 2, which is why it won't present after age 2.

Swallowed maternal blood presents as **painless effortless regurgitation** of bright red blood in a newborn with no evidence of volume depletion. Remember to check mom's breasts for cracks that would lead to blood ingested by the infant.

An **Apt Test** will help you determine if the blood is the mother's or the infant's. A NEGATIVE Apt test would signify blood of maternal origin.

In infants and children, the bleeding is classified by the source of the UGI bleed:

Esophagus: Common causes include esophagitis (due to acid reflux or pill-ingestion) and Mallory-Weiss tears, which are tears in the mucosal lining where the esophagus meets the stomach caused by either prolonged or forceful vomiting, coughing, or convulsions. Uncommon causes include portal hypertension.

Stomach: Gastritis due to NSAIDs or stress/ acid/ infection.

Intestine: Crohn's disease.

Esophagogastroduodenoscopy (EGD) is the preferred study to identify the source of UGI bleeding. It should be conducted after initial stabilization and in the first 24 hours of presentation.

Lower GI Bleed (LGB)

Infants and Toddlers

Hirschsprung's disease can present as lower GI bleeding when there is an **associated colitis**.

Malrotation with midgut volvulus presents with bilious vomiting and sometimes **melena**.

NEC, especially if they describe a preemie.

Anal fissures are the most common cause of a lower GI bleed in this age group, and they are quite benign. They are usually secondary to **constipation**.

Intussusception typically presents in a child 9 months of age or older.

> ### Guaic pitfalls
>
> Some situations may give you either a false-positive or a false-negative in guiac testing for occult blood.
>
> **False-positive** results may be seen with recent meat ingestion, horseradish, and ferrous sulfate administration.
>
> **False-negative** results may be seen with Vitamin C ingestion, outdated cards or improper storage of specimen.

Hematochezia	Melena[11]
The passage of **bright red** or **maroon stools**. It suggests either **distal bleeding** or **massive proximal bleeding**. Diagnoses to consider are allergic proctocolitis, infectious colitis, intussusception, Meckel's, rectal fissures/ tears, ingestions, and bleeding disorders.	The words **dark tarry stools** will be described. It is usually due to an **upper GI bleed**. Melena can also be **associated with Meckel's diverticulum**, so consider this diagnosis when melena is described instead of the classic painless bleeding.

---

[11] They won't use the word melena; they will instead describe tarry stools (hopefully not just before the lunch break).

Meckel diverticulum

Meckel diverticulum (MD) is a very common cause of lower GI bleeding. It is present in 2-3% of newborns. It manifests as **painless rectal bleeding** during the first 2 years of life (let's say age 2) and is **diagnosed by technetium 99m pertechnetate scintigraphic study**.[12]

I remember it because **pertechnetate is close enough to the word "petechiae."** MD consists of ectopic gastric mucosa, which takes up the material and lights up.

Treatment is surgical.

Rule of 2 — It typically presents around the **age of 2**, with **2 types of tissue** (gastric and intestinal). In addition, it is usually found **2 feet from the ileocecal valve**, it is **2 inches in length**, and it occurs in **2% of the population**.

> ### Down for Down Syndrome
>
> Down Syndrome has an increased risk of Hirschprung disease, duodenal atresia, Meckel diverticulum, and pyloric stenosis.

Think of it as Meckel's **diverTWOculum** to help associate it with **the rule of two's**.

School Age

Constipation is the most common cause of rectal bleeding at this age, and is usually associated with painful defecation.

Polyps are the most common cause of painless bright red bleeding and one minor bleeding episode with negative family history for polyposis syndromes and GI cancer does not warrant further work up.

Crohn's and ulcerative colitis can also present with blood in stools.

Infectious diseases can present as fever, crampy abdominal pain, and bloody stools.

> ### Beware Red Cefdinir
>
> Cefdinir can cause red stools because it binds iron.

Diarrhea

No matter what scenario they give you, no matter how old the child, no matter how sick the child is, no matter how severe the diarrhea, no matter how mad the dad is, no matter the season of the year or the phase of the moon, **antidiarrheal medications are not to be used in children**.

- If the question asks for treatment of diarrhea, antidiarrheal medications will be the incorrect choice.
- If you are presented with a patient with GI distress who has been given antidiarrheal medications, then these medications will be the cause of the symptoms.

---

[12] Whatever the heck that is.

Watery Diarrhea

Watery diarrhea derives from the small intestine and will be described as being **high volume** but **not bloody**.

No specific tests are needed when presented with a patient with *watery* diarrhea. The exceptions to the rule would be suspicion of *Clostridium difficile* or diarrhea due to *cholera*.

Picture watery diarrhea complicated by the presence of a "C" (sea) of diarrhea to remind you that in this case specific studies would be indicated for diarrhea due to *Clostridium difficile* or *cholera*.

Inflammatory Diarrhea

Inflammatory diarrhea is small and frequently **contains blood, mucous, and white blood cells.** In addition, a more **toxic** picture will be described.

Diarrhea and Feeding

Many pediatricians tell parents to limit the diet of children with diarrhea, even in the absence of dehydration. This is not the policy of the AAP;[13] according to them, children who have diarrhea should continue to be fed **age-appropriate diets**.

If a child is moderately to severely dehydrated, the optimal mixture of oral rehydration solution should be **2% glucose and 90 mEq NaCl**. Pedialyte is NOT a rehydration solution, per se. The AAP recommends **avoiding fatty foods and foods high in simple sugars**, such as sweetened tea, juices, and soft drinks to help the diarrhea resolve faster.

The AAP states that the **BRAT** diet, which we all recite like a Pediatric mantra, contains well-tolerated foods, but it is too limited and does not supply optimal nutrition. In fact, "bowel rest" is considered to be "unnecessary starvation."

Anything that reduces intestinal motility is also dangerous, since it results in pooling of fluids, with dehydration going unnoticed. In addition, it is important to note that oral rehydration fluids do not reduce ongoing stool losses.

By the way — tea is not part of the BRAT diet.

---

[13] Guess whose policy dictates the correct answers on the exam.

Infectious Diarrhea

Viral Diarrhea

Viral diarrhea will present with **low grade fever, vomiting,** and **large loose watery stools**.

Risk increases with daycare attendance and in hospital settings (nosocomial).

Soap and water are better than alcohol gels for eradicating GI pathogens. Norovirus in particular is more resistant to chlorine and ethanol than other viruses.

Diagnosis is made by PCR antigen testing of stool.

Stool WBC

Neutrophils in the stool are more indicative of a diarrhea secondary to bacteria than occult blood. **You use methylene blue to find white blood cells.**

Go Go ! Norovirus !

Thanks to the advent of rotavirus vaccines, Norovirus is now the most common cause of viral gastroenteritis in the U.S. and is often seen in epidemics in schools, institutions, cruise ships, and restaurants as well as on board exams !.

Bacterial Diarrhea

Bacterial diarrhea often presents with **high fever, small frequent stools,** and **mucous or blood** and several were already covered in the ID chapter. Here we will cover the E. coli family.

E. coli Diarrhea

Enteropathogenic *E. coli* (EPEC)

Enteropathogenic *E. coli* results in acute and chronic diarrhea in **neonates** and children **under age 2**. It is more common in areas where there is **poor sanitation**.

Diarrhea is mild, watery, and **non-bloody**, but **fever and vomiting** are commonly seen.

Enterotoxigenic *E. coli* (ETEC)

Presents with **severe watery, nonbloody diarrhea and cramping** and is self-limited. This is known as **traveler's diarrhea** (as in travelers to Mexico). ETEC also affects young infants.

Entero-**TACO**-genic (Enterotoxigenic) *E. coli* causes traveler's diarrhea.

If diarrhea does not improve after several days of supportive care and assays for Shiga toxin are negative, antimicrobial therapy can be considered.

Treatment can include trimethoprim-sulfamethoxazole, azithromycin, or ciprofloxacin, depending on the age of the patient they present.

Enterohemorrhagic/Shiga toxin *E. coli* (STEC)

This type of *E. coli* has changed its name several times like Prince, to the point that it has now been assigned an impossible to remember number instead. **O157:H7.**

The most important point to remember here in addition to the O157:H7 serotype ID card is the fact that it is a "Shiga toxin" -producing bacteria, and all the problems occur when the Shiga hits the fan.

Stools usually start as watery diarrhea and **become bloody after 3 or 4 days.** Severe abdominal pain and cramping are typical but **fever is rare.** This presentation can mimic intussusception.

It can result in **hemorrhagic colitis** and **hemolytic uremic syndrome** (HUS).

Antibiotics are contraindicated in enterohemorrhagic *E. coli* diarrhea. This is because it can result in the release of *shiga toxins* and increase the risk of hemolytic uremic syndrome.

> ### Where's the Shiga?
> Risk factors for contracting the dreaded Shiga toxin producing *E. coli* (STEC) include:
> - unpasteurized milk and apple juice
> - petting zoos: feces of cattle, sheep, deer, and other ruminants
> - raw/ undercooked ground beef
> - raw fruits and vegetables

> ### Hemolytic Uremic Syndrome
>
>
>
> **FAT RN**
>
> **F**ever
> **A**nemia (microangiopathic hemolytic)
> **T**hrombocytopenia
>
> **R**enal insufficiency (AKI)
> **N**euro issues (seizures)

Enteroaggregative *E. coli* (EAEC)

These organisms cause prolonged watery diarrhea and are common in people of all ages in industrialized as well as developing countries.

It gets this absurd name because the bacteria stack up on each other. The bacteria aggregate and colonize the intestinal mucosa, releasing enterotoxins and cytotoxins that destroy the cells lining the intestines.

Enteroinvasive *E. coli* (EIEC)

Enteroinvasive diarrhea presents with a clinical picture similar to dysentery, i.e. *Shigella*. Stools may be **blood- and mucous-tinged**, and **tenesmus** may be present.

Patients are usually **afebrile.**

Protozoal Diarrhea

Giardia intestinalis[14] Infections (Giardiasis)

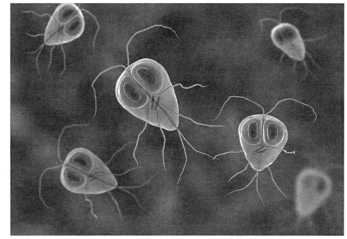

May present with **acute watery nonbloody diarrhea** with **abdominal pain,** and **foul-smelling stools** associated with **flatulence.** Immunocompromised patients may develop chronic infection with **anorexia, weight loss, failure to thrive,** and **anemia.**

Giardiasis is the most common cause of parasitic diarrhea worldwide. **Humans** are the principal reservoir of infection. People become infected **directly from an infected person** or through **ingestion of fecally contaminated water or food.**

Diagnosis is by use of **enzyme immunoassay (EIA)** and **direct fluorescence antibody (DFA) assays in stool.** Under the microscope, Giardia trophozoites are binucleated and look like a happy face.

Some infections are self-limited and treatment is not required. If treatment is needed, **tinidazole, metronidazole,** and **nitazoxanide** are the drugs of choice.

Cryptosporidium

Cryptosporidium species are intracellular parasites that are chlorine tolerant (i.e. not easily killed by your local municipality water treatment plant) and are transmitted **via the fecal-oral route.**

In immunocompetent patients, infections can be asymptomatic but usually cause 1-2 weeks of **watery nonbloody diarrhea.** It is similar to viral diarrhea, but it lasts a lot longer.

In **immunocompromised** patients however, infection can be severe, disseminated, and life-threatening with protracted watery nonbloody diarrhea, abdominal pain, vomiting, and weight loss without fever.

Outbreaks have been associated with **contaminated drinking and recreational water.**

Outbreaks have also been associated with farm livestock, especially petting zoos.

Person-to-person transmission is common in childcare centers due to poor hygiene after diaper changes.

> ### CCSP
>
>
>
> • **C**ryptosporidium
> • **C**hildcare Centers
> • **S**wimming Pools
> • **P**etting Zoos
>
> And just imagine a daycare taking a field trip to a petting zoo and then to a city pool. Your chance to be on the evening news and go viral so to speak !

---

[14] Formerly *Giardia lamblia* and *Giardia duodenalis.*

Diarrhea: Putting it all Together

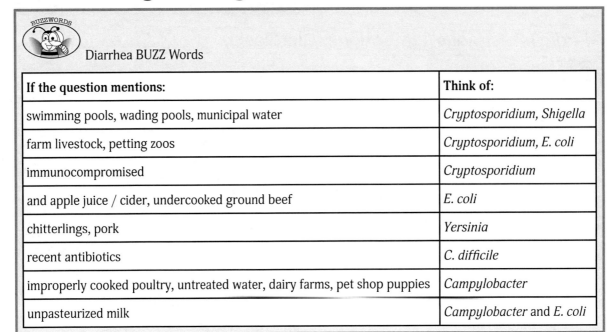

Diarrhea BUZZ Words

If the question mentions:	Think of:
swimming pools, wading pools, municipal water	*Cryptosporidium, Shigella*
farm livestock, petting zoos	*Cryptosporidium, E. coli*
immunocompromised	*Cryptosporidium*
and apple juice / cider, undercooked ground beef	*E. coli*
chitterlings, pork	*Yersinia*
recent antibiotics	*C. difficile*
improperly cooked poultry, untreated water, dairy farms, pet shop puppies	*Campylobacter*
unpasteurized milk	*Campylobacter* and *E. coli*

Protracted Diarrhea

Protracted diarrhea is defined as diarrhea **beyond 2 weeks** that cannot be attributed to an acute gastroenteritis.

The causes vary with the age of the child. **Newborns** will have anatomical causes such as short gut syndrome; for **infants**, think of viral infection and protein intolerance; in **toddlers** (see Toddler's diarrhea) and in **older kids**, think of lactose intolerance.

Passing through the Screen: Screening Tests for Malabsorption		
Malabsorbed Substance	**Test**	**Comments**
Sugars	Clinitest® (Quick Screen)	**Tests for reducing substances,** which are all dietary sugars except for sucrose. The presence of these reducing substances in stool would correlate with sugar malabsorption.
Sugars	Hydrogen Breath Test	A positive hydrogen breath test would correlate with **sugar malabsorption.** This is because the normal gut flora "ferments" the sugar, resulting in hydrogen production, which is absorbed in the blood and excreted in the lungs.

Malabsorbed Substance	Test	Comments
Fat	Fecal Fat Measurement	A single stool specimen for fat is not a valid verification. A **3-day fecal fat determination is necessary.**
Fat	Serum Carotene and Prothrombin Time	These are indirect tests since they correlate with **vitamin A and vitamin K absorption.**
Protein	Albumin level, total protein	Typically occurs along with fat malabsorption. When it occurs as an isolated clinical finding, edema and other clinical findings will be noted.

The description of loose stools does not necessarily suggest or confirm "chronic diarrhea." Keep in mind that a child with **steatorrhea** may only have a couple of large firm stools a day yet still be suffering from chronic malabsorption.

Neuroblastoma can produce **vasoactive intestinal peptides** that can cause diarrhea.

Protracted Diarrhea

Diarrhea can be seen with the following predisposing factors:

- Malnutrition
- Chronic infection
- Systemic Disease
- Immunodeficiency

Transient Lactase Deficiency

This typically occurs after an acute gastroenteritis, and can take up to 3-6 months to return to normal.

Toddler's Diarrhea (Chronic Non-Specific Diarrhea)

This is the most common cause of chronic diarrhea in children up to age 3, and it is often due to excess fruit juice intake. The high sugar content of fruit juices acts as an osmotic laxative.

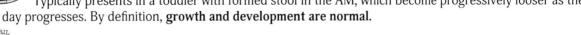

Typically presents in a toddler with formed stool in the AM, which become progressively looser as the day progresses. By definition, **growth and development are normal.**

Poor growth, fever, and melena are not *seen* with chronic nonspecific diarrhea.

Treatment consists of **limiting carbohydrates** in the diet, and increasing intake of **high fiber foods** such as fruits and vegetables.

A Liver Runs Through It/
Liver Diseases

Cholestatic Jaundice

This presents with **elevated direct bilirubin, pale stools** and **hepatomegaly**, and is caused by **liver/hepatocellular** disease or **anatomical/obstructive** disease. Intervention is required to prevent severe liver disease.

Hepatobiliary scintigraphy is a good first step to establish the diagnosis.

With liver disease, the isotope is taken up and it makes its way to the biliary system.

With obstruction, there will be uptake in the liver but no excretion down the biliary tree.

Neonatal hepatitis will present later (months after birth), whereas **obstructive disease** can present at **birth or within weeks**, not months, later.

Biliary Atresia

They will describe an **elevated direct bilirubin** and possibly **acholic (clay-colored) stools** in a child over **one month of age**. The *Kasai* procedure, which essentially joins the liver to the intestine, can be done if the infant is **younger than 2 months**.

When biliary atresia is suspected, the first test should be an **ultrasound**, followed by a **HIDA scan** and ultimately a biopsy.

The most common cause of cholestatic jaundice in a newborn is TPN (especially if they tell you it is a preemie).

If you need to distinguish **cholestatic jaundice** from **hepatocellular-caused jaundice**, remember:

- Cholestatic disease has a very high alkaline phosphatase
- Hepatocellular has a very high ALT/AST.

Bronze Babies

Remember **direct** hyperbiliru-binemia should not be present if you choose **phototherapy** for an infant with jaundice.

If you light the cholestatic babies, you will turn yellow babies into "bronze" babies, which really look more like green-blue babies and they'll stay that color for months.

And it may surprise you, but most parents don't really want babies that look like the Statue of Liberty.

Hyperalimentation (HAL)

An important point to remember is that HAL-induced cholestasis is due primarily to protein intake associated with TPN, and this should be limited to 2 g/kg/day.

If all else fails, phenobarbital can be used to stimulate bile secretion and decrease serum bili levels.

Choledochal Cyst (CDC)

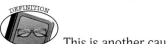 This is another cause of extrahepatic biliary obstruction and presents similarly to biliary atresia. It is also diagnosed with **abdominal ultrasound.**

 CDC presents as **neonatal jaundice, fever, acholic stools, RUQ pain** and a **palpable mass.**

Gilbert Syndrome

Gilbert syndrome is a harmless familial condition due to **glucuronyl transferase deficiency,** and this results in an **intermittently** elevated **unconjugated** serum bili, particularly with fasting illness or other stressors.[15] They will also likely drop a hint of a **similar history in other family members.** That will be your clue to pick Gilbert syndrome as your answer.

"Gil- bili" syndrome. Picture a "hill Bili" unable to transfer his yellow bananas because he lacks a truck (transferase), and his whole family is involved due to all that inbreeding.

This is normally **recognized after puberty.** So consider Gilbert syndrome if they present you with a **teenager** who gets **jaundiced** when he has an **upper respiratory infection** or **is fasting.**[16] Another presentation could be **jaundice in the morning** resolved by the afternoon.

Other than the **elevated indirect bilirubin,** the **LFTs are normal.** There is NO hemolysis. No treatment is necessary.

Reye's syndrome

This should be an easy one to figure out on the exam, since they will have to drop hints all over the place. They will likely mention a **recent influenza-like disease or varicella,** during which **aspirin** was given. The child typically presents comatose with **elevated LFTs** and **serum ammonia levels.**

If they tell you this is the **second such episode,** Reye's syndrome is not the correct answer, although it will definitely be one of the choices given. In this case, consider an **inborn error of metabolism.**

Wilson's Disease (Hepatolenticular degeneration)

 An **autosomal recessive** disorder of **copper metabolism.**

---

15 Like what you are experiencing right now.
16 Like when you ordered fasting labs and can't understand why the bili is elevated.

This is due to a **lot of copper floating around** and getting deposited, like unwanted pennies at a Floyd Mayweather yachting extravaganza. They get deposited in the eyes (**Kayser Fleischer rings**), the liver, the brain (basal ganglia), and the kidney (renal tubular acidosis is the result).

WIlson disease presents as **liver disease in children and teenagers** and as **neuropsychiatric disease in adults**.

Diagnosis is made clinically along with finding **significantly elevated hepatic copper** and **decreased ceruloplasmin**. Ceruloplasmin is a "carrier vehicle", and all vehicles are "taken" going around depositing copper around. **Serum copper levels are low** because most of the copper is **accumulated in the tissues**. There is often **increased copper in the urine**.

Treatment is with **D-penicillamine** to chelate the copper along with a low copper diet. Wilson's disease is **fatal** if not treated.

Think of yourself as "**rec**eiving" a copper penny, and you will remember that this is a **rec**essive disorder. If you remember the copper **penny**, it will be easy to remember that **penicillamine** is the treatment.

Remember Copper ➔ Penny ➔ Cillamine. **Penicillamine can result in aplastic anemia**, so picture a fistful of pennies clogging up the bone marrow.

Excess copper can also be seen in **chronic active hepatitis**.

Alpha-1 Antitrypsin (A1AT) deficiency

Persistent jaundice in the newborn period is a very common presentation of alpha-1 antitrypsin (A1AT) deficiency.

A1AT deficiency affects 3 main organ systems: **the lung** (COPD), **the liver** (neonatal hepatitis with cholestasis), and **the skin** (necrotizing panniculitis and psoriasis in adults).

Recent studies suggest that A1AT deficiency is under-recognized and may be as prevalent as cystic fibrosis. Therefore its prevalance on the boards is also likely to increase as well.

Portal Hypertension (PH)

Either a portal venous pressure of more than 5mm Hg, or a portal to hepatic vein pressure gradient of more than 10 mm Hg.

It is usually suspected with a combination of clinical and laboratory data. The venous congestion then leads to the development of collateral circulation (varices) at the junction of the high pressure and the low pressure venous system(esophagus and stomach).

Children with a history of **instrumentation of the umbilical vein** during the neonatal period (leading to portal vein thrombosis), think preemies and other critically ill infants, and children with chronic liver disease (biliary atresia being the most common) are at risk for portal hypertension. Portal Hypertension presents with **splenomegaly** and **hematemesis** from either esophageal or gastric varices. The causes may be pre, post, and intrahepatic and the liver size may be large, normal, or small.

Abdominal U/S with Doppler is the best noninvasive test to identify the cause of the portal venous obstruction.

Laboratory studies will be helpful if the portal pressure gradient is enough to cause hypersplenism. **Leukopenia** and **thrombocytopenia** are common and splenic requestration of RBCs may also be described in the history.

LFTs may be relatively normal if it is not due to primary liver disease. Don't be fooled by normal LFTs.

Splenomegaly is the most sensitive indicator of portal hypertension and varices.

The Alphabet Soup of Hepatitis

Somewhere in the exam you will be called upon to decipher hepatitis A from hepatitis B, HBe antigen vs. core antigen vs. Auntie Jean from Ellie May vs. Non A, **"non-B, Non C and sometimes D"** and "tomorrow something else but today Non A." Well, here is the ABC of hepatitis for today's Board candidate.

Most of the diagnostic lab tests in hepatitis, and in many other conditions as well, will be measuring antigen and antibodies. Remember that **IgM-specific antibody is positive only acutely and then resolves. IgG however, persists for life**: once it turns positive, it is always positive, but tells you nothing about recent disease.

IgM is **iMMediate** and IgG is **for Good**.

Hepatitis A (HAV)

The presentations will be **"flu-like symptoms,"** along with **jaundice** and **elevated liver function tests**. Also included in the history might be a recent trip to a place where hepatitis A is endemic.

It is transmitted via the **fecal-oral route**. It is prevalent where there is **poor hygiene and poor sanitation**. It is contracted from household contacts and daycare centers by **drinking contaminated water** or by **ingesting** contaminated foods such as **raw or undercooked shellfish from contaminated waters**.

90% of children younger than 5 years have asymptomatic infection and will not be jaundiced.

HOT TIP

Hepatitis A is prevalent among Native Americans and Alaskan Natives.[17] However, **hepatitis A is not commonly seen in Asians.**

Children and adults with HAV **who work in food service** or **in child care centers** should be excluded from work for **one week after the onset of symptoms.**

TAKE HOME MESSAGE

Diagnosis of acute infection is via serum **IgM** which can remain elevated for 6 months. Elevated **IgG** confirms previous infection and immunity against the disease.

TREATMENT

Treatment is **supportive.** Hepatitis A is self-limited and does not lead to chronic disease. Immune globulin against HAV is available for pre and post-exposure prophylaxis.

Hepatitis B

It is spread via contact with bodily fluids, so the main modes of transmission are **blood transfusions, sexual contact,** and **perinatal transmission.** HepB is a HepaDNAvirus. The only DNA hepatitis virus. (The others, A, E, C, D are RNA viruses).

With hepatitis B, you need to keep track of the antigens and antibodies—and be familiar with their rise and fall.[18] Sort of like being a hepatitis historian on a serological archaeological dig.

Phase	Serological Test	Meaning[19]
Acute	HBsAg (surface antigen)	A marker of active infection but does not differentiate between acute and chronic infection
	HBeAg (e antigen)	Indicates "high viral load," **infectivity**, and replication
	HBV-DNA	A sensitive marker indicating "viral replication"
Recovery	Disappearance of HBV-DNA and HBsAg	This occurs around 6 months after its appearance
	Appearance of HBsAb, HB$_c$Ab, and HB$_e$Ab	**Antibodies** to Hepatitis B surface antigen, core antigen and HBe. Shows resolution of disease.
Chronic infection	The persistence of surface antigen HBsAg beyond 6 months indicates chronic infection	It is detected in the serum lifelong in those with chronic infection.

HOT TIP

In a patient with no hepatitis B disease, but having had the hepatitis B vaccine, you will find a **positive HBsAb** (Hep B surface antibody) but **every other antigen and antibody will be negative.** Patients with previous natural disease will have positive HBsAb but also HBcAb (Hep B core antibody).

MNEMONIC

Think **E** as in Evil, or very infectious. You can also think of the "E" antigen as "Excess" because it can spread to Everyone.

---

[17] The old politically incorrect term that may still appear on the exam is "Eskimo".
[18] Insert your own rise and fall of the Roman Empire joke.
[19] Or added confusion depending on how many times you read it and the state of mind you are in while reading it.

When HBeAg is positive, the mother is highly infectious. Almost ALL kids born to mothers with HBeAg positivity will develop chronic hepatitis B. **The earlier the age of infection, the higher the incidence of chronic HBV** (90% for infants, 10% for adults).

Fulminant hepatic failure and **hepatocellular cancer** are the most feared complications of chronic HBV infection.

Hepatitis C Virus (HCV)

During my third year of medical school, this was called *"non-A, non-B."* During my residency it was known as "Clifford the Clip-haired Cutie." Now it is just known as **hepatitis C**. It can result in **liver disease** and **cirrhosis**, and is associated with an **increased incidence of hepatocellular carcinoma**.

It is the most common bloodborne infection in the United States and the most common cause of **chronic viral hepatitis**. It is transmitted by the same route as hepatitis B. Most infections in children are asymptomatic.

Hepatitis **C** is associated with Liver **C**ancer and **C**irrhosis.

Hepatitis D Virus (HDV)

If they mention "**Delta Agent**," they are either referring to hepatitis D or Gene Hackman in *Mississippi Burning*. Remember, this is a virus that cannot replicate by itself. **It requires the presence of HBsAg to provide its outer coat.**

D represents **D**ependent or **D**eficient.

Hepatitis E Virus (HEV)

Hepatitis E is transmitted via the **fecal-oral route** and is most common in parts of Asia, Africa, and Mexico and is associated with **exposure to contaminated water.**

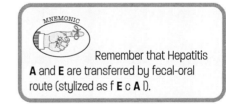

Remember that Hepatitis **A** and **E** are transferred by fecal-oral route (stylized as f **E** c **A** l).

It does not lead to chronic hepatitis.

Liver Failure

The most important findings in a child with impending liver failure are an **elevated serum ammonia level** and **change in mental status**.

However, if you are presented with a patient with **chronic tremor and anxiety**, and lab findings consistent with liver disease, you will want to rule out **Wilson's Disease** by measuring a **serum ceruloplasmin level**.

Pancreas

Acute Pancreatitis

This is characterized by **mid-epigastric pain radiating to the back** with **guarding and rebound**, coupled with **diminished bowel sounds** and **vomiting**. They could describe a child more comfortable lying on his side, with his knees to his chest. In more severe cases, they could also describe signs of volume depletion, including decreased urine output and even pulmonary edema and pulmonary effusions.

Remember that Pancreatitis can be associated with Pulmonary edema and Pleural effusion.

Abdominal ultrasound, not serum amylase, **is the most specific test in diagnosing pancreatitis.** ERCP (endoscopic retrograde cholangiopancreatography) is used to follow recurrent pancreatitis, not to diagnose acute pancreatitis.

A normal amylase does not rule out pancreatitis. Lipase is a more specific test for pancreatic disease. Additional lab findings could include **hyperglycemia, hypocalcemia, elevated BUN/ creatinine, and anemia, as well as evidence of coagulopathy**.

Recurrent / Chronic Pancreatitis

Familial dyslipidemia is an important cause for recurrent pancreatitis in children. They could hint at this by noting a family member had died of premature atherosclerosis. You might be fooled into believing the cause of the abdominal pain is cardiac.

If you are asked which test to order to reveal the underlying cause of the abdominal pain, the answer will be **serum lipid levels (especially triglycerides)**, not the myriad of imaging or cardiac studies you will be offered.

Hypercalcemia is another known cause of acute or recurrent pancreatitis. Keep this in mind if presented with a child with **hyperparathyroidism** or **kidney stones** who is presenting with acute or recurrent abdominal pain.

Acute Sporadic vs Recurrent Chronic

In case you are tested on it, there **is** a difference between *acute, sporadic pancreatitis and recurrent, chronic pancreatitis.*

Acute sporadic is more common and usually due to **blunt abdominal trauma** or just plain "we don't know," i.e. **idiopathic**.

Chronic, relapsing pancreatitis is usually caused by infection, autoimmune disease, inherited conditions, or medications. The most common cause of recurrent pancreatitis is **hereditary pancreatitis**.

Bad Gall Bladder

Cholecystitis

Although it is not a cardinal sign in adults, **jaundice is a presenting sign in over one fourth of children with cholecystitis.**

Therefore, if they describe a child who is jaundiced with fatty food intolerance and has **fever, pain radiating to the right scapula**, and a **palpable mass in the right upper quadrant**, think of cholecystitis.

Referred Visceral Pain

Abdominal pain that **radiates to the shoulder** is likely to be gallbladder pain, which is a result of diaphragm irritation. The **diaphragm and shoulder** share common pain pathways.

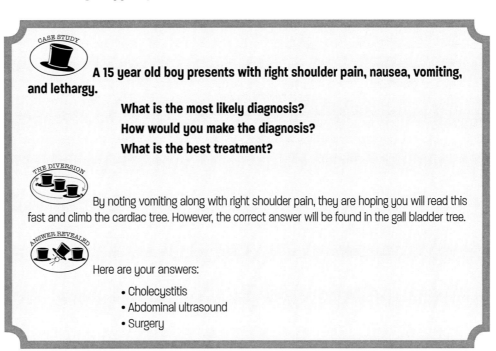

CASE STUDY

A 15 year old boy presents with right shoulder pain, nausea, vomiting, and lethargy.

What is the most likely diagnosis?

How would you make the diagnosis?

What is the best treatment?

THE DIVERSION

By noting vomiting along with right shoulder pain, they are hoping you will read this fast and climb the cardiac tree. However, the correct answer will be found in the gall bladder tree.

ANSWER REVEALED

Here are your answers:

- Cholecystitis
- Abdominal ultrasound
- Surgery

Sticks and Stones

Cholelithiasis refers to stones in the gallbladder. Gallstones have a peak incidence during adolescence.

There is a current increase in gallstones in children most likely due to the rise in childhood obesity.

Conditions that predispose children to gallstone formation (choledocholithiasis) include:

- cholesterol stones (radioluscent): obesity, Hispanic ethnicity, family history, parity, and female sex
- pigmented stones (black): hereditary hemolytic anemias such as sickle cell and hereditary spherocytosis
- infection-related (brown): seen with bacterial or parasitic infections
- calcium carbonate stones: unknown mechanism

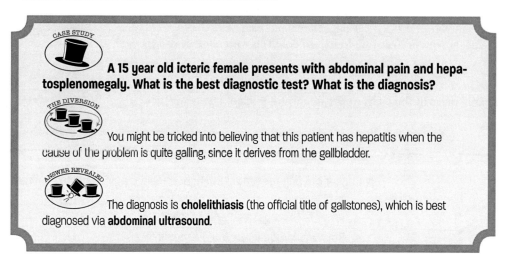

CASE STUDY

A 15 year old icteric female presents with abdominal pain and hepatosplenomegaly. What is the best diagnostic test? What is the diagnosis?

THE DIVERSION

You might be tricked into believing that this patient has hepatitis when the cause of the problem is quite galling, since it derives from the gallbladder.

ANSWER REVEALED

The diagnosis is **cholelithiasis** (the official title of gallstones), which is best diagnosed via **abdominal ultrasound**.

COIN FLIP

Notice the similar presentations of cholelithiasis and cholecystitis. Both are diagnosed by ultrasound, but the presentations are slightly different.

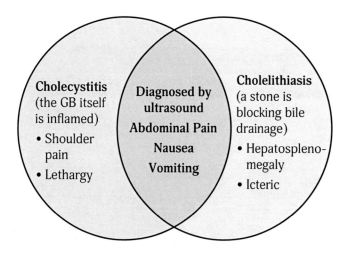

Cholecystitis (the GB itself is inflamed)
- Shoulder pain
- Lethargy

Diagnosed by ultrasound
Abdominal Pain
Nausea
Vomiting

Cholelithiasis (a stone is blocking bile drainage)
- Hepatosplenomegaly
- Icteric

Chapter 23

Catching Your Breath: Pulmonary

Just as in clinical practice, pulmonary problems are commonly encountered on the boards. This is where we begin our breathtaking journey through the world of pulmonary disorders.

Wheezing

All that wheezes is not asthma, especially in an infant. You've already learned all about asthma in the Allergy chapter. For other causes of wheezing, consider **foreign body aspiration, swallowing dysfunction,** and **bronchiolitis.** To put it another way:

❑ Aspirated **Drinks**
❑ Babies with **Kinks**
❑ Swallowed **Thinks** (=Things)[1]
❑ Vascular **Rinks** (=Rings)

Foreign Body Aspiration

This is seen most commonly in **infants and toddlers.** Another possibility is **a child with a developmental disability, or any child with CNS depression.** Most foreign body aspirations manifest within 24 hours.

The classic **triad** is **cough, wheeze,** and **unilateral decreased breath sounds.** Infants and toddlers typically aspirate **food**, especially hot dogs and popcorn, and older children typically aspirate **objects.**

There is virtually no chance they will give you a clue that an object was aspirated. In fact, they often try to throw you off the trail by mentioning a history of asthma and/or giving signs of croup with x-ray findings consistent with croup.

Whether or not they mention a history of asthma, signs of croup, or any other red herrings for that matter, the clues to foreign body aspiration will be **unlabored breathing with nonproductive cough** with an **expiratory wheeze** heard best **on the right side.** They may, if you are lucky, describe the symptoms occurring just after the child was playing with a toy, but that hint would be a gift. They will often include a history of a **cough of sudden onset.** Chest x-ray may show unilateral hyperinflation.

---

[1] Aspirated things (foreign bodies) are more likely in older children who are mobile, but it is still a consideration in an infant.

PERIL

In nearly 50% of cases, **there is no recollection of an actual aspiration.**

CASE STUDY

You could be presented with yet another long-winded description of a one-year-old child with acute onset of coughing coupled with a right-sided expiratory wheeze. Then, just as you pat yourself on the back for making the correct diagnosis, they provide you with the suspected diagnosis and then simply ask you to pick the best test to confirm your suspicions.

THE DIVERSION

Plain chest x-ray will be one of the choices. However, while the x-ray may hint that a foreign body was aspirated (unilateral hyperinflation), this cannot *confirm* the diagnosis, since the foreign body may be radiolucent. It may show hyperexpansion, but nothing else. Then, sitting right there for the taking is what you believe to be the juicy correct answer: "inspiratory/expiratory films" – right out of the textbook that is your brain. This will be incorrect, since it is impossible to have a child this age cooperate with such a test.

ANSWER REVEALED

Oddly enough, the correct answer will be **airway fluoroscopy.** This is the safest and most effective way to confirm foreign body aspiration in this age group. **Bronchoscopy** would also be a correct diagnostic option, and a method of retrieval of the foreign body.

Vascular Rings and other Things causing vascular compression

Vascular rings and other entities such as bronchogenic cysts, tracheal stenosis, and a double aortic arch, which can cause external tracheal or esophageal compression, should be suspected in an infant with **recurrent wheezing** that **increases with feeding and neck flexion.** In addition to wheezing, the infant can also present with **stridor** and/or **dyspnea during feeding.**

HOT TIP

Diagnosis is established with CT or MR angiography.

Swallowing dysfunction

BUZZWORDS

If you are presented with an infant with recurrent coughing associated with wheezing, the underlying problem might be a result of recurrent cough and wheezing during feed that is due to a swallowing dysfunction. This would be confirmed by a **barium swallow study** with **video fluoroscopy.**

TREATMENT

Treatment of swallowing dysfunction consists of **thickened feedings**. These infants also require **feeding therapy.** Severe swallowing dysfunction may require placement of a **G-tube.**

Congenital Malformations of the Lung

DEFINITION

Congenital malformations of the lower airway include pulmonary sequestrations, bronchogenic cysts, congenital adenomatoid malformations, and congenital lobar emphysema. They either present with recurrent respiratory symptoms, or are incidental findings on chest XR. Treatment usually involves surgical removal.

Respiratory Failure

Respiratory failure is present when the lungs are unable to perform adequate gas exchange.

The evaluation of **respiratory effort** is more important than any lab value.

Signs of respiratory failure include **hypoxemia, grunting, agitation, decreased mentation, poor tone, cyanosis, and signs of fatigue**.

If you are presented with a patient with an underlying neurological disorder who is in respiratory distress, elective intubation might be a correct answer since such patients are an aspiration risk.

The first thing to do in deciding whether to intubate is to **assess respiratory effort**.

The difference in blood pressure during inspiration and expiration should not be greater than 10 mmHg. **Pulsus paradoxus** is defined as a decrease in systolic blood pressure by more than 10 mm Hg during inspiration. It is a sign of severe respiratory distress or decreased cardiac output.

Obtaining an ABG, or any other time-consuming lab, is **not the "first thing" to do** and would not be the correct choice in assessing a child in respiratory distress. You can almost never be wrong in choosing "assess airway" - the "A" in the ABC of managing acute situations.

They could present you with a child in respiratory distress and ask you the best way to assess and confirm this.

Assessing respiratory distress can be tricky. The diversionary answer will be to assess the respiratory rate. This is frequently the incorrect answer in ruling out respiratory failure since the "normal" respiratory rate may only be a transition from tachypnea to apnea.

When asked for the best way to assess the severity of respiratory distress, the correct answer will often be to watch for signs of anxiety (tachycardia).

Chronic Hypoxemia

Any persistent condition that compromises the ability to oxygenate blood results in chronic hypoxemia.

They won't come right out and hit you over the head with a hammer and tell you the patient has chronic hypoxemia; it will be hinted at in the history.

"How can this Happen?" You Ask

There is no memorization here, just cool explanation of the physiological facts, nothing but the facts.

When the kidneys see hypoxemia, they respond by producing erythropoietin (the only thing they can do) so red cells get produced, and the HCT goes up. A Hct of 65 is fine, but greater than that can result in **headaches, joint pain, clots** (leading to **pulmonary emboli**), and **hemoptysis**. Any of the above can be clues that chronic hypoxemia is the underlying problem.

For some reason, the platelet shelf life also goes down, so there is also an **increased risk of bleeding**.

In addition, the **respiratory drive** of patients with chronic lung disease is often **driven by hypoxemia**, rather than acidosis and hypercapnia. You are expected to know that **correction of hypoxemia (by administration of oxygen) in a patient suffering from chronic lung disease may put the patient at risk for respiratory arrest**. Therefore, oxygen supplementation should be provided at the lowest concentration needed to maintain an oxygen saturation of 90%. CO_2 measurements via ABG should be followed as well.

> ### Let's go Clubbing
> If you are presented with a patient with clubbing of the fingers or the toes, depending on other information presented, consider a diagnosis of *cyanotic heart disease, chronic lung disease*, or *cirrhosis of the liver*. It can also be a familial trait, in the absence of any other disorders.

> ### Hypoxia vs. Hypercarbia
> Hypoxia will be described as **cyanosis** with **depressed sensorium**.
>
> Hypercarbia is often described as **flushing, agitation** and **headaches** because of elevated CO_2 leading to cerebral vasodilation. If severe, hypercarbia causes somnolence and coma.

Pulse Oximetry / What It Can and Can't Do

We have all become reliant on pulse oximetry without knowing its limitations. You will have to know these limitations. The easy part is to make sure the **pulse is correlating,** and that there are **no mechanical or artifactual problems**. That is for the real world; now for the Board world.

Pulse oximetry **estimates** the saturation of hemoglobin with oxygen by measuring the differential light absorption of oxyhemoglobin and deoxyhemoglobin.

> ### What's your Pulse Ox score?
> Know that under normal conditions, hemoglobin is:
> - 95% saturated at PaO_2 of 80 torr
> - 90% saturated at PaO_2 of 60 torr
> - and only 50% saturated of PaO_2 of 27 torr.

Pulse oximetry is limited by:

- decreased signal from motion
- external light
- severe anemia
- cold skin
- decreased perfusion and pulsatility

HOT TIP

Any given arterial pressure of oxygen (PaO_2) would lead to a **lower SpO_2** in the face of acidosis, increased body temperature, and increased levels of 2,3-BPG which cause Hgb to dump oxygen. The reverse is also true.

Carbon Monoxide Poisoning

Carbon monoxide poisoning leads to elevated levels of carboxyhemoglobin. Carboxyhemoglobin absorbs light in the same wavelength as oxyhemoglobin, so SpO_2 may appear falsely normal.

TAKE HOME MESSAGE

If you can't trust the pulse oximeter, who can you trust? If you are asked for the best measure of hypoxemia, the correct answer will be **arterial blood gas measurement (ABG)**.

PERIL

Do not be fooled into choosing capillary or venous blood gas; it HAS to be arterial for the oxygen component to be valid.

Methemoglobinemia

DEFINITION

Be on the lookout for methemoglobinemia, a condition in which the iron in the hemoglobin molecule is in the oxidized ferric (Fe^{+3}) state, making it unable to effectively unload oxygen to the tissues. This can be congenital or acquired. **It results in cyanosis in the absence of cyanotic heart disease.**

BUZZWORDS

Symptoms include **fatigue**, **dizziness**, and **nausea** leading to life-threatening **arrhythmias**, **seizures**, and **altered mental status**. One clue to diagnosis would be if the patient has mild hypoxemia (SpO_2 85%) that does not improve with supplemental oxygen.

HOT TIP

Watch for mentioning babies who have been given **topical anesthetics (like benzocaine for teething)**, history of gastroenteritis, exposure to nitric oxide, or ingestion of nitrite-containing well water.

TREATMENT

Treatment consists of eliminating the triggering agent and/or IV methylene blue.

CO-oximetry is Cooler

Carboxyhemoglobin and Methemoglobin are best diagnosed with **co-oximetry** which involves blood gas analysis of oxyhemoglobin, deoxyhemoglobin, methemoglobin, and carboxyhemoglobin. It's like a fancy sophisticated pulse oximeter.

Methemoglobin Messes with SpO_2

PERIL

Methemoglobinemia will lead to unreliable SpO_2 readings because pulse oxymetry recognizes all hemoglobin as oxygenated or deoxygenated but methemoglobin absorbs light in both wavelengths of the pulse oximeter. SpO_2 will be reported around 85% regardless of the true SpO_2.

Cyanosis

DEFINITION

Cyanosis is defined as a **central blueish discoloration of the skin** due to poorly oxygenated blood. It has a myriad of causes including, but not limited to, heart and lung conditions.

PERIL

Anemia does NOT cause cyanosis. Cyanosis is visible at 5 g/dL of desaturated Hgb, so it is actually more readily seen at higher Hgb levels (polycythemia).

Left-to-Right intracardiac shunts alone DO NOT cause cyanosis.

TAKE HOME MESSAGE

The **hyperoxia test** helps distinguish pulmonary from cardiac cyanosis. After 20 minutes of 100% inspired oxygen, PaO_2 would **increase to >250 in most pulmonary diseases** (except PPHN) but would remain <150 in cardiac diseases.

Out of the Blue Causes of Cyanosis

These are some causes of Cyanosis that are a bit out of the box !

- intracardiac shunts
- shock
- methemoglobinemia
- CNS depression
- cold exposure
- polycythemia
- breath holding spells

CASE STUDY

A frantic mom presents in your office with her 6 month old infant, whose hands and feet are blue and have been this way on and off since birth. Five minutes later, the grandmother comes in carrying 14 pounds of blankets because of the draft she detects from the open window in the office 140 feet down the hall. The baby is otherwise normal. They both note that, when the hands and feet are not blue, they are mottled. You try to hide your own mottled and cyanotic appearance and figure out what's going on.

THE DIVERSION

You might be diverted into doing a workup for methemoglobinemia, obtaining an EKG, or something simple like an oxygen saturation reading.

ANSWER REVEALED

This is nothing more than episodic acrocyanosis, which requires no workup at all other than reassurance to all involved (including you). If this were a case of true cyanosis, they would have described central blueness of the lips or face.

Calling All Chronic Coughs

Sometimes coughs present early without a lot of other clues, and you need to pick out the etiologies. Here is your roadmap.

Working Up a Chronic Cough

A cough is considered chronic if it persists for more than 4 weeks. Common causes include asthma, aspiration, bronchiectasis and protracted bacterial bronchitis (PBB).

It is important to assess for specific "cough pointers" to help point you in the right direction. Some useful pointers include a dry vs. wet cough, hoarse voice, recurrent infections, or wheeze.

All patients with chronic cough should undergo chest x-ray and spirometry (if age appropriate). Further testing is directed by the presence of specific cough pointers. If the cough is non-specific and chest x-ray and spirometry are normal, no further testing is required.

And don't forget pertussis, the "100-day cough".

When a Cough is Not Effective

Cerebral palsy, muscle weakness, vocal cord dysfunction, CNS disease, thoracic deformities, and pain **all impair the effectiveness of coughing**.

TNT: **T**horaco **N**euro (Cerebral Palsy/ CNS Disease) **T**ied up with weakness and pain. It takes TNT to clear lungs when coughing isn't effective.

Psychogenic Cough

"Loud, brassy barking and/or honking that can be **produced on command**." If they note that it **disappears during sleep**, you have your answer.

More Serious Considerations

TB, fungal infections, parasitic infections, and even chest malignancies, can produce persistent coughs. If they include the combination of **fever, weight loss,** or **night sweats** along with a chronic cough, further testing is indicated.

Cough Meds

Despite parental pressure, **cough suppressants in children have no benefit over a placebo**. For purposes of the Boards, just say NO to cough suppressants.

Cystic Fibrosis (CF)

Signs and symptoms consistent with CF include **anemia, failure to thrive, chronic diarrhea, steatorrhea, recurrent sinopulmonary infections, low serum albumin, low sodium,** and **pseudomonas infections**. Congenital absence of vas deferens can be a finding in CFTR mutations.

The Sweat Test: 60 mmol/L chloride or greater is diagnostic. This number is critical in case they throw in a normal value, implying it is abnormal simply by including it in the description.

In early childhood children with cystic fibrosis Staph aureus predominates as a source of infection. In late adolescence pseudomonas is more common.

> **CASE STUDY**
> **They can present you with a child suspected of having cystic fibrosis, and ask for the best next step.**
>
> **THE DIVERSION**
> The diversion will be DNA analysis or genetic testing. You will be tempted to take the bait, believing that modern methods must trump the old.
>
> **ANSWER REVEALED**
> Sometimes an oldie but a goodie is better than new technology. This is the case in confirming a diagnosis of cystic fibrosis. DNA analysis has not replaced sweat testing as the gold standard. While genetic analysis for CFTR mutations is necessary to guide therapy, the first step in diagnosing CF is always the chloride sweat test. False negatives are rare on the sweat test. When it occurs, it is usually due to an inadequate sample or technique.

Genetics of CF

PERIL

The gene is inherited in an **autosomal recessive** pattern. Carriers show no signs, so any physical findings they tell you about are red herrings.

HOT TIP

"What are the odds of a **healthy sibling** of someone with CF being a **carrier**?" The answer is **2/3**.

HOT TIP

They could ask "If a sibling of someone with CF marries someone from the general population, what are the odds of them having a kid with CF?"[2] Using the formula that oddsmakers in Las Vegas use, you can easily answer this question.

In the general Caucasian population, the carrier rate is **1 in 25 (1/25)**. Memorize this fact!

- If 2 carriers are married,[3] the risk of having a child with a double recessive trait is 1/4.

Therefore, the answer to the typical question they ask above is:

- **(2/3)**[chance of a sibling carrier] × **(1/25)**[chance of picking a carrier out of the general Caucasian population] × **(1/4)**[chance of child being double recessive] = 1 in 150.

Neonatal Screening for CF

Know that the Newborn Screen (NBS) is only 95% sensitive for the detection of CF. 95% would be an extraordinary batting average but not reliable for questions on screening on the boards!

PERIL

So if you are presented with a newborn with symptoms suspicious for CF, **don't let the fact that the infant had a normal NBS rule out CF completely.**

Alternately, know that newborn screening is not diagnostic of CF. Only one in 20 infants with an abnormal NBS for CF, actually has CF after further testing.

TAKE HOME MESSAGE **Sweat chloride testing is the only true diagnostic test.**

Vitamins in CF

Vitamin E deficiency is a major problem with CF. **Vitamin E supplementation should be started before age 5.**

Any sign of fat-soluble vitamin deficiency should prompt consideration of CF diagnosis.

---

2 They should tell you they are both Caucasian; otherwise, the risk is too low to bother with.
3 And of course, some people have been known to have children even without being married. The same odds would apply.

GI Manifestations of CF

During infancy, GI symptoms are more prevalent than respiratory symptoms.

GI manifestations of CF in the neonatal period could be **meconium ileus, meconium peritonitis,** and/or **unconjugated hyperbilirubinemia.**

Meconium ileus may present with a history of **polyhydramnios.** Abdominal films would show a **ground glass** appearance due to decreased bowel gas.

Meconium peritonitis might present as a **pseudocyst** (which is **calcified meconium**) on x-ray.

Pulmonary Manifestations of CF

Even though the GI manifestations may present sooner, and both GI and pulmonary manifestations cause chronic problems, it's the pulmonary exacerbations that are acutely life-threatening and land most of these kids in the hospital.

Popular bacteria in CF patients include *S. aureus, H. influenzae,* and *P. aeruginosa*. With advanced CF, you see *Burkholderia cepacia* which is associated with worsening lung function and poor overall outcome in some CF patients.

Acute exacerbations present with worsening cough, sputum production, dyspnea and decreased FEV1.

Mainstay of treatment for acute exacerbations is with antibiotics, using prior respiratory cultures to guide therapy. Other important aspects of treatment include aggressive pulmonary hygiene and use of inhaled mucolytic agents.

Lung manifestations of CF include bronchiectasis, pulmonary hypertension, pneumothoraces, and hemoptysis. Additionally, patients are at risk for **allergic bronchopulmonary aspergillosis (ABPA).**

Pulmonary Hypertension (PHTN)

Either heart disease or chronic lung disease may lead to pulmonary vasculature remodeling, which will increase pulmonary arterial pressure.

Distal intestinal obstruction syndrome (DIOS)

Occurs mainly in older children and adolescents. The obstruction typically occurs at the ileocecal junction, resulting in right lower quadrant pain.

Management includes either contrast enema or surgery, depending on the severity.

Growing Up with CF

Know that infants now diagnosed with CF are expected to live well into adulthood, so planning for their future is important.

You need to know that they should be encouraged to complete high school and pursue college and careers.

Infants and children with CF should receive all routine immunizations, including yearly influenza vaccination.

Exciting new **CFTR modulators** have been developed in recent years that are poised to be game changers. It is important to know that these medications will prevent worse disease but will NOT repair existing damage.

Important aspects of CF maintenance therapy include fat soluble vitamin (A,E,D,K) and pancreatic enzyme supplementation, anti-inflammatory medications (azithromycin or ibuprofen), exercise, regular pulmonary hygiene, CFTR modulators, and aggressive nutritional support.

Causes can include **primary pulmonary** conditions, sickle cell anemia, idopathic pulmonary hypertension, medications, and congenital heart disease. PHTN is also associated with several syndromes, especially Down Syndrome. Important neonatal causes of PHTN include persistent pulmonary hypertension of the newborn (PPHN) and congenital diaphragmatic hernia.

Cardiac causes of PHTN include lesions that cause excessive pulmonary blood flow (left-to-right shunt) over a long period of time, as with a large unrepaired VSD. If pulmonary pressures exceed systemic vascular resistance, the shunt reverses and becomes right to left and blood bypasses the lungs. This is called **Eisenmenger syndrome** and it results in severe hypoxemia.

For the classic pulmonary presentation, they might present a newborn with persistent fetal circulation who **develops respiratory distress shortly after a C/S or meconium delivery, with oxygen saturations in the lower extremities lower than that seen in the upper body.** This is because of right-to-left shunting through a PDA, resulting in desaturated blood reaching the descending aorta and below. In addition, because of the **increased workload of the right ventricle, a precordial lift,** or at least a prominent precordial impulse, may be described. Classic echocardiogram findings of PHTN are right ventricular hypertrophy and flattening of the interventricular septum.

> **PHTN signs and symptoms**
>
> HOT TIP
> Toddlers and older children will be expected to have a loud P2 component to their second heart sound (S2) with decreased exercise tolerance.

Cor Pulmonale

Cor pulmonale refers to **right ventricular dysfunction** caused by PHTN related to chronic lung disease, and not caused by congenital or left sided heart disease.

Lower body edema, hepatomegaly, gallop rhythm, and clubbing are all signs of cor pulmonale.

Since cor pulmonale in most cases is caused by **pulmonary hypertension**, it is not reversible. However, when severe upper airway obstruction is the cause, it is surgically correctable and reversible.

Cor pulmonale may be seen in many chronic lung diseases, including cystic fibrosis.

Primary Ciliary Dyskinesia (PCD)

Primary ciliary dyskinesia, also known as **dysmotile cilia syndrome**, is an **autosomal recessive condition** in which the cilia do not function normally.

If you ever wondered how important cilia were to your life, ciliary dysfunction leads to **chronic sinusitis** and **bronchiectasis**. Cilia are also responsible for the **heart "swimming" to the left side** of the chest during fetal development. Cilia dysfunction may also result in **male infertility**.

The classic presentation is unexplained respiratory distress during the newborn period, early onset chronic cough and rhinorrhea, and recurrent sinopulmonary infections.

> **Kartagener Syndrome**
>
> Kartagener syndrome is a type of PCD associated with a mirror-image orientation of the heart and other internal organs (situs inversus).
>
> HOT TIP
> If they note heart sounds on the right side of the chest, they are clearly noting this for a reason and situs inversus and its association with Kartagener syndrome is the reason.

Initial diagnostic test involves measuring exhaled nasal nitric oxide after a diagnosis of CF has been excluded.

The new way to diagnose PKD in children 5 years of age and older is exhaled nitric oxide.

Plowing through Pleural Collections

You will have to decipher different pleural fluids and their countries of origin based on the clothes they wear (color) and what they say (contents). Here is your travel guide.

In general, I remember pleural fluids as "transitional," meaning that "the source of the problem lies elsewhere." Causes of pleural effusions in children include:

- Pneumonia
- Liver failure
- Renal disease, including nephrotic syndrome
- Congenital heart disease
- Trauma
- Viral disease
- Malignancy
- Sickle cell anemia

Chylothorax

 In a chylothorax, electrolyte concentrations are **close to those found in serum**.

Triglyceride greater than 110, elevated lymphocyte count, and protein greater than 3 are consistent with chylothorax. Typically they will describe it in a **post-op** patient, especially after cardiac surgery.

Transudates vs. Exudates

Exudate is seen with inflammation. This can be expected when you are presented with a pleural effusion in the context of pneumonia, cancer, trauma, or inflammatory disease.

With an exudate, the **pleural lactate dehydrogenase (LDH) concentrations are at least 2/3 of the concentrations in serum, and protein value will be at least 3 grams/dL.**

> ### Checking the pH
> Pleural fluid pH is the most accurate test for determining if a parapneumonic effusion is an **exudate** or **transudate**.
>
> A pH over 7.45, or greater than the blood pH, is indicative of a transudate. Exudates have pH <7.3.

In contrast, **transudates** will have **less than 2/3 pleural LDH concentration than serum and less than 3 grams/dL of protein.** Transudates are typically seen with **congestive heart failure and nephrotic syndrome.**

Empyema

Empyema is the collection of pus in the pleural space.

If pneumonia is not improving despite treatment with appropriate antibiotics, think of **empyema**. This is especially true if there is some **initial** clinical improvement after treatment followed by deterioration.

Imaging (either ultrasound or CT scan) should be performed to determine whether the empyema is loculated or not.

If loculated, either video-assisted thoracoscopic surgery (VATS) or chest tube with fibrinolytic agent are required.

If not loculated, indications for chest tube insertion include significant respiratory symptoms or clinical worsening despite antibiotic therapy.

IV antibiotics should be continued **until the patient is afebrile for 48 hours after the chest tube has been removed**.

Pneumothorax (PTX)

You should suspect a pneumothorax if you are presented with a patient with **tachypnea, tachycardia, and unilateral decreased breath sounds**.

A small spontaneous PTX can occur with **marijuana smoking in tall, thin adolescents,** and this may be a clue they are handing you that drug use is an issue.

Risk factors include smoking, asthma, CF, connective tissue disorders (Marfan syndrome), and chronic lung disease of prematurity. It can also occur in the context of mechanical ventilation.

For a small pneumothorax, **watchful observation** with **oxygen administration** is the first thing to do. For a large pneumothorax in a stable patient, needle aspiration with placement of a pigtail catheter by the Seldinger technique may suffice.

If there is a **tracheal shift** with **decreased blood pressure,** you should suspect a **tension pneumothorax.** This is a medical emergency requiring **immediate needle decompression.** Only when the patient is stable, insert a chest tube.

The degree of pain does not correlate directly with the extent of the pneumothorax. **Intubation is rarely the answer they want with a pneumothorax.**

> ### Be Mechanical Fanatical
>
> Remember that mechanical issues can be the cause of clinical findings.
>
> To remember the possible causes of respiratory deterioration in an intubated patient, remember the mnemonic TOMB.
>
> - **T**ension pneumothorax
> - **O**xygen source interruption
> - **M**oved ET tube
> - **B**roken equipment.
>   - Is the tube blocked?
>   - Did the O2 tubing fall off the wall?
>
> Choices involving "mechanical failure" are often hinted at in the question buried in a can of red herrings.

Bronchiectasis

This is basically inflammation with **permanent dilation of a small segment of airway**. The most common causes are recurrent pulmonary infections and **cystic fibrosis**.

The most common symptom is chronic wet cough. Watch for repeated **lower respiratory tract infections** with a specific area of atelectasis on CXR (e.g., they might say R middle lobe atelectasis). In addition, the **coughing symptoms are made worse with changes in position (e.g., after lying down)**.

Diagnosis

The MOST helpful diagnostic test is **CT of the chest**.

Think bronchie**CT**asis.

The causes of bronchiectasis in addition to cystic fibrosis can be remembered with the following mnemonic

- **D**yskinesia (primary ciliary dyskinesia)
- **I**mmunodeficiency and **I**nfection
- **L**obar pneumonia, right middle **L**obe syndrome
- **A**spergillosis and disorders typically prevented by **A** vaccine, such as measles or pertussis
- **T**B
- **E**xtinsic compression caused by enlarged lymph nodes or masses

Hemoptysis

The most likely causes of hemoptysis in children are:

1. Infection (pneumonia, TB)
2. Bronchiectasis (cystic fibrosis)
3. Foreign body aspiration

More rare causes of hemoptysis that may be tested:

- Systemic vasculitis can also cause hemoptysis, so be on the lookout for signs of conditions such as lupus, granulomatosis with polyangitis, or Henoch Schonlein purpura.
- Pulmonary hemosiderosis causes recurrent hemopytsis in children. Chest x-ray will show multiple infiltrates.

If you are presented with a patient with acute hemoptysis and are asked for the best next step, the answer will be any choice which is diagnostic, since the most important task when faced with a patient experiencing hemoptysis would be to identify the source of the bleeding.

Correct choices would include **pH of the bloody fluid** to determine if it is acidic (stomach content) or alkaline (from the lungs), **CBC,** and **coagulation studies. Chest Xray, CT,** and **bronchoscopy** would also be appropriate choices.

Pneumonia through the Ages

The pneumonias of Neonates (the first 3 weeks of life) are covered in the Neonatal chapter.

Children with asthma, congenital heart disease, and tobacco smoke exposure are at increased risk for developing pneumonia of any type.

Infants (3 weeks through 12 months)

- **Chlamydia** transmitted during delivery. They will be afebrile, with interstitial infiltrates on CXR.
- Viruses can cause bronchiolitis or pneumonia in infants. Causes include **RSV, rhinovirus, human metapneumovirus,** and **parainfluenza.**
- **Pertussis,** with paroxysmal cough and no fever. This may also lead to aspiration pneumonia.

Pre-school (1-4 years of age)

- **Viral,** including RSV, parainfluenza, human metapneumovirus, influenza, and rhinovirus. **Viral pneumonia is much more common than bacterial pneumonia in children less than 5 years old.**
- *S. pneumoniae* which is the most common treatable form of pneumonia in preschool children

School age

- *Mycoplasma pneumoniae* is the most treatable form of pneumonia in this age group
- *Chlamydophilia pneumoniae* presents similarly to mycoplasma pneumonia
- *S. pneumoniae* in this age group can lead to complications, including empyema
- *Mycobacterium tuberculosis* if they present a child among the high risk pool.
- *S. aureus* is a rare but known complication of influenza

> **No Studies for Pneumonia**
>
> Unless there is something compelling in the presented history, lab studies would not be necessary in establishing a diagnosis of pneumonia.
>
> Chest x-rays in general would not be indicated if the pneumonia is minor enough for outpatient management.

Pneumonia By Etiology

S. pneumoniae

S. pneumoniae or pneumococcus typically presents with **abrupt onset of productive cough and fever,** with a somewhat toxic picture preceded by URI symptoms. **Abdominal pain with vomiting** can be part of the picture, possibly even mimicking an acute abdomen.

> **Recurrent pneumonia**
>
> If you see a child with recurrent pneumonia, think:
> - anatomic defects
> - immunodeficiencies
> - systemic illnesses

Those with sickle cell disease, immunodeficiency, and cochlear implants are at risk for severe pneumococcal infections.

High risk patients should receive both the 13-valent pneumococcal vaccine, followed by the 23-valent pneumococcal vaccine.

Mycoplasma pneumonia

Characterized by insidious onset of fever, myalgias, and fatigue. Sore throat is common. Chest x-ray will show diffuse interstitial infiltrates.

Infection may be associated with extrapulmonary symptoms such as rash, anemia, and encephalitis.

Viral Pneumonia

The patient will have upper respiratory symptoms including nasal congestion and rhinorrhea. Onset of symptoms will be gradual, and findings on lung exam will be **bilateral**.

Complications of Pneumonia

Necrotizing pneumonia

Necrotizing pneumonia occurs as a result of toxins produced by bacteria, leading to necrosis and liquification of lung tissue. Strep pneumoniae is the most common cause. Patients are ill appearing. Diagnosed with chest x-ray or CT scan.

Treatment requires broad spectrum antibiotics, including coverage for MRSA.

Lung Abscess

This will typically be described in a child at risk for aspiration, including a child with a **seizure** or **neurological disorder**. It is diagnosed with CT scan. Treatment should include coverage for anaerobic bacteria.

Effusions

A pleural effusion associated with pneumonia is called a **parapneumonic effusion**. The classic presentation is a child being treated for pneumonia with antibiotics who fails to improve after 48 hours of treatment. Management depends on the size of the effusion. **Purulent effusions** (empyema) may be described as having dullness on chest percussion and decreased air movement, planted in a sea of general findings (including **ill appearance**, **tachypnea**, and **chest discomfort**).

Musculoskeletal Conditions and Pulmonary Function

Scoliosis

Childhood-onset scoliosis can impair pulmonary function. Therefore, if severe, treatment is indicated to minimize the impact on pulmonary function.

Adolescent-onset scoliosis does not necessarily carry the same concerns.

Pectus Excavatum

Pectus excavatum does not typically result in any pulmonary issues. It is primarily a cosmetic concern, although I've been told by a friend with this condition that this is offset by the fact that it serves as a nice spot for guacamole dip when lying on the beach.

Although pectus excavatum is not a "typical" cause of pulmonary issues it can cause shortness of breath in severe cases. Put that in the back of your mind.

Chapter 24

Don't Go Breaking My Heart: Cardiology

Cardiology, although it can often be a difficult subject, is only a small part of the exam. What you need to know is limited to a set of core areas which, if mastered, should earn you easy points on the exam. There is some overlap, and some cardiology topics are covered in other chapters. This chapter will focus on specific core topics in cardiology.

Critical Congenital Heart Defects Screening (CCHD)

Different hospitals have different protocols to try to catch the CCHD conditions before infants leave the hospital. These conditions present with hypoxia and include Tetralogy of Fallot, total anomalous pulmonary venous return, transposition of the great arteries, tricuspid atresia, truncus arteriosus (together these you know as the 5 Ts of cyanotic heart diseases) and well and hypoplastic left heart syndrome and pulmonary atresia.

 The core principles are:

- the test is done 24 hours after birth
- a passing score involves a oxygen saturation in the right hand and either foot >95% with a difference between the 2 sites of less than 3%
- the screen is more reliable after 24 hours of age (after PDA closure and other non-cardiac problems resolved)
- O_2 less than 90% in the right hand / either foot is immediate failure
- if it is between 90-95%, or > 3% discrepancy , then you can repeat the test an hour later, twice
- if it is still less than 95% on the 3 screens, 3 strikes and you are out !

 Confirmation of CCHD is done with echocardiogram.

I say Murmur, you say Mummur

Evaluating and distinguishing innocent murmurs is an important component of general practice, and one you will need to navigate with ease on the exam as well. Here are the guidelines to getting the answer correct on the exam.

Up to 90% of children will have a murmur at some point in their lives; more than that if they are appearing on the Board exam. *Less than 5% of these will actually represent pathology.*

Here are some of the typical descriptions of innocent murmurs:

"Vibratory," "Venous hum."

V's: **V**ery good, **V**enous hum, **V**ibratory.

Any description of associated physiological problems suggests a pathological murmur. If they mention any of the following in the question, you are **not** dealing with an innocent murmur: **tachypnea, exercise intolerance, feeding difficulties, dyspnea, cyanosis, syncope, or wheezing and hacking like a diesel engine when seeing what pictures of you were posted on Facebook.**

Watch for any family history of cardiac disease. If they describe any — and I mean *any* — associated physical findings, that could be your clue that the murmur is not innocent and is probably part of a syndrome.

Auscultating[1] the Murmur (Described in Plain English)

The nice thing about the exam (aside from the fact that it will eventually end) is that it will describe the murmur for you, using buzz words and you won't actually have to listen[2] and decode the murmur yourself, at least not at this point in time.

Since these buzz words are very specific for their associated disorders, and we're about to give them to you, you should get all the answers correct.

You, on the other hand, might get the question wrong if you don't commit these descriptions to memory.

Any of the following terms should raise a flag:

- ❏ Harsh sounding
- ❏ Intensity greater than 3/6
- ❏ Pansystolic/ holosystolic or late systolic
- ❏ Diastolic murmur
- ❏ A fourth heart sound is not normal, nor is an S4 gallop
- ❏ Ejection and/or mid systolic clicks are not normal

If they describe a 3rd heart sound, check the position.[3] **If the child is lying down, it could be normal.** If it is a normal finding, when the child sits up, the 3rd heart sound should disappear; if it does not, you could be dealing with an abnormal sound.

Picture a number 3 lying down, murmuring, and stopping when it sits up, which is normal for a 3.

---

[1] Auscultating means "listening" to the rest of the non-medical world.
[2] Or auscultate.
[3] Of the child, not you.

Sounds for Musing

ASD Sounds

Patients with an ASD will present with specific auscultatory findings (also known as heart sounds). This would include a **fixed split 2nd heart sound**. They might describe this in a patient with **decreased exercise tolerance**.

Know that the murmur described in an ASD is NOT from flow across the ASD, because the pressures are roughly equal in both atria. The murmur is from the **relative increase in flow through the pulmonary valve and sometimes the pulmonary artery branches** so it is heard best at the **left upper sternal border** just like pulmonic stenosis. Watch for this description in the history.

If they hint that an ASD is missed, it may lead to **Eisenmenger syndrome** with eventual **right-to-left flow** due to **pulmonary hypertension**.

They could present a patient from another country with limited medical care where they have not been evaluated before.

VSD Sounds

The murmur associated with a VSD is best heard at the **left lower sternal border,** and is typically **blowing/harsh and holosystolic**.

Suddenly, at your 2 week or 2 month wellness check, this murmur is clearly audible and you wonder how you possibly could have missed it at all your previous visits. The answer: you didn't miss it. The right and left ventricular pressures were roughly equal, so there was no interventricular flow to create a murmur previously.

Infants with VSDs do NOT typically have murmurs in the immediate newborn period.

It is important to note what age the patient is to help determine which is the likely cardiac defect. For example, for a 2 month old presenting with heart failure, a left to right lesion is most likely, (usually VSD).

Interestingly, the larger the VSD, the softer the murmur because there is less turbulence. But the baby will have **tachypnea** and **sweating with feedings** and have a **hyperdynamic precordium**. So watch out for the symptoms of VSD even with no mention of a murmur.

Conversely, a patient with a small muscular ventricular septal defect will have a loud murmur. Patients with small muscular VSDs are asymptomatic and the VSDs spontaneously close most of the time.

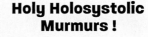

Holy Holosystolic Murmurs !

A "blowing" or "harsh" holosystolic murmur is a **VSD**.

A "high pitched" holosystolic murmur is **mitral regurgitation**.

Pulmonary Stenosis

Pulmonary stenosis will often be described with a **systolic (ejection) click** that **varies with respiration** and normal splitting of S2.

In this case there would be **right ventricular hypertrophy** due to the ventricle having to push against the narrowed pulmonic valve.

The murmur they will describe would be at the **LUSB** just like was described with ASD. It may also have a **thrill** and **radiate to the back**.

Critical or severe pulmonary stenosis is ductal dependent (PDA needs to remain open) and will likely need neonatal cardiac catheterization for balloon valvuloplasty.

Aortic Stenosis

Aortic stenosis would have a **systolic (ejection) click** heard at the apex (really close to S1) that **does NOT vary with respiration**, regardless of position.

There will also be a **murmur best heard at the upper right sternal border** and **with a thrill at the sternal notch** and **left ventricular hypertrophy** due to the ventricle having to push against the narrowed aortic valve.

Patent Ductus Arteriosus (PDA)

The classic murmur of a PDA is a **to-and-fro or continuous machinery-type murmur**. It can present with **bounding femoral pulses**.

AV Canal Defect

This is a condition that should instantly and automatically make you think **Down Syndrome**.

AV Canal has a **"Superior" QRS axis** (e.g., 30°–90°) because the conduction system has to go around the large defect in the middle of the heart. It also has left axis deviation.[4]

Humming cousins

Still's vibratory murmur and the venous hum are benign "cousin" murmurs.

Still's will be louder supine and softer on standing and the **venous hum** will disappear with pressure on the jugular vein.

Hypertrophy vs. Deviation

In general, left ventricular hypertrophy (LVH) leads to left axis deviation on EKG, but the two are not always directly associated.

Disorders like hypertrophic cardiomyopathy that result in LVH **DO NOT result in left axis deviation on EKG**.

Left axis deviation without hypertrophy will be seen with tricuspid atresia and AV canal defects because of its effect on the conducting system's orientation.

Right-sided Aortic Arch

If you are presented with ANY infant with a right-sided aortic arch, think 22q11 deletion.

Right sided arch is highly associated with vascular rings.

---

[4] Not to be confused with the axis of evil.

Congestive Heart Failure

 Inadequate delivery of oxygen to the tissues.

 Congestive heart failure (CHF) will present differently in infants than in older children.

CHF in Infancy would present as **difficulty feeding**, **weight loss** or **failure to gain weight, tachypnea, tachycardia, wheezing, cardiomegaly,** as well as **hepatomegaly.**

Many times this presentation could be confused with respiratory/ viral illness.

Think CHF if you see infants that are the 4 **Ss**: **s**mall, **s**weaty, **s**urly and **s**ick.

CHF in Older Children will present with **fatigue**, especially with **exertion** or **exercise.** This would include activities they enjoy, not just chores (for those of us who have asked our kids to take out the garbage, only to be told they are too tired).

Subtle signs could include **poor appetite** and **coughing** as well as **nausea/ vomiting, shortness of breath** and/or **diaphoresis.**

On physical exam, they could describe **hepatomegaly, cardiomegaly,** a **gallop rhythm, distended jugular veins,** or **peripheral edema.**

 Whenever possible, CHF treatments that **rest the heart** like diuretics, vasodilators, and beta-blockers are preferred over treatments like inotropes [Digoxin] that overexert the heart.

With cardiogenic shock, fluid boluses with make the patient worse!!

Systemic AV Malformation

Systemic arteriovenous shunting of blood (as might be seen in the case of an AV malformation in the brain or liver) results in left to right extracardiac shunting, and ultimately leads to right-sided congestion.

If you hear a cranial bruit on exam, think of systemic AV malformation.

This is because the blood can move directly from the higher pressure arterial side to the lower pressure venous side. The end result is volume overload to the right side of the heart, leading to jugular vein distension and hepatomegaly in cases of significant congestion.

If you are presented with high output cardiac failure in a fetus or newborn with hydrops this is likely due to a systemic AV malformation.

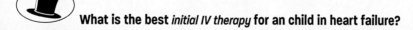

What is the best *initial IV therapy* for an child in heart failure?

Among the choices you will be given are diuretics, steroids, epinephrine, and digoxin. Even if you decide that a diuretic is appropriate, you might be presented with two choices: furosemide or an ACE inhibitor. Both of these are used to treat heart failure - but which one is used **immediately** in acute failure?

The correct answer will be furosemide, which acts within minutes and may yield rapid clinical improvement. ACE inhibitors are more appropriate for *long- term* treatment. Digoxin onset is much slower. Steroids would be helpful for myocarditis. Epinephrine would increase cardiac afterload by increasing peripheral vascular resistance.

Coarctation of the Aorta

BUZZWORDS

The classic findings of coarctation of the aorta are a **systolic murmur** heard in the left axilla sometimes with radiation to the upper back and sometimes with an early diastolic component, **systolic hypertension** and **decreased perfusion/pulses in lower extremities.**

HOT TIP

Coarc is the only cardiac murmur heard **louder in the back!**

PERIL

They are unlikely to present you with the classic description of **differential (greater than 10 mm Hg) blood pressures** between the arms and the leg or **brachial/femoral pulse delay.** They might just present you with classic signs of **congestive heart failure** and nothing else. This would include signs of **shock** and **acidosis,** in addition to an infant who is **lethargic** and **not feeding well.** Physical findings could also include a **non-specific gallop, nasal flaring,** and **sweating while feeding.**

PERIL

Coarctation of the aorta in newborns presents with right ventricular hypertrophy because, in a fetus, the RV is the dominant pumping chamber.

TREATMENT

The goal of treatment is to maintain a PDA[5] with a **prostaglandin drip,** thereby increasing blood flow to the descending aorta. Coarctation of the aorta is ultimately treated surgically.

Even after coarctation correction, **recurrences and hypertension** can occur.

> ## Differential Cyanosis
>
> Both aortic obstruction (from either a coarctation or interrupted aortic arch) with a PDA and pulmonary hypertension can lead to differential cyanosis, which is a pulse oximetry reading that is higher in the right hand than the lower extremity.

Hypoplastic Left Heart Syndrome

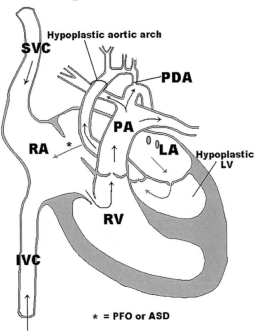

Hypoplastic Left Heart Syndrome

---

[5] Patent Ductus Arteriosus not Public Displays of Affection.

Infants with hypoplastic left heart syndrome look like normal healthy babies at birth. But the trouble starts **when the PDA closes** and they develop signs of **severe congestive heart failure** with marked **cardiomegaly** on chest radiography in the immediate newborn period.

Additional findings include **precordial hyperactivity** and a **loud S2.**

You must have a patent foramen ovale or ASD in HLHS, otherwise this is incompatible with life.

A 10 day old newborn is brought to your office. You immediately notice that the infant is tachypneic with thready peripheral pulses and an enlarged liver. You accompany the infant to the emergency room and obtain an ABG, which reveals marked metabolic acidosis. From a list of dobutamine, epinephrine, prostaglandin, and IV fluids, you are asked which therapy should be used immediately.

Since you are being presented with an infant with signs of *cardiogenic shock,* you might be tempted to pick IV fluids, or a pressor like dobutamine, or even epinephrine. The key to remember is that hypoplastic left heart syndrome presents after the immediate newborn period, and presents with a picture of cardiogenic shock.

Since cardiogenic shock is the primary problem and started with the closing of the ductus arteriosus, keeping it opened is the most important step to ameliorate the cardiogenic shock. In other words, fix the pump, and the hoses and water will take care of themselves. Therefore, *prostaglandin E_1* would be the correct answer to this question.

There is no murmur associated with **hypoplastic left heart syndrome,** even though the ductus remains open. This is because pulmonary and aortic pressures are equal, resulting in **no turbulence across the patent ductus.**

This is why an **EKG and cardiac echo** are important parts of a workup of a child presenting in shock.

Blue vs gray? No ! We are not talking about the American Civil War!

The presentation of a sick infant as blue is likely to imply cyanosis, and possible cyanotic heart disease.

But if they describe the infant as grey, start thinking one of the causes of shock instead (septic, cardiogenic, hypovolemic, etc)

Cyanotic Congenital Heart Disease

If you are presented with a newborn with hypoxemia whose oxygen saturation does not improve significantly with 100% oxygen, you are likely dealing with cardiac rather than pulmonary disease.

This is an important piece of information they could present in the question.

Infants with **cyanotic heart disease** and **polycythemia** are at high risk for cerebrovascular accidents.

Cyanotic at Birth

There are 3 causes of **severe cyanosis in the immediate newborn period**:

1. Transposition of the Great Arteries TGA
2. Pulmonary atresia
3. Ebstein malformation

All 3 will have **central cyanosis** with **no respiratory distress** and with **no significant murmur**. All 3 will fail to correct with administration of 100% oxygen (hyperoxia test).

Chest X-Ray will help separate between the three because TGA has increased pulmonary blood flow and the other two have decreased pulmonary blood flow.

Initial treatment for all 3 is **infusion of prostaglandin E1[6]** to maintain patency of the ductus arteriosus.

Persistent pulmonary hypertension of the newborn (PPHN) presents similarly, but will improve with oxygen administration.

The Tease of the 5 Ts

Here are the 5 Ts of cyanotic congenital heart disease:

- Truncus Arteriosus
- Transposition of the Great Arteries

Cyanotic Heart Disease and Anemia

You will be expected to determine the presence or absence of cyanotic heart disease when provided with a hematocrit value.

If an infant is anemic, he may not show signs of cyanosis on physical exam, even with O_2 sats around 88%. Infants have high fetal Hgb levels, so cyanosis may not be clinically apparent until O_2 sats are quite low.

Silent but Deadly

Cyanotic heart disease with no murmur:

- Transposition
- Tricuspid atresia
- Pulmonary atresia
- TAPVR

Ductal Dependent Lesions

They may describe an infant with good Apgars who was pink and well-perfused initially and then some time during the first or second day of life, the infant gradually became **cyanotic due to the closing PDA**, which resulted in diminished mixing at the ductal level. In addition, **tachypnea** might be described. They might also describe the **lack of increased vascular markings** on CXR, ruling out pulmonary disease.

Treatment consists of **prostaglandin** to maintain a patent ductus arteriosus.

---

[6] Main side effects of PGE1 are fever and apnea.

- Tricuspid Atresia
- Tetralogy of Fallot
- Total Anomalous Pulmonary Venous Return

PERIL

However, these are not always described with the T prominent in the description, i.e. total anomalous venous return might be described as anomalous venous return.

HOT TIP

Of these, transposition of the great vessels is the only cyanotic heart lesion which presents with severe cyanosis in the **first few hours of life**. The rest turn blue after the ductus closes.

> ### Three Things you Should Know about the Tricuspid Valve
>
> 1. It's found between the right atrium and the right ventricle.
>
> 2. Tricuspid Atresia is one of the "T"s of cyanotic congenital heart disease.
>
> 3. Abnormality of the Tricuspid valve leaflets (Ebsteins' anomaly) may be due to lithium or benzodiazepine use in pregnancy. So watch for maternal use of these meds during pregnancy or disorders that require treatment with these medications.

Total Anomalous Pulmonary Venous

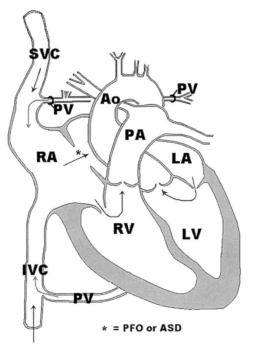

* = PFO or ASD

©Medhumor Medical Publications, LLC

Return (TAPVR)

DEFINITION

With Total Anomalous Pulmonary Venous Return, none of the four veins that drain blood from the lungs to the heart is attached to the left atrium. The oxygenated blood leaving the lungs returns to the right atrium and then back to the lungs. There must be a connection to the left side of the heart or the condition is incompatible with life.

BUZZWORDS

TAPVR will often present in a full term infant as **increased right ventricular activity** with **cyanosis, hypoxia, hypercarbia,** and **pulmonary edema.**

The **CXR** will be significant for findings consistent with **pulmonary congestion** (because of the increased venous return), along with a **normal to small heart**. The ABG will have an increased PCO_2.

TAPVR and RDS can present in similar ways; however, if they are describing **a full term baby, consider TAPVR first** even though RDS <u>can</u> occur in full term infants.

Tetralogy of Fallot (TOF)

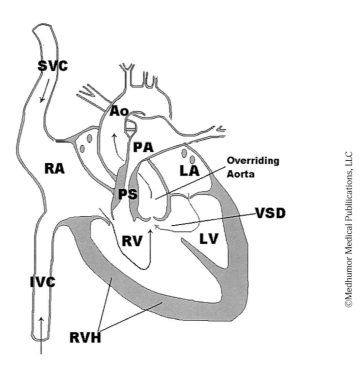

©Medhumor Medical Publications, LLC

Tetralogy of Fallot (TOF)

You might be asked to pick out the 4 components of TOF from among a list of 5:

1. Pulmonary Stenosis
2. Overriding Aorta
3. Insatiable desire to sing 50s R and B songs with lyrics containing the word Fallot, as in "I Will Fallot You", or Judy Garland Show tunes: "Fallot the Yellow Brick Road"
4. VSD
5. Right Ventricular Hypertrophy with right axis deviation on EKG

In most instances choice 3 will be incorrect.

> **Common Blues**
>
> TOF is the most common cyanotic heart defect overall. However, in newborns, transposition of the great arteries is the most common cyanotic lesion seen because TOF does not usually present in the newborn period.

Children with Tetralogy of Fallot have a **palpable right ventricular impulse** and a **single 2nd heart sound** (the pulmonary component is absent). The EKG shows **right ventricular hypertrophy** and the CXR shows a **"boot-shaped" heart** with **decreased pulmonary vascularity**.

Remember, this is **often asymptomatic in early infancy**, especially on the Boards. The typical presentation is **in an infant of 3-5 months of age**. These "pink Tets" present with CHF because of left-to-right flow across the VSD.

After surgical repair there is a chance for **arrhythmias and episodes of syncope**.

The Tet Offensive Redux: Under a "Tet Spell"

Recognizing a Tet spell is worth a point or two. These are basically **hypercyanotic hypoxic episodes**, similar to a prima donna athlete being denied his big contract. Common triggers are **anemia** and **dehydration**. It is a result of **increased R to L shunting during an acute episode**.[7]

During a "Tet spell", the infant will **suddenly turn blue** and will develop a **deep rapid respiratory pattern** (hyperpnea).

Infants with TOF, usually have a systolic murmur **from flow across the pulmonic stenosis**, not across the VSD because it is too big. But during a Tet spell, the murmur suddenly disappears because flow to the lungs decreases and that's why there is cyanosis. **The inability to hear a previous murmur is an important feature of a tet spell.**

> ## Cognitive Effects of Cyanotic Heart Disease
>
> This is a ripe topic for the exam. Factors that worsen the cognitive prognosis are:
>
> ❏ **Decreased neurological baseline before surgery**
>
> ❏ **Seizures occurring after surgery** (especially early)
>
> ❏ **Coexistent problems** such as a chromosomal abnormality
>
> ❏ **Duration of intraoperative circulatory arrest** (e.g., greater than 75 minutes makes for a worse prognosis)

Correcting Your Tet Spelling

If they describe a classic spell in the question (**the acute onset is often the clue**), then the treatment consists of placing the child in a **squatting position** (to increase peripheral vascular resistance) just like a free agent baseball catcher. And if they are real little, don't pick them up and simulate a squat on the table or bed – just do a **knee to chest move** – but you knew that, right?

In addition, **morphine, phenylephrine, IV propranolol** (to slow the heart and increase filling), and **volume expansion** are given. Oxygen will not hurt or help.

Elective repair of TOF in the first postnatal year is now the rule.

---

[7] Shunting deoxygenated blood through the VSD to the left side.

Transposition of the Great Arteries

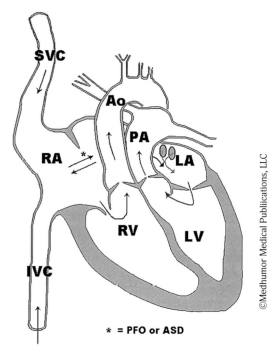

* = PFO or ASD

Transposition of the Great Arteries

Transposition of the great arteries is the most common congenital heart lesion presenting with **cyanosis at birth**. It is due to the connection of the aorta to the right ventricle and the pulmonary artery to the left ventricle. The result is two circulations in parallel.[8]

Blood mixing must occur either through the foramen ovale (at the atrial level), the ventricular level, or through the PDA; thus, it is "ductal dependent."

Transposition of the great arteries should be your first thought when presented with any cyanotic newborn. They typically present with tachypnea and a **single 2nd heart sound**. On CXR the **heart appears like an egg on a string** (which can be absent in the first week of life) and **increased pulmonary vascularity**.[9]

Both Tetralogy of Fallot and transposition of the great arteries present with a **single 2nd heart sound**. However, transposition of the great arteries presents with **increased** pulmonary vascularity, while Tetralogy of Fallot presents with **decreased** pulmonary vasculature.

What's the S2 to you ?

S2 is composed of A2 and P2 and represents the closure of the aortic and pulmonic valves.

HOT TIP Whenever they mention "normal split S2", you may breathe a sigh of relief, because you've essentially ruled out cyanotic heart disease.

TAKE HOME MESSAGE On the contrary, if they mention "single S2", start looking for prostaglandin among the choices.

A "fixed split S2" is seen with ASD.

Arms vs legs

A differential O_2 saturation [high SaO_2 in the lower extremities but low SaO_2 in the right hand] is seen in TGA when either aortic arch obstruction or pulmonary hypertension is present because the upper extremities are dependent on the right ventricle while the lower extremities are dependent on the left ventricle via the duct.

COIN FLIP But do not confuse this with a differential BP in arms vs legs as is seen in Coarctation of the Aorta.

---

[8] Sort of like a couple not on speaking terms.
[9] Some now say that the egg shaped heart is a non-specific finding. However, on the exam it would be wise to still consider it to be an association with transposition of the great vessels.

Treatment consists of **IV prostaglandin E₁** to maintain the PDA and, if this does not work, a **balloon septostomy** to maintain a patent ASD. Ultimately, surgical correction is needed (the specifics of which should not be tested on the general pediatric board exam).

> ### Genetic Echo
>
> There is a strong association between chromosomal abnormalities and congenital heart disease.
>
> Therefore, cardiac echo is routinely done in infants with atypical physical features even with a normal initial cardiac exam.

Finding the Heart in the Genes

Genetic conditions and the heart defects that love them	
22q11 deletion syndrome[10]	Conotruncal defects and VSD
Down Syndrome	AV canal defect and VSD
Marfan Syndrome	Aortic root dilation and dissection, mitral valve prolapse
William Syndrome	Supravalvular aortic stenosis
Noonan Syndrome	Supravalvular pulmonic stenosis
Turner Syndrome	Coarctation of the aorta
CHARGE and VACTERL syndrome	VSDs

Arrhythmias

The following are some of the basic arrhythmias that can appear on the exam.

Sinus Arrhythmia

This is another name for a **normal variant**.

Sinus arrhythmia is a normal variation in the heart rhythm caused by breathing. It is fairly common in perfectly healthy, normal children.

Sinus Tachycardia

Sinus Tach

Sinus tachycardia is **secondary to conditions**, some more benign like fever and dehydration, or more pathologic as in hyperthyroidism or pheochromocytoma.

You may consider the MAX normal sinus rate as **220 minus AGE in years**, ie. 210 for a 10 year old. A HR higher than this and you should consider a diagnosis of SVT.

---

[10] Previously known as DiGeorge syndrome

Premature Atrial Contractions (PACs)

When we refer to a PAC, we are not referring to the folks who hang around the corridors of Congress, syphoning money to our poor and humble politicians, called "Political Action Committees."

Remember that 4% of all beats every day can be PACs and PVCs and be benign (much unlike their political counterparts) and may be due to **caffeine intake, drug use** and **electrolyte imbalances**. Benign PACs and PVCs will go away when children exercise and return when the HR returns to baseline.

Beware of PACs in children on **digoxin** and **children less than 1 year old**. They are at risk of PACs progressing to atrial flutter.

Atrial Flutter/Fib

Atrial fib has a more structured tracing. **Saw tooth waves** are the classic EKG pattern for atrial flutter.

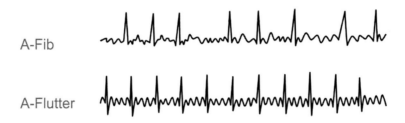

A-Fib

A-Flutter

Wolff Parkinson White Syndrome (WPW)

Wolff Parkinson White Syndrome was named after Bernard Wolff Parkinson, an eccentric dog physiologist and part-time canine couple's therapist who did all his research in the Alaskan Tundra. His obsession with white snow earned him the moniker "White." He also discovered, and later designed, the first Parka coat. Rumor has it that Frank Zappa had him in mind when he wrote the lyrics, "Don't go where the huskies go, don't you eat that yellow snow."[11]

They will show or describe a **shortened PR interval** and/or a **delta wave**[12] that distorts the QRS upstroke. These kids are also **at risk of SVT**. Therefore SVT might be one of the presenting signs of WPW you are provided with on the exam.

Treatment WPW

Adenosine can be used with WPW but must be done with extreme caution. The definitive treatment is ablation. However, Symptomatic WPW (those who have SVT due to WPW) could be treated with a beta blocker.

---

[11] My editor says that this story is not factually accurate. Yes we confirmed this is not accurate but we are leaving it in anyway.
[12] The wave on the EKG – not the sleep stage you are in right now.

Supraventricular Tachycardia (SVT)

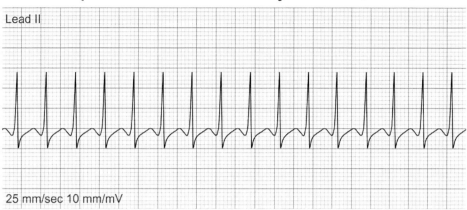

Supraventricular Tachycardia (SVT)

Lead II

25 mm/sec 10 mm/mV

SVT is **the most common symptomatic arrhythmia in children.** Infants may just be fussy and tachypneic, while older children may describe chest pain or palpitations or palpitations. Normal heart rate varies with age and condition (fever, exercise, etc) but a **narrow complex tachycardia over 200-220,** is considered SVT.

If they ask what is the first thing to do in a cardiovascularly stable patient in SVT (HR greater than 220), the correct answer is **obtain a 12 Lead EKG.**

In a stable child, you would then try **vasovagal maneuvers,** such as brief facial stimulation (cold, wet cloth or ice bag); to induce the "diving reflex" that normally slows down the heart.

Adenosine is the drug of choice to slow the heart down. If the adenosine works but the SVT returns right after the adenosine is given, then the appropriate treatment is **amiodarone or procainamide.**

The effects of adenosine are **diminished by methylxanthines** such as caffeine and theophylline.

If you are presented with a patient in SVT who is demonstrating signs of **cardiac failure,** vasovagal maneuvers would not be the correct choice. In this case, **adenosine** would be appropriate immediately. If IV adenosine is unavailable, **cardioversion** would be the most appropriate next step.

Digoxin is sometimes used in the long-term management of children with SVT. **Digoxin is contraindicated in children with Wolff-Parkinson White syndrome.**

Verapamil is not indicated for SVT in children, especially those younger than one year, because it can cause cardiac arrest, and, to quote *Ghostbusters*, "that would be bad."

Prolonged QT (Cutie) Syndrome

The QT interval is the time it takes the heart muscle to recover between beats. When a new beat starts before the old beat has had time to end, this could be bad. By bad here we mean arrhythmia bad, sometimes "dead bad", which is as bad as it gets. **A QTc >460 ms is considered prolonged.**

They will typically describe a **family history of sudden death, near drowning, one-person car accidents,** etc. Presentation may include a previously healthy person who has unexplained syncope. The syncope may be associated with emotions, like a **sudden fright**, or surprise, or an alarm clock going off, rather than exercise. It may be **followed by a seizure**, but the clue in the history is that **the syncope happens first** and then the seizure.

Prolonged "Cutie:" If someone dies young, he/she is forever young and "cute," and thus a "prolonged cutie."

CASE STUDY

You are presented with a child who collapses or is resuscitated after passing out in a pool. They will then note a history of a close family member who died suddenly and had a history of epilepsy. What is the most likely test to confirm the abnormality in this patient?

THE DIVERSION

Of course, among the choices will be an EEG. If the answer were that simple, anybody with a pulse and an EEG above a flat line could pass the exam. Cardiac echo, angiography, as well as a simple EKG, will be included in the choices.

ANSWER REVEALED

If you did not know anything and simply picked the least invasive of the cardiac answers, you would get it correct. If you knew that *congenital long QT syndrome* is caused by a variant of ventricular tachycardia, and can result in brief generalized seizures, you would realize that epilepsy may be a misdiagnosis in the close relative. A simple EKG would be the correct answer; it would illustrate a long QT measurement, which is the underlying problem.

CASE STUDY You are presented with a patient who has recurrent episodes of syncope, usually while standing for prolonged periods of time. There is no family history of sudden death in anyone younger than 50 or other premature cardiac disease. What is the most likely diagnosis?

THE DIVERSION You might be fooled into picking prolonged QT syndrome. However, the clue here will be the absence of a family history of sudden death in anyone younger than 50 or other significant cardiac disease.

ANSWER REVEALED The correct diagnosis when presented with recurrent syncope, particularly with prolonged standing, would be **neurocardiogenic syncope**.

CASE STUDY You are taking care of a very athletic teenage boy. He has been playing varsity level basketball and is in great condition. In the past 6 weeks he has passed out twice during practice, despite maintaining adequate hydration. His drug screen is negative. There is no known family history of any cardiac arrhythmias and no known history of sudden death in anyone younger than 50. What would be the most appropriate management at this time?

THE DIVERSION The diversion here is the lack of "known" history of sudden premature death. Read the question carefully. Even in the absence of a known history, long QT syndrome could exist in the family. The key here is the history of syncope during exercise, as opposed to occurring with prolonged standing.

ANSWER REVEALED The correct answer here would be to obtain a cardiology consultation. In addition, the patient should not be allowed to return to sports until cleared by a cardiologist.

By the way, had they asked for the most important additional history, the answer would have been to uncover the true family history.

AV Block

DEFINITION When the P waves and the QRS complexes are working independently of each other.

HOT TIP The important thing to remember is that **a widened QRS complex** is more ominous than a narrow one. With the widened complex, blood flow to the brain can be compromised, resulting in risk for **seizure** and **syncope** (the double S).

Picture a double S falling through a wide QRS.

 Often the mother of a **child with complete (3rd degree) heart block** is diagnosed with **SLE** retrospectively.

 AV block can be associated with **viral myocarditis**.

Ventricular Tachycardia (VT)

PVC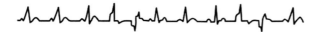

 VT is defined as **3 or more continuous PVC's**. The rate will be 120-250 bpm and is confirmed by EKG.

 Symptoms of VT include **pallor**, **fatigue**, and **palpitations**.

The majority of patients with VT have **underlying heart disease**.

 The most likely cause of VT with loss of consciousness is **torsades de pointes VT**, which is lethal if untreated.

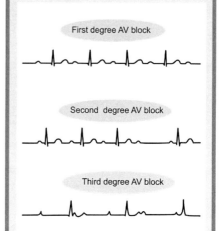

- **First Degree heart block** - note the increased PR interval.
- **Second Degree (Wenkebach) heart block** - note the normal PR interval with dropped QRS complexes.
- **Third Degree AV block** - note the PR interval varies since there is no P and QRS relationship. The block is complete.

First degree AV block

Second degree AV block

Third degree AV block

Synchronized cardioversion is the treatment of choice for **sustained VT longer than 30 seconds**.

Syncope

 Most causes of syncope in children are not cardiac. They are usually vasovagal or due to dehydration and treated with fluid and salt intake (pretzels, potato chips, popcorn, pickles, and pepperoni).

Commotio Cordis

 Occurs when there is a direct blow over the chest (such as occurring during a baseball game) and the hit occurs during upstroke of T wave causing ventricular fibrillation.

Cardiac causes of syncope include:

- Long QT syndrome
- Cardiomyopathy
- WPW syndrome
- Coronary anomalies
- Arrhythmias (late post-op)
- Valvar aortic stenosis
- Lyme disease (AV block)
- Bradycardia/Asystole

Neurologically Mediated Syncope:

- Neurocardiogenic (vasovagal) syncope
- Postural Orthostatic Tachycardia syndrome (POTS)
- Convulsive Syncope
- Breath holding spells

Rheumatic Fever (RF)

Getting your Jones on

The criteria for the diagnosis of RF were first proposed by original Rolling Stones founder Brian Jones, in the late 60s, two hours before he was found dead in his swimming pool with a copy of Nelson's Pediatrics. That and the constant bickering with Mick Jagger and Keith Richards are his greatest legacies.[13]

You will need to commit the Jones criteria—both **major and minor**—to memory and know them cold. Again, you need proof of a **recent group A strep infection,** as well as:

2 major symptoms

or

1 major <u>and</u> **2 minor** symptoms

It is easy to forget that a recent group A strep infection is a part of the requirement.

Major Jones Criteria

J – Joints = Polyarthritis – occurs in 75% of cases

♥ – Carditis (CHF, new murmurs, cardiomegaly)

N – Nodules (subcutaneous) – firm and painless on the extensor surfaces of wrists, elbows, and knees

E – Erythema marginatum

S – Sydenham chorea – rapid, purposeless movements of the face and upper extremities

Minor Jones Criteria

The minor criteria are much less specific:

❏ Arthralgia
❏ Fever
❏ Elevated acute phase reactants (ESR, C-reactive protein)
❏ Prolonged PR interval

To **help** remember the **minor** criteria, remember the word **help,** since the minor criteria by themselves are not adequate (they need *help*):

H (hot) – as in fever
E (elevated) – as in elevated acute phase reactants
L – to help remember that this minor criterion is arthra–L–gia, and not arthritis
P (prolonged) – as in prolonged PR interval

Splitting Hearts in RF

Mitral valve regurgitation, which is the **most common murmur in RF**, will be described as a murmur **heard best at the apex.**

If they describe **a new murmur** along with **mild congestive heart failure**, this may be **aortic regurgitation**.

 Emotional lability, coupled with purposeless rapid movements of the extremities and muscle weakness, is either Alec Baldwin fighting over a parking spot in lower Manhattan, or a patient with **Sydenham's chorea**.

Sydenham's chorea ALONE is enough to diagnose RF.

Strep Mining and Mining for Strep

The following are some of the tests they want you to order when you suspect a diagnosis of rheumatic fever.

If they just hint at a recent strep infection, it isn't enough to make a diagnosis of rheumatic fever. You also need to document the infection.

Rapid Strep/Throat Culture
A positive throat culture will not distinguish chronic carrier state from recent infection. A negative rapid strep does not rule out a recent infection.

ASO Titers and Streptozyme

ASO titers and positive streptozyme correlate very well with a recent strep infection. Definitive documentation of a recent strep infection is usually the answer they are looking for.

---

[13] Folks, that is a joke. Please do not send us letters that the Jones Criteria were proposed by T. Duckett Jones; we know that.

Boning up on the Jones Criteria

Let's take a closer look at the specific aspects of the Jones Criteria.

Arthritis: Remember that arth**ritis** is one of the major criteria and that arth**ralgia** one of the minor. The arthritis is "migratory," and usually involves the larger joints (knees, ankles, elbows, and wrists). Each episode lasts from a week up to one month.

The rash is called erythema **marginatum**, but the arthritis is **migratory**. Do not confuse erythema marginatum (RF) and erythema migrans (Lyme).

There are 3 primary treatment goals:

1) Eliminate Group A strep infection
2) Alleviate symptoms
3) Prophylaxis to prevent recurrence

Elimination of the Strep infection is best accomplished with **penicillin**. It is an empiric, prudent measure that does not alter the course of the disease. Penicillin is also used for prophylaxis.

Aspirin is used to treat the **migratory arthritis**, and to some degree the **fever**.

Steroids would be indicated to treat **carditis** (although this is increasingly controversial for mild carditis).

Haloperidol may help with chorea.

Digoxin is used in heart failure.

Endocarditis, Myocarditis, Hiscarditis, Pericarditis and Theircarditis

Infective Endocarditis (IE)

This is self defined, basically an infection of the endocardial surface of the heart, usually involving the valves. **Congenital heart disease** (whether repaired or not) and **dental work** are major risk factors for infective endocarditis.

Look for a history of **unexplained fever** along with **hepatosplenomegaly, petechiae,** a new or **changing murmur, myalgias, arthalgias, headaches** and **generalized malaise.**

- **Osler Nodes** are the "<u>tender</u> nodules on the pads of fingers and toes."
- **Janeway Lesions** are the <u>non-tender</u> red nodules on the palms or soles.

Envision the Osler nodes as gigantic Os on the toes causing pain ("Ooooowwwww").

If they give you the classic description of endocarditis and ask what is the **best** study to **confirm the diagnosis**, the answer will be **blood culture**, not cardiac echo or the other decoys waiting for you. This is because the infection can only be identified by isolating the pathogen in the blood.

Staph aureus is the most common cause of acute bacterial endocarditis in children.

For *S. aureus* infective endocarditis, initial IV antibiotic regimen includes **vancomycin plus a ß-lactamase-resistant antibiotic (i.e. nafcillin, oxacillin, or cefazolin)**. Treatment is for 2-8 weeks.

Dental Plan

Dental prophylaxis is no longer done **routinely** for all congenital heart disease.

Routine antibiotic prophylaxis is now reserved for patients with congenital heart disease in specific situations including:

- Unrepaired cyanotic heart disease
- Heart disease surgically corrected with hardware and other devices within the previous 6 months
- Any residual defect near a prosthetic cardiac device
- Prosthetic cardiac valve
- Previous infective endocarditis
- Cyanotic congenital heart disease
- Repaired CHD
- Cardiac transplant

When prophylaxis is indicated, **oral amoxicillin** [50 mg/kg] 60 minutes prior to the procedure is appropriate. If the child is penicillin allergic, **clindamycin** and **azithromycin** are the alternatives.

Myocarditis

Myocarditis will typically follow a **viral illness**. If myocarditis is the correct answer, they will usually slip in something about a **recent URI** that precedes the current presentation. They will likely describe **a new murmur**.

The symptoms can range from **fatigue and lethargy** (similar to what you are experiencing while reading this material), to **tachypnea**, **tachycardia**, and **chest pain**, and in extreme cases to **shock, CHF, pulmonary edema, arrhythmias,** and **death**.

EKG will show diffuse low voltages. Diagnosis is by MRI.

Many viruses can cause myocarditis, but **coxsackie group B virus** is the most common cause.

Treatment of myocarditis is supportive. Use of steroids to treat myocarditis is controversial and, therefore, very unlikely to be the correct answer.

Pericarditis

Pericarditis is the inflammation of the pericardial sac, typically involving the epicardium and pericardium. The more common causes are **viral,** as in URI, or **collagen vascular disease**, for example, JIA. When pericarditis is caused by bacteria, it is usually due to a preceding or concurrent bacterial infection elsewhere, i.e., pneumonia. *Staph aureus is the most common bacterial cause of pericarditis.*

If a definitive cause is needed, then it must be done by obtaining a sample via cardiocentesis. Viral serology and cultures are needed to document the etiology.

Children with pericarditis tend to **lean forward** and may have a **pericardial friction rub** on auscultation. ECG would demonstrate **ST segment elevation**. Additional findings could include **nonspecific chest and epigastric pain**. There may also be a **low grade fever** and **jugular venous distention**. If the patient has an **underlying rheumatological disorder**, this is further information pointing to pericarditis.

The fact that the pain is worse when lying down could lead you to believe it is musculoskeletal, but the **EKG findings** and **muffled heart sounds** would tell you that pericarditis is the most likely cause.

Penny Carditis. Envision a penny on the chest causing pain. When you sit up, the penny falls off and the pain is gone.

The most important study to order when pericarditis or effusion is suspected is a **CXR.**

> ## Pulsus Paradoxus
>
> A drop of systolic blood pressure of more than 10 mm Hg seen with inspiration in certain conditions including pericardial effusion, tamponade, pericarditis, some cardiomyopathies, and severe asthma.

Pericardial Effusion

Presentation may include a child with chest pain and possibly **shoulder pain** which is referred from diaphragmatic irritation. They may have general malaise and an **enlarged heart on CXR** with **no heart failure clinically.** Echocardiogram will show **pericardial fluid.**

Causes include **metabolic conditions** (uremia, hypothyroidism), **infections** (with or without carditis), and **autoimmune conditions** (SLE, JIA, acute rheumatic fever).

Cardiac Tamponade

DEFINITION

When a pericardial effusion builds up enough pressure to collapse the right atrium and ventricle. Signs include tachypnea, rales, pulsus paradoxus, muffled heart sounds, jugular venous distention, hepatomegaly, peripheral edema, and hypotension.

PERIL

Diuretics here would be dangerous because they would lower the circulating blood volume making compression of the right ventricle more severe and acutely lowering the systolic output. Fluid boluses might help while a more definitive treatment is arranged.

Chest Pain

BUZZWORDS

If you are presented with one of the less than 1% of cases of chest pain that is cardiac in origin, it will be described as pain that **radiates to the neck, back, shoulders,** or **left arm**.

Additional findings that tip you off to a cardiac origin include pain that is **constant/frequent, dull, pressure-like,** is **associated with exercise** or interferes with sleep.

Cardiac pain may be associated with dizziness, palpitations, syncope, and/ or shortness of breath.

EKG and CXR would be indicated and consideration should be given to referral to a cardiologist for further evaluation and testing.

Pain that is infrequent and brief, sharp that increases with a deep breath would be consistent with **musculoskeletal** or **pleuritic pain**.

Precordial Catch Syndrome (PCS)

BUZZWORDS

PCS will likely be described as brief episodes of sharp chest pain which is well localized over the cardiac apex. The onset of pain is acute, and can occur during rest or with activity.

HOT TIP

It causes a lot of anxiety for parents and board candidates. It is considered to be benign.

TREATMENT

Treatment is only reassurance, rather than EKG , cardiac echo or referral to a cardiologist.

Pain in the Chest !

You will be expected to be familiar with the possible cardiac causes of chest pain in children, which include:

- Precordial Catch Syndrome
- Pericarditis/Myocarditis
- Aortic stenosis and severe pulmonic stenosis
- Anomalous origin of coronary arteries
- Mitral valve prolapse
- Kawasaki disease
- Arrhythmias (SVT and VT)
- Hypertrophic (Obstructive) Cardiomyopathy

Chapter 25

Heme Onc

This chapter will deal with diseases of the blood and neoplastic disorders, otherwise known as "heme-onc." Basically, the focus is on the ABCs of RBCs and WBCs, and of course, oncologies...

Disorders of Red Cells

Anemia Mania

Anemia of the newborn

A physiological drop in the H/H is to be expected by the 2nd or 3rd month of life (8-10 weeks of age) in term infants and even a Hgb of 9 may be normal at this age.

If they describe garden-variety asymptomatic **physiologic anemia of infancy**, the correct answer will likely be **no further laboratory evaluation is necessary**.

In premature infants, the nadir may actually happen at 1-2 months (7-8 weeks).

Should they ask for the "etiology" of physiological anemia in newborns, the answer is **low erythropoietin production**.

> **Guesstimating MCV**
>
> Normal MCV is roughly
> 70 + 2 (age in years).

Sizing It All Up

The best approach to questions concerning anemias is to break them up into size order. Note the MCV, and note whether it is **micro-, macro-, or normocytic**. It shouldn't be subtle. Remember that the **normal MCV for children is 70-90**, as opposed to 80-100 for adults.

Since these are not the Heme-Onc Boards, there are only a limited number of anemias you need to know, and a limited number of ways they can present them. So here goes:

Microcytic Anemia

The primary considerations here are the **thalassemias**, **too little iron** and **too much lead**. The MCV will be less than 70.

Thalassemia

The usual hemoglobins are:

- Hemoglobin F (2 alpha and 2 gamma chains)
- Hemoglobin A (2 alpha and 2 beta chains)
- Hemoglobin A_2 (2 alpha and 2 delta chains)

Thalassemias are caused by defects in the genes that code for hemoglobin chains so that the proper **quantities** are not produced. This is in contrast to hemoglobinopathies which are errors in the sequencing (ie. **quality**) of the hemoglobin chains.

Diagnosis is made either by the NBS or later by hemoglobin electrophoresis or a thalassemia panel.

> ## Watch That Iron
>
> Any patient who undergoes **regular transfusion therapy** (thalassemia, sickle cell, aplastic anemia, vampires) will eventually have **iron overload.**
>
> These patients must begin chelation therapy to remove excess iron, or they will have toxic buildup in their livers (hemosiderosis) and hearts. This is a significant cause of morbidity and mortality in chronically transfused patients.

Alpha Thalassemia

There are two alpha globin genes on chromosome 16 (thus 4 alleles = aa/aa), and alpha thalassemia results from mutations in one to all four of these alleles. With the defect, the alpha chains are in short supply.

Trading Traits

If only one ("silent carrier") alpha allele is defective, patients are completely asymptomatic. If two ("alpha thalassemia minor" or "trait") alpha alleles are defective, children will be asymptomatic and picked up on routine screening with a mild **microcytic hypochromic anemia** that had normal iron and lead studies.

Diagnosis may be made by exclusion (as above) or via **hemoglobin electrophoresis** (EP, which will be normal) with a **thalassemia panel.**[1] No treatment is necessary for the traits.

> ## Where's the Thal?
>
> The thalassemia panel cannot diagnose alpha thalassemia trait in the presence of iron deficiency. So the iron must be replenished first.

More than Traits

When there are three defective alpha genes, the result is **Hemoglobin H disease**, or "alpha thalassemia intermedia", which leads to **hemolysis** and **hepatomegaly**.

At birth, it will present as **Hemoglobin Barts** (tetramers of gamma chains) on newborn screening. It may be treated with **transfusions**, but usually is treated with **splenectomy**.

Four defective alpha genes causes **hydrops fetalis**, or "alpha thalassemia major" and results in a **stillbirth** or **death soon after birth**. Those who survive thanks to intrauterine transfusions, require **transfusions for life** and eventually bone marrow transplantation.

Needless to say, these patients should be referred for genetic counseling.

---

[1] The thalassemia panel is key, the EP alone will be normal.

Beta Thalassemia

Beta Thalassemia Minor (a.k.a. **Beta Thalassemia Trait**), is caused by a **defect in one of the beta globin gene alleles**. These patients are **asymptomatic**, and usually diagnosed when a **mild microcytic anemia** is noted on incidental testing. Diagnosis is made by **hemoglobin electrophoresis** with **elevated A2** and normal iron studies.

Beta thalassemia intermedia results from a mutation in **both beta globin gene alleles** when one of the mutations yields a mild phenotype.

With **Beta thalassemia major** (a.k.a. Cooley's anemia), they can describe a **small-for-age** Greek child with anemia, fatigue and an **enlarged liver or spleen**.

The newborn screen will have an **F only** pattern. These patients present in the first year of life with **progressive severe microcytic, hypochromic anemia**. **Hepatosplenomegaly** will also be present. They could also describe or show an x-ray that has **thickened bone**. The skull x-ray will often have the classic **"hair-on-end" appearance**, as one would see in hair exposed to static electricity (this is secondary to extramedullary hematopoiesis).

The mainstay of treatment is **chronic transfusion therapy** or **transplantation.**.

The two **long-term complications** seen with beta thalassemia major are

1. Cholelithiasis[2]
2. Hemochromatosis (iron deposition in the heart, liver, and pancreas).

Sickle cell anemia and **beta thalassemia** can be distinguished on **hemoglobin electrophoresis** as follows:

- sickle cell anemia ➜ hemoglobin F and hemoglobin S
- beta thalassemia ➜ low or no hemoglobin A_1, elevated hemoglobin A_2 and hemoglobin F

You are presented with a 10 week old infant of Mediterranean descent with a hemoglobin of 9.0 and an MCV of 89. What is the most likely explanation for the anemia?

The diversion here is the child of Mediterranean descent. If your eyes were drawn to this word and you ignored the numbers and picked thalassemia, you would be adrift in the Mediterranean.

This is an example where "putting numbers into words" would be helpful. You would have noted that this is a normocytic anemia, and given the age of the infant, the most likely cause of the anemia is *physiologic anemia of infancy*.

---

[2] Known as gallstones to the rest of humanity.

Iron Deficiency Anemia

Infants

The risk for iron deficiency anemia in infants begins **after 4 months**, particularly in breast fed infants. It begins earlier in preterm infants that have not had iron supplementation.

How now Bad Cow

Because of the low amount of iron absorbed, **infants** given cow's milk (versus formula or breast milk) before 12 months of age are also at increased risk for **iron deficiency anemia**.

Toddlers

Even though most times iron deficiency anemia is completely asymptomatic, look for this common scenario – An 18 month-old kiddo with **pallor** and **tachycardia**. The **hemoglobin** may be very **low** (<6) and the MCV will also be low (<60). The tip-off for iron deficiency anemia in this child will be a history of drinking **lots and lots and lots of cows milk** (over 32 oz per day) and probably **still on the bottle**, to the exclusion of anything else containing iron.

This is also why **obesity** is a risk factor for iron-deficiency anemia.

Low iron is responsible for more than anemia. Even without frank anemia, low iron causes mild **delays neurodevelopment**.

Once you find microcytic anemia in the right setting, you may go ahead and give a **trial of iron**. If the anemia improves in one month, you may continue the iron treatment. If it does not, then you must investigate for other causes of microcytic anemia (ie. lead toxicity or thalassemia) or of chronic iron deficiency (ie. celiac disease).

Iron deficiency anemia is treated with **ferrous sulfate** until 2 months after hemoglobin levels are normalized. This is to replenish iron stores. Think of it as paying off all your bad debts first (resolving the anemia) and then putting some savings away in the bank (building up iron stores). And improve their **diet**, and **get them off the bottle**!

Parenteral iron administration will never be the right answer, unless 1) the kid cannot take oral iron, or 2) in very extreme social circumstances.

> ## RDW, the Road to Passing
>
> You can be presented with a grid with at least five forms of anemia, along with their associated lab findings. At one point, you will narrow down the choices to two microcytic anemias: one with a **high RDW** and one with **a low or normal RDW**.
>
> Iron deficiency and lead toxicity will have the increased RDW. Thalassemia will have the lower RDW.[3]
>
> This is easy to remember since
> - Iron deficiency has the higher RDW
> - Thalassemia has the lower RDW

> ## Ferritin is your friend
>
> The H/H will tell you if you have anemia, but a low ferritin can tell you if you have early iron deficiency before it reaches anemia levels.

---

3 There are NO conditions associated with a low RDW.

You are doing a routine sports physical on a 16-year-old female. She has a hemoglobin of 11 and an SMR of 5. She proudly notes that she is a strict vegetarian.

What other physical findings would you expect to note in this patient?

You will be tempted with choices such as tachycardia, marked pallor, weakness, and perhaps oral lesions. You will be tempted to pick these choices because they note that she is a vegetarian.

The correct answer will be that no other physical findings should be expected. Vegetarians in general tend to have low iron stores. However, in this specific case, her hemoglobin is only consistent with mild iron deficiency anemia, and no other physical findings would be expected.

Lead Poisoning

Lead poisoning is **the most common environmental illness** in kids. It acts by interfering with various enzyme systems; most notably it can **affect the production of heme**.

Measuring a **whole blood, NOT fingerstick, lead level** is the gold standard test.

A **ringed sideroblast** (immature red blood cell with iron-bloated mitochondria surrounding the nucleus) could be an important clue that lead poisoning is the diagnosis, although the much rarer sideroblastic anemia should also be considered.

> **FEP**
>
> FEP (free erythrocyte protoporphyrin) is elevated in both lead poisoning and Fe deficiency. It is normal in thalassemia. Although not very common in clinical practice, it might creep up in a question.

Macrocytic Anemias

The MCV in macrocytic anemias will be >100, often around 110.

We will discuss B12 and folate deficiency here and Fanconi and Diamond-Blackfan macrocytic aplastic anemias in a later section in this chapter.

Remember that hypothyroidism has also been associated with macrocytic anemia.

Vitamin B12 Deficiency

Frequently this is due to **poor absorption of B12**, often as a result of a gastrointestinal disorder such as Crohn's disease.

B12 deficiency can also be due to

- Intrinsic factor deficiency, ie. "pernicious anemia"
- Bacterial overgrowth
- Bowel resection
- Vegetarian diets

Often they will drop a hint as to the etiology of the deficiency in the question. Vitamin B12 deficiency will frequently be the underlying problem if a compromised gut is combined with a heme question.

Remember the **B** Rule: **B**12 deficiency, **B**acterial overgrowth, **B**owel resection, HLA-**B**27 (Crohn's), and of course **B**egan and **b**egetarian diets.[4]

Folate Deficiency

Got Goat Milk? – If you see the words "goat milk" in the question, it is probably a macrocytic anemia caused by folic acid deficiency. That points you to the treatment.

Remember, goats are "foolish animals;" therefore, drinking their milk results in **"foolate"** deficiency. Don't pick B12 deficiency, even though that trap will be waiting for you.

B12 and folate deficiency often coexist. If you treat with folate and forget to correct the B12 deficiency, this will make your CBC look prettier, but may lead to irreversible neurologic damage.

Normocytic Anemias

When you see a normocytic anemia, consider (1) the patient is **bleeding**, (2) the patient has a **chronic disease**, or (3) there is a **hemolytic process**. For obvious reasons, we will only walk you through the last one.

Breaking up is Hard to Do:
The Hemolytic Anemias

There are a few types of hemolytic anemias, each with its own unique characteristics and descriptions. These should be easy-to-answer questions once you have them down straight. They each have different inheritance patterns, a subject ripe for the matching section. Follow the bouncing memory aides and you won't go wrong.

Pesky Parvo

Hemolytic Anemias result in an **elevated reticulocyte count (normal is 1%)**.

One exception to this would be a parvovirus infection leading to an aplastic crisis in a patient with a chronic hemolytic anemia, like sickle cell and hereditary spherocytosis.

Therefore, if you have a question that points to a hemolytic anemia, but there is **no elevated retic count, parvovirus** could be the correct answer regarding etiology.

---

[4] OK maybe we're getting s little carried away here, but if it works, go with it.

Consider the reasons that a red cell might be destroyed. There could be enzyme problems (G6PD), structural problems (HS), or a weird shape that causes its removal from the circulation (sickle cell).

With all these red cells breaking open, the remnants have to go somewhere. You will find them in the **urine**, usually in the form of **hemosiderin** and **bilirubin**.

Serum haptoglobin will be low because it is used up transporting the released hemoglobin.

Autoimmune Hemolysis

If they tell you the **Coombs test is positive**, then they have just given you a gift. The direct Coombs identifies antibodies on the surface of the red cell. This is a dead giveaway that a hemolytic process is **immune-mediated**.

In disorders like this with increased destruction of RBCs you would expect an increased reticulocyte count. On the other hand, disorders associated with decreased production of RBCs would be associated with a low reticulocyte count.

Autoimmune Hemolytic Anemia (AIHA)

The primary treatment is with glucocorticoids. However, transfusion would be indicated if you are presented with signs of end organ impact. These could include CNS (mental status change or seizures), cardiac (chest pain), or lab findings suggestive of acute renal failure

G6PD Deficiency

Glucose-6-phosphate dehydrogenase protects the red cell from oxidative stress which can lead to hemolysis. There may be a reference to "**Heinz Bodies,**" which are small, purple granules in the red cell that form as a result of damage to the hemoglobin molecule.

> **G6PD Star POWER!**
>
> G6PD is the most common RBC enzymopathy worldwde.

Memorize Heinz body as "Hein6" body to keep this straight. Another way to remember this association is that **6** year olds like **Heinz**® ketchup on everything. You can also picture the cells as "Heinz®" bottles of ketchup ready to explode (hemolyze).

Infants may present with **jaundice in the first few days of life**, obviously mostly in **boys** since it is **X-linked**, but girls can also develop symptoms since carriers can exhibit decreased expression of G6PD due to lyonization.

To remember that this is **X linked**, remember G-si**X**-PD deficiency.

Postnatally, **most individuals are asymptomatic** but they could describe an **African American** or **Mediterranean boy** with **fatigue, back pain, jaundice, anemia and dark urine.** There is **NO hepatomegaly or splenomegaly.**

HOT TIP

Watch for a trigger in the history that would cause the oxidative stress, such as treatment with a **sulfa-containing antibiotic (ie. trimethoprim-sulfamethoxazole), nitrofurantoin, moth balls, antimalarial meds,** or **ingestion of fava beans**. G6PD patients also cannot use EMLA anesthetic cream.

PERIL

When testing for G6PD deficiency, **testing right after or during an episode is not reliable,** because reticulocytes have a large amount of G6PD and can lead to a false negative test. Testing should be done several weeks after the episode. **Therefore, if the question includes a negative test right after an episode, G6PD deficiency has not necessarily been ruled out.**

Besides the Heinz bodies mentioned above, other clues in the blood smear will be **helmet cells**[5] and **blister cells**.

MNEMONIC

Heinz, Helmets and Blitz !

TREATMENT

Treatment involves appropriate hemodynamic support with fluid and/ or RBC transfusions as well as **removal of the oxidant stressor.** Newborns may also require phototherapy and/or exchange transfusion to resolve the indirect hyperbilirubinemia.

Long term treatment involves family education on trigger avoidance as well as recognition of the signs and symptoms of hemolysis and possible folic acid supplementation.

Hereditary Spherocytosis (HS)

DEFINITION

HS is the most common inherited cause of hemolytic anemia in individuals of European ancestry. HS is due to **defects in the surface of red cells** resulting in loss of erythrocyte surface area. The most common form is **autosomal dominant.**[6]

BUZZWORDS

The hallmark of HS is **chronic hemolysis**. HS typically presents **with mild or moderate anemia, reticulocytosis,** and **splenomegaly,** but rarely jaundice since it is a low-level hemolysis. **Gallstones** are also common.

HOT TIP

It is a nonimmune hemolysis so the **DAT test will be negative**. These cells will break open more easily than normal erythrocytes when subjected to hypotonic solutions, and therefore **osmotic fragility testing**

> ### Watch the stones
>
> Upper abdominal pain in patients with hemolytic disorders should prompt consideration of cholelithiasis.
>
> Cholecystectomy could be a correct answer, since recurrence and complications (including pancreatitis) are common.

> ### Splenectomy
>
> Patients who have hemolytic anemias may require partial or total splenectomy to resolve the chronic hemolysis.
>
> It is important to **vaccinate these children against H. flu, S. pneumoniae, and N. meningitidis a few weeks before the surgery.**
>
> Post-splenectomy patients remain at risk for these bacteria after surgery and consideration should be given to antibiotic prophylaxis until adolescence.
>
> Fever in these patients requires CBC, blood culture, and IV ceftriaxone.
>
> Patients with asplenia at highest risk for sepsis are:
>
> - those who underwent splenectomy for hematologic disorders
> - those who were younger at the time of splenectomy
> - those whose splenectomy was more recent

---

[5] Helmet cells are seen in mechanical hemolytic anemias. Just remember when everything is being destroyed, you need helmets on your cells!

[6] But an autosomal recessive form can also occur.

has classically been the diagnostic method of choice. However, because of the relatively poor sensitivity and specificity of this test, **EMA flow cytometry** is being used more now. Therefore this could be a correct choice on the exam.

Parvovirus B19 is the most common cause of aplastic crisis in children with hereditary spherocytosis and is the most common reason for these children to require a blood transfusion.

If the hemolysis is not severe (Hgb remains above 5-6 g/dL), monitoring until recovery is usually sufficient. Severe hemolysis would require transfusion. **Splenectomy** is sometimes done and is usually **curative**.

Folic acid supplementation is recommentation.

Sickle Cell Anemia (SCA)

Sickle cell disease is caused by a substitution at **amino acid six of the beta globin chain**. In the abnormal gene, a **valine is substituted for a glutamic acid**.

They could ask you which diseases are a result of **amino acid substitution**. This fact would come in handy for such a question.

Sickle cell anemia **does not usually present clinically until after 6 months of age**, but children are usually diagnosed when their newborn screens come back abnormal.

CBC usually shows a **normocytic anemia with a high reticulocyte count**. Indirect hyperbilirubinemia is also present from chronic hemolysis.

Most states screen newborns for sickle cell disease, so there are fewer and fewer diagnostic surprises. However, you may be faced with a child newly emmigrated from a developing country who has never been diagnosed with sickle cell, so you must still maintain an index of suspicion.

A Time of Crisis

Vasoocclusive Crisis: This will present with **acute pain secondary to ischemia and infarction**. Infants can have **dactylitis** – pain and swelling of the hands and feet. **Rehydration** and **aggressive pain control** are the staples of management.

Form vs. Function

Defects of structure (e.g., membrane) are dominant traits.

Enzyme defects are usually recessive.

Sickle Cell Amongst Us

1:12 African Americans (8%) in the US have sickle cell trait (FAS or similar) on newborn screening. Hemoglobin electrophoresis is indicated after 3 months of age.

Those with sickle cell trait have some symptoms such as trouble concentrating urine so may dehydrate more easily when playing vigorous sports like football.

In addition, they may demonstrate microscopic or gross hematuria, increased risk of kidney disease and renal medullary carcinoma, splenic infarction, rhabdomyolysis, and glaucoma after hyphema.

Sequestration Crisis: They will describe signs of **shock**. This is due to pooling of blood in the **liver and spleen**, often in response to an **infection**. This is a **medical emergency** and requires aggressive medical intervention, including **hospitalization and transfusion. Splenectomy** is usually indicated after the second or third sequestration episode.

Aplastic Crisis: Aplastic crises are typically due to **parvovirus infection**. A person with sickle cell (or HS for that matter) needs to keep a high reticulocyte count to keep up with increased red cell destruction. If this is turned off, the patient is in dire straits indeed, and their hemoglobin will plummet. Treatment involves **blood transfusions** as needed.

Hyperhemolytic Crisis: Usually they will describe an **infection** as well as a history of SCA. It can often precede an aplastic crisis or sequestration crisis.

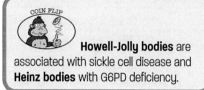

Howell-Jolly bodies are associated with sickle cell disease and **Heinz bodies** with G6PD deficiency.

Priapism may be seen in sickle cell disease, particularly on the boards.

Infection was the leading cause of death in infants prior to prophylaxis. **Antibiotic prophylaxis** with **penicillin VK (alternative is amoxicillin)** is recommended for all children with sickle cell disease from 2 months of age at least through age 5. These children should also receive the **pneumococcal vaccine series described in the Preventive chapter of this book** (both Prevnar and PPSV 23).

All routine vaccines, including the meningococcal vaccines, are crucial.

Spleen Truth

By age 5, children with SCA have **functional asplenia**, and many will have a small, hard, non-palpable spleen.

Children with functional asplenia are at the same risks as the post splenectomy patents listed in the previous section.

Any older child should be **considered asplenic** and treated as such (antibiotics and a septic workup for fevers). The spleen removes **Howell-Jolly bodies** from the red cells, so once asplenic, you will expect to find these nuclear particles.

Can't Get Me Malaria!

Children with SCA and thalassemia are resistant to **malaria**, which is thought to be how these abnormal genes have selectively remained in the gene pool.

Acute Chest Syndrome (ACS)[7]

Acute chest syndrome is defined as **chest pain**, **infiltrate on x-ray**, and **hypoxia**.

If they describe a sickle cell patient with these symptoms and signs, the next study to get would be an **ABG to confirm the hypoxia** –the oxygen saturation, especially if borderline, is usually not good enough to make the diagnosis of ACS.

The treatment for ACS is **transfusion**. If the starting hematocrit is low, a simple transfusion may suffice. But if the hematocrit is relatively high to start with, the patient may require an **exchange transfusion**.

---

[7] As an intern, I once dictated this diagnosis and the transcriptionist typed it out as "A Cute Dress" Syndrome. Of course this was in the pre-EMR days and I just dated myself.

Chest pain in a child with SCA is difficult to distinguish between **pneumonia** and **pulmonary infarct**. Therefore, **fever, cough and chest pain** should be treated for both.

Cerebrovascular accident (CVA)

If they were to describe an African American child with symptoms of a stroke, treatment would consist of **transfusion first**, followed by an MRI. You want to treat before you diagnose because you don't want the CVA to progress on the MRI table.

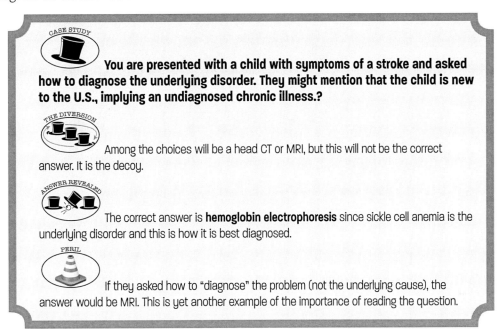

CASE STUDY

You are presented with a child with symptoms of a stroke and asked how to diagnose the underlying disorder. They might mention that the child is new to the U.S., implying an undiagnosed chronic illness.?

THE DIVERSION

Among the choices will be a head CT or MRI, but this will not be the correct answer. It is the decoy.

ANSWER REVEALED

The correct answer is **hemoglobin electrophoresis** since sickle cell anemia is the underlying disorder and this is how it is best diagnosed.

PERIL

If they asked how to "diagnose" the problem (not the underlying cause), the answer would be MRI. This is yet another example of the importance of reading the question.

Cholelithiasis

Cholelithiasis, or gallstones (as they are commonly called), is associated with sickle cell disease. Consider this diagnosis and order an abdominal ultrasound in a child with sickle cell disease presenting with right upper quadrant tenderness.

Hypoplastic and Aplastic Anemias

In general these are anemias due to **suppression of the red cell line in the bone marrow**.

Aplastic anemia and acute leukemia can look very similar. They will have to give you something to help differentiate them. **Hepatosplenomegaly, lymphadenopathy, depression of the WBC or PLT counts, a high LDH or uric acid**, as well as **fevers** and **bone pain** (and, of course, **circulating blasts**), make the diagnosis of leukemia more likely. Diagnosis for both is confirmed by **bone marrow biopsy**.

Just because **chloramphenicol** is rarely used in practice does not mean it will not make an appearance on Boards. It is still used in the Board's world, and be responsible for an **aplastic crisis.**

Fanconi's Anemia (A Fan Made up of Ice Cream Cones)

In addition to Fanconi's Anemia being the most common form of inherited bone marrow failure (pancytopenia), there are **chromosomal structural abnormalities**, as well as distinct **congenital malformations** often associated with it. Usually presents **after age 3.**

It is a **macrocytic anemia** (MCV >100%) with **elevated fetal hemoglobin.**

The following **physical characteristics** are associated with Fanconi's Anemia:

❑ Abnormal skin pigmentation
❑ Growth retardation short stature and microcephaly
❑ Renal abnormalities
❑ Abnormal thumb and forearm – orthopedic surgeons sometimes sometimes see these kids first for "radial ray" defects
❑ Developmental Delays
❑ Eye and ear anomalies

We already established that we would think of a **"fan made up of ice cream cones."**

❑ First, the fan chops off the **thumbs**, then the **feet**, which results in **short stature**. Ironically it does result in elevated FEET-al-Hemoglobin.
❑ Because the fan is made up of ice cream cones, picture the cones spraying odd-colored pigment all over the room, resulting in **abnormal skin pigment.**
❑ The pigment turns into hard plastic. You can't go to the bathroom covered in hard plastic. This results in **urinary retention** and a plastic kidney (**renal abnormalities**).

Yeah, this one is a stretch but still better than free association and rote memory.

> **BIG FAN Anemias**
>
> Fanconi anemia and Diamond-Blackfan anemia are both macrocytic anemias.
>
> Picture the large Red Blood Cells as a giant electric fan, and you will remember that FANconi's and BlackFAN are both macrocytic anemias.

It is **recessive**. Remember this by picturing the fan in the **"recess"** of the ceiling. Fanconi's anemia is a cancer predisposition syndrome. These patients are also **at risk of transformation to AML or myelodysplastic syndrome.**

Patients invariably require **transfusions of red cells and platelets**. The only **cure is a bone marrow transplant**, although medical therapy with immunosuppressants or, less commonly, androgens, can lead to a prolonged remission (it takes a muscle builder on androgen to take down the fan).

Diamond-Blackfan Anemia (DBA) vs. Transient Erythroblastopenia of Childhood (TEC)

Both DBA and TEC are **profound isolated red cell anemias** that **present in infancy/toddlerhood**. Differentiating them can be tricky, but you will be given some important clues to help with this differentiation.

 Diamond-Blackfan Anemia (DBA) is due to an **arrest in the maturation of red cells**.

 Transient Erythroblastopenia of Childhood (TEC) is a consequence of a **suppression of erythroid production**.

In both TEC and DBA, **the reticulocyte count and hemoglobin will be low at the start**. Both may have gradual onset, though **DBA often presents with anemia at birth**. Both are likely to be relatively asymptomatic.

Both TEC and DBA **affect the red cell line exclusively**, and you will be expected to distinguish them. As noted, **DBA affects infants**, so if they describe a 2 or 3 year old they are NOT describing DBA. Also, DBA is chronic, while transient erythroblastopenia is, of course as the name implies, transient.

It is very important to look for clues suggestive of **DBA**. If you see mention of **thumb abnormalities, urogenital defects,** or **craniofacial problems** in a **kid with severe anemia**, they are probably talking about DBA.

Features of DBA can be remembered as :

- **D**ysmorphic facies (unlike Fanconi's anemia)
- **B**abies (unlike TEC), with
- **A**nemia

	TEC	DBA
Incidence	Common	Extremely rare
Spontaneous recovery	Almost always	Rarely
Dysmorphology	Uncommon	Common
Transfusions	Uncommon	Common
Steroids	Not indicated	Often helpful
Median age of onset	18-26 months (TEC=**T**oddler)	2-3 months (DBA=**BA**by)

You could be presented with a child with **fairly severe anemia** (hemoglobin 3-5), who has a **reticulocytosis** (retic count 5-10%). They may even give you the history of a **recent viral illness**. Unless there are other clues, this is probably someone who had TEC and is now in the recovery phase.

TEC resolves spontaneously **within several months**. Transfusion is rarely warranted. **Steroids** are used with DBA and **not in TEC**.

Also, Blackfan is **MACRO** (remember the big fan). **MCV** in TEC will usually be normal, unless the patient has already started to recover and there is a reticulocytosis, in which case the MCV may be slightly elevated.

Remember to watch for signs of hemolysis. **If they describe dark urine or a positive Coombs test (DAT), and an elevated reticulocyte count, you should put DBA and TEC aside and think about a hemolytic process as a cause of the anemia.**

Transfusion Confusion

To avoid confusion regarding the ill effects of **transfusion reactions**, keep the following in mind.

Febrile Nonhemolytic reactions

These present as **fever and chills**. Risk is reduced by using **leukocyte-filtered blood**.

Pre-medicating with antipyretics does not help prevent this reaction.

Hemolytic reactions

These occur when blood is **not properly cross- matched**.

Allergic reactions

These typically present with **urticaria**. Cessation of transfusion and administration of an **antihistamine** is the correct response. If the urticaria resolves rapidly, the transfusion may resume.

Neutropenia Encyclopedia

Neutropenia is a deficit of the innate immune system and places the child at risk for invasive infections.[8]

Neutropenia is further classified by severity with:

- **Mild** being an ANC between 1000-1500 neutrophils/μL
- **Moderate** being an ANC between 500-1000 neutrophils/μL

---

[8] ANC is calculated by multiplying the WBC by the % of segs plus bands.

- **Severe** being an ANC less than 500 neutrophils/μL
- **Very severe** being less than 200 neutrophils/μL

Classic presentations includes **recurrent mucosal ulceration** (from mouth to perirectal), **gingivitis, cellulitis, abscess formation, pneumonia**, and **septicemia**. They may present with abdominal pain and failure to thrive from GI irritation. Kids with neutropenia are most commonly infected with endogenous organisms including *S. aureus, S. epi,* **gram-negatives**, and **enterococci**.

If **recurrent mucosal ulcerations** are described in the history, your brain should immediately jump to **neutropenia**.

Very few labs are necessary besides a CBC with smear review by a hematologist. Diagnosis will require bone marrow evaluation and specific genetic tests

Congenital vs. Acquired

The congenital neutropenias have a wide spectrum of presentation and include cyclic neutropenia, severe congenital neutropenia (**Kostmann syndrome**), chronic benign neutropenia, and the ones where you look weird (like **Shwachman-Diamond**).

The most common cause of **acquired neutropenia** is **infection. Many, many, many drugs cause neutropenia,** but the ones to know for the Boards are the **antibiotics and the anticonvulsants.** Other causes are autoimmune and bone marrow infiltration, ie malignancy.

Transient Neutropenia

Once again don't forget the ever-present "**viral suppression**" that usually follows a cold and lasts a **couple of days** (not quite as long as in cyclic neutropenia). **No treatment or monitoring is needed.**

Ethnic Neutropenia

Some African American patients and other ethnic groups may have a normal baseline ANC of under 1,000 and be symptom-freem.

Antibiotic Neutropenic Panic Button

A patient known to have neutropenia (from any cause) needs to have a blood culture and antibiotics when they have a fever.

If they give you a kid with an ANC<500 and a fever, the treatment is IV antibiotics and admission to the hospital.

Isoimmune Neonatal Neutropenia

This is a situation similar to Rh hemolytic disease where maternal antibodies against the infant's neutrophils cross the placenta.

It usually presents as a mild neutropenia in a healthy infant and resolves without treatment.

CASE STUDY **You are presented with a previously well child with a febrile illness with no hepatosplenomegaly or lymphadenopathy. They provide you with the results of a CBC, with the only significant result being a WBC of 3.5. You are asked for the next step in the management of this apparent leukopenia.**

THE DIVERSION The diversion here is the neutropenia and your call to manage it. You will be provided with several decoy choices including *antibiotics, bone marrow, referral to a hematologist-oncologist, a call to the man on the moon, whatever!*

ANSWER REVEALED The correct answer will be to repeat the WBC in a few weeks (when it will of course be normal). This is *transient neutropenia due to a viral illness.*

Cyclic Neutropenia

Cyclic Neutropenia is a rare inherited **autosomal dominant** disorder. Picture someone dominant whipping the white cells into submission in the marrow.

The low WBC count (ANC near zero) **lasts around a week** and **reappears every month or so**. Often they will describe **oral ulcers, fever, malaise** and **enlarged lymph nodes**, and it will be in a child **younger than 10 years old**. Invasive infections are less common. The diagnosis can only be made by genetic testing or with **serial CBCs** (2-3 times per week for 6 weeks) in order to document the cycle.

They often ask how long the neutropenia lasts and how long the cycles are. It is easy to remember that it is similar to a **menstrual period**, since it lasts around **one week** and occurs on a **monthly cycle**.

Oral lesions are common: picture white blood cells sharp around the edges cycling around the mouth causing oral lesions

Clostridium perfringens and **gram-negative organisms** are responsible for most deaths in untreated patients.

Treatment is to manage infections and to start patients on **daily rhG-CSF** (recombinant human granulocyte colony stimulating factor) to reduce the number of neutropenic days.

Chronic Benign Neutropenia

This condition is far the most common. It is also known as chronic autoimmune neutropenia because of the presence of anti-neutrophil antibodies.

These children usually present because the pediatrician did a CBC in a 1-5 year-old and discovered it as an incidental finding. These children rarely have oral ulcers or other signs of infection, but when they do, G-CSF may be helpful. Management is usually supportive with IV antibiotics when febrile if they have an ANC below 500.

Distinguishing chronic benign neutropenia from cyclic neutropenia can be done with serial CBCs. Children **usually outgrow chronic benign neutropenia by the age of 5**.

Severe Congenital Neutropenia (SCN)

Also known as **Kostmann syndrome, or Kostmann agranulocytosis,** this is an **autosomal recessive** disorder that results in an **arrest in the development of neutrophils**. The consequence of this neutropenia may be severe, and may lead to life-threatening infections.

These infants present early in life with recurrent and severe infections.

It can be difficult to distinguish Kostmann syndrome from cyclic neutropenia (both in real life and on the Boards).

- In babies with **cyclic neutropenia**, the **ANC will rise to normal as the cycle ends.**
- In **Kostmann syndrome**, the **ANC will remain low.**

Be careful – in BOTH disorders, the ANC may rise in response to G-CSF.

As in cyclic neutropenia, **rhG-CSF is life-saving.** Those who do not respond to rhG-CSF often benefit from **bone marrow transplantation.**

> ### From BAD to UGLY
>
> Patients with SCN are at increased risk for transformation to **myelodysplastic syndrome (MDS) and AML** and must be followed closely, including annual bone marrow evaluations.

Shwachman-Diamond Syndrome (SDS)

In addition to **pancreatic exocrine insufficiency** (which leads to steatorrhea), these kids all have some degree of **pancytopenia.**

Patients usually present with **short stature, diarrhea/steatorrhea, and recurrent infections,** especially those of the **upper respiratory tract and skin.** They may also have **skeletal abnormalities** like **clinodactyly** and **syndactyly.**

Change the name to "**Squashman Diamond**" syndrome. Picture a hammer smashing the bone marrow and diamonds falling out and forming the shape of the pancreas. Squashed bones would remind you of the bone abnormalities.

You can also remember it by its initials Shwachman-Diamond Syndrome, which can stand for:

Substandard neutrophils,
Dumb pancreas,
Steatorrhea and Skeletal abnormalities.

Since Cystic Fibrosis also has pancreatic insufficiency, you may have to distinguish between the two. Of course, Shwachman-Diamond Syndrome is the one with the **decreased cell lines (neutropenia, anemia, thrombocytopenia).** Remember that Shwachman-Diamond Syndrome also has **normal electrolytes, no history of chronic pulmonary problems,** and the **sweat test will be normal.**

The treatment of SDS is to control/prevent infections, give pancreatic enzyme supplementation, prevent orthopedic abnormalities, and to monitor for leukemic transformation.

> ### Neutropenia and Fever
>
> When they present you with an immunocompromised child with fever and /or neutropenia, you need broad-spectrum antibiotics, especially for gram-negative organisms.
>
> **Zosyn® (piperacillin-tazobactam)** plus an **aminoglycoside** or **ceftazidime** monotherapy are reasonable choices.
>
> A first- or second-generation cephalosporin as monotherapy will never be the answer in treating an immunocompromised child with fever and neutropenia.

Bleeding Anomalies:
Platelet and Clotting Issues

Thrombocytopenia

Thrombocytopenia is defined as a platelet count lower than 150,000/cubic millimeters and just like with anemia, it is either the result of **decreased production** or **increased destruction of platelets**.

Children will present with a history of **easy bruising** and **bleeding**, particularly **mucosal bleeding**.

With thrombocytopenia, look for **recent meds** in the question and note it, since it may be the key to the question. Certain meds like **sulfas, seizure meds**, and **vancomycin** can lower platelet counts. Platelet counts return to normal approximately one week after removal of offending drug.

Aspirin and ibuprofen result in abnormal platelet function; however, the platelet count will be normal.

Both **thrombocytopenia** and or **functional platelet disorders** can cause bruising, petechiae, epistaxis, or gastrointestinal bleeding.

However, **deep muscle or joint bleeding** will likely be due to a **coagulopathy**, not a platelet problem. Remember, "dinner" plates (platelets) are too big to penetrate a joint or a muscle.

Neonatal Thrombocytopenia

Thrombocytopenia is the most common hematologic abnormality in neonates admitted to the ICU. And, of course, thrombocytopenia may be present with neonatal sepsis. The most common cause of true neonatal primary isolated thrombocytopenia is related to maternal factors such as allo- or autoantibodies. But the MOST COMMON reason for a low platelet count is clumping from improper collection.

Neonatal alloimmune thrombocytopenia is an isolated, transient but severe thrombocytopenia in a well-appearing neonate in the first 48 hours of life due to platelet destruction by maternal antibodies. It is **similar to Rh disease** in that it occurs when fetal platelets display the antigen inherited by the father, which triggers maternal antibodies to attack them. In this case, **the mother is asymptomatic, and her platelets are normal**.

Unlike Rh disease, this **may occur in the first pregnancy** and is is usually more severe in subsequent pregnancies.

Neonates may also develop **autoimmune thrombocytopenia**. In this case, the mother has antibodies to her own platelets as well as the infant's, and **both mother and child have low platelets**.

Immune Thrombocytopenic Purpura (ITP)

ITP previously stood for Idiopathic Thrombocytopenic Purpura, but now that we know that it is caused by **destruction of platelets by antibodies**, its name was changed. Good thing "idiopathic" and "immune" both start with "I" so the acronym ITP still applies.

They will describe an otherwise healthy 3-year-old with a **recent viral illness**, a **platelet count under 100,000 with the other cell lines intact, ecchymoses**, and perhaps **petechiae**.

If you are presented with a patient with ITP who has new onset **headaches or neurological changes**, you are expected to realize that the patient may be experiencing an **intracranial hemorrhage**. Risk factors include being male, age under 3 years, and history of trauma.

Children with **persistent ITP, mucosal bleeding**, or those with atypical features like **other cell line deficits**, should be **referred to hematology** for possible treatment.

Prognosis is worse if it presents in an older kid, i.e., older than 10 years. In such cases it can become a chronic problem. The younger the patient, the more likely it will be a single occurrence.

> ## Purpura with a Purpose
>
> Recognize that vasculitic disorders may be a cause of purpura. If they describe bruising or purpura in a child, but there is a normal or perhaps increased platelet count, then do not bark up the Heme Tree. They are pointing you in the direction of Henoch-Schönlein Purpura or other forms of vasculitis.
>
> Alternatively, they may drop hints of abuse. But bruising of shins in a 2 year old is a normal finding. This is an important normal finding to keep in mind.
>
> Occasionally, they will try to trip you up with the nomenclature. **Anaphylactoid purpura and Henoch-Schönlein purpura are the same thing.**

Most children with mild ITP will require **no treatment**. IVIg may be an option for extremely low platelet levels or significant bleeding (usually seen with platelet counts under 20,000). With chronic ITP, splenectomy may be the only option, although it should be avoided in children younger than 5.

Steroids are an excellent treatment but if you are actually dealing with leukemia instead of ITP, the consequences may be fatal, so resist the temptation, especially on the Boards.

Kasabach-Merritt Syndrome

Here you have a hemangioma that serves as a "sand trap" for platelets. Thrombocytopenia is caused by a localized consumptive coagulopathy. **The bone marrow is normal.** Patients are at risk for DIC.

If you had a "sand castle on your back," your back would be black and blue and your platelets would be destroyed.

Treatment is to control the hemangioma and provide hemodynamic support via blood transfusions.

TAR Syndrome

This is an autosommal recessive condition and the name says it all—**T**hrombocytopenia **A**bsent **R**adius. Often they just hand this to you either by describing it or showing you the x-ray. You won't miss the absent radius.

In addition to the upper and ower limb defects, renal agenesis may also be seen and the WBC is usually elevated. **50% are symptomatic in the first week of life and 90% have symptoms by 4 months.**

Platelet transfusions are usually necessary in the first year, and there is often spontaneous recovery thereafter.

There is really no excuse for getting this wrong.

Thumbs Away! – You may have noticed that there are three disorders associated with upper limb abnormalities and low blood counts.

	Upper Limb Abnormalities	Platelets	Hemoglobin	Presents
DBA	Thumb	Normal	Low	at 2-3 months
Fanconi	Thumb	Low	Low	after age 3
TAR	Radius	Low	Normal	first month

Coagulopathies

Vitamin K Deficiency

The Vitamin K dependent factors are II, VII, IX, X which, if you're not fluent in Roman, are **2, 7, 9, and 10**. Committing this to memory could be worth at least one correct answer on the exam.

The letter K looks like 2 Sevens (7) stuck to each other and turned around; 7 + 2 = 9 plus one "fact" = 10.

In **early onset** vitamin K-dependent bleeding, consider maternal factors, such as **medications** that interfere with her vitamin K stores (anticonvulsants, warfarin, some antibiotics). Common sources of bleeding are at **venipuncture sites, penis after circumcision, mucous membranes and the GI tract.**

A classic presentation for this disorder is a baby **born at home** who is **exclusively breast-fed**. The baby will present **at a week or less** with the bleeding described above.

Take the K Train

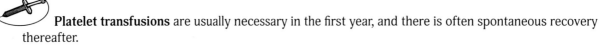 The classic 1 week time frame for Vitamin K deficiency in newborns isn't absolute. Therefore consider Vitamin K deficiency if you are presented within the following time frame

Early - within 24 hours

Classical - within 1 week

Late - 2 weeks to 6 months

The "born at home" is important because the baby may not have gotten the Vitamin K injection after birth. The "exclusively breastfed" is important because formula is fortified with Vitamin K.

Deficiency in the vitamin K factors (i.e., **hemorrhagic disease of the newborn**) results in **elevated PT**.

Remember, "**KEPT**" – Vitamin **K**, **E**xtrinsic pathway, **PT**.

Treatment is to give Vitamin K along with fresh frozen plasma if there is active bleeding.

Hemophilia

The main types of hemophilia to know are Hemophilia A (factor VIII deficiency or "Classic Hemophilia") and Hemophilia B (factor IX deficiency, Christmas disease). They are both se**X-linked recessive**.

"A" and "8" sound alike. "B" and "9" both come right after "A" and "8".

Santa Claus is a "benign" fellow; therefore, it is easy to associate "B9" with Christmas disease. Call it X-mas disease and you will remember it is X-linked recessive. Whoosh!

There may not be a family history, but if there is, it will be of **uncles and boy cousins on mom's side**.

Like Vitamin K deficiency, kids with hemophilia often present in the neonatal period with **bruising, bleeding from their circumcision,** or **bleeding at the site of venipuncture**. Unlike Vitamin K deficiency, the **PTT is prolonged**, and the diagnosis is made by **measuring factor levels**.

Older kids are subject to **deep joint bleeds**. Mortality can occur from **intracranial bleeding**.

Treatment is with **factor supplementation**. Those with severe disease, may need replacement 2-3 times a week.

Venipuncture in Hemophiliacs

If you are presented with a patient with hemophilia who has bleeding in the antecubital area following a blood draw, this is serious. It can lead to nerve compression and is considered to be a medical emergency.

Blood should not be drawn from the jugular or femoral veins of individuals with hemophilia who have not received replacement therapy. It could be fatal to both the patient and your chances of passing the boards.

Persistent oozing

If they describe a child with persistent bleeding after a heelstick or circumcision, a workup for a congenital factor deficiency is the answer.

PT/ PTT

Prolonged PT: think extrinsic factor (VII) or common pathway (II, V, X).

Prolonged PTT: think intrinsic factor VIII, IX (hemophilias) and XI, XII or common pathway (II, V, X).

Remember that normal values for PT, PTT and platelets do not rule out other coagulopathies such as platelet function disorders and dysfibrogenemia.

If you are presented with a patient with hemophilia who suffers significant head trauma, replacement therapy is indicated even in the absence of clinical signs.

 If they give you a girl with bleeding, it is NOT hemophilia (but it may be von Willebrand's disease).

You could be presented with a child who develops a hematoma from the vitamin K shot. The reason the child got the hematoma may be hemophilia. They are trying to hypnotize you by mentioning vitamin K – don't let them!

Von Willebrand's Disease

Von Willebrand's Disease (vWD) affects boys and girls equally and is due to an **abnormal von Willebrand factor**, which is required for normal Factor VIII function as well as normal platelet aggregation.

They will commonly present a child who has (1) excessive bleeding after a **dental procedure or tonsillectomy,** (2) **epistaxis,** or (3) **a girl with menorrhagia.**

The hallmark of vWD is a normal PT. PTT is often normal, but may be slightly prolonged in some cases.

Levels of **von Willebrand factor activity should be low.** If it is a girl, you are done – the diagnosis is most likely vWD. If it is a boy, you need to measure Factor VIII and IX levels to establish the diagnosis.

To rule out the condition with a typical history, you should check vW factor levels three times.

Most of the time, **no treatment** is indicated. For minor bleeding, **intranasal or intravenous DDAVP** (desmopressin, Stimate®) can be used, as it stimulates endogenous release of stored vWF and factor VIII. For major surgery or life-threatening bleeds, **replacement with a factor VIII concentrate** should be administered.

Amicar® (aminocaproic acid) helps with mucosal bleeding by inhibiting fibrinolysis, and is often used in vWD.

Hereditary

With bleeding disorders, even if they **do not describe** or specifically mention the presence of a **family history** for bleeding disorders, **"hemophilia" cannot be ruled out.**

In addition, if they specifically mention that the **mother** has a **family history** of a bleeding disorder, they are hinting at an **X-linked recessive** disease.

Male offspring (also known as boys) of a **mother** who is a carrier have a 50% chance of being born with the disease.

Bleeding time

Bleeding time test is no longer done. It is unreliable due to operator variability.

Bleeding where?

 Von Willebrand's Disease – mucosal bleeds.

Hemophilia – bleeding into joints and muscles.

Disseminated Intravascular Coagulopathy (DIC)

With disseminated intravascular coagulopathy, there will be a history of **sepsis** or other major illness such as **malignancy** or **severe burns.** The **platelets will always be low.** Other supporting labs are a **low fibrinogen, elevated fibrin degradation products** and **elevated D-dimers.** PT and PTT are unpredictable. **Thrombin time will be prolonged.**

Treatment of the underlying condition is the most important factor in management. Support with blood products as needed - platelets, fresh frozen plasma (if clotting factors are low), cryoprecipitate (if fibrinogen is low), and/or RBCs.

Oncology

Bone Tumors

The two types of bone tumors they will ask you about are **Ewing** and **osteogenic sarcoma**. Each has its own very distinct characteristics, and they love to focus on these for a few questions. Invest in some of the easy-to-remember details below and you will be rewarded with a few slam-dunk lay-ups.

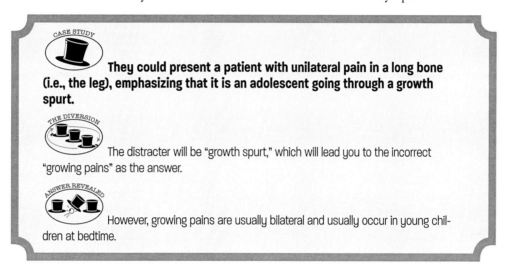

CASE STUDY

They could present a patient with unilateral pain in a long bone (i.e., the leg), emphasizing that it is an adolescent going through a growth spurt.

THE DIVERSION

The distracter will be "growth spurt," which will lead you to the incorrect "growing pains" as the answer.

ANSWER REVEALED

However, growing pains are usually bilateral and usually occur in young children at bedtime.

Osteogenic Sarcoma (a.k.a. Osteosarcoma)

BUZZWORDS

Any time a child presents with **weeks of unilateral limb pain**, an xray would be indicated looking for malignancy. Especially watch for the child **no longer participating in their sport, limping, or waking up at night with pain**. Peak incidence is in the second decade of life (teens) during the adolescent growth spurt.

Laboratory studies may show **elevated LDH, alkaline phosphatase, and sedimentation rate**.

TREATMENT

Treatment is **surgery** with **chemo** in all cases.

HOT TIP

Mets go to the lungs.

> ### Bad to the Bone !
> Osteosarcoma is the most common malignant bone tumor in children and adolescents.

MNEMONIC

Picture a teen with an **amputated leg trying to run**. Well, he will be **out of breath** pretty fast, which should remind you that mets go to the **lungs**.

They can try to throw you off by including a history of trauma, followed by bone pain or swelling. Don't go for this distractor if there are other signs of a possible tumor, such as **preceding recurrent persistent pain and swelling.** They are likely describing osteogenic sarcoma despite the mention of trauma.

Ewing Sarcoma vs. Osteogenic Sarcoma (OS)

Ewing Sarcoma	Osteogenic Sarcoma	Both
• Soft tissue component • Ewing Sarcoma is not usually seen in African Americans • X-ray shows **"onionskinning"** representing layers of periosteal reaction	• OS is more common in African Americans • **Teenager, usually going through a growth spurt, who presents with pain** • X-ray shows **"sunbursting"** representing calcified blood vessels	• Both can occur in long bones • **Treatment for both is chemotherapy, radiation, and surgery** • **Both can metastasize to the lungs, but this is the main site of OS mets**

Osteoid Osteoma

Questions on osteoid osteoma are very easy to get correct because the history is as unique as are the x-ray findings. For a typical picture, look at your favorite Atlas. They will describe **tibia pain** or **femur pain, worse at night, relieved by ibuprofen.**[9]

The picture will have a **central radiolucent (white area) surrounded by thick sclerotic bone.**

Leukemia

Leukemia is the **most common childhood malignancy.**

There are 4 types of childhood leukemia:

      1. Acute lymphocytic leukemia (ALL)

      2. Acute nonlymphocytic leukemia (ANLL)

      3. Chronic myelogenous leukemia (CML)

      4. Chronic lymphocytic leukemia (CLL)

Treatment is dependent on the type.

> ### Linked with Leukemia
>
> Certain conditions are associated with an increased risk of leukemia. **The most common congenital condition associated with leukemia is Down syndrome.**
>
> Increased risk is also seen with SCID, ataxia telangiectasia and other immunodeficiency syndromes, Fanconi anemia, Bloom syndrome, Klinefelter syndrome, Noonan syndrome, and neurofibromatosis.

Acute Lymphocytic Leukemia (ALL)

ALL is by far the most common (80%) of all childhood leukemias and its highest incidence is in children **2 to 5 years of age.** Both genetic and environmental factors are believed to contribute.

---

[9] In past years this was described as pain relieved by aspirin. However it seems that finally this has been updated to reflect that the use of aspirin in children has been phased out with 1970s rotary phones.

They could present you with a child with **pallor, fatigue, bruisability, lymphadenopathy, bone pain** and/or **joint pain or swelling**. There will often be **fevers**. Labs may show **pancytopenia**, though the WBC count may also be normal or elevated.

To be fair, they will have to include something in the history to differentiate ALL from aplastic anemia, such as an **enlarged liver** or **spleen**. Leukemia should not be diagnosed without a **bone marrow examination**.

Infection

Infection is a major cause of death in kids with leukemia. Indwelling catheters and neutropenia combine to increase the risk for infection. **Therefore, children receive broad-spectrum parenteral antibiotics with all febrile episodes.**

> ## Atypical Limps and Lymphs
>
> **Watch for a CBC with the term "atypical lymphs"** to throw you off the trail, with some choices consistent with mono. In the context of a clinical picture of ALL, the **"atypical lymphs" are actually "lymphoblasts,"** incorrectly reported in the CBC as atypical lymphs.

The treatment goal in kids with ALL is to induce remission with one course of chemotherapy.

The **5 year survival rates** for children with newly diagnosed ALL in the US is now **over 80%**. Current chemotherapy regimens have a greater than 99% probability of achieving a complete remission.

Even after treatment, children who have had ALL are at risk of **relapse**. In ALL, the **CNS and testes** are sanctuary sites of ALL which are more resistant to therapy. These are **common sites of relapse**. Early relapse has a worse prognosis.

Survivors of ALL are also at increased risk of subsequent **neuropsychological abnormalities** with **cognitive defects** that can affect education and future employment for life.

Lymphoma

Lymphoma can be confusing. Basically, there is **Hodgkin's lymphoma** (Hodgkin's disease) and "everything else" (**non-Hodgkin's lymphoma**).

 A chest x-ray would be the correct choice if you are presented with a patient with **unexplained lymphadenopathy**, especially if there are symptoms suggesting **chest pathology** (including cough, new-onset wheezing, trouble swallowing, facial or neck swelling, chest pain, or shortness of breath).

Another hint to lymphoma is the presence of **unexplained pruritus**.

Hodgkin's Lymphoma

Hodgkin's lymphoma typically presents in **teens as non-tender enlarged cervical or supraclavicular lymph nodes.** Patients often have **weight loss**, **fevers** and **night sweats**. It is a slow-growing malignancy.

The white count will be high with a **relatively low lymphocyte** count. **Lymph node biopsy may reveal Reed Sternberg cells.**

In general, younger children are more likely to have infection as an explanation for their enlarged lymph nodes, and lymphoma is more likely in adolescents.

Atypical mycobacteria may present with a cervical node, but there will be other signs, i.e., a positive PPD, and there will be no supraclavicular nodes.

> ## Supraclavicular adenopathy
>
> Supraclavicular adenopathy means **lymphoma** until proven otherwise.
>
> You must always, always, always, get a **CXR**. Did we say always? This will likely be the answer to the question "What is the next step?"

Non-Hodgkin Lymphoma

Non-Hodgkin lymphoma is more likely if they present you with a **small child rather than a teen**. It has a much more **rapid presentation**, usually with **airway compression** rather than painless cervical adenopathy. It can also present in the **abdomen as a non-tender mass**. Keep this in mind in addition to **Wilms tumor and neuroblastoma.**

Neuroblastoma

This is the **most common solid tumor of infancy**, and the second most common solid tumor of childhood, after brain tumors.[10]

It presents initially in the adrenal glands in 50% of cases. It is most common in children under 5 years of age. **When neuroblastoma occurs before 12 months of age, the survival rate is 95%.** In fact, neuroblastoma has the highest rate of spontaneous regression of any human malignancy.

Diagnosis

Typical presentations of Neuroblastoma include

- ❑ **Persistent bone or joint pain**
- ❑ Non-tender hard smooth abdominal mass
- ❑ Weight loss, anorexia, night sweats, fever
- ❑ UTI from obstructing abdominal mass
- ❑ **Raccoon eyes** and proptosis (due to metastases)

---

[10] Leukemia is not a solid tumor.

❏ Horner syndrome (due to a mediastinal tumor compressing the recurrent laryngeal nerve[11])

❏ Irritability, hypertension, and diarrhea all due to catecholamine production

❏ **Opsoclonus-myoclonus** ("dancing eyes") paraneoplastic syndrome

Laboratory evaluation may be relatively normal, or may include pancytopenias (from bone marrow involvement), elevated ferritin, LDH and alkaline phosphatase.

Diagnosis of neuroblastoma is made either by:

(1) **Biopsy** of tumor

(2) **Elevated urine VMA and HMA** along with **neuroblasts** found in bone marrow and in this case, biopsy is not necessary

If you are asked to choose what to order, **DO NOT order Urine Catecholamines**, because they will measure epinephrine and norepinephrine. You will need to order specifically urinary VMA and HMA.

Prognosis

The most important prognostic feature is age.

• If younger than 1 year, the prognosis is excellent

• If older than 1, the prognosis is poor

Raccoon Eyes

Raccoon eyes are most commonly associated with basal skull fractures or basilar head bleeds and should raise a flag for child abuse.

But in the right setting, they are also a sign of neuroblastoma.

They could also be outside your home going through your garbage.

Either way, raccoon eyes are always BAD.

Big News on MIBG

Now there is also an MIBG scan that finds neuroendocrine tumors (like pheochromocytomas and neuroblastomas) better.

If it's an option on the test, you may choose it.

Hepatoblastoma

Hepatoblastoma is the most common primary malignany of the liver in childhood.

Risk is increased with prematurity and low-birth-weight infants and children with Beckwith-Wiedemann syndrome.

Children present with a painless abdominal mass or with slowly increasing abdominal distention.

Diagnosis is suspected on US and serum alpha-fetoprotein concentration is usually increased.

---

[11] Which would affect speech.

Retinoblastoma

BUZZWORDS This tumor usually occurs in **children under age 5**, and presents with either **leukocoria** ("white pupil") or **strabismus**.

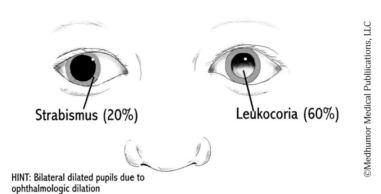

Strabismus (20%)   Leukocoria (60%)

HINT: Bilateral dilated pupils due to ophthalmologic dilation

©Medhumor Medical Publications, LLC

BUZZWORDS A typical presentation would be a mom who brings in a family photo showing the **normal red light reflex in only one eye**.

TAKE HOME MESSAGE Despite the genetic association of retinoblastoma, **only 5% will have a family history.**

In general, try to avoid CT for diagnosis since the radiation may increase the risk of second primary cancers. If among the choices, pick ultrasound or MRI instead.

TREATMENT The mainstays of treatment are **surgical excision, chemotherapy, and radiation**. If the tumor is limited to one eye, cure rates are greater than 90%.

HOT TIP In cases of hereditary retinoblastoma, there is a risk for **pineal gland tumors**. The combination of pineal gland tumor PLUS bilat retinoblastomas is known as **trilateral retinoblastoma**, and these children are at risk for osteosarcoma, other sarcomas, and malignant melanomas as adolescents and adults.

PERIL Children with disease in one eye need to be monitored for **disease in the other eye**, although one would think that was so blatantly obvious that it didn't need to be said. Therefore you can cross this paragraph out if you would like to!

Genetics of Retinoblastoma

There is a heavy genetic component to this, and they like to harp on this point.

COIN FLIP When retinoblastoma is sporadic, it is usually unilateral and unifocal. When it is genetic, it is usually bilateral or multifocal and the inheritance is **autosomal dominant with incomplete penetrance**.

VERY BORING MATERIAL WARNING! The gene for retinoblastoma (RB1) is on the long arm of chromosome 13 and laboratory investigation is often recommended for prognosis and genetic planning.

Remember, if a parent had it in **2** eyes, there is a 1/2 **(50%)** chance of any child having it.

However, if a parent had only **1** eye affected, then there is only a **1/20 (5%)** chance of a child having it. The same odds apply if one sib has unilateral disease.

Rhabdomyosarcoma

Rhabdomyosarcoma is the **most common soft tissue sarcoma** in children and is a Board favorite.

They could describe a child with **constipation**. On rectal exam a mass is **visible or palpated**. This description should tip you off to the diagnosis.

They may show a **grape-like mass protruding from the vagina**. This is classic rhabdomyosarcoma. Change it to "grape-domyosarcoma" and you won't forget that image if they present it to you on the exam.

Young patients (2-6) tend to have **head and neck** rhabdo, while older patients (teenagers) are more likely to have **truncal or extremity** tumors. Diagnosis is made by biopsy. Treatment is with **chemotherapy, surgery,** and **radiation**.

When rhabdomyosarcoma occurs in an extremity, they **often describe a history of trauma to throw you off**. Don't be fooled, and don't go for the distractor. What will tip you off is that the area of trauma **is getting worse after a couple of weeks**. This is a typical presentation of rhabdomyosarcoma, as is "atypical" pain following routine trauma.

Two disorders that can get worse after trauma injury are **rhabdomyosarcoma** and **osteogenic sarcoma**. Don't be deceived by the mention of the trauma.

Craniopharyngioma

Craniopharyngioma presents with central hypothyroidism, hypocortisolism, hypogonadism, GH deficiency and central DI.

If the tumor is large enough it put pressure on the optic chiasm, resulting in bitemporal hemianopia. They will described impaired peripheral vision.

Treatment consists of surgical resection and possibly radiation. This is followed by life long hormone replacement of all missing hormones.

Oncologic Emergencies

Tumor Lysis Syndrome

Tumor Lysis Syndrome occurs with the rapid breakdown of a large number of tumor cells. It is most common at the **initiation of chemotherapy** for **large tumors, lymphomas, or leukemia**.

Bad Bad Steroids!

Tumor Lysis syndrome is the reason you want to make super-sure NEVER pick systemic steroids to treat a symptom that could really represent a malignancy unless they specifically state that a malignancy has been ruled out.

Examples of traps would be ITP, JIA, new onset wheezing, and mononucleosis.

PERIL

This may be **triggered by systemic steroids** and it is a serious consideration when giving steroids for a condition like wheezing or thrombocytopenia which could turn out to be malignancy instead of asthma or ITP.

MNEMONIC

If you end up with tumor lysis, you go to the PICU- **PKU** to help remember elevated Phosphate, Potassium, and Uric acid. Calcium is low, but is sodium affected, you ask? "Naaaa"

PERIL

The high potassium can lead to dysrhythmias. You can also end up with **renal insufficiency with increased creatinine and decreased urine output. LDH is elevated** as a marker of cell breakdown.

TREATMENT

It is prevented and treated with **hydration, alkalinization,** and **allopurinol.**

Spinal Cord Compression

Any tumor in or around the spine can cause cord compression, which often presents with **neurologic symptoms including bowel/bladder dysfunction and flaccid, bilateral paralysis of the lower extremities.**

HOT TIP

Emergent MRI of the spine is the most important first step in management.

TREATMENT

This emergency is usually treated with **steroids** and/or **radiation**.

> ### Superior Vena Cava (SVC) Syndrome
>
> Superior Vena Cava Syndrome is usually due to extrinsic **compression of the SVC by an anterior mediastinal tumor,** most commonly **lymphoma**.
>
> BUZZWORDS
>
> Superior Vena Cava Syndrome typically presents with **red face (plethora), facial swelling, cyanosis, distended neck veins,** and, if bad enough, **neurologic symptoms**.
>
> MNEMONIC
>
> Think about a big heavy Donald Trump type at Christmas after a few drinks – big red swollen face. That is plethora.

Anterior Mediastinal Mass

The primary symptoms here is **respiratory distress**, especially when **supine**.

PERIL

Intubation is NOT the answer because the airway compression is BELOW the vocal cords, and once the patient is anesthetized, there will be no way to maintain oxygenation and ventilation.

MNEMONIC

Any of the four **T**s can result in the symptoms associated with anterior mediastinal masses: Thymoma, Teratoma, Thyroid carcinoma and Terrible lymphoma. Of these, lymphoma is the one that most commonly results in airway compromise.

TREATMENT

Treatment is to make the diagnosis and treat the underlying condition, usually with chemotherapy. In an emergency, **steroids and radiation** can be used.

Side Effects of Chemotherapeutic Agents

This is an excellent topic for the matching section. Having these at your fingertips will provide you with a few easy lay-ups if you need them.

Alkylating Agents: Gonadal Dysfunction

Cyclophosphamide: Hemorrhagic Cystitis

 Cyclophosphamide and **C**ystitis both begin with **Cy**. Or you can picture somebody riding a **Cy**cle in your bladder, causing bleeding.

Management includes serial urineanalysis to monitor for cystitis as well as bleeding. Management is through hydration to increase urine output.

Cisplatin: Hearing Loss and Peripheral Neuropathy

CisBLASTin should remind you of a blast leading to hearing loss and it probably would knock you down and keep you from feeling your hands and feet.

Bleomycin: Pulmonary Fibrosis

"**Blow My Icing:**" When you take this medication, your **lungs are so bad**, you "**blow icing**" instead of air.

Anthracycline (Doxorubicin, Daunomycin) – Cardiac Toxicity

One way to remember this is to remember that rubies and hearts are both red, so the ruby drug attacks the heart. Or picture "**anthrax cycling in your heart**," causing toxicity.

Vincristine/Vinblastine

Neurotoxicity and **SIADH** are the side effects here. Picture a drunk guy named Vinny staggering around and constantly urinating.

Methotrexate: Oral and GI Ulcers, Bone Loss

 "**Moutho Tray X:**" Picture a mouth **filled with trays of sharp Xs** resulting in oral and GI ulcers.

Chapter 26

Renal

Hematuria

To paraphrase the Byrds, who paraphrased Ecclesiastes, "there is a time to reassure, a time to work up, and a time to follow-up." Here is "the way" to know which. First, some definitions.

Microscopic Hematuria

5 or more red blood cells per high-powered field (hpf) in 3 centrifuged samples of freshly voided urine. The 3 separate samples are collected during a 3 week period of time. The urine is **not discolored** when there is microscopic hematuria.

0-4 cells per high-power field (hpf) is not hematuria.

Transient hematuria may be caused by minor trauma, exercise, or fever.

Family history is important in assessing hematuria. If other family members have a history of hematuria without complications, then **benign familial hematuria** is a strong possibility.

Other than **monitoring for hypertension and proteinuria**, no further workup or intervention is necessary.

Heeding Hematuria

If you are only told that the urine dipstick is positive for blood, then the next step will be to obtain a urinalysis with microscopy since a dipstick that is positive for blood could be positive for:

• Hemoglobin

• Myoglobin

• Porphyrins

Patients with **hemoglobinuria** may also be jaundiced and present with anemia. There will be no RBC in the urine, and, therefore, no hematuria.

CASE STUDY

You could be presented with a child who engaged in vigorous activity and presents with "gross hematuria." He is otherwise asymptomatic, and they note 0-2 RBCs on microscopic urinalysis. What is the most likely diagnosis?

THE DIVERSION

Here the diversion is the description of "gross hematuria," which is really red urine. If you assume that hematuria is present, then you might pick transient hematuria or other disorders associated with hematuria, including renal stones, as the diagnosis.

ANSWER REVEALED

You need to remember that 0-2 RBCs per hpf is not hematuria. If you are given a patient who engaged in vigorous exercise, has grossly bloody urine and a U/A with 0-2 RBC per hpf, you are dealing with a patient with myoglobinuria.

Your Workup

When you are presented with a patient with hematuria you should immediately note if the following are also part of the presentation:

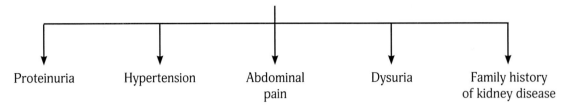

| Proteinuria | Hypertension | Abdominal pain | Dysuria | Family history of kidney disease |

 Microscopic hematuria is seen normally in **2-3% of school-aged children**. At 6 months follow-up, only 1% remain positive. In the absence of any of the above, the correct answer will simply be to repeat the urinalysis in a few weeks.

Persistent microscopic hematuria

If the UA is still positive on repeat, then the next step is to **check a urine Ca/Cr ratio** looking for **hypercalciuria**, which is a common cause of microscopic hematuria.

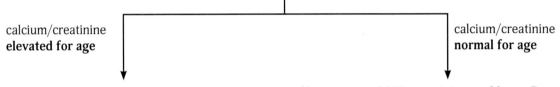

calcium/creatinine **elevated for age**

calcium/creatinine **normal for age**

Check the **24 hour total calcium excretion**. A value **> 4mg/kg/day** would confirm hypercalciuria and would need further evaluation.

Obtain serum BUN, creatinine, and lytes. Based on other findings in the history, it may be necessary to order C3, C4, ANA, double-stranded DNA, CBC, sed rate, urine protein-to-creatinine ratio, ASO titers, ANCA, as well as a renal/bladder ultrasound to check for UPJ obstruction.

Keep in mind that **sickle cell disease** as a cause of hematuria.

Cystoscopy would **never** be indicated in a pediatric patient, since bladder carcinoma will be unlikely and not worth the trauma of a cystoscopy.

> ### Red Diaper !
> In newborns, a **red or pink discoloration in the diaper** is likely to be due to urate crystals, not hematuria, and no treatment is needed once a UA is normal.

Myoglobinuria

These children will present with muscle pain and weakness along with dark urine from muscle breakdown (rhabdomyolysis).

Triggers include viral infections, trauma, excessive exertion, drug overdose, seizures or metabolic/ electrolyte disorders, especially hypokalemia.

Gross Hematuria

The finding of RBCs in a urine sample **that is discolored**.

Remember possible causes as:

H   Henoch Schönlein Purpura and Hereditary nephritis

E   Easy benign familial hematuria

M   Membranoproliferative glomerulonephritis

A   Alport syndrome and IgA nephropathy

T   Trauma

U   Ureteropelvic junction obstruction

R   Renal stones and crystals

I   Infectious (i.e. post strep)

A   Abnormal blood cells
     (i.e. sickle cell) and other
     bleeding disorders

Kidney Stones

In addition to hematuria, children with kidney stones will often be described with **abdominal/flank pain, urinary frequency, dysuria**, and possibly **fever**.

The most common stones in children are **calcium stones**. Children with **distal RTA** are at particular risk, as are children with **hypercalciuria** from any cause, including **hyperparathyroidism, hypercalcemia**, and those on **loop diuretics**.

The initial diagnostic study would be **plain x-ray** and/or **ultrasound**.

Finding Stones

Non contrast CT is the most sensitive modality to confirm kidney stones. **Ultrasound** might be the first test ordered. Read the phrasing of the question carefull.

X-ray is the least sensitive

Who Gets Stones?

Watch for a history of multiple and recurrent UTIs, family history, and metabolic conditions that predispose to kidney stones ie, cystinuria, hyperoxaluria.

Orange urine

Don't forget that **rifampin**, turns urine, as well as tears and sweat, orange. Don't confuse this with the red or tea-colored urine of gross hematuria.

Shades of Red

The color of the urine described can be a clue to the correct diagnosis.

Painless tea or coke colored urine, with RBC casts and deformed RBCs but without clots is typical of glomerular disease.

Bright red urine with clots is usually due to non-glomerular disease. Often this is due to a structural anatomical abnormality, including kidney stones, Wilms tumor, or even cystic kidney disease.

REDRUM

Red urine that is dipstick positive but **RBC negative on micros-copy** is due to **pigmenturia** (hemoglo-binuria and myoglobinuria).

After spinning, the the urine in pigmenturias has a **clear sediment** and a **red supernatant**.

Patients with glomerular disease or lower UTI bleeding would have **red sediment** due to RBCs in the urine and **clear supernatant** after spinning.

Rolling with the Stones

Unlike adults, children with kidney stones should undergo a full metabolic workup.

All will also need an ultrasound to look for stone burden as well as renal and urologic abnormalities.

Additional hints in the history would be parents who are " into " megadoses of vitamins such as C and D. Certain diuretics increase the risk of renal stones and acyclovir would be another one.

The X-ray will catch calcium, struvite, and cystine stones but miss radioluscent uric acid stones, small stones, and stones overlying bone.

CT is more sensitive but has the radiation risk. MRI misses even more than CT!

Stones smaller than 5mm usually pass on their own. Larger stones may require percutaneous nephrolithotomy.

Long-term treatment for children with kidney stones involves **increasing fluid intake** and **restricting salt intake**. Children who do not respond to these modalities, may require a **thiazide diuretic**.

Proteinuria

Proteinuria, in the **absence of hematuria** or other clinical findings, is most likely benign. Proteinuria may be a benign finding in **alkali urine** as well as in **concentrated urine**.

Orthostatic Proteinuria

Orthostatic proteinuria is a benign normal variant in which proteinuria is **present during the daytime**, but disappears when the patient has been lying down, which typically occurs when they are asleep.

> **Transient Proteinuria**
>
> **Fever, exercise,** and **dehydration** can all cause temporary proteinuria. So if they give you a patient who is doing gymnastics and is febrile, keep these causes in mind.

This is best confirmed by a **first void spot urine** right after waking up.

- If the proteinuria disappears with the night's sleep, then a **serum creatinine** is checked. If the serum creatinine is normal, then a **3 month follow up is fine.**
- If the proteinuria does not disappear on a first morning specimen, then the urine should be checked with a **protein/creatinine ratio, which, if greater than 0.2,** suggests **renal disease.**

If they mention **edema, a history of a UTI,** and/or possible **exposure to toxins**, then you are probably looking at something other than benign transient proteinuria.

A 24-hour urine collection is generally not used in children. Serial spot checks for proteinuria are the standard.

Hereditary Nephropathy

Alport Syndrome (Familial Nephritis)

Alport is inherited primarily as an **x-linked dominant** disorder (so this means it is seen mostly in boys). Hematuria is the earliest manifestation and is universal,usually seen by age 6. Other findings include **bilateral sensorineural hearing loss, ocular defects** and ultimately **renal failure**.

Renal ultrasound is initially normal.

Progression to renal failure is associated with the development of proteinuria, elevation of serum creatinine, hypertension, and anemia.

Think of someone skiing on the Alps who can't see because he is blinded by the snow and can't hear because of the strong winds. The same person has to urinate but can't because there are no bathrooms around.

Renal Masses

The most commonly palpated masses in infants are **hydronephrotic kidneys** (most commonly due to UPJ obstruction) and **multicystic dysplastic kidneys (MCDK)**.

Ureteropelvic Junction Obstruction (UPJ)

One scenario could be a child presenting with **microscopic hematuria after an MVA or sports injury**. Another scenario could be a newborn with **hydronephrosis on prenatal U/S** or a **palpable flank mass**.

Multicystic Dysplastic Kidney Disease (MCDK or MCDKD)

MCDK is an **enlarged kidney** with **non-communicating cysts** along with **thin or no parenchyma** and, of course, **dysplasia**. The **kidney does not function** and there is **no treatment**.

A "**unilateral flank mass**" is a clue to renal dysplasia. The diagnosis (especially if bilateral) can be suspected prenatally with the presence of **oligohydramnios** and **minimal fluid in the bladder**.

It is usually **unilateral**, with other **urinary tract anomalies** occurring around **50%** of the time, including:

- UPJ obstruction
- Vesicoureteral reflux
- Posterior urethral valves
- Megaureter and duplication

A **renal ultrasound** is necessary to confirm the diagnosis, followed by a **VCUG** to rule out these comorbid anomalies. If they ask you which is the best study to order, read the question carefully to see if the diagnosis was confirmed with renal ultrasound already.

Autosomal Recessive Polycystic Kidney Disease (ARPKD)

The typical presentation in infancy is **bilateral flank masses,** along with a history of **oligohydramnios.**

Older children with ARPKD will be described as having **bilateral kidney masses** and signs of **chronic portal hypertension,** due to congenital hepatic fibrosis. Signs of portal hypertension include **hematemesis, palpable liver, thrombocytopenia** and/or **splenomegaly.**

Autosomal Dominant Polycystic Kidney Disease (ADPKD)

Even though this is primarily an adult disease, it could make its way onto the pediatric boards.

It is important to know the following:

- The workup for autsomal dominant polycystic kidney disease should include a **renal ultrasound**
- Adult polycystic kidney disease is associated with **intracranial aneurysms**
- They will almost always include the **history of adults in the family** who died of renal disease and/or cerebral aneurysms

Wilms Tumor (Nephroblastoma)

Wilms tumor is **the most common pediatric kidney tumor**. The median age for diagnosis is 3 years.

The most common presentation is an **asymptomatic abdominal mass.**[1] Sometimes it causes **hypertension** and/or **gross hematuria. Aniridia** and **hemihypertrophy** are other important findings. Diagnosis is made by histology.

Think of Wilma from the Flintstones, who had no iris.[2]

---

[1] 10% are bilateral.
[2] If you do not know who this is, check it out on YouTube®, but don't get carried away unless you have met your study quota for the day.

Wilms tumor is easy to recognize on X-ray. Wilms tumor **does not calcify**. Remember this since Wilma Flintstone lived in the Stone Age, not the Calcium Age. **If you do see calcification on an abdominal mass X-ray, think neuroblastoma.**

Following possible nephrectomy, the patient receives **chemotherapy and radiation** according to the stage of their disease. Today, close to 90% of children with Wilms tumor stage 1 and 2 may be cured, although 15-50% develop recurrent disease (often in the lungs).

Nephrotic Syndrome (NS)

Nephrotic syndrome is not in itself a disease as much as it is a presentation of many conditions. This presentation consists of the triad of

1. **Hypoproteinemia**
2. **Proteinuria**
3. **Edema**

Most cases in children are **primary**, although NS may be **secondary** to conditions such as infections, drugs, malignancies, lupus, and diabetes. Several glomerulopathies may also be associated with nephrotic syndrome.

Most cases of nephrotic syndrome in children are **idiopathic, with minimal change disease found in histologic analysis.** It occurs primarily between the ages of **2-8** and **primarily in males (2:1).** Important findings include **decreased urine output, abdominal pain, diarrhea,** and **weight gain.**

Renal function is normal.

Chaos everywhere

The triad of **hypoproteinemia, proteinuria** and **edema** are related, and it flows logically:
spilling of protein in the urine ➜ low serum protein ➜ low oncotic pressure ➜ resulting in edema.

The low oncotic pressure does not make the **liver** too happy, and it begins to act out in a variety of ways:

VLDL[3] production increases ➜ resulting in a high LDL/HDL Ratio.

Fibrinogen, Factor V and VII increases ➜ and combines with decreased volume ➜ and increased platelet count ➜ resulting in **hypercoagulability.**

Even though it started all the trouble, the **kidney** won't be undersold by its rival, the liver, and it too begins to act out.

Since protein is spilling out of the kidneys, **important proteins are lost,** including:

❏ **Immunoglobulins** ➜ Complement levels decrease as well ➜ **Immunodeficiency**
❏ **Albumin** ➜ low albumin decreases bound and available calcium, resulting in ➜ **Hypocalcemia**
❏ **Thyroxine Binding Globulin** ➜ resulting in functional hypothyroidism

---

[3] Very low density lipids.

Complications

3 Important complications of nephrotic syndrome are:

- **Hyponatremia**
- **Vascular thrombosis**
- **Peritonitis** (pneumococcal) and other forms of pneumococcal disease due to their hypogammaglobulinemic state

Vascular thrombosis should be suspected in a child with a diagnosis of minimal change disease who then develops **hematuria**.

> **Pneumococcal infections**
>
> Children with nephrotic syndrome are at risk for invasive pneumococcal infections, not only peritonitis, but others as well, because of their hypogammaglobulenemic state.

TREATMENT

Hospitalization is only necessary in cases of **incapacitating edema or infection.** Initial treatment includes **sodium restriction and prednisone.**

PERIL

In the absence of severe edema, fluid restriction is unnecessary.

A **worse prognosis** and a **renal biopsy** are indicated if there are **two or more** of the following:

- Age over 10 years
- Persistent or gross hematuria
- Hypertension
- Renal insufficiency
- Low C3 complement levels

If proteinuria persists after 4 weeks of daily prednisone, then a **renal biopsy** is indicated. 1-2 relapses per year are not uncommon and this usually ceases during adolescence.

Prognosis in nephrotic syndrome is often based on response to treatment. **Most important is the response to steroid treatment.**

Specific Nephropathies/Nephrides

When I was in medical school (back when dinosaurs and Ronald Reagan still roamed the earth), I recall not so fondly poring over renal histopathology slides. Each one looked strangely familiar to the woody grain seen in cheap paneling, and I tried to distinguish them — only to discover they are all treated with steroids.

Here are a few salient points that will get you through this section of the Boards.

Glomerular disease is suggested by the presence of **RBC** casts.

HOT TIP

ASO and C_3 levels, blood pressure, lytes, BUN/Creatinine, and serum albumin are important values to note in the question.

BUZZWORDS

The following words, values, or smoke signals in the question will tip you off as to the cause of hematuria: **positive family history, recent trauma, abdominal pain or mass, recent strep infection,** or **sickle cell disease.**

We all remember what the glomerulus looks like all coiled up. Now picture a bad glomerulus where the coil is made up of "**rope,**" which would not work well. The word ROPE will help you remember the **symptoms of nephritic syndrome.**

R ed urine (hematuria)
O liguria
P roteinuria
E levated BP and BUN (azotemia)

Hematuria with proteinuria indicates glomerulonephritis. So isolated hematuria can be benign, and isolated proteinuria can be benign, but both together says "You better get looking for more."

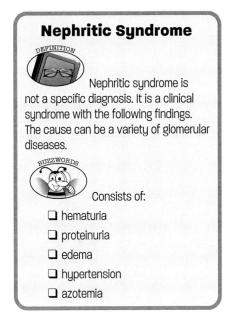

Nephritic Syndrome

Nephritic syndrome is not a specific diagnosis. It is a clinical syndrome with the following findings. The cause can be a variety of glomerular diseases.

Consists of:

❑ hematuria
❑ proteinuria
❑ edema
❑ hypertension
❑ azotemia

Kidney Punch: The Causes of Glomerulonephritis (GN)

These can be divided into 2 camps:

1) Those with low complement levels

2) Those with normal complement levels

FSGS, MPGN, MSNBC, PSGN, IgA, CNN, ESPN

Once again, the different glomerulonephropathies are difficult enough to spell, let alone keep straight. The good news is there is a limit to what you need to know about each. Knowing the basics will allow you to score easy points on the exam.

Normal Complement

IgA Nephropathy

IgA Nephropathy, who also goes by the alias **Berger's Disease**, is associated with elevated serum IgA with IgA deposits noted on renal biopsy, the same as **Henoch Schönlein purpura**.

IgA nephropathy will rarely occur in any child younger than 10. The typical presentation is **recurrent gross painless hematuria with, or days after, upper respiratory infections.** While the hematuria is usually painless, **mild abdominal pain can be part of the history.**

The hematuria may recur with subsequent minor illnesses.

CASE STUDY You are presented with a patient who you figure out has IgA nephropathy. However, the diagnosis is not what they are after. Instead, they present you with a variety of clinical findings, all consistent with the disease. You are asked to determine which one correlates with worsening disease.

THE DIVERSION Since you already figured out that this is IgA nephropathy, your eyes will zero in on the choice that includes IgA levels. They know this, so this decoy choice will be sitting there for you, drawing you away from "A" passing grade.

ANSWER REVEALED The correct answer would be **persistent proteinuria** which correlates with worsening or progressive disease.

HOT TIP C3/C4 are normal in IGA nephritis.

Focal Segmental Glomerulosclerosis (FSGS)

FSGS is typically seen in teenagers. It may present as nephrotic syndrome. Remember, FSGS usually **leads to progressive renal failure**. You would expect to see low serum albumin and edema. In addition, look for normal C3 levels.

Low Complement

Membranoproliferative Glomerulonephritis (MPGN)

MPGN results in **low C_3** (you knew this because it is part of "PMS").

TREATMENT Aggressive treatment is necessary to prevent renal failure.

Post Strep Glomerulonephritis (PSGN)

DEFINITION Post Strep Glomerulonephritis (PSGN) is a nonsuppurative sequelae of an infection with a nephritogenic strain of group A beta hemolytic strep. Both **throat and skin infections** can lead to PSGN. It is due to the **deposition of immune complexes** in the kidney.

BUZZWORDS They always describe the triad of **hypertension, edema,** and **hematuria**. They may not mention a recent strep infection, just a subtle hint that the patient was "recently ill."

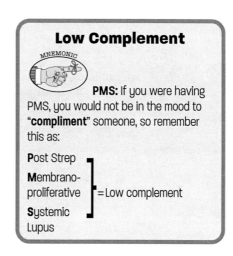

Low Complement

MNEMONIC **PMS:** If you were having PMS, you would not be in the mood to "**compliment**" someone, so remember this as:

Post Strep

Membrano-proliferative

Systemic Lupus
= Low complement

The edema will typically be described in the **eyelids and/or the face**, often noticed by the family rather than the physician.[4]

The hematuria will typically be described as **tea- or cola-colored**, rusty, or smoky.[5]

PSGN does not typically lead to renal failure.

In case they get technical, the **low serum albumin levels** are due to hemodilution rather than proteinuria.

C_3 levels are lowered for up to two months, but then go back to normal.[6] **Therefore, documentation of the C_3 returning to normal differentiates it from the two disorders that result in more sustained low C_3 levels,** lupus and membranoproliferative GN. (Remember, they are part of "PMS" - low complement).

Treatment of PSGN is largely supportive, including **fluid restriction** and **BP control**. The long-term outcome of PSGN is excellent. Hypertension and edema (secondary to fluid/sodium retention) is best treated with a diuretic like furosemide.

The gross hematuria in PSGN is not recurrent. If you see **recurrent gross hematuria, think IgA nephropathy.**

> ### The Throat and the Urine
>
> If you see a glomerulonephritis WITH a pharyngitis, think IgA nephropathy.
>
> If it appears AFTER a pharyngitis, think PSGN.

> ### Timing of PSGN
>
> PSGN usually occurs 1-2 weeks after Strep throat and 6 weeks after impetigo.

Hemolytic Uremic Syndrome (HUS)

Questions on HUS will usually include the **classic triad**, making it one of the easier questions to answer. The triad is implied in the name:

- **Hemolytic anemia**
- **Uremia (elevated BUN)**
- **Thrombocytopenia**

Think of **H.U.T.S** instead: Hemolytic Uremic Thrombocytopenic Syndrome.

Anemia and **pallor** are the typical initial signs, followed by **abdominal pain** and **decreased urine output**. **Purpura** and **ecchymoses** will also be typically described. CNS signs (seizures, lethargy, and even coma) and hypertension may also be part of the clinical scenario of HUS.

---

[4] Which is pretty scary.
[5] Not unlike the way single malt scotch is described.
[6] C4 levels remain normal.

Because it is often contracted from contaminated food or water (*E. coli*), exposure to **poorly cooked meat, unpasteurized apple cider,** or **cow and goat milk** may be included in the question.

Sometimes these kids can be mistaken for new leukemias. They will be anemic with low platelets. The white count is variable. An elevated BUN/Creatinine can also be seen in new onset leukemia, so look to your history for more clues. Your main clue to HUS will be the presence of **diarrhea** and **hematuria**.

Treatment for H.U.S. is **supportive**.

Antimicrobials are not indicated and may even worsen the course.

Serum complement levels are normal in HUS, and the Coombs test will be negative.

Acute Renal Failure (ARF)

ARF is defined as a **rapid worsening of renal function** along with an **increase in BUN and creatinine** and often **hyperkalemia, metabolic acidosis,** and **hypertension**.

Acute renal failure is divided into 3 forms: **pre-renal** (the most common), **intrinsic renal**, and **post-renal**. You must get a UA and check urine indices to differentiate between them.

In patients with **prerenal causes** of ARF

- the urine specific gravity with be >1.020
- the urine/plasma osm >1.5
- the BUN/Cr ratio will be >20
- the urine sodium will be <10

In those with intrinsic **renal causes** of ARF

- the FeNa will be high (>2%)
- the urine spec grav <1.010
- the urine/plasma osm <1.5
- the urine sodium will be >40

If you are presented with a patient in acute renal failure taking medications that require renal clearance, the **dosages have to be adjusted** accordingly.

If the creatinine level is 2x normal, the GFR is cut in half. The right answer will probably be to **increase the dosing interval of the drug,** but the loading dose remains the same.

Causes of Acute Renal Failure

Pre-renal:
- ❏ blood or fluid losses
- ❏ cardiac disease

Intrinsic renal:
- ❏ acute tubular necrosis
- ❏ interstitial nephritis
- ❏ hemolytic uremic syndrome
- ❏ glomerulonephritis
- ❏ nephrotoxic drugs

Post-renal:
- ❏ urologic obstruction

Hyperkalemia

Regardless of the cause, **hyperkalemia** is also a problem with acute renal failure.

Calculating FeNa

$$FeNa = \frac{U\ Na/\ Serum\ Na}{U\ Cr/\ Plasma\ Cr}$$

Just Say No

NSAIDs and aspirin are contraindicated in patients with renal disease.

Treatment of ARF requires correction of the underlying insult (hypovolemia, medications), management of hypertension, acidosis and electrolyte abnormalities, vitamin D supplementation, proper nutrition with careful management of fluid intake, and if necessary, dialysis.

Patients with prerenal causes of acute renal failure typically need **isotonic fluid replacement** to maintain intravascular volume.

> ## Azotemia
> Azotemia is another term for Renal Failure, as in Renal Azotemia or PreRenal Azotemia.

Drugs and the Kidney

Watch for a history that suggests include decreased intravascular volume, underlying renal insufficiency, and use of multiple nephrotoxic medications

The key to reducing the risk of nephrotoxicity is adjusting doses to renal function

Recognize the importance of hydration prior to giving these medications (for example, give fluids before IV acyclovir because crystals may precipitate in the renal tubules and lead to nephrotoxicity and acute renal insufficiency).

Drug induces interstitial nephritis is commonly causes by NSAIDs, and most patients improve once the drug is stopped. Therefore, don't miss an easy point in the exam when asked what the first step in treatment should be. Additional treatment, would include fluid and electrolyte management.

Chronic Kidney Disease

They might tell you a child has chronic kidney disease, or they might work backwards by letting you know that a child has some of the common features of kidney disease listed below.

The most common causes of chronic kidney disease in children are **urologic abnormalities** and **glomerulopathies**.

Failure to Thrive and Growth Failure

If they present you with a child with failure to thrive or with growth failure, chronic kidney disease should be in the differential. The cause of this is thought to consist of many factors, including acidosis, nutrition status, and problems with bone mineralization.

Anemia

This is due to **decreased erythropoietin production** by the kidney.

> ## What drugs hurt the kidney?
> Nephrotoxic drugs include **aminoglycosides, cyclosporine, tacrolimus,** and the chemotherapeutic drugs **cisplatin, carboplatin,** and **ifosfamide**.

Treatment with exogenous erythropoietin is indicated when the **Hgb level drops below 8**. The anemia will be **normocytic.**

However, the downside to erythropoietin therapy is that **polycythemia** may occur, and it is associated with **hypertension** and **thrombosis**.

Metabolic Acidosis

Metabolic acidosis is a result of bicarbonate loss, decreased production of bicarbonate by the renal tubules, and decreased acid excretion. This is a contributing factor to growth failure in chronic kidney disease.

Uremia

Elevated BUN is an important component of renal failure and obstructive uropathy.

 Restricted protein intake is a key component of management.

Hypertension

Hypertension in renal failure is due to **salt and water retention**, and sometimes increased renin levels.

Neurological abnormalities

Changes in mental status, seizures, and peripheral neuropathies can all be manifestations of kidney disease.

Secondary Hyperparathyroidism

In chronic kidney disease, 1,25-dihydroxyvitamin D3 production decreases. As you no doubt recall, this is the active metabolite of Vitamin D and it's made in the kidneys. This results in decreased calcium absorption (causing hypocalcemia), resulting in **elevated PTH**.

Increased serum phosphorus

The faulty kidneys cannot excrete phosphorus, so it accumulates in the serum. This further suppresses calcitriol production, resulting in additional calcium losses, increased PTH levels and a snowball effect.

Dermatological abnormalities

Dry skin, pruritus, and easy bruisability can all be a part of kidney disease.

Immunizations in Chronic Kidney Disease

Maintaining the recommended immunization schedule in children with chronic kidney disease is important.

Creating Creatinine

HOT TIP — Serum creatinine levels correlate with muscle mass. Therefore, serum creatinine levels are higher with increasing pediatric age, since older patients generally have more muscle mass due to growth. After adolescence, males usually have higher creatinine levels than females.

TAKE HOME MESSAGE — On the other hand, creatinine is typically elevated in the newborn period, which is a reflection of maternal creatinine levels. It has also been shown that premature babies tend to have higher creatinine levels than full term babies.

Preterm neonates —> lower GFR compared to term neonates.

GFR reaches adult values by age 2.

It takes 1-2 weeks for the creatinine to decrease to the neonatal level from the adult/maternal level.

If they are not up to date on immunizations, children may not qualify for a kidney transplant. **Live vaccines should be given prior to transplant**, since these vaccines would be contraindicated once patients are on immunosuppressive therapy.

Children undergoing dialysis must have their hepatitis B titers checked regularly, since these antibodies may be removed by dialysis.

Kidney Transplantation

Kids with renal transplants for chronic renal failure have increased linear growth and better qualities of life after the transplant.

There are many factors that determine long term kidney graft survival, including cardiovascular risk factors, medication compliance, and acute rejection episodes.

Kids with kidney transplants (and other solid organ transplants) are at increased risk for contracting invasive pneumococcal disease.

Prognosis after transplantation is good but complications include **rejection** and **infection**. The drugs needed to prevent rejection lead to a decrease in ability to fight infection.

Besides the burden of compliance with taking daily medications, post-transplant children also are at risk for **poor growth** and may qualify for growth hormone.

Hypertension (HTN)

Hypertension is defined as BP **greater than the 95th percentile for age and sex, taken on 3 separate occasions**. Routine BP screening should start by age 3 at all healthcare visits, and earlier if at risk for HTN.

CASE STUDY

You are presented with a child who is noted to have high blood pressure. You won't have to know the definition of what that is, since they will clearly state that everything is normal except for the blood pressure. What is the next best step in the initial management?

THE DIVERSION

Well, Well, Well — there could be all kinds of seemingly innocent non invasive choices, such as the "urinalysis" and "culture." Seemingly innocent, but if you pick these choices, you have overanalyzed yourself into picking the wrong answer.

ANSWER REVEALED

The correct answer could be to repeat the blood pressure two more times on two separate occasions. Remember to read the question and to remember the definition of hypertension. One elevated reading is not enough for any workup beyond confirming that the diagnosis is real.

PERIL

Look for a hint in the question that the **wrong cuff size** has been used. This is often the answer they are looking for.

HOT TIP

With hypertension in childhood, **the heart and the kidneys** are always the main suspects. So **check 4 extremity pulses and BPs and UA as well as BUN/ creatinine**. Another relatively common cause is **hyperthyroidism**.

Children who are obese are more than three times more likely to develop hypertension than children who are not. The younger the child, the harder you have to look for a cause of the hypertension and not assume it's primary (essential).

> ### Cuff' Em
> The proper BP cuff size is a must to get an accurate BP reading.
> - The width of the cuff bladder should be 40% of the arm circumference midway between the olecranon and the acromion.
> - When in place, the cuff will cover 80-100% of the arm circumference and 2/3 of the length.

Pressure Elevators

In addition to pure renal etiologies, there are other causes, and often the clues in the question are obvious.

HOT TIP

To remember the causes of hypertension in children, link it to the phrase **"Pound Hard,"** since high blood pressure "pounds hard."

Polycystic Kidney Disease
O (Zero) Enzyme (11 hydroxylase deficiency)
Urinary Reflux Nephropathy
Neonatal Problem (Renal Artery Stenosis) Neurofibromatosis
Deficiency (17 Hydroxylase Deficiency)

Heart = Coarctation of the Aorta
Adrenal = Pheochromocytoma
Rheumaologic disorders (Lupus)
Due to Endocrine issues, like Cushings and hyperthyroidism

> ### Drugs and Hypertension
> Medications that may cause HTN include albuterol, contraceptives, corticosteroids, and decongestants.
>
> *HOT TIP*
> If they describe a child with HTN and hint that he/she is using illicit drugs, this can also be the cause.

Historical Clues/Hypertension

Here, more than anywhere, the clues will be in the wording of the question.

BUZZWORDS

If the question includes the following terms and buzzwords on the left side, then think of the etiology on the right side.

"Family history of hypertension"	**Renal or endocrine problems that run in families**
"Prematurity"	**Renal artery stenosis secondary to umbilical catheterization**
"Joint pain, swelling"	**Connective tissue disorder like lupus**
"Flushing," "palpitations," "fever," "weight loss"	**Either a teenager in love or pheochromocytoma**
"Muscle cramps, weakness"	**Hypokalemia secondary to hyperaldosteronism**
"Onset with sexual development"	**One of the enzyme deficiencies**

HOT TIP

Children placed in prolonged traction after orthopedic procedures are at increased risk for acute hypertension.

Physical Evidence/Hypertension

BUZZWORDS

In addition to the history, the physical findings may also include clues pointing to the cause of the hypertension. If the physical findings include the descriptions on the left, then think of the diagnosis on the right:

"Pale color, edema"	Kidney disease (pallor is due to poor erythropoietin production)
"Pale color, increased sweating even at rest, flushing, abdominal mass"	Pheochromocytoma
"Wide spaced nipples, webbing of the neck"	Turner syndrome (coarctation of the aorta)
"Elfin facies, high serum calcium, friendly personality"	Williams syndrome; supravalvular aortic stenosis
"Decreased femoral pulse or low BP in legs vs. arms"	Coarctation of the aorta
"Short obese"	Cushing syndrome

TREATMENT

The most important non-pharmacological intervention is **weight reduction** if obesity is a problem.

Pharmacological treatment of hypertension may include the following:

- **Calcium Channel Blockers**: nifedipine or amlodipine
- **Vasodilators**: hydralazine or minoxidil
- **ACE inhibitors**: enalapril or lisinopril
- **Angiotensin Receptor Blockers**: losartan
- **Beta Blockers**: propranolol or atenolol
- **Alpha 2 Agonists**: clonidine
- **Diuretics**: thiazides, furosemide, or spironolactone

Pheochromocytoma

Pheochromocytoma is associated with von Hippel-Lindau Syndrome, MEN (multiple endocrine neoplasia) type 2, and NF (neurofibromatosis) type 1.

Symptoms due to excessive catecholamines, such as: tachycardia, sweating, and headaches.

Before surgical resection, patients with pheochromocytoma must have their blood pressure under control via **alpha adrenergic blockade,** an example of which is **phenoxybenzamine.**

Even though tachycardia can be a problem, **initial treatment via beta blockers alone is contraindicated since it would lead to unopposed alpha effect and paradoxical increase in blood pressure.**

Renal Causes of Hypertension

When a renal cause of hypertension is suspected, the next step is a **renal arteriography with differential central venous renin determination.**

For example, when renal stenosis is the suspected cause, **renin** levels will be higher in the renal vein of the involved kidney.

Renal scars can also cause hypertension.

Chapter 27

Urinary Plumbing Issues

Collecting System Pathology

Ureteroceles

Ureterocele presents with symptoms that mimic **UTIs,** such as **dysuria, hematuria,** and/or **abdominal pain.**

Ureteroceles are a common cause of **urinary retention in females**, and can present as a mass protruding from the urethral meatus or a **round filling defect on IVP**. It can lead to **urinary tract obstruction**.

Vesicoureteral Reflux

The **earlier** a UTI presents in life, **the more likely** that reflux is a contributing factor. The diagnosis is confirmed with **VCUG**.

Management depends on the grade of reflux and with the knowledge that reflux significantly improves over time. **The goal of management is to avoid hypertension and renal insufficiency and/or ultimate failure**.

Prophylactic antibiotics are no longer routinely recommended. They may be indicated for certain children with high grade VUR, but this is usually decided in conjunction with your favorite urologist.

For purposes off the exam, you expected to pick answers consistent with knowing that immediate urine evaluation is indicated for future febrile illnesses to make sure all UTIs are caught and treated without delay.

Urethral Strictures

Urethral strictures usually result from urethral trauma. Of course, this can be iatrogenic (as in the placement of catheters). Therefore, watch for a history of a recent surgical procedure that may be unrelated to the urinary tract.

Other causes of urethral strictures are infections, including GC.

Insertion of a catheter is contraindicated in a patient who is experiencing gross urethral bleeding following trauma.

Posterior Urethral Valves (PUV)

Typical presentation in a newborn male with a **palpable bladder** and delayed urination or a **weak urinary stream. Ultrasound** would show **bilateral hydronephrosis, hydroureteronephrosis, distended bladder, and reduced renal parenchyma.**

The most appropriate next step will be to pass a urine catheter and schedule a VCUG.

Immediate urological consult for surgical correction is indicated.

- **Renal failure** can occur even **after surgical correction of posterior valves.** Therefore, long-term followup of bladder function is important.
- Posterior urethral valves occurs exclusively in males.

Prune Belly (Eagle Barrett) Syndrome

Not many disorders present with a baby with an abdomen looking like a prune. These children are prone to chronic UTIs, dilated ureters, and large bladders.

Posterior urethral valves are the cause of the problems.

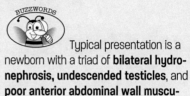

Typical presentation is a newborn with a triad of **bilateral hydronephrosis, undescended testicles**, and **poor anterior abdominal wall musculature.**

VCUG Now !

Know that the presentation of males with **bilateral hydronephrosis** warrants immediate VCUG to rule out PUV.

Dysuria

Age of Dysuria

Pay close attention to the age of the patient presenting with dysuria:

Age	Possible causes of Dysuria (not comprehensive)
Pre-adolescent female	Pinworms Poor hygiene Trauma Vaginitis Urinary tract infection
Adolescent female who is not sexually active	Urinary tract infection
Adolescent female who is sexually active	Urinary tract infection Chlamydia or gonococcal infection
Adolescent male	Chlamydia or gonococcal infection

CASE STUDY You are given the scenario of a teenage girl treated empirically for a urinary tract infection who is still experiencing dysuria. What is the most appropriate next step?

THE DIVERSION Among the tempting diversions would be a change of antibiotics or addition of other medications.

ANSWER REVEALED In this setting, additional treatment would not be correct. Additional history, physical exam, or lab tests would be appropriate. If you were provided with any of these choices, including pelvic exam, these would be correct.

Urinary Frequency and Incontinence

You may be tested on causes of urinary incontinence other than UTI. This could include:

Ectopic urethral opening in females

BUZZWORDS This would be presented as a girl who, despite a thorough negative work up, is always wetting her pants.

Urinary Tract Infections (UTI)

DEFINITION A UTI would be diagnosed by a culture result of **greater than 50,000** colonies of a single organism grown from a reliable sample, ie. a catheterized or a suprapubic tap specimen.

Etiology

Remember, a UTI is not always due to a bacterial infection. It can be caused by **adenovirus**. However, most UTIs *are* caused by bacteria.

E. coli is the most common organism associated with UTI. Other less common organisms are *klebsiella* and **enterococcus**. Remember that urinary tract infections may be seen more commonly in children with constipation.

MNEMONIC Picture the bladder as a cave. You "**club**" *(klebsiella)* your way in, and **enter** (enterococcus), and then you hear a loud **echo** *(E. coli)* that repeats itself over and over (to remind you *E. coli* is the most common cause).

Who Gets UTIs

The following information can come in handy on the exam:

During the first 3 months of life, boys are at higher risk for UTIs than girls (especially boys who are uncircumcised). After that time, UTIs are more common in girls.

In adolescence, UTIs are more common in sexually active females and homosexual males than in other demographic groups.

Positive leukocyte esterase is only suggestive of a UTI, but not diagnostic. Positive nitrites on a UA is a more specific test for UTI. Even though we often treat empirically, UA alone is not enough to diagnose a UTI; **a positive urine culture is needed to make the diagnosis**.

Asymptomatic bacteruria can be something they present on routine screening and will require no further intervention.

Most children with febrile UTI may be treated with **oral antibiotics** unless they appear toxic, have problems with oral intake, or have compliance concerns. Treatment duration is 7-14 days.

Oral antibiotic choices include **amoxicillin-clavulanate, trimethoprim-sulfamethoxazole,** and certain cephalosporins such as **cephalexin, cefixime, and cefuroxime**.

Parenteral antibiotic choices include **ceftriaxone, cefotaxime, gentamicin, tobramycin,** and **piperacillin**.

This is, of course, until sensitivities come back.

UTI prophylaxis, when indicated, usually involves **amoxicillin** (especially in infants), **trimethoprim-sulfamethoxazole,** and **nitrofurantoin**.

To VCUG or not to VCUG?: That is the question

The guidelines for management of febrile UTIs used to recommend a VCUG after the first febrile UTI to find VUR as soon as possible and start prophylactic antibiotics. However, that has all changed.

The first febrile UTI now only deserves a **renal and bladder U/S** and if that's normal, wait and see if they get another febrile UTI.

A VCUG is now indicated only after a **second febrile UTI**, or of course **if the U/S is abnormal in any way**.

GU Bulges

Inguinal Hernia

Inguinal hernias will be described as a bulge either in the suprapubic or in the scrotal area that increases in size with crying or straining.

Inguinal hernias eventually need to be repaired surgically. **Umbilical hernias** can resolved without surgery. Waiting until age 4 would be an appropriate answer for umbilical hernia.

Incarcerated Inguinal Hernia

In addition to the symptoms of a reducible inguinal hernia, an incarcerated inguinal hernia will present with **irritability**, **a tender abdomen**, and **vomiting**. The mass will appear tense, and attempts to reduce it will be unsuccessful.

Reactive **lymphadenopathy** is a very common cause of inguinal masses in older children and adolescents.

Incarcerated versus Strangulated Hernia:

- **Incarcerated** hernias cannot be reduced back into original location
- **Strangulated** hernias are already ischemic due to constricted blood flow

 If you are presented with a female infant with an inguinal hernia, the next step will be an ultrasound to make sure there isn't an ovary in the herniated tissue.

You will be expected to differentiate an incarcerated hernia from other inguinal masses. A **hydrocele** can mimic an incarcerated hernia, since they both present as scrotal enlargement.

Another diagnostic possibility is **inguinal lymphadenitis**. This too will present as a tender mass; however, it will also present with the skin over the mass being **red** and **warm to touch**, and there likely will be an infection distal to the node noted in the history.

You are called in to the ER to evaluate a 2-year-old girl on peritoneal dialysis for progressive abdominal pain. The child has been afebrile, and her immunizations are up to date. On physical examination, you do not notice anything in the dialysis drainage that is abnormal. In addition to some crusted edges around the catheter site, you note a large mass in the left lower abdomen just lateral to the catheter, but no guarding or rebound tenderness.

What is the most likely cause of the patient's symptoms?

You could be provided with several diversionary choices including bacterial peritonitis, cellulitis, incarcerated omentum, and incarcerated inguinal hernia. Noting that the child is on dialysis is not necessarily a diversionary tactic, although it could be if you automatically assume some of the worse case scenarios implicated in these choices. For example, picking incarcerated omentum will only impede your momentum en route to passing the exam.

Clearly an afebrile child with a benign abdominal exam is unlikely to have any of the diagnoses noted. The only correct answer would be "hernia." This should be the logical choice without even knowing that children on peritoneal dialysis frequently develop abdominal hernias because of increased intraperitoneal pressure.

Hydrocele

A hydrocele will typically be described as an infant with **painless swelling** of the scrotum. It **transilluminates** on exam.

Management is **watch and wait** until age 1 or 2. If unresolved then surgical correction is indicated.

Varicocele

A varicocele typically presents on the **left side**, and will be described as a **heavy sensation** or a "**bag of worms.**" The swelling will **decrease when the patient lies down** and will be **painless**.

The "Boy Parts" and What can go Wrong

Undescended Testicles

The following are some important tips and points to remember:

- The longer the testicle remains uptown, the lower the chances of having a baby downtown.
- Bringing the testicle downtown may improve fertility, but it does not completely eliminate the risk of malignancy. The reason to bring it down is so that it's palpable and increase your chances of finding the cancer early.
- The descended testicle on the other side also has a higher malignancy risk, but not as high as the one stuck uptown.
- It is very important for these boys to start testicular self-exams at puberty.
- Undescended testis are at an increased risk for testicular torsion.

Neither **human chorionic gonadotropin** nor **testosterone** are considered to be effective treatment, and will likely therefore be the incorrect choice.

Ultrasound is not typically performed to evaluate for undescended testis due to low specificity and sensitivity

You should refer infants whose testicles have **not descended by 3-6 months. Orchiopexy by 12-18 months** is the appropriate treatment for an undescended testicle.

Spontaneous descent after 4 months of age is uncommon, and is rare beyond 6 months of age.

Treatment before 2 years of age is associated with improved testicular growth and fertility.

Big Sack

Other **causes of scrotal swelling**:

- Kawasaki Disease
- Henoch-Shonlen Purpura
- Idiopathic scrotal edema

Circ or No Circ?

The stand of the AAP is that the preventive health benefits of circumcision in newborns outweigh the risks of the procedure.

A subcutaneous ring block or dorsal penile block should be used during circumcision.

Topical anesthetics and oral sucrose may also be helpful in pain relief.

Contraindications to circumcision include anatomical penile abnormalities and medical conditions, such as connective tissue disorders.

CASE STUDY

You are performing a routine physical on a 3-year-old boy who is new to your practice. You are having difficulty palpating the right testicle. You review his previous record, and bilateral descended testicles have been documented in the past. What is the most appropriate next step?

THE DIVERSION

You could be presented will several diversionary choices, such as testicular ultrasound, pelvic ultrasound, referral to Urology, and genetic studies.

ANSWER REVEALED

Well, all of these steps will be incorrect. If the previously documented bilateral descended testicles wasn't considered authentic, they would have placed it in quotes. Therefore, they are describing retractile testicles secondary to an overactive cremaster muscle. The correct answer would be related to re-examining the patient, usually in the "tailor position," or "frog-leg" position, which is the cross-legged position (knees out, ankles crossed). We are not sure why this is the tailor position, but this would be the correct answer.

PERIL

Even if you are absolutely sure that you noticed that both testicles were in the scrotum previously, there IS such a thing as **retractile testes that re-ascend and stay there**, so you must always follow these patients up and be sure that both testicles are present in the scrotum or refer to Urology for further evaluation.

A patient with retractile testis shoudl be evaluated annually to see if will descend or not.

Patients with retractile testis do not have the same complications and outcomes as those with undescended tesits in terms of malignancy and fertility.

TAKE HOME MESSAGE

Nonpalpable testes in a newborn require a **urologic evaluation and testicular ultrasound prior to discharge** to home, as it may be a presentation of **ambiguous genitalia/congenital adrenal hyperplasia**.

Hypospadias

DEFINITION

Hypospadias is a congenital condition in males in which the opening of the urethra is on the underside of the penis.

Can be associated with a chordee, which is a fixed ventral curvature of the penis. Hypospadias is also associated with undescended testis and inguinal hernias.

BILATERAL Non Palpable Testes/ Newborn

UPDATED & NEW
BREAKING NEWS
INFORMATION If you are presented with a newborn with "non palpable testes" you must consider Differences in Sexual Development (DSD).[1]

Work-up includes:

- Karyotype testing
- Pelvic Ultrasound
- Labs (DHEA, 17-hydroxyprogesterone, testosterone, cortisol, renin, ACTH, FSH, LH,)

For an older child with undescended testes bilaterally, similar evaluation with lab-work, urology referral, and possibly exploratory surgery for definitive diagnosis (absent vs undescended testes) if the ultrasound findings are equivocal.

---

[1] This is the latest terminology.

With a distal hypospadias, the incidence of renal anomalies is low and no specific intervention is needed.

However, hypospadias can be associated with <u>some</u> syndromes.

Because someone with hypospadias is likely to urinate all over the floor, he would be a **slob**. That is an easy way to remember the syndromes associated with hypospadias:

Silver Russell Syndrome (Russell Silver Syndrome)
Laurence-Moon-Biedl Syndrome
Opitz Syndrome
Beckwith Wiedemann Syndrome

When indicated, surgical correction should be done between 6 months to 1 year. Circumcision should **not** be done in a patient with hypospadias, because the foreskin will likely be needed for surgical revision.

Micropenis

If you are presented with boy with the following triad

1. **Micropenis**
2. **Poor feeding**
3. **Hypotonia**

You are most likely dealing with a boy with **Prader-Willi syndrome**.

In addition to Prader-Willi syndrome, **micropenis** is also associated with **Kallmann syndrome,**[2] **growth hormone deficiency, septo-optic dysplasia,** and **hypoglycemia**.

Hypogonadotropic hypogonadism can also be seen with hypopituitarism, Klinefelter syndrome, Noonan syndrome, and gonadal dysgenesis.

If they present you with an infant whose penis length is at least 2.5 cm whose father projects his own inadequacies by expressing concern over his son's penis length, the answer is to reassure the father (well, at least reassure him that his son's penis length is normal).

With a penis length **less than 2.5 cm (one inch)**, an endocrine and/or genetic workup **would be** indicated.

> ### Beware the Fat Pad
>
> Size may or may not be important, but you have to make sure you are measuring what you should be measuring.
>
> If they hint at a large suprapubic fat pad, accurate measurement requires pushing down the fat pad and gentle stretching of the penis to its full length, measured from pubic symphysis.

---

[2] Hypogonadism (delayed puberty) and anosmia.

Painful Scrotal Conditions

Epididymitis

The typical presentation is **unilateral scrotal pain, dysuria,** and/or **fever**. Pertinent negatives will include no testicular masses or urethral discharge. The cremasteric reflex will be present.

They may describe **Prehn sign** which is the alleviation of pain with scrotal elevation This would be your hint that the diagnosis is epididymitis rather than torsion. However, if the questions asks how to distinguish the two then ultrasound is the correct answer.

If **sexually active** ceftriaxone and doxycycline would be correct. If **not sexually active**, then conservative support measures then cephalexin or trimethorprim/sulfa could be correct choices.

In sexually active males epididymitis is usually due to **Chlamydia** or *Neisseria gonorrhea*.

Epididymitis must be distinguished from other conditions with similar presentations. **Orchitis**, for example, can be similar in presentation, but they will **not describe dysuria**.

Testicular Torsion

Torsed testicles will present with sudden severe scrotal pain.

When the testis is torsed, it already is elevated with no place to go, so **you will not be able to elicit a cremasteric reflex**.

Torsion of the Appendix Testis

Would be described as focal tenderenss of the superior testis with the classic blue dot sign, where the scrotal skin will be described as having a blue hue.

After confirmation with ultrasound or on the exam based on the above description, treatment is primarily supportive.

Epididymitis vs. Testicular Torsion

Epididymitis	Testicular Torsion
❏ The cremaster reflex is maintained.	❏ Any manipulation makes the pain worse.
❏ The testicle will be described as low lying.	❏ The cremaster reflex is not maintained.
❏ White cells will be noted in the urine.	❏ The testicle will be described as being "high" or retracted.
❏ Milder more insidious pain often after activity.	❏ Abrupt onset of severe pain.
	❏ Higher risk in cases of Bell Clapper deformity.[2]

Testicular torsion can be bilateral. Testicular torsion needs to be evaluated urgently. If the diagnosis is unclear, ultrasonography with Doppler flow is indicated. **If the diagnosis is clear from history and exam, imaging is unnecessary and urology should be consulted immediately, if not sooner.**

---

[3] Congenital failure of the normal posterior anchoring of the testis in the scrotum so it is free to swing and rotate within the tunic vaginalis.

Orchitis

Look for a description of pain, edema, erythema, and marked tenderness of testis/scrotum.

Mostly viral in origin and therefore treatment is primarily supportive.

> **CASE STUDY**
>
> **You are presented with a 16 year old patient from Panama, who is febrile and presents with a 2 day history of right testicular pain. The testicle is swollen and diffusely tender, with erythema of the overlying skin. There is no urethral discharge or history of dysuria. He is Tanner Stage 4 and he denies any sexual history. Testicular ultrasound is negative, with normal bilateral blood flow. The most appropriate next step would be to order a:**
>
> **THE DIVERSION**
>
> You might be tricked into picking non-specific lab studies such as an ESR, a CBC, or even a blood culture. Chlamydia cultures might be another you could be tricked into picking, since perhaps his denial of sexual activity is unreliable and he could be asymptomatic.
>
> **ANSWER REVEALED**
>
> We rarely if ever see mumps anymore given widespread immunization in the United States. However, if you remembered to read the question carefully and noted that they mentioned his coming from abroad, you would have made a note to consider 1) *diseases we immunize for here in the US* or 2) *an undiagnosed chronic illness.*
>
> In this case, the patient's symptoms are consistent with orchitis, which occurs in mumps 30% of the time. The appropriate next step would be **mumps serology**.

Phimosis

Phimosis is the inability to retract the foreskin. In order for this to be considered clinically significant, they should present this in a boy **older than age 3**, since this can be a normal finding up to age 3.

Treatment would consist of a **topical steroid cream**, along with periodic gentle retraction and maintenance of good hygiene. If it does not improve, circumcision might be indicated.

Paraphimosis

Paraphimosis is foreskin that, once retracted, cannot be brought back to its normal position, resulting in constriction and severe pain. If it cannot be reduced with routine retraction attempt, it is a **surgical emergency**.

Urethritis

This is usually due to either **gonorrhea** or **Chlamydia**.

> **A 3rd year medical student presents a 15 year old boy who has recently had unprotected sex. He is complaining of dysuria and swelling of the foreskin. His urinalysis is positive for 3+WBC, and the Gram stain is negative. In addition, you also note conjunctivitis on physical exam. Additional physical findings would most likely include which of the following?**
>
> The negative gram stain noted would point away from gonococcal urethritis. However, with conjunctivitis included in the description you might be tricked into thinking it is chlamydia, and that, therefore, pneumonia is probably the correct answer. After all, this occurs in infants exposed to chlamydia and this must be what they are alluding to.
>
> You would need to know that **reactive arthritis**[3] is felt at times to be due to an **autoimmune response** to chlamydia infections, which is very possible given the history of unprotected sexual activity. Since **reactive arthritis** can be remembered as "It hurts where you see (conjunctivitis), where you pee (urethritis), and your knee (arthritis)," the correct answer for additional physical findings would be **arthritis**.

Treatment for GC / Chlarmyidia urtethritis is IM Ceftriaxone and PO Doxycycline for 7 days.

Azithromycin is no longer used, due to increased resistance.

Another common mnemonic is:

> Can't see, Can't pee, Can't climb a tree

Urethral instrumentation following a surgical procedure is a common cause of non-sexually transmitted urethritis. If a bladder infection is suspected, then a urinalysis and culture should be obtained.

---

4 Formerly known as Reiter syndrome. The term "reactive arthritis" is increasingly used as a substitute for this designation due to Dr. Reiter's 3rd Reich connections.

"Pus" on Mr. Penis

CASE STUDY A 4 year old boy who is not circumcised is brought to the office by his mother because she noted tiny white bumps on the tip of his penis. You are then asked to determine the cause of this.

THE DIVERSION Well, you might jump to conclusions that the boy needs medical treatment because of infectious balanitis, candida, or herpes.

ANSWER REVEALED This is nothing more than "inclusion cysts," which require no treatment beyond reassuring the mother.

PERIL They might also present you with a boy whose grandmother or parent noticed "pus" around the head of the penis.

The accumulation of white debris (smegma) under the prepuce in an uncircumcised child up until age 3 is a normal finding and requires no treatment.

Testicular Cancer

BUZZWORDS Any **firm painless solid scrotal mass** is testicular cancer until proven otherwise.

You are expected to be familiar with some important points regarding risk and diagnosis of testicular cancer. This includes:

- Testicular masses should be evaluated using **bilateral ultrasound,** even when the mass is unilateral
- Lab studies include **lactate dehydrogenase, B-HCG,** and **alpha-fetoprotein**
- Most common among white males followed by Hispanic followed by African American males.
- High risk factors include **cryptorchidism, gonadal dysgenesis, previous testicular cancer, family history,** and **Klinefelter syndrome**
- Two peaks of incidence in pediatric population: around age 2 and post-pubertal
- The mass will not transilluminate
- Initial imaging would be ultrasound

Chapter 28

The Neuro Bureau: Neurology

With Neurology, you have to pay close attention to the details in the wording of the question. Many of the disorders are quite similar, with only fine differences that distinguish them. We will call attention to these fine differences, and by committing them to memory, you will be on the road to getting these potentially tricky questions correct each time.

Encephalitis

You will be expected to diagnose and understand the underlying causes for a child presenting with symptoms consistent with encephalitis. The time of year and other epidemiologic information in the history will be critical. The following are important considerations to keep in mind on the exam:

- **Arboviruses** - typically occur in **warm climates** and are carried by **insects**, especially mosquitos. This would include California (La Crosse), St. Louis and West Nile viruses. Diagnosis is via *acute* and *convalescent* antibody titers specific to each subtype.

- **Enteroviruses** - present with **generalized neurological findings** and are transmitted from **human to human**. Watch for non-specific findings preceding confusion and irritability.

- **Herpes encephalitis** - often presents with non-specific findings **without** a history of oral lesions. It is best diagnosed by **DNA PCR**.

- **Mumps encephalitis** – presents with or after development of parotitis. Watch for a child or teenager who is **from another country**, or other hints that the patient **wasn't immunized**. Late winter and early spring are the typical times of presentation.

CASE STUDY

You may be presented with a febrile toddler who is lethargic one hour after a seizure. Additional information might include a CBC that is unremarkable, and results of a lumbar puncture may show a negative gram stain and a moderate amount of WBCs, consistent with viral meningitis. You will be presented with several treatment choices.

THE DIVERSION

This clinical vignette could be consistent with a typical febrile seizure. However, the fact that the child is lethargic one hour later and has WBCs in the CSF suggests otherwise. Therefore, reassurance would be the incorrect choice. Anticonvulsants such as phenobarbital would also be incorrect, since the seizure is not ongoing.

ANSWER REVEALED

The correct answer would be acyclovir to cover for the possibility of HSV encephalitis. If they were to present IV antibiotics as one of the choices, this too could be correct, since you would want to cover for bacterial meningitis as well as HSV encephalitis. The key point is that HSV encephalitis can present with non-specific findings. Don't look for a history of HSV lesions either; that will never be part of the presentation of HSV CNS infections on the boards.

What a Headache

You will need to know how to distinguish different types of headaches and their etiologies — which shouldn't be hard, considering that you will have many headaches yourself while studying for the boards. Keep in mind: the correct answers are often hidden in the specific phrasing of the questions.

DEFINITION **Primary** headaches: occur in the absence of an organic cause. **Secondary** headaches: occur secondary to an underlying condition.

Tension Headaches

Non-specific headaches that usually occur in a band-like distribution across the head. Patients typically describe a sensation of pressure in the affected area. These should be easy to distinguish, because they will be describing what you are experiencing at the moment.

BUZZWORDS Tension headaches may be caused by stress, depression and anxiety. Look for other hints in the history such as malaise, excessive sleeping, and/or declining school performance.

TREATMENT Treatment consists of pain relievers and eliminating stressors (in your case, passing the boards and getting on with your life).

PERIL If they describe a headache without a history of trauma or evidence of increased intracranial pressure, **complicated studies are usually not indicated.**

Migraine Headaches

BUZZWORDS **Throbbing or pulsatile** headaches in the frontal , retro-orbital or temporal regions, often associated with nausea and/or vomiting. They may also describe sensitivity to light (photophobia) or sound (phonophobia), which make the headache worse. Headaches are usually episodic, with no symptoms in between episodes. Watch out for a description of a symptomatic child **who stops all activities** and **wants to lay down**.

HOT TIP "Hard" neurological signs, including **hemiparesis** and/or **temporary visual deficits** may be seen with certain migraines.

PERIL The boards most likely will **not** include hints such as an aura in the description of a migraine headache. That would be too easy.

A vicious cycle

DEFINITION Chronic daily headaches occur at least 15 days a month for more than 3 months.

They usually have no organic cause. However, they may be the result of medication overuse (i.e., pain medications used to relieve the headache). Medications should be limited to 2-3 days a week to prevent these "rebound headaches."Watch for their mentioning medication use in the history you are presented with.

Headache Prevention

The most important recommendations for prevention of recurrent headaches are not pharmacologic.

Lifestyle modifications that should be encouraged include:

- regular exercise and activities
- regular sleep patterns
- regular eating patterns
- good hydration

Treatment usually includes **ibuprofen, acetaminophen, fluids,** and **rest**. Other treatments include **ergotamine and oral or intranasal triptans**.

Once again, ibuprofen and acetaminophen should be limited to no more than 2-3 days a week to reduce the risk of rebound headaches.

Narcotics for migraine pain will always be the wrong answer.

Frequent migraines will require both **abortive** therapy (to immediately stop the headache), and **prophylactic** therapy (to prevent future episodes).

The most commonly used medications for migraine **prevention** are **cyproheptadine** and **topiramate**.

Depression on its own can trigger headaches. However, these headaches will be described as **chronic daily headaches**, without the other commonly associated signs of migraines.

You are presented with a patient who suffered a minor head injury a few months ago. He now presents with daily headaches that are not relieved despite frequent acetaminophen, ibuprofen, or naproxen. The headaches are frontotemporal. What is the most appropriate next step in managing this patient?

If you are not careful, you will go down the path leading to a headache caused by picking the wrong answer. The answers will include "obtain a head CT." By noting that the head trauma was minor, and that the patient "now" presents with headaches, they are implying that the patient was asymptomatic until this point. Therefore, a head CT would not be appropriate.

They might provide additional medications among the choices. However, the vignette is not consistent with a migraine headache, most notably because migraine headaches are not daily headaches; they are episodic.

The key to the diagnosis: the medication is being used chronically and its effect is blunted. Rescue medications such as ibuprofen should not be used chronically. The correct step in this case would be to stop all medications.

Increased Intracranial Pressure (ICP)

Visual disturbances, worsening headaches, abnormal eye movements, deteriorating school performance and/or **ataxia** are clues to increased ICP.

Vision changes occurring **only before** the headache are more typical of visual auras preceding a migraine.

Headaches due to a space-occupying lesion may also cause other **red flags**, including **headaches worse in the morning, vomiting with no nausea,** or **headaches relieved by vomiting.**

A **lumbar puncture (LP) is contraindicated** in any patient showing signs and symptoms of increased ICP.

The diagnostic test of choice is an **urgent CT with contrast**; followed by an MRI later when stable.

Treatment consists of osmotic agents such as mannitol, and 3% hypertonic saline (while waiting for the neurosurgeon to show up).

Pseudotumor Cerebri (aka Idiopathic or Benign Intracranial Hypertension)

This condition causes **increased intracranial pressure with no known organic causes.** It is considered benign - it does not involve an actual "tumor," or cause herniation of the brain. However, it can lead to **papilledema**; and eventual **optic disc atrophy** and **blindness** if left untreated. This is an important consideration and often shows up on the exam.

Take the Pressure?

The clinical signs for increased intracranial pressure in **infants** include: irritability, decreased PO intake, and failure to thrive. Other signs include macrocephaly due to hydrocephalus (rapid head growth with widening sutures and a bulging fontanel).

Look for clues such as the "setting sun" sign: downward deviation of the eyes with hydrocephalus.

The clinical signs for increased intracranial pressure in **children** include: hypertension, papilledema, bradycardia, and abducens nerve (CN VI) palsy.

Cushing's Triad

Cushing's triad includes

1. hypertension
2. bradycardia
3. abnormal respirations.

These are late findings of increased intracranial pressure and usually indicate impending herniation.

Say NO to LP

LP is contraindicated with signs/symptoms of increased ICP.

Additional **contraindications to performing an LP** include focal neurological signs, history of a coagulopathy, and cardiorespiratory instability.

Remember that your ABCs come before an LP.

Say Uncal

Uncal herniation is characterized by unilateral pupil dilatation due to compression of the oculomotor (3rd) cranial nerve. This is classically known as the "down-and-out" pupil.

Pseudotumor cerebri will typically present with headache and tinnitus (evidence for increased ICP), as well as diplopia due to abducens nerve (CN VI) palsy. Papilledema (optic disc swelling) and potential vision loss are usually late findings.

The headache tends to **get worse when laying flat and/or with Valsalva maneuvers**. There should be something in the question to suggest this.

Pseudotumor cerebri is commonly caused by megadoses of **Vitamin A** and its derivatives (such as Retin-A).

Other **medications** known to cause pseudotumor cerebri include:

- Isotretinoin
- Steroids
- Thyroxine
- Lithium
- Some antibiotics (i.e., tetracycline)

Pseudotumor cerebri may be treated with **carbonic anhydrase inhibitors (acetazolamide)** and **diuretics**. Severe cases may require steroids, serial lumbar punctures and possibly surgery with CSF shunting to relieve optic nerve pressure.

Yes - steroids can both cause *and* treat pseudotumor cerebri; just like alcohol can be the cause of, and solution to, all of life's problems, in some cases.

Hydrocephalus

Accumulation of excessive amounts of CSF in the brain. It is usually associated with **increased intracranial pressure** and dilation of the ventricles.

Major risk factorz for developing hydrocephalus is a **neural tube defects** (especially myelomeningocele), Chiari and other brain malformations. It may also be seen with congenital infections, intracranial bleeds, and spaceoccupying lesions blocking CSF flow.

There are two main types of hyrocephalus:

1. **Communicating (or non-obstructive)** - cerebrospinal fluid (CSF) can flow between the ventricles, but it cannot be reabsorbed properly; causing excess buildup of CSF.

2. **Non-communicating (or obstructive)** - blocked flow between ventricles, leading to build up of CSF. This is commonly seen in premies with intraventricular hemorrhage where bleeding leads to ventricular obstruction..

SHUNT problems

Most shunt infections occur in the first 6 months after shunt placement.

Shunt infection should be suspected in any patient with a shunt who presents with symptoms of hydrocephalus and persistent fever. In addition to IV antibiotics, the infected shunt should be removed.

Shunt malfunctions present with symptoms of increased ICP but without fever.

Brain Tumors

Infratentorial Tumors

BUZZWORDS

2/3 of brain tumors in children are infratentorial and located in the **posterior fossa**. Look for the the triad of **headache, vomiting**, and **ataxia** in an **afebrile** child. Also look for mention of **head tilt** and **torticollis** along with evidence of cranial nerve dysfunction, such as decreased upward gaze from abducens nerve (CN VI) palsy.

Medulloblastoma

BUZZWORDS

Across all ages, **medulloblastoma is the most common malignant brain tumor of childhood**. It derives from tumor stem cells in the cerebellum and presents with a triad of **headache, ataxia**, and **obstructive hydrocephalus**.

Bad Brain BooBoo

Brain tumors, taken as a whole, are **the most common type of SOLID tumors in children**. More importantly, brain tumors are the **number one cause of death** among all childhood cancers.

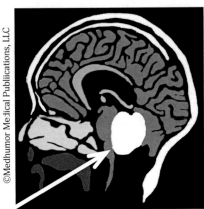

Contrast MRI scan showing midline, posterior-fossa medulloblastoma
- Contrast-enhancing 4th ventricle mass
- Hydrocephalus

CASE STUDY

You are presented with a child just under 1 year old who is vomiting, but not experiencing diarrhea. Among the physical findings (which will be consistent with dehydration, including dry oral mucosa and decreased urine output), they note a full anterior fontanel. He is provided with two normal saline boluses, after which he postures by fully extending his arms and legs. You are asked what would be the best next step.

THE DIVERSION

If you do not read the key words carefully[1] you might mistakenly read "full fontanel" as "flat fontanel." This is the key to the question. If you read it as flat fontanel, you might pick the diversionary choice of continued boluses and IV fluids. If you misinterpreted this as a seizure, you would have picked anticonvulsants incorrectly.

ANSWER REVEALED

The history is consistent with a **space occupying lesion**, most likely a brain tumor. The full fontanel is what gives this away. The posturing with arms and legs extended is secondary to increased intracranial pressure, *not a seizure*. Therefore, IV dexamethasone and other steps to reduce increased intracranial pressure would be the correct response.

---

[1] Again, sounds like a cliché, but it is important to read the key words carefully.

Supratentorial Tumors

In general, supratentorial tumors present with **headaches**, **seizures** and **hemiparesis**.

Craniopharyngioma

Craniopharyngioma is one of those diagnoses that you will probably never run into in real life, but afflicts many, many children on the boards.

Craniopharyngioma shows up **gradually** (over 1-2 years), with a triad of **endocrinopathies** (i.e., diabetes insipidus, short stature, premature or delayed puberty), **behavior changes**, and **visual disturbances** (due to pressure on the optic tracts). **Obstruction of the 3rd ventricle may lead to hydrocephalus**.

They could also show or describe a skull film with **calcification in the sella turcica**. These classic descriptions should make it an easy question.

This tumor is technically not malignant, it's just in a very unfortunate location leading to the mass effects described above. You've heard the realtor's expression: "location, location, location."

Surgery and possibly **radiation** are the treatments. Most patients respond well.

These kids need close endocrine follow-up.

Please see Heme Onc chapter for additional information on craniopharyngioma.

Optic nerve Gliomas

Optic nerve gliomas can lead to decreased vision (imagine that).

25% of cases are associated with **neurofibromatosis**.

Brain Abscess

Watch for a child with sinusitis symptoms, who also has severe headache and vomiting. They could also present with encephalitis-like symptoms including focal neurologic deficits, papilledema, and seizures.

You would think fever is a common symptom, but you would be wrong.

HOT TIP

Remember that patients with **bacterial rhinosinusitis, pulmonary disease and cyanotic heart disease** are at **increased risk** for developing a brain abscess.

BUZZWORDS

Ring enhancing lesion is a classic description of the lesion on CT.

TREATMENT

There is a witch's brew of potential bacterial causes of brain abscess, with S. aureus being the most common. Initial treatment involves empiric IV antibiotics directed towards the expected organisms based on the source of infection. **Nafcillin/vancomycin, metronidazole, and ceftriaxone** is a common combination; **ceftazidime/cefepime** would be a good alternative if *Pseudomonas* is suspected. Therapy should be adjusted as necessary based on culture results obtained via **CT-guided aspiration or surgical excision.**

California, Oregon, and Other Altered States of Consciousness

If you are presented with a patient with an "altered state of consciousness," pay particular attention to the **age** of the child, since this will help determine the etiology and should make these questions some of the easiest ones on the exam (leading to a euphoric state of consciousness in yourself).

> ## Vein of Galen Malformation
>
> they describe a cranial bruit in a neonate with hydrocephalus and a history of congestive heart failure, they are referring to a Vein of Galen malformation.

> ## Neo Poetry Night
>
> If they describe a non-responsive neonate, don't automatically jump on the "sepsis" bandwagon. They may want you to measure **serum ammonia** and **organic acid levels**. In other words, keep an open mind with your differential for this: include Inborn Errors of Metabolism on that list.
>
> *MNEMONIC*
>
> Remember this with the following poem: "Neo Coma Order Organic Ammonia.".

Differentials for Unresponsiveness and Altered States of Consciousness in Older Infants and Kids

 HOT TIP

1. Encephalopathy.
2. Toxic ingestion. Consider this if symptoms rapidly progressed over several hours. The hints in the history will often be subtle, such as a **family member with a condition that requires medication** (i.e., depression, seizures, or heart disease).
3. Head trauma. This is a strong possibility, especially if the onset was abrupt.

Even if the question specifically states "no *history* of head trauma," you would be correct in choosing **head CT** as an initial study. This is because the head trauma might have been **unwitnessed or undisclosed (i.e., non-accidental trauma or NAT)**. What the question is really stating is, "no *known* history of head trauma."

Narcolepsy

This condition is characterized by excessive and uncontrolled daytime sleepiness, with sudden mid-day "sleep attacks." It is frequently experienced by pediatricians preparing for the boards. Episodes are significantly reduced by using this book.

Additional manifestations include **cataplexy** (sleep attacks precipitated by strong emotion such as laughter), **sleep paralysis**, or **hypnagogic** (almost asleep) **hallucinations**.

These children can fall asleep in the midst of doing everyday activities - even while riding their bikes! **Academic problems are common.**

Onset is typically during adolescence. Diagnosis is made by clinical history, **overnight polysomnography and a sleep latency test**.

Treatment is mostly supportive, and includes behavioral and environmental changes. Referral to a sleep specialist and medication-based management may be necessary for severe cases.

Wilson's Disease

To recap from the GI chapter, this is an **autosomal recessive** disorder involving excess copper buildup in tissues. Common neurologic manifestations include tremors, emotional problems, difficulty with handwriting, depression, and abnormal eye movements *without* visual abnormalities.

As we've already discussed previously:

- **Younger patients** mostly present with **symptoms of liver disease.**
- **Older patients** have more **neuro/psych symptoms.**

If they describe evidence of **acute hepatic failure** coupled with **dystonia** and **mental status changes,** think of Wilson's disease.

By the time neurologic or psychiatric symptoms are present, there will almost always be **Kaiser-Fleischer rings** in the eyes (yellow-green ringlike copper deposits encircling the iris. These are best seen on slit-lamp exam and in close-up shots on the board exam).

Supportive labs for diagnosis include **low** ceruloplasmin and serum copper levels; and **high** tissue and urine copper levels. Confirmatory diagnosis is via liver biopsy.

Ataxia Attackia

You need to distinguish different forms of **ataxia** from each other. A systematic approach that looks at the clues in the question will help you avoid getting "tripped up."

Acute Ataxia

There are multiple causes for childhood ataxia with **acute** onset. Your first thought should be a **post-infectious** etiology (aka **acute cerebellar ataxia**). They may mention a recent viral illness such as chickenpox[2], Epstein-Barr virus, parvovirus B19, or mumps. They may also hint at other culprits like Borrelia burgdorfeli (Lyme disease), Mycoplasma pneumoniae, and typhoid fever.

The prognosis of acute cerebellar ataxia is generally excellent.

Additional causes of acute ataxia would include toxic ingestion, neoplasm, trauma, metabolic problems, CNS infections and neurodegenerative disorders.

Ataxia Telangiectasia

Ataxia Telangiectasia (AT) is an **autosomal recessive** disorder due to a defect in DNA processing and repair. Telangiectasias are capillary dilatations that cause red blotches which blanch on pressure (aka dioscopy); they are located on the skin and conjunctiva. The disease has **CNS effects, skin and eye findings, immunologic effects,** and sometimes **intellectual disability.**

The immunologic effects lead to both decreased levels of immunoglobulins IgA and IgG, and T-cell dysfunction; manifesting as **frequent upper and lower respiratory tract infections and malignancy** later in life.

Ocular telangiectasias that become advanced over time can **mimic conjunctivitis.**

Despite these eye findings, both **acuity and pupillary reflexes are often normal.**

There is a high incidence of **malignancy** in ataxia telangectasia, especially **Hodgkin lymphoma** and **leukemia.** Look for elevated Alpha-Fetoprotein (AFP) levels.

Tin walk

To remember the possible causes of ataxia, remember the stilted walk of The **Tin** Man in The **Wizard** of Oz.

Toxic ingestion
(e.g., ethanol, pesticides)

Infection
(including Guillain Barré)

Neoplasm
(e.g., glioma, medulloblastoma)

Additional causes would include a cerebral hemorrhage and a variety of metabolic disorders.

Meds that Move

You should be familiar with various medications that can cause movement disorders.

Ataxia can be caused by anticonvulsants, alcohol, and thallium.

That's easy to remember: a**taxia**, **anticonvulsants**, and **alcohol** all begin with the letter **A.**

You will just have to remember that **thallium** is also associated with ataxia.

Tremors can be caused by amphetamines, valproic acid, phenothiazines, and tricyclic antidepressants.

Methylxanthines such as caffeine and theophylline may also cause tremors.

---

[2] Always referred to by its formal title, varicella, or sometimes as nom de-Guerre chicken pops. While this is seen more and more rarely out there in the real world, it is another example of something that is still seen on the boards (much the same way old Hollywood has-beens are seen in Las Vegas).

Recognizing this condition should be a piece of cake because the question will likely include a description of the pigmentation in the eye. Otherwise, they may give information on high AFP and/or decreased immunoglobin levels coupled with a description of ataxia.

Friedreich Ataxia

Friedreich ataxia is an **autosomal recessive** disorder accounting for about half of all cases of **inherited ataxia**.

It typically presents in **late childhood** or **early adolescence**. Children tend to present initially with a **slow and clumsy gait**. This ataxia is due to both cerebellar impairment and loss of proprioception.

Watch for signs of spinal cord and peripheral nerve problems. This could be described as **decreased strength** in the feet, as well as **decreased reflexes** in the lower extremities.

Clinical features that distinguish **Friedreich ataxia** from other forms of ataxia are:
- **Elevated plantar arch (i.e. pes cavus)**
- **Absence of lower extremity deep tendon reflexes**
- **Myocardial fiber degeneration leading to cardiomyopathy and CHF**
- **Glucose intolerance leading to diabetes mellitus**

Friedreich ataxia presents later than ataxia telangiectasia.

Remember *"Fried Arch"* (= Friedreich) ataxia and picture the elevated arch. If you ate "fried" arches or any fried food for that matter, you would have "high blood sugar and heart problems," too.

The only treatment for Friedreich ataxia is **supportive**.

Charcot-Marie-Tooth disease

This disorder belongs to a group of **hereditary motor/sensory neuropathies** involving mutations in the myelin gene. It has multiple inheritance patterns, the most common being **autosomal dominant (CMT1)**.

Initial signs include:
- Clumsiness, distal muscle weakness, absence of lower extremity deep tendon reflexes,
- High plantar arch (i.e., pes cavus), foot drop.

Later signs include:
- Weakness and sensory deficits in all extremities
- Distal calf muscle atrophy (aka "stork leg" deformity)

Definitive diagnosis is via genetic testing; nerve conduction studies and nerve biopsy can support the diagnosis. Treatment is supportive.

Strange Movements (in D Minor)

Chorea

Relatively **random** and **purposeless** movements. These writhing movements usually affect the distal extremities, and appear "dance-like."

The two main types of chorea to know for the boards are **Sydenham chorea** and **Huntington chorea**.

Sydenham Chorea

As you no doubt recall, this is one of the **major Jones criteria** of **rheumatic fever**.

If they mention normal antistreptococcal antibody titers, that does **not** automatically rule out Sydenham chorea. As in, this condition can be a stand-alone diagnosis.

Sydenham chorea is essentially self-limited. However, low dose haloperidol would also be correct if listed among the choices.

Huntington Chorea[3]

Huntington chorea (Huntington disease) is an **autosomal dominant** disorder that involves the **triad** of:

1) Chorea
2) Hypotonia
3) Emotional lability

Most of the time, symptoms are not apparent until adulthood (after age 35), but about 10% will have juvenile Huntington chorea (which more commonly presents with **rigidity**). This differentiation is important to keep in mind for the exam.

> ### Gangly Gait
> The part of the brain most often affected in movement disorders is the **basal ganglia**.

> ### Treating Chorea
> You could be questioned on the appropriate treatment of chorea in general.
>
> **Dopamine-blocking agents** in the antipsychotic category, especially **haloperidol**, are very effective.
>
> Other medications that could be considered correct choices include **fluphenazine, risperidone,** or **tetrabenazine.**

---

[3] By the way, this is what Woody Guthrie died of. (He wrote *This Land is Your Land.*)

Dystonic Reactions

CASE STUDY

You are presented with a 2 year old who has a fixed upward gaze. Throughout the exam, he remains alert and appropriately frightened. His parents and the paramedics who brought him confirm that he has remained alert. His airway is patent and his vital signs are stable. A toxic ingestion is a possibility. You are asked to pick a pharmacological treatment until ingestion can be confirmed. Which would you use?

THE DIVERSION

You could be provided with choices such as rectal diazepam, which will lead you to believe this is a seizure, even though the wording of the question serves as a neon beacon that says "NO SEIZURE." NG tube, activated charcoal, and even syrup of ipecac can be among the choices, since ingestion is a possibility.

ANSWER REVEALED

If they tell you or strongly hint that there was no seizure, then treatment of a seizure is not the answer. If they specifically state that ingestion is suspected, then a simple answer like charcoal or NG tube placement will probably be incorrect, since everyone taking or even proctoring the exam will get it right. No, they want you to identify the specific toxin ingested and treat it specifically. That is what it takes to grab the brass ring of board certification.

In this case, the upward gaze is a dystonic reaction, which is probably due to ingestion of promethazine, metoclopramide or a related drug. Therefore, treatment with *diphenhydramine* would be most appropriate.

TAKE HOME MESSAGE

If you are presented with a patient with an acute dystonic reaction characterized by **neck hyperextension** and **decreased extraocular movements**, watch for certain medications (especially neuroleptics) as the cause. Medication-induced acute dystonic reaction can be reversed with diphenhydramine.

HOT TIP

Metoclopramide Reglan® is in fact a neuroleptic, though not typically thought of as one. **Promethazine Phenergan**® is also associated with acute dystonic reactions.

Tips on Tics

CASE STUDY

You are presented with a 10 year old with ADHD who has been on methylphenidate for the past 3 years. He briefly experienced eye blinking, which has since resolved with no intervention. You will be asked for the most likely explanation for the eye blinking, and for appropriate further management.

THE DIVERSION

The combination of the eye blinking and a child with ADHD on methylphenidate (or other stimulant medication) may trigger you to consider a diagnosis of a tic disorder such as Tourette syndrome. This is exactly the diversion they want to lead you to.

ANSWER REVEALED

However, in this patient the tic was limited and resolved spontaneously, despite the continuation of methylphenidate. Therefore, the correct explanation would be a simple motor tic and no additional intervention.

Distinguishing a Tic from a Toc

The following will help you distinguish tics from other movements on the exam.

COIN FLIP

Tics follow a **specific pattern, are repetitive, improve or disappear during purposeful movement, and may be voluntarily suppressed**, at least for short periods of time.

Choreiform movements are **random and purposeless movements, increase during deliberate movement** and **cannot be voluntarily suppressed**.

Rocking and **hand flapping** are examples of **stereotypies**, which may sometimes be seen in normal children; but are more commonly associated with children with autism and Rett syndrome.

Simple Motor Tics

BUZZWORDS

Simple motor tics typically present as **eye blinking** and **movements of the head, face,** and/or **shoulders**. They are common and transient in many children without underlying conditions.

Unmasking Tics

PERIL

Stimulant medications **do not** cause tics. However, they may unmask an underlying tic disorder in predisposed patients.

PERIL

In the past, the presentation of tics meant that stimulant medication for ADHD had to be discontinued. This is no longer the case.

However, parents need to be made aware of the fact that stimulants may unmask an underlying tic disorder.

Tourette Syndrome

Tourette syndrome is part of a continuum of tic disorders that, involve multiple motor and one or more vocal tics in a waxing and waning course over at least one year. Onset of symptoms must be before 21 years of age and cannot be attributable to an underlying medical disorder or medication use.

There is often co-occurrence between Tourette syndrome and **ADHD**. Tourette syndrome also occurs frequently in children with **obsessive-compulsive disorder (OCD)**.

> ### Treatment for Tourette Syndrome
>
> **Habit reversal training** is currently advocated for Tourette syndrome. It consists of recognizing when tics are about to occur, and starting a voluntary movement that will not allow the tic to occur.
>
> Pharmacotherapy is only indicated when tics interfere with daily activities.

Weakness and Hypotonia

CNS causes of hypotonia include cerebral palsy [specifically the dyskinetic (aka athetoid) and ataxic subtypes], genetic disorders (i.e., Prader Willi, Angelman, and Down syndromes), or metabolic problems (i.e,, leukodystrophies, peroxisomal disorders).

Spinal Neurology

If you are presented with a patient whose symptoms are consistent with a spinal cord lesion, then the best study to order is a a **MRI of the spine**.

Epidural Abscess

An epidural abscess compresses the spinal cord and can cause **pain, paresthesias, weakness** and/or **paralysis**. Most people have fever and **localized back pain as their initial symptoms**. Other signs of localized spinal compression include **decreased bowel and bladder tone, reduced sensation in the lower extremities**, and **increased** reflexes.

> ### The shifty spine: a clear and present danger
>
> For any child with a spinal cord lesion or other condition involving progressive weakness, paralysis, and/or loss of tone (i.e. muscle, bowel, bladder); your **first step** is to **assess respiratory function!**
>
> • Respiratory compromise is a serious consequence
>
> • Look for clues in the question...
>   o Tachypnea
>   o Shallow respirations
>   o Grunting
>   o Abdominal breathing/accessory muscle use
>
> • Check your ABCs, and determine if **intubation** is needed

Infection can occur by direct extension from the paraspinal tissues or seeding from a distant infection (i.e., UTI, dental abscess, central venous catheter). **IV drug users** are particularly susceptible.

Urgent spinal imaging is mandatory. If **MRI** is not available, a **CT** should be performed.

Treatment involves IV antibiotics with good **anti-staphylococcal** activity, and IV steroids to reduce inflammation and further compression. In addition, **emergency surgical decompression** should be performed.

Acute Transverse Myelitis (aka Post-infectious Myelitis)

This condition is due to **lymphocytic infiltration** and **demyelination** of nerves/spinal cord secondary to **inflammation.**

They may describe a child presenting initially with **fever** and an **abrupt onset of muscle weakness and low tone.** This is followed **later** by *increased* **motor tone** and *increased* **reflexes. Bowel and bladder dysfunction** are also common. Patients often report pain on palpation of the spinous processes.

Diagnosis is by a gadolinium-contrast MRI showing cord swelling. A lumbar puncture, typically done after the MRI, shows increased neutrophils (PMNs) in the CSF and a negative gram stain.

Most cases have **spontaneous recovery** over a few months. However, respiratory compromise or arrest is a concerning sequelae.

This is one of the many "serious" presentations triggered by a virus that they want you to know.

Extrinsic Spinal Cord Mass Lesion

If you are presented with a question about a patient with an extrinsic spinal cord lesion, the most **immediate** treatment should be **high dose IV dexamethasone** to reduce pain, edema, and potential ischemia.

Spinal Muscular Atrophy (SMA) Type 1 (aka Werdnig-Hoffmann Disease)

This condition is due to the degeneration of **anterior horn cells**; therefore, **only motor function is affected**, and there are no sensory deficits. It is usually inherited in an **autosomal recessive** fashion.

The typical presentation **in infancy** includes **severe hypotonia, weakness** and **poor suck. Tongue fasciculations** are also common. This latter symptom is what distinguishes SMA Type 1 from botulism. Know these key differences.

Diagnosis is made by **muscle biopsy**. There is no treatment, and most kids die by two years of age due to impending respiratory failure.

Neural Tube Defects (NTD)

These defects occur when the spinal vertebrae fail to form normally, around the 3rd and 4th weeks of gestation. Both environmental and genetic factors play a role in their development. Maternal folate deficiency and maternal anti-convulsant use also increase the risk.

Diagnosis is made by spinal ultrasound or MRI.

There are three main subtypes (listed in order of severity):

1) **Spina bifida occulta**

- There is only a minimal opening between the vertebrae; so the spinal column and nerves are in tact.
- Patients typically have no visible openings on the back; except for a possible hair tuft or sacral dimple.
- Most are asymptomatic; with occasional incontinence or mild sensory issues. 80% have normal intelligence and often do well during preschool years. However, in later years they may have difficulty with organization, memory, or other learning skills.

2) **Meningocele**

- This one has a larger vertebral opening, allowing for the meninges to herniate out of the spinal column.
- Patients may have a cyst-like protrusion in the back, with CSF and meninges; but without the spinal cord. Again, the nerves are in tact.
- Patients may have the same symptoms on occasion as listed above for spina bifida occulta.

3) **Myelomeningocele**

- This one is serious. The vertebrae are widely split, allowing for both the meninges and the spinal cord to herniate.
- Patients have the above-mentioned symptoms plus some paralysis, as well as orthopedic and urologic complications (i.e., urinary incontinence or retention, UTIs). Multi-specialty management with Neurosurgery, Orthopedics and Urology is usually required.
- These patients have a poor prognosis and often die by two years.

If they present a patient with a suspected myelomeningocele, make sure to get a head CT to rule out a Chiari II malformation, as this is a very common association. Look for an image or description of downward displacement of the cerebellar tonsils through the foramen magnum, and a non-communicating (obstructive) hydrocephalus. These children frequently require ventriculoperitoneal (VP) shunt placement.

Spinal Cord Dysfunction

You are expected to recognize the different **clinical manifestations** of spinal cord dysfunction. The question stem may mention a **lipoma, hair tuft, hemangioma, discoloration**, and of course a **sacral dimple**.

You should also be able to differentiate the **specific causes**: whether it be **occult spinal dysraphism** (such as a NTD, or incomplete fusion of the spinal vertebrae) or **tethered cord**. Both conditions can present with back and leg pain, diminished sensation in the perineal area, and/or bowel and bladder incontinence. Later, patients may show neurologic and orthopedic abnormalities including gait disturbances, high plantar arches, progressive scoliosis, leg length discrepancy, contractures or limb atrophy.

MRI of the spine is the diagnostic test of choice.

Spinal Trauma

This will typically be described as **focal pain along the spine following trauma**. They may also describe **weakness** and/or **sensory deficits**. **Bladder and bowel function** can be lost as well.

If there is a high index of suspicion for **spinal trauma**, then in addition to immobilizing the cervical and lower spine, **IV methylprednisolone 30 mg/kg** should also be administered over an hour.

Know which steroids to use! **IV dexamethasone** would be indicated for **spinal cord compression**, but not spinal trauma.

Rhyme it up. "<u>Methyl</u> is for sp<u>inal</u> trauma; <u>Dex</u> is for com-<u>press</u>-ion."

If mannitol is among the answer choices you are given in this setting, it would only be indicated with signs of increased intracranial pressure. Remember that manitol is an osmotic diuretic, so its main job is to drain the fluid causing the pressure.

Peripheral Nerve Conditions

Bell's palsy

An acquired **idiopathic unilateral facial paralysis** presumed to be due to **post-infectious inflammation of the facial (CN VII) nerve. The most common causes are HSV and VZV; as well as Lyme disease.**

The unilateral facial paralysis develops abruptly and includes forehead weakness manifested as decreased forehead wrinkling; and decreased smiling on the affected side.

Patients with unilateral facial weakness and forehead **sparing** should be immediately evaluated for a stroke.

Treatment options include **prednisone** for 5 days, best when started in the first 3 days of symptom onset. For severe cases, antivirals like **acyclovir** and **valacyclovir** may also be used.

> ### Ramsay Hunt Facial Paralysis
>
> Ramsay Hunt Syndrome occurs with reactivation of the **varicella zoster virus. It manifests as facial paralysis** associated with **painful vesicles in the ear canal.**

Guillain Barré Syndrome (GBS)

This is also known **Acute Inflammatory Demyelinating Polyneuropathy (AIDP)**. It is a **pure motor neuropathy**; sensation, bowel and bladder function are completely preserved.

Patients often present with fever and back pain; followed later by proximal muscle weakness., including **leg weakness and/or an unsteady gait**. The muscle weakness **starts in the lower extremities** and **progresses upward in a symmetric fashion** (aka "ascending paralysis"). **Loss of reflexes of the lower extremities** is also a key manifestation. On physical exam, there will often be cranial nerve findings (i.e., facial palsy) and dysautonomia (i.e., tachycardia, orthostatic hypotension, dizziness).

GBS is often preceded by **infections** such as viruses, or GI bugs like *Campylobacter jejuni.* Other causes include back surgery, bone marrow transplantation and trauma.

Don't get fooled by the question. **Areflexia is always seen in GBS**. If reflexes are present in the lower extremity, it is not GBS they are describing.

On lumbar puncture, there is **increased protein in the CSF** with a normal cell count. This finding is also known as **albuminocytologic dissociatio**n.

Remember that **proximal muscle weakness** is a classic sign. They will rarely come right out and say "proximal muscle weakness." Instead, they will simply describe it. They might note a child who has **difficulty rising from a sitting position or cannot shrug his/her shoulders**. Sometimes they will present a child who **becomes clumsy or starts falling**.

Just as in spinal cord pathology; the **biggest risk for GBS and other neuropathies involving weakness and/or paralysis is respiratory failure.** They definitely expect you to know that lung function must be followed closely.

You need to **measure pulmonary function tests**; pulse oximetry is inadequate and will be the incorrect answer since O2 saturations only decline once the patient is severely compromised. Correct parameters or studies to follow would include "vital capacity," "negative inspiratory force," or "pulmonary function tests" – never "oxygen saturation" (unless it is the only choice relating to pulmonary function).

GBS is treated with supportive measures (including intubation if needed), as well as **plasmapheresis** and **IVIG**. Most patients who survive have a full recovery, but there is permanent disability in about 10% of cases.

Paralysis by Analysis

Tick paralysis is caused by a neurotoxin secreted by the tick. It is seen during the summer months.

It can present exactly like GBS with ascending paralysis,[5] but progresses much faster (hours to days), with *no fever* and *normal CSF* findings.

Botulism,[6] in contrast, causes descending paralysis, and is due to ingestion of a neurotoxin that blocks acetylcholine release. This toxin is produced by Clostridium botulinum, a bug that can brew in contaminated canned foods (including home-made) and honey.

Look for infants < 6 months with acute proximal muscle weakness and:

- poor suck, progressive ptosis
- constipation, urinary retention

In older infants and children, also look for the "D-symptoms:"

- **d**isconjugaye gaze
- **d**iplopia
- **d**ysphgia
- **d**ysarthria

---

[4] This is easy to remember since ticks usually bite your leg while you are walking in tall grass.
[5] For more information on botulism see corresponding section in the ID Chapter.

Steroids have no proven benefit in the treatment of Guillain Barré syndrome.

This should be easy to remember: a tick usually hangs out on tall grass and bites you on the legs, so the symptoms go up. If you ingest a toxin with your mouth, symptoms would go down.

Acute Flaccid Myelitis (AFM)

A polio-like or GBS-like weakness seen often in summer and early fall in alternating (even) years.

Presentation often includes a 3-6 yo child with a prodrome of a URI, asthma exacerbation, or GI illness with fever followed about days to weeks later by neurologic symptoms such as limb weakness or paralysis, hypotonia, hyporeflexia, facial droop, ophthalmoplegia, and dysphagia. Paralysis is rapid, within hours to days, asymmetric, with a preference for the upper extremities.

The cause is unknown but enterovirus EV-68 has been proposed to play a role.

Diagnosis is made by appropriate history with MRI of the spine showing lesions in the grey matter spanning one or more vertebral segments. Respiratory and stool specimens should be sent for PCR and viral cultures. CSF fluid shows pleocytosis.

The best treatment is still evolving but will also require years of physical and occupational therapy. Recovery is often incomplete, with children still showing deficits more than a year after onset of symptoms.

Neuromuscular Junction disease

Myasthenia Gravis

This is an **autoimmune disorder** in which the patient develops **antibodies against the acetylcholine receptor** in the neuromuscular junction. The etiology of myasthenia gravis is unknown. **Penicillamine** may be a known iatrogenic cause. Other drugs, as well as illnesses, can exacerbate symptoms.

Proximal muscle weakness from myasthenia gets worse with activity and **improves with rest**. Patients report feeling good in the morning, but tire out as the day goes on.[6] Ptosis is a very common finding in myasthenia gravis. Many patients present when someone else notices their droopy eyes – look for this in the question.

 Myasthenia gravis is strongly **associated with thymoma**. A diagnosis of myasthenia gravis should prompt chest imaging (X-ray, CT, MRI) to evaluate for a thymoma.

---

[6] Of course, this describes everyone with a job, family, kids, or anyone who is alive. On the boards it will likely be noted and emphasized in the question.

Tensilon it in

When suspected, myasthenia gravis can be confirmed by the **Tensilon test** which uses **edrophonium**, a short acting **acetylcholinesterase inhibitor**.

Tensilon (edrophonium) is NOT a treatment for myasthenia gravis – it is very short acting and is only used for testing.

Adjunct tests for supporting the diagnosis include the presence of **anti-acetylcholine receptor antibodies, anti-Smith antibodies** and an **electromyelogram (EMG)**.

The mainstay of chronic therapy is **pyridostigmine (Mestinon®)**, a long-acting acetylcholinesterase inhibitor that increases the quantity of acetylcholine available at the neuromuscular junction. **Plasmapheresis** and **plasma exchange** are also used. **Prednisone** and other immunomodulating agents are less commonly used. **Thymectomy** is often done (especially in kids), and can be curative.

Botulism

We have already covered botulism in detail in the ID chapter and above, so we will just take a moment here to differentiate it from the other neuromuscular conditions.

The botulism toxin blocks the release of acetylcholine at the neuromuscular junction.

The paralysis of **botulism** is **descending**, while those of **Guillain Barré syndrome** and **tick paralysis** are **ascending**.

Infantile botulism can look similar to **myasthenia gravis**; but botulism has a rapid onset (within hours) while myasthenia gravis is more progressive, occurring over the course of weeks.

Muscular Diseases

The dystrophinopathies include Duchenne and Becker muscular dystrophies.

Duchenne muscular dystrophy (DMD)

This is an X-linked recessive disorder (<u>only</u> boys get it). The **absence of dystrophin protein** is the underlying cause (duh!). The diagnosis is made by **muscle biopsy**.

Children with Duchenne muscular dystrophy are usually not symptomatic at birth. In fact, they often achieve their baby milestones at the right times.

> ### Becker muscular dystrophy
>
> Becker muscular dystrophy involves *reduced* (but not absent) dystrophin protein. It is very similar to DMD; but with **later** onset, **milder** severity, and **slower** deterioration.
>
> Children may report **severe muscle cramps** on exertion and have even more serious **cardiac** involvement than with DMD.

PERIL

Poor head control may be the first sign in infancy. Toddlers have **weakness in the hip muscles** as well as a **lordotic posture** to compensate for their gluteal weakness. They **cannot walk up stairs** and usually crawl up or cry to be carried up.

BUZZWORDS

Look for a child with a "waddling gait." He may also attempt to stand up by "walking" his hands up his legs for support. This is the infamous **"Gower sign,"**[7] associated with proximal muscle weakness. Look for **enlarged calves** or the term, **"pseudohypertrophy."** This is not true muscle hypertrophy; it is actually fat deposition and proliferation of collagen.

> ### Carrying the Heart
>
> *UPDATED & NEW*
> **BREAKING**
> **NEWS**
> *INFORMATION* Female carriers of Duchenne's muscular dystrophy are now reported to have mild muscle weakness and dilated cardiomyopathy. Therefore cardiac surveillance is recommended for female carriers.

Most kids with DMD have mild **intellectual disability**. They are also at high risk for cardiomyopathy, pneumonia and impending respiratory failure; all of which are frequent causes of death in these patients. They often die by the third decade of life (somewhere in their 20s).

CPK is elevated at all times in kids with DMD, **even at birth. Therefore, CPK levels can be elevated before weakness appears.** Genetic testing is confirmatory, and assesses for **Xp21 gene** abnormalities.

MNEMONIC

Remember that DMD is carried on the X chromosome to avoid being confused by other choices on the exam. Think of it as DuXchenne muscular dystrophy to remember that it is X-linked recessive. Think of it as **DuXchenne** muscular dystrophy to remember that it is **X**-linked recessive.

COIN FLIP

An item that distinguishes DMD from other neuromuscular disorders is the **absence of tongue fasciculations** (rule out SMA Type 1) **and eye muscle involvement** (rule out myasthenia gravis).

HOT TIP

Remember that DMD has a significant spontaneous mutation rate. They could try to trick you by providing a choice that states that the mother is *always* a carrier. In 1/3 of the cases, the mother is NOT a carrier.

Asymptomatic Carriers: The CPK level can be elevated in asymptomatic female carriers.

Myotonic Muscular Dystrophy (MMD)

DEFINITION

This is an **autosomal dominant** condition that affects **both striated and smooth muscle**. It therefore impacts multiple systems in addition to skeletal muscle; including the **heart** and **GI tract**.

BUZZWORDS

MMD typically presents around 4-5 years of age with **distal muscle weakness**. The **hand muscles** are particularly affected, and display **"slow relaxation after contraction."** This abnormality is known as **myotonia** (hence its name). Patients may also have **cardiac, endocrine and GI problems**.

---

[7] Gower sign is also seen in other conditions with proximal muscle weakness, such as Guillan-Barre and dermatomyositis. Watch for the details in the description.

Remember: the muscle wasting in MMD is <u>distal</u>, compared to proximal for most other neuromuscular disorders. In contrast to Duchenne muscular dystrophy, **CPK may be normal in MMD.**

Confirmatory diagnosis for MMD is **by muscle biopsy.**

They might describe MMD and casually tell you the mother also has it - so what are the chances of subsequent children getting it? They will say "mother" to trick you into believing it is X-linked recessive. However, if it were an X-Linked recessive disorder, Mom wouldn't have it.

MMD is also known as *Steinert* disease. Think, "Stein-heart" to remind you that this disorder can affect the heart.

The following table helps organize your approach to diagnostic differentials when presented with a child with weakness:

Type of Disorder	Presentation	Examples
Brain Lesion	• Contralateral face and body weakness	• Tumor • Abscess
Brainstem Lesion	• Ipsilateral facial weakness • Contralateral body weakness • **Weak eye movements**	• Tumor
Spinal cord lesion	• Loss of motor and sensation function • Loss of bladder and bowel function • **Increased reflexes** • There is **no eye involvement**	• Transverse myelitis • Anterior spinal artery infarction • Spinal cord compression (tumor, epidural abscess) • Tethered cord • Trauma
Acute Peripheral Nerve Processes	• Loss of deep tendon reflexes	• Guillain Barré • Lead poisoning • Polio • Bell's palsy • Diphtheria • Tick paralysis
Chronic Peripheral Nerve Processes	• Loss of deep tendon reflexes	• Chronic demyelinating polyneuropathy • Hereditary neuropathies • Leukodystrophies
Neuromuscular **Junction Disorders**	• **Reduced, not absent,** deep tendon reflexes, descending weakness • Gradual onset, waxing and waning	• Myasthenia gravis
Toxic Ingestion	• Rapidly progressing, descending weakness	• Botulism
Muscular Disorders	• Proximal Weakness	• Muscular Dystrophy • Mitochondrial myopathies • Congenital myopathies • Polymyositis • Dermatomyositis • Electrolyte disturbances

Hail Seizure

When you are presented with a patient that *appears* to have a seizure, make sure it is actually a seizure and not a "pseudoseizure," or other medical concern such as syncope or tics.

If you follow these guidelines, you are less likely to be, ahem, "shaken" off the trail to the correct answer.

Pseudoseizures (aka paroxysmal non-epileptic events) are psychogenic by nature. They appear like true seizures but typically occur during the day, often with other people around. The key differentiating factors are **the lack of abnormal neuronal activity on the EEG during episodes; and the absence of the post-ictal state.**

A **seizure**,[8] by contrast, results from **abdnormal electrical discharge by neurons**, which have a measurable effect on the innervated organ. It typically occurs suddenly and cannot be controlled. At most, the patient might describe an "aura" that preceded the event.

You need to distinguish different categories of seizures based on the history and physical findings. They will not simply just ask what kind of seizure it is. Instead they will ask you to pick the prognosis and treatment based on the associated features they describe.

> ## What's the shake up?
> Not all shakes are the same !
> - **Seizure:** sudden, uncontrollable, abnormal EEG, possible post-ictal state
> - **Pseudoseizure:** psychogenic, daytime with audience, normal EEG, no post-ictal state
> - **Tics:** specific patterns, repetitive, purposeful, voluntarily suppressed, no post-ictal state
> - **Syncope:** typically preceded by dizziness, pallor, blurred vision, "blacking out"

There are a myriad of names for different types of seizures. This can get confusing, but most can be put into one of the following categories.

SEIZING SEIZURE NOMENCLATURE	
1. Neonatal seizures	These occur within the **first month of life**. They have a variety of causes, including sepsis/infection, inborn errors of metabolism, perinatal hypoxia, birth defects and drug effects.
2. Febrile seizures	These are very common10 (2-5% of all children); especially between 6 months to 6 years of age. They typically occur during a rapid rise in body temperature, usually in response to a common infection such as acute otitis media or URI.
3. Partial seizures	These are **focal** and only involve part of the brain. They come in two main flavors. 1. **Simple partial seizures** have a localized motor component (limited to one part of the body). This can progress, or "march" to other parts of the body. Children remain awake and **conscious** during episodes (i.e., Jacksonian seizure). 2. **Complex partial seizures** also involve motor activity; but the child is unaware and **unconscious** of what they're doing, thus making it more "complicated."

---

[8] It is also defined as the illegal or forceful attainment of land or property (as in seizure of property), but this is the Board exam, not the Bar exam.

[9] You guessed it, even more common on the boards.

---

4. Generalized seizures	These are **non-focal** (as the name implies), and have even more flavors: 1. **Absence seizures (aka petit mal seizures)** are short episodes where the child is mentally "checked out."[11] They are described as **staring into space**, fidgeting, lip smacking or fumbling with their clothes (aka **automatisms**); with no awareness of their environment. 2. **Infantile spasms** usually occur in children less than 1 year of age. They are commonly associated with intellectual disability and certain genetic conditions like **tuberous sclerosis**. The prognosis is very poor. 3. **Generalized tonic-clonic (GTC) seizures, (aka grand mal seizures)** are the "classic" seizures your non-physician friends witness while watching *Grey's Anatomy* and munching on stale popcorn. These seizures typically last a few minutes and have a **post-ictal period** during which the patient is unarousable.
5. Status epilepticus	This is defined as seizure activity **greater than 30 minutes in duration**, or repeated seizures without a return to normal in between episodes. This is a **medical emergency**.

Apparently the nomenclature was selected to maximize confusion and to increase the chances of actually experiencing a seizure while trying to memorize and remember the appropriate associations. Let's face it, using the term "partial seizure" to describe a focal seizure is quite bizarre.

We go into greater detail further down. First we go over some general principles.

EEGs

They will not show you EEG tracings. For most non-neurologists (and many neurologists, for that matter), EEG printouts are indistinguishable from the Richter scale printouts by the Geological Society. However, they will describe the EEG pattern. Becoming familiar with the EEG "descriptions" associated with different disorders will allow you to often recognize the diagnosis based on this alone.

HOT TIP

If they describe a child who still has a seizure despite being on anticonvulsant medication, the initial step is to **obtain drug levels**, - especially in adolescents - since **poor medication compliance** is a known cause for these **breakthrough seizures**.

Weight gain resulting in a child **outgrowing their dose** and/or factors interfering with medication absorption are other common causes.

Metabolic Seizure

Common **metabolic** causes of seizures, especially in the newborn period, include:

- Hypoglycemia
- Hyponatremia
- Hypocalcemia
- Pyridoxine deficiency
- Inborn errors of metabolism

EEG Not that Easy

HOT TIP

A normal EEG does not rule out epilepsy. This is because it only captures a snapshot of brainwave activity that might fall within the "normal" window (between abnormal episodes). **Conversely, some kids may have an abnormal EEG without actually having seizure episodes**. These are also known as **subclinical seizures**.

---

10 Kind of like what you're doing right now while reading this.

Generalized Seizures

Febrile Seizures

DEFINITION

These are the most common type of seizures overall in children. They typically occur in children ages 6 months - 6 years. They are associated with a febrile illness, but **not** caused by CNS infections, or related to previous neonatal[11] or other pathologic childhood seizures.

HOT TIP

Approximately 1/4 of children with febrile seizures have a known family history of febrile seizures. Watch for this in the presenting history.

Febrile seizures have two subtypes: **simple febrile** vs. **complex febrile seizures**.

Simple Febrile Seizures

These are the most common type of febrile seizure, characterized by:

1. Generalized seizure type
2. Duration less than 15 minutes
3. Only one episode per 24 hour period

Complex Febrile Seizures

These are the less common type of febrile seizure, characterized by:

DEFINITION

- May be focal seizure type
- Duration longer than 15 minutes
- Multiple episodes within 24 hours

Patients experiencing a complex febrile seizure initially (rather than simple febrile seizure), are at increased risk for developing epilepsy.

Recurrence of Febrile Seizures

About 1/3 of kids will go on to have a second febrile seizure.

Risk factors for recurrence include:

- A low fever at time of first seizure
- A short period of time between onset of fever and the seizure
- Young age
- Family history of febrile seizures

First Things First
Seizures

MYTH

You might be tricked into believing a variety of myths, both medical and non-medical, regarding first generalized seizures in well-appearing children.

Medications are not indicated after only one seizure.

Other than a dextrose stick, routine labs and EEG are not indicated.

Parents are to be educated on safety, including wearing a helmet while biking and no bathing without supervision, which really should be guidelines for ALL parents, right?

The risk of swallowing the tongue during a seizure is a myth; therefore, sticking a spoon or other object in the mouth is incorrect.

Seizures in and of themselves do not cause brain damage unless they last longer then 20-30 minutes.

Seizing the Pharm

A variety of medications are known to cause seizures, including:

1. **Chemotherapeutic agents**
   - Cyclosporin
   - Intrathecal methotrexate
2. **Other medications**
   - Isoniazid
   - Insulin/ oral hypoglycemics
   - Bupropion and other psych meds
   - Theophylline

Recreational drugs such as **cocaine** are also known to cause seizures. Know this.

---

[11] Neonatal seizures were covered in the Neonatal Chapter.

Approximately 5% of children with febrile seizures eventually develop epilepsy. Risk is increased in **children with family history of epilepsy, children with complex febrile seizures, and children with neurodevelopmental abnormalities.**

EEG, LP, CT, To Be or not to Bee

Blood tests, EEG and head CT are not indicated in simple febrile seizures. Doing a full workup for complex febrile seizures is more subjective and at the discretion of individual clinicians. This is therefore something they should not ask you.

A lumbar puncture should be strongly considered in neonates and **infants**; those with **complex partial seizures** or **febrile status epilepticus**; and in children **partially treated with antibiotics.**

Absence Seizures

These involve **brief staring spells**. The child is **not responsive** during the episode, and there is **no postictal period**.

Key words include **spacing out** with **blinking, lip smacking or other automatisms**. Afterwards, patients have **no recollection** of the event.[12] The EEG will be described as "**3 Hz per second spike and wave**" – whatever that is – but if you see that phrase in the question, they are talking about an absence seizure. Absence seizures are also called "potato chips" seizures because you can't stop with one (i.e., they come in clusters).

"**3 Hz per second spike and wave**"- picture a surfer spiking a wave 3 times and then "spacing out" into the horizon.

Absence seizures are generalized seizures; but have a lot of similarities with complex partial seizures. Knowing the differences below is key to scoring big points on the exam:

The Absence Seizure	The Complex Partial Seizure
• Abrupt onset, abrupt ending	• May start off as "simple" partial seizures (child is aware) before progressing to "complex" type
• Short duration (< 30 seconds)	• Longer duration (minutes)
• No post-ictal state (child goes back to "normal" without recollection of events)	• Gradual ending, progressing to post-ictal state
• 3 Hz per second spike and wave activity on EEG	

---

[12] Reminds me of one of those cult leaders who ask for donations and subsequently direct deposit the money into their Cayman Islands account after rolling their eyes back and communicating with Satan's Secretary.

Hyperventilating can induce an absence seizure, and this maneuver is diagnostic.

Absence seizures are treated with **ethosuximide** (specific for absence seizures), **lamotrigine**, or **valproic acid** (a more general anticonvulsant). The younger the child, the more likely that they will respond to therapy and remain seizure-free, even after discontinuation of therapy. In other words, younger kids have a better prognosis.

Valproic acid may depress platelet counts and elevate liver function tests and pancreatic enzyme levels, so blood levels must be monitored along with complete blood counts, liver and pancreatic function tests.

Generalized Tonic-Clonic (GTC) Seizure

These patients can have an aura or prodrome for minutes, hours, or even days before the onset of the seizure. A key component of a tonic-clonic seizure is the **loss of consciousness and possibly bowel or bladder control** with **full body tonic-clonic movements**.

GTC seizures occur in three phases: 1) tonic, 2) clonic, and 3) post-ictal. These are outlined in more detail below:

Tonic Phase

This phase is characterized by **tonic flexion of the trunk** and **extension of the back, arms, and legs,** which typically lasts less than 30 seconds. There is **no loss of bowel or bladder control** during this time.

Clonic Phase

This phase is characterized by **clonic convulsive movements with thythmic jerking of extremities**. These clonic movements alternate with short periods of **atonia, during which the person may void or stool without control**. The child is **apneic** at this time, which usually lasts for 1-2 minutes.

Post-ictal Phase

During this phase, patients are **initially unconscious** and subsequently **sleepy** and **confused** upon slowly awakening. They gradually become more oriented as the phase resolves. They are **unable to recall** the events of the seizure.

Taking the bad with the good...

Valproic acid is one of the most effective and resiliant anticonvulsants used for a variety of seizure disorders. It comes with a price, however. Known side effects are:

- Myelosuppression, aplastic anemia, thrombocytopenia, hepatotixicty, pancreatitis
- Teratogenicity in pregnancy (i.e., meningomyelocele)

Blood levels must therefore be monitored, including complete blood counts, liver and pancreatic function tests.

Other popular anticonvulsants with adverse effects include:

Tomiramate: glaucoma (look for acute eye swelling, pain and redness on a child)

Lamotrigine: Stevens Johnson syndrome

Phenytoin: teratogenicity in pregnancy (i.e., fetal hydantoin syndrome). Look for a constellation of defects:

- Cardiac (aortic stenosis, pulmonic stenosis, Tetrology of Fallot)
- IUGR, microcephaly, prominent wide anterior fontanel, widened metopic ridge
- Dysmorphic facies, hypertelorism (widened space between eyes), broad nose, anteverted nostrils
- Cleft lip/palate, fingernail hypoplasia, skin necrosis (i.e., "purple glove syndrome")

Treatment options include **valproic acid, phenytoin, lamotrigine and levetiracetam. Phenytoin** is being used with less frequency due to its side effect profile (as mentioned above), but you should still be familiar with it for the boards.

Juvenile Myoclonic Epilepsy (JME)

JME is a type of generalized idiopathic epilepsy that starts in the adolescent years and often persists for life.

> ### Myoclonic Seizures
>
> These are brief, single or repetitive "jerks" of an isolated group of muscles. Also known as myoclonic jerks, these are relatively rare outside of JME and Lennox-Gastaut syndrome.

Classic presentation of JME involves:

1. Myoclonic jerks of bilateral upper extremities **upon awakening** (think of a teen knocking over stuff while getting out of bed)
2. Generalized tonic-clonic seizures in most patients
3. Absence seizures in 1/3 of patients.

The EEG pattern for JME is characterized by "**4-6 Hz polyspike and wave discharges.**" However, many episodes of JME are not associated with an abnormal EEG finding. If you are presented with a normal EEG and a classic description of JME, then it will still most likely be the correct diagnosis.

Treatment is with **valproic acid** or **levetiracetam**. Most patients will require lifelong therapy.

Infantile Spasms (aka West Syndrome)

Look for a **triad** of:

1. Infantile spasms
2. Hypsarrhythmia (on interictal[13] EEG)
3. Developmental delay

Infantile spasms represent only 2% of all epilepsy, but account for 25% of epilepsy seen in the first year of life (and likely more than that on the exam).

Most patients present between **3 and 9 months**. The spasms occur in **clusters**, sometimes 20 or 30 in a row. They appear as a **startle response** with **sudden flexion or extension of the body** - sort of like a Moro reflex in a child too old to be demonstrating the Moro reflex. **Almost all patients have developmental delay.**

Repetitive flexing of the head, trunk, and extremities,[14] with an EEG finding that includes the word "hypsarrhythmia," is a classic giveaway for infantile spasms.

---

13 This would be "in between seizure episodes," for those who prefer English to Latin Medicalese.
14 These were called Salaam movements in the pre-politically correct days when ethnic and religious traits were attributed to children (e.g., kids with Down syndrome were called mongoloids). The term still helps with memorizing the movement and passing the Boards.

Where the Tube Grows

It is important to note that there is a **definite association between Tuberous Sclerosis (TS) and infantile spasms.** Remember that TS is an **autosomal dominant** disease that can present with periventricular or cortical tubers (causing infantile spasms, seizures); various **tumors** (cardiac rhabdomyomas, renal angiomyolipomas), **shagreen patches, ash-leaf spots** and **angiofibromas.**

Recall that babies love their sweet potato "tubers," so you can easily remember the association between **infantile spasms** and **"tuberous"** sclerosis.

Treatment is primarily with ACTH or **vigabatrin.** Additional therapies include valproic acid, topiramate, **steroids, benzodiazepines** and a ketogenic diet. Focal resection may be indicated in severe cases. Despite these treatments, most children eventually develop other seizure types.

Prognosis is dependent on the patient's developmental status prior to the onset of the seizures. If developmental delay was present at that time, then the prognosis is poor.

Partial Seizures

Remember: **"partial** seizures" = **focal** seizures.

Simple Partial Seizures

"**Simple**" means **consciousness is maintained.**

They may describe **motor activity starting in the face or upper extremities, which can possibly "march" to other locations.** Episodes often occur **as the patient just wakes up or falls asleep.**

Other simple partial seizures may present as **sensory seizures or autonomic seizures.**

Remember: **"simple"** partial seizure means **consciousness is maintained.** Therefore, if they note that the patient is conscious, then a **complex** partial seizure is essentially ruled out.

Simple partial seizures are treated with **carbamazepine.** Many cases remit during adolescence, and **treatment is not always necessary.**

Complex Partial Seizures

"**Complex**" means **alteration in consciousness.** The description will include **facial movements.**

Consciousness is not be impaired completely; patients may still be able to respond to simple commands. Patients may also have **automatisms** - movements like "lip smacking" or vocalizations (i.e., moaning, mumbling) that accompany *both* absense seizures and complex partial seizures. Auditory and/ or visual hallucinations are also possible during episodes.

EEG and **head MRI** are part of the workup.

Anti-epileptic drugs are the treatment of choice. Surgery is rarely used for severe or refractory cases.

Once again, complex partial seizures can present similar to absence seizures. This is a classic example where knowing the subtle differences between the two can win you points on the exam. With **absence seizures**, patients "just snap out of it," and resume normal activity as if nothing had happened. With **complex partial seizures**, patients are "post-ictal" afterwards.

Benign Rolandic Epilepsy

This is also known by its long name, **Benign Childhood Epilepsy with Centrotemporal Spikes (aka BCECTS)**. Benign rolandic epilepsy has **autosomal dominant** inheritance (so look for a mention of family history). It is **the most common type of partial seizure in childhood**. Episodes involve the face; and may include twitching, grunting, tongue rolling and a choking sensation. Patients often cannot speak if episodes occur during wakefulness, although they are conscious the entire time. Luckily for them, **most episodes occur during sleep and are self-limited**.

Picture a child rolling (Rolandic) around in bed, making weird facial movements. Certainly anyone rolling around like that would dominate the bed, which helps recall that this is a dominant trait.

About 1/2 of BCECTS kids will go on to develop generalized tonic-clonic seizures. Some will also have learning disabilities.

As the long name implies, the EEG has "**biphasic focal centrotemporal spikes and slow waves**." Hopefully this will be described as a gift to you.

BCECTS is self-limited; and usually resolves by age 16. Treatment is indicated only **after 3 or more seizures**. It responds well to most anticonvulsants.

Complex partial seizures can also involve weird facial movements; however, most complex partial seizures occur at daytime with the child

---

Cyanotic Breath Holding Spells

These are typically seen in 6-18 month olds; and involve **cyansis and apnea** triggered by an **emotional stressor** (i.e., anger, fear, pain, frustration).

While this is not a seizure, all choices will lead you to believe it is. They will describe a toddler having a temper tantrum, turning blue, passing out, and then coming to. It is a benign, although frightening, process. Parental reassurance is the answer they want.

There is NO post-ictal phase with breath-holding spells... at least not in the child. The parents, however, are often in a state of shock closely mimicking a post-ictal state.

---

unconscious. **Rolandic seizures**, by contrast, take the **"simple"** route, may occur at daytime with the **child aware but unable to respond**; though most are during the night when the child is asleep.[15]

Status Epilepticus

Repeated or continued seizures for 30 minutes without recovery.

Remember your ABCDs. Attend first to the airway, breathing, and circulation and check dextrose. **Ativan® (lorazepam)** is used because of its rapid onset of action.

If the seizure continues after lorazepam administration, then **IV *fosphenytoin*** should be administered. This "prodrug" (inactive precursor) has a much more favorable side effect profile than phenytoin (mentioned previously).

If IV access is not available, give **rectal diazepam (Diastat®)**.

The Facts and Nothing but the Facts

Patients with active epilepsy can bathe and swim, but they must be supervised by an adult. In cases of water recreation, try to pick a sober adult who knows how to swim.

They should not participate in contact sports that can cause head injury.

They may ride bicycles but with helmets, just like all other children.

They should not climb trees.

Teenagers can drive unaccompanied even while on anticonvulsant medication, provided that they have been seizure free for 3-12 months. The exact period varies from state to state, so on the boards, the child presented will likely have been seizure-free for over 12 months.

In general, withdrawal from medication can be attempted if the patient has remained seizure-free for 2 years.

Cerebral Palsy (CP)

This is a topic that will show up in several questions.

CP is a **static encephalopathy** characterized by **non-progressive gross and fine motor abnormalities** evident early in life. There are dozens of proposed etiologies.

Contrary to popular belief, birth trauma and asphyxia are not the leading cause of CP; they compromise only about 10% of cases. While neonates with prematurity, IUGR and intrauterine infections have a higher risk for CP; in most cases, the etiology is unknown.

---

[15] Rolandic seizures can occur during both sleep and wakefulness, with up to 2/3 occurring exclusively during sleep. However, this rate is closer to 100% on the exam, which is why we state this as such.

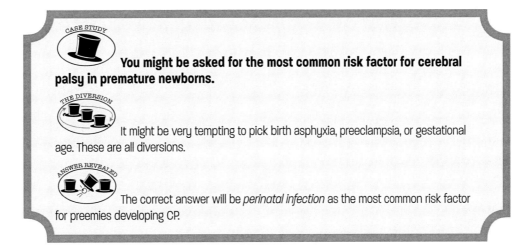

You might be asked for the most common risk factor for cerebral palsy in premature newborns.

It might be very tempting to pick birth asphyxia, preeclampsia, or gestational age. These are all diversions.

The correct answer will be *perinatal infection* as the most common risk factor for preemies developing CP.

Do not automatically pick "birth asphyxia" as the answer – consider the clinical scenario and look at the other etiologies that may have affected the developing brain. **A specific cause of CP is often not found**.

Another myth is that children with CP are always intellectually disabled. On the contrary, many children and adults with CP have normal (or above normal) intelligence. **Unless the question specifically states that the child is intellectually disabled, do not assume this.**

Cerebral palsy can be broken down into several types as noted in the table below:

CP Subtype	Buzz Words	Associations
Spastic diplegia	• Bilateral spasticity of legs • **Walking is delayed** • **Tip-toe walking**	• Normal cognitive function • No seizures • Involves mostly lower extremities
Spastic hemiplegia	• Ipsilateral spasticity (entire one-half of the body) • Same-side arm, trunk, and leg • Diagnosed as CP if onset < 2 yrs	• 1/4 are cognitively impaired • Upper > lower extremity involvement
Spastic quadriplegia	• Increased tone in **all extremities** • Lower > upper extremity involvement	*More likely* to be associated with: • Intellectual disability • Seizures • Feeding difficulties • Speech difficulties • Visual difficulties
Dyskinetic (aka athetoid) CP	Similar to spastic quadriplegia *plus*: • **Dystonia and strange movements**	• Same as spastic quadriplegia
Ataxic CP	• Hypotonia in the trunk and extremities.	• **Delay in motor and language milestones** • **Retention of primitive reflexes and/or hyperactive reflexes**

Cerebrovascular Accident (CVA)

The typical presentation would be an **afebrile child** with a **headache and neck pain**, who then develops **focal paralysis**.

Vascular malformations (including arteriovenous and cavernous malformations) are the most common causes of **hemorrhagic stroke** in children. Watch for severe **headache** and/or **mental status change as the initial presentation**.

If you are presented with a patient with a CVA **suspected by a head CT**, then **cerebral angiography** would be the next step to identifying a specific diagnosis.

> **You are presented with a child who comes in with acute unilateral hemiparesis. Other than blunt trauma to the chest yesterday during football practice, his history is benign. Which diagnostic study would be most helpful in making the diagnosis?**
>
> You might be tempted to pick a head CT, which will be conveniently listed among the choices for your diversionary pleasure. However, if you remember the "don't pick an answer so obvious that your next door neighbor, the hospital CFO, would pick it," you won't be diverted towards the incorrect answer.
>
> The CVA or stroke in this case was caused by the blunt trauma to the chest, which resulted in *carotid dissection*, leading to an *embolic stroke*. This would be best diagnosed via *carotid angiography*.

If they present you with a clinical history consistent with a stroke, and also mention an **elevated lactate level** and **sensorineural deafness**; they are describing a patient with a **mitochondrial disorder**. Your differential in this case should include **MELAS**, the acronym for **Mitochondrial Encephalopathy, Lactic Acidosis, and Stroke-like Episodes**. Lucky for you, the name has all of the info you need to pick the right choice.

If they ask for the best diagnostic step to establish the underlying diagnosis, the answer will be molecular analysis of mitochondrial DNA. If you read the question carefully, you won't be tricked into picking head CT.

Neurodiagnostic Testing

Please note some of the indications for head imaging in the table below:

Diagnostic Test	Acuity Level	Indications
Head CT	Urgent	• Hemorrhage • Tumors • Abscesses
Head MRI	Non-urgent	• Partial seizures • Herpes encephalitis (confirmed by DNA PCR)
Head Ultrasound	Non-urgent	• Infants with accelerating head circumference across percentiles

Chapter 29

Skin Deep: Dermatology

The old summary of the field of Dermatology - "if it's dry, wet it; if it's wet, dry it; and if all else fails, use steroids" - could apply to any field in medicine.

There will be many dermatology questions that are not depicted as a picture. In these cases, you will need to recognize the disorder or symptoms of a larger disorder based on the key words in the clinical history. This is the focus of this chapter.

You will either have to recognize a typical rash based on the description or based on it's appearance in photo. Knowing the fine differences between similar rashes is the key to this section.

Neonatal Lesions

Neonatal Herpes

Neonatal herpes could be described as **clustered or grouped vesicles on an erythematous base.**

Lesions frequently appear on the **buttocks** or **scalp** since these are often the presenting parts closest to the maternal lesions. Watch for lesions that were **not present at birth** but appeared sometime in the first 3 weeks of life, and the mention in the question of the use of a **scalp pH monitor.**

Wright stain would contain multinucleated giant cells and eosinophilic intranuclear inclusions. Diagnosis is made by surface culture of conjunctiva, nasopharynx, mouth, rectum, blood, CSF, or skin vesicles or by PCR of blood or CSF.

IV acyclovir would be the treatment if this were **suspected**, even before confimation of diagnosis.

If they tell you the infant's mother has a history of herpes, they are probably trying to trick you. Most cases of neonatal herpes occur without a known history of maternal herpes.

Incontinentia pigmenti would also present as vesicles, but in a **linear pattern (along the lines of Blaschko) without an erythematous base.**

Transient Neonatal Pustular Melanosis

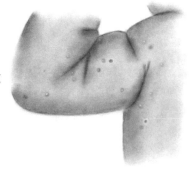

Multiple pustules, brown macules, vesicles, and pustules on a non-erythematous base. Another possible buzz word would be **"leaving a collarette"**. It is **present at birth** and is more common in **African American infants**.

No treatment is necessary. Think pustular "Leave-Em-Alone-osis".

If the rash starts out as pustules, they generally become **hyperpigmented macules** within a few days. Gram stain or Wright stain will show **PMNs or they may only say neutrophils without organisms**.

A **staph infection**, usually involving hair follicles, will reveal **both PMNs and gram-positive cocci** on gram stain.

Erythema Toxicum Neonatorum (ETN)

A very common rash that presents as **yellow pustules on an erythematous macule**, or possibly generalized erythmatous macules with solitary papules or vesicles in the center.

The rash is frequently **not present at birth** but appears within a few days of birth.

Wright stain will reveal eosinophils, which makes sense: ETN and Eosinophils both begin with the letter "E." Tzanck smear will also show eosinophils and perhaps some neutrophils, but otherwise it will be negative.

ETN does not appear on the palms or soles. In addition, it is rarely seen in preterm newborns. Remember that it is not present at birth — this is important in differentiating it from other newborn rashes, especially on the boards.

Mongolian Spots

Mongolian spots (dermal melanocytosis) are very common in dark skinned infants and would likely be a normal finding rather than bruising.

 If extensive, consider some Inborn Errors of Metabolism like GM1 Gangliosidosis and Hurler syndrome.

They could present a one-day-old infant with *erythematous macules* **with an** *occasional vesicle* **in the center. What is the most likely diagnosis?**

Well you might be tempted to pick herpes simplex by going for the decoy of the description of a vesicle.

However, the correct answer would be erythema toxicum, since this is a classical description. Remember a central vesicle in a macular lesion would be consistent with erythema toxicum.

Reassurance. No treatment is necessary and the rash will fade within the week.

Cutaneous Candidiasis

 Cutaneous candidiasis will present as **diffuse scaling** and **erythematous papules** and **pustules**.

The key point to diagnose cutaneous candidiasis is the presence of satellite lesions. It will usually occur in moist, warm areas, such as the diaper area or other areas with skin folds. The border will have a peripheral scale.

Candidiasis and contact dermatitis can both be seen in the diaper areas of infants. They will differ, however, in that contact dermatitis should not reach into deep inguinal folds as the diaper doesn't touch there. Diaper candidiasis will reach any and everywhere thanks to the appropriately named satellite lesions.

Dry and/or Scaly Skin

Atopic Dermatitis

"**Lichenification with scratching**" is a key phrase that tells you they are talking about atopic dermatitis. They could describe a distribution pattern **behind the knees** and **in the antecubital areas** with dry and chapped hands. **Itching is a crucial component of atopic dermatitis.** It is often referred to as "the itch that rashes."

Heredity plays a big role. If the family history is emphasized in the question, then they are pointing you to atopic dermatitis. The mention of **allergic rhinitis** and **asthma** are classic co-existing conditions. If both parents have any of these disorders, and if they should happen to mention a **high IgE** level in the cord blood, you have been given a gift. Unwrap it.

Factors that can worsen atopic dermatitis include allergens such as food, chemical irritants, heat, physical trauma, and drying elements.

Food Triggers

When presented with an infant with eczema, there is up to a 30% chance that food allergy is a factor. **Milk, eggs, soy, wheat, and peanuts** are likely culprits and the eczema will flare after eating this food.

Pulling Your Footing

If you are presented with patient who has a rash on the foot, it is very easy to slip up and immediately pick tinea pedis (or "athlete's foot," as it is called in the locker room).

 Tinea pedis will be described as a pruritic rash with scaling and peeling. It will involve the plantar aspect and sometimes the lateral aspect of the foot. However, the dorsal aspect will be spared. There will typically be maceration.

Atopic dermatitis *that involves the foot* will be scaly, but instead of maceration will be described as being dry, with lichenification. The dorsal aspect of the foot will be involved.

Juvenile plantar dermatosis - this spares the interdigital tissues

Pitted keratolysis - white clusters of punched out pits on the soles of the feet . They might also describe a very foul odor that might make you nauseated in the "pit" of your stomach!

PERIL Negative testing helps rule out a food allergy, but a positive result is not as diagnostic. Verification will require either a food challenge or skin testing.

HOT TIP Without allergy testing, **eliminating these foods is not usually recommended**, since food allergy is not a factor in up to 70% of cases of atopic dermatitis. Unnecessary food elimination is not recommended because of the potential negative impact on nutrition.

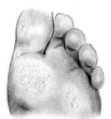 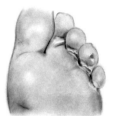

Pitted Keratolysis   **Tinea Pedis**

Superinfection

BUZZWORDS Watch for a description of **oozing and crusting**, in the context of eczema that is not responding to usual treatment modalities.

Just remember not to ever use the word "superinfection" when talking to a parent since they are likely to envision some Godzilla-like microbe that is unstoppable and will kill their baby and most of their family in days.

TREATMENT Treatment should be directed to *Staph aureus*.

Eczema Herpeticum

As the name implies, this is invasion of eczematous skin by herpes. If they describe **inflamed eczema which is not responding to steroids and antibiotics**, consider this diagnosis if it is among the choices.

BUZZWORDS The classic description will include the words **vesicles, punched out lesions** and **crusted erosions**. This often occurs on the face, in which case it is usually a primary herpes infection. As with (most) primary herpes infections, expect fever within 2-3 days and a child who seems rather uncomfortable. It is also seen in the occasional young child who sucks his/her thumb or finger.

TREATMENT Treatment is with **acyclovir**.

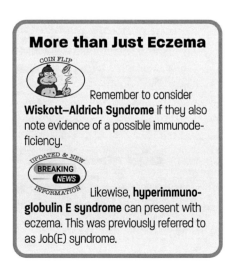

More than Just Eczema

COIN FLIP Remember to consider **Wiskott–Aldrich Syndrome** if they also note evidence of a possible immunodeficiency.

UPDATED & NEW **BREAKING NEWS** *INFORMATION* Likewise, **hyperimmunoglobulin E syndrome** can present with eczema. This was previously referred to as Job(E) syndrome.

Seborrheic Dermatitis

 This could be described as **greasy yellow patches** on the **scalp**[1], **face, behind the ears** and **in the skin folds** during the first few months of life.

 Treatment is with regular **antifungal washes** and **topical steroids**.

 If they include other features like profuse **ear discharge** and/or profuse **urine output**, then consider **Langerhans cell histiocytosis X**.

Eczema

By definition, eczema is a rash that involves **erythema, edema, vesicle formation, exudate, and scaling**.

Technically speaking, even though the two are used interchangeably by physicians, atopic dermatitis and eczema are not synonymous. Nummular eczema and contact dermatitis would be considered forms of **non-atopic eczema**.

Contact Dermatitis

Contact dermatitis is divided into two types: **allergic** and **primary irritant**.

Allergic contact dermatitis

This is a **delayed hypersensitivity** reaction that **requires multiple exposures**. It results in a rash, which is **red, vesicular,** and sometimes **crusting**.

Jewelry and **poison ivy** are typical examples.

Because it can require multiple exposures, they may try to trick you by stating that the child has "worn this necklace for years," etc. It can still be allergic contact dermatitis.

> ### Primary irritant contact dermatitis
>
> Here there is **no delay in reaction**. Soaps and detergents are typical agents that can trigger this reaction.

---

[1] Cradle Cap.

CASE STUDY You are presented with an 8-year-old girl who has a pruritic rash on the soles of her feet. Symptoms of the rash include minimal scaling, thickening of the skin, and hyper-linearity of the distal soles. The interdigital skin is normal. You have to choose the proper treatment.

THE DIVERSION It might be quite tempting to assume this is athlete's foot, or tinea pedis, and pick an anti-fungal cream such as clotrimazole or miconazole. But if you did that, you would have picked the wrong answer and the patient would still be picking at her feet.

ANSWER REVEALED The key to answering this question correctly is noting the minimal scaling and noting that the interdigital skin is not involved. In addition, athlete's foot rarely occurs before puberty. This rules out tinea. The description is of **juvenile plantar dermatosis**, which is a form of contact dermatitis. It is a result of occlusive shoes and synthetic socks. Appropriate treatment is with a steroid cream such as **triamcinolone**.

Poison Ivy (Toxicodendron radicans)

BUZZWORDS Poison ivy would typically be described as **linear vesicles and papules**.

MNEMONIC It is a Type 4 hypersensitivity reaction. This is easy to remember because "**IV**" is the Roman numeral for 4. Type 4 hypersensitivity reactions are **D**elayed, taking over 12 hours (or days) to begin occurring. **D** is the fourth letter of the alphabet.

HOT TIP The rash appears to spread, but in reality it's just the slower appearance of lesions in the areas that had a milder exposure. The rash may be limited by washing with soap and water immediately after exposure. In severe cases, oral steroids may be required for up to 21 days.

MYTH There are lots of myths around poison ivy that are ripe for diversionary tactics on the exam. Keeping the following facts in mind will be worth at least a point or two:

- Exposure to poison ivy during the winter **can** result in a rash, so can exposure to aerosolized poison ivy if someone is raking it up even a distance away.
- Fluid from the vesicles does not spread the rash. The rash is not contagious. Once the urushiol (oily resin from the plant which causes the allergic reaction) is washed off, there should be no further spreading of the rash.
- Barrier preparations can protect from exposure, but there are no desensitization treatments available.

Psoriasis (the Heartbreak of)

They could describe or show **silvery** lesions on the **elbows** or **knees**. When these silvery plaques are picked off, or come off, they leave behind "bleeding spots" the size of pins: this is called **Auspitz sign.** Typical buzzwords could include: **erythematous plaques surrounded by thick adherent scales, pinpoint areas of hemorrhage, and/or thick scales on the scalp.**

Psoriasis needs to be differentiated from rashes that can sound quite similar to it when described. If you pay close attention to the buzzwords, you will not be misled.

> ## Gutte Check!
>
> *Guttate psoriasis* is a form of psoriasis which usually occurs after strep infection and is spread more diffusely on the trunk and extremities.
>
> *Guttate* is latin for "drop", so *guttate psoriasis* looks like rain drops over the body. Treatment is the same as regular psoriasis, start with topical steroids.

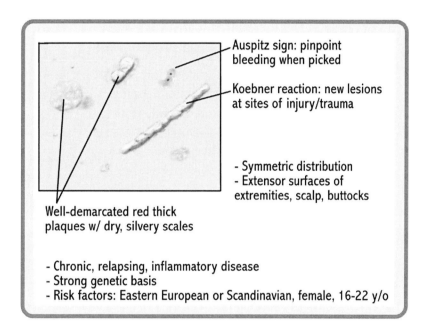

Auspitz sign: pinpoint bleeding when picked

Koebner reaction: new lesions at sites of injury/trauma

- Symmetric distribution
- Extensor surfaces of extremities, scalp, buttocks

Well-demarcated red thick plaques w/ dry, silvery scales

- Chronic, relapsing, inflammatory disease
- Strong genetic basis
- Risk factors: Eastern European or Scandinavian, female, 16-22 y/o

Pityriasis Rosea (PR)

Look for **small oval scaling patches of rash on the trunk and back** and the classic **herald patch** in a **Christmas tree pattern** with the **long axis of the lesions parallel to the lines of skin stress (you knew that already).**

Treatment is not necessary, but **exposure to the sun or other light** improves symptoms and may hasten resolution.

This is easy to remember when you think of "Christmas lights," and link that to the Christmas tree pattern of the rash, and "Hark the Herald (patch) Angels Sing" while you're at it!

Pityriasis can be confused with, and must be distinguished from, the following other rashes:

- **Secondary Syphilis** – The rash may appear similar, but patients with secondary syphilis will also present with **fever** and **generalized lymphadenopathy.** Secondary syphilis often **involves the palms** and **soles but PR does not.**

- **Tinea corporis** and **Ptyriasis (formerly tinea) versicolor**

- **Nummular eczema** and **tinea corporis** – The herald patch can be confused with these two other rashes. So keep in mind that tinea corporis will be described as having an **elevated border with central clearing.** Nummular eczema will be described as **crusting erosions,** which will distinguish it from the herald patch of pityriasis rosea.

- **Tinea versicolor aka pityriasis versicolor** – may mimic pityriasis because of a similar distribution on the trunk and back. This rash, rather than being described as plaques, will be described as **hyper- or hypo- pigmented scaling macules.** Other buzz words associated with versicolor: Malassezia furfur or globosa, spaghetti and meatballs (the fungal hyphae and spores on microscopy), and fluorescence on Wood's lamp.

- **Tinea incognito** – this is actually tinea corporis that has been (mis)treated with steroids so now is unrecognizable, like an individual in the Witness Protection Program.

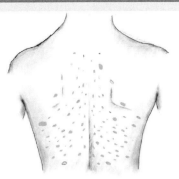

"Christmas tree" pattern on back

- Oval lesions oriented along dermal lines
- Lesions may be macular, raised, or scaly

- "Herald patch"
--Signals onset, appearing on trunk/thigh
--Large, isolated, salmon-colored, scaly
--Often mistaken for tinea corporis

Come One, Come All!

You might see a single oval lesion and diagnose *tinea corporis.* You could be given a history of a patient returning and stating the cream did not work and the rash "spread" all over his back.

Now you might say, "My bad, that was actually the herald patch of PR." This could be an easy slam dunk on the exam.

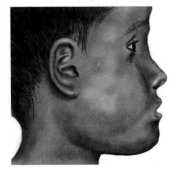

Pityriasis Alba

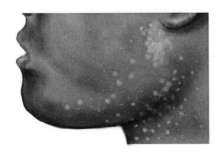

Tinea Versicolor

Granuloma Annulare (GA)

 GA is a benign inflammatory condition that manifests as **non-scaling annular lesions without epidermal involvement**.

We really don't know what causes it.

 The key phrase is **non-scaling**.

 Swimming pool granuloma (a papule caused by atypical mycobacteria and found on the sole of a child who likes walking barefoot) presents with a break in the skin; with **granuloma annulare** the skin will be <u>intact</u>.

Skin Infections

Impetigo

This can be caused by *Strep* or *Staph*. However, you are expected to know that *Staph aureus* is the most likely cause of both bullous impetigo and crusted impetigo.

 Treatment is with mupirocin ointment for localized lesions. For more extensive/widespread areas, oral antibiotics targeting *Staph* and *Strep* are recommended (Cephalexin, clindamycin, amoxicillin-clavulanate).

 Treatment of the Strep skin infection **does not prevent post-strep GN**.

Cellulitis

Cellulitis requires 4 key elements

1. **red**
2. **hot**
3. **tender**
4. **swollen**

The most common causes are ***Strep pyogenes* aka Group A *Strep*** (GAS) and ***Staph aureus***.

Treatment will depend on several factors as follows:

- Cephalexin or amoxicillin-clavulanate may be used empirically if there is low likelihood of MRSA.
- If the cellulitis is more advanced or if they note that MRSA is prevalent in the community, then clindamycin, trimethoprim-sulfamethoxazole, or doxycycline (in a child older than 8) would be indicated.

Toxic Dumps

The following are caused by **toxin-producing bacteria**:

Staph Scalded Skin Syndrome	Due to an exotoxin produced by *Staph aureus*
Toxic Shock Syndrome	Caused by toxin production either by *S. aureus* or *Strep*; the mortality of *Strep* TSS is much higher than *Staph* TSS
Scarlet Fever	Also due to a toxin caused by *Strep*

Skin Conditions that can "Burn" you

You will need to know about several skin conditions that are easily confused with each other. Here are the distinguishing points of each.

Staphylococcal Scalded Skin Syndrome (SSSS)

This is typically described in a preschooler. It starts out **very tender and red**, and spreads to become a **sheet-like loss of skin**.

The exotoxins (exfoliatoxin A &B) cleave desmosomes (the protein which attaches neighboring skin cells) resulting in blisters, Nikolsy sign, and eventual skin peeling.

A **toxin** causes all of this, and **antibiotics** are the treatment of choice.

They may throw in earlier treatment with an antibiotic to lead you into thinking it is erythema multiforme.

Erythema Multiforme

Erythema multiforme is **a hypersensitivity reaction** in response to a variety of triggers. There are two forms: erythema multiforme minor and major.

Erythema Multiforme Minor

Rarely will a child younger than 3 present with erythema multiforme minor. The most likely trigger will be a primary or recurrent infection with **Herpes Simplex** but **medications** may also cause it. The rash appears abruptly on the **extremities** and then spreads to the trunk.

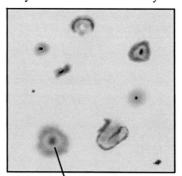

Erythema Multiforme Major

Pathognomonic target lesion

©Medhumor Medical Publications, LLC

Mycoplasma pneumoniae is another common cause of EM.

Treatment is geared toward the triggering agent, i.e., stopping the medication or treating the infection.

CASE STUDY **You could be presented with a child who, after completing an antibiotic regimen, develops a rash on the distal extremities described as "maculo–papular, with some lesions appearing to be *dusky* in the center." There may be 1-2 lesions on the mouth. The child is otherwise well *appearing*. What is the diagnosis?**

THE DIVERSION Well, with what sound like target lesions, 1-2 lesions appearing on the mouth, and a recent course of antibiotics, you might be tempted to pick erythema multiforme major, or Stevens Johnson syndrome.

ANSWER REVEALED However, the description given in this vignette (especially the fact that the child is *well appearing*) makes the correct diagnosis erythema multiforme minor, not major.

Stevens Johnson Syndrome

SJS typically involves <10% of the body surface area.

BUZZWORDS With Stevens Johnson Syndrome, the rash is preceded by **fever, muscle aches,** and **joint aches**. Initially the rash is similar to EM minor with bullous or target lesions which sometimes coalesce, but it **spreads more quickly**, progressing from primarily cutaneous to **mucous membrane involvement,** including **conjunctiva, oral mucosa, and anogenital mucosa**. The lesions involving the mucosa frequently become **encrusted**.

UPDATED & NEW BREAKING NEWS INFORMATION Previously EM, SJS, and TEN were thought to be a spectrum of diseases. More recently, however, the three can be differentiated in that EM will have typical target lesions, will likely be post-infections. SJS and TEN are typically thought to be more often related to a drug-induced process with high morbidity. SJS and TEN will always have mucosal involvement.

Typical medications triggering SJS are **sulfa drugs, anticonvulsants,** and **NSAIDs**.

TREATMENT Treatment begins with stopping the offending agent then is geared toward preventing dehydration and superinfection, and patients are frequently managed in burn units.

There is no separation of the skin in sheets as there is in scalded skin syndrome.

Toxic Epidermal Necrolysis (TEN)

TEN involves >30% cutaneous involvement.

Here, too, the **sunburn-like erythema** and **sheet-like separation of skin** can be seen. In addition to the lesions described above, one would see **widespread bullae** as well as **denuded necrotic skin.**

If they ask you how to distinguish scalded skin syndrome from TEN, the answer is biopsy. That is because **TEN involves the dermis (as does Stevens Johnson) and SSSS is high in the epidermis.** SSSS usually affects infants and younger children, whereas TEN involves older children. Mortality is much higher for TEN than for SSSS.

Toxic epidermal necrolysis (TEN) is **not** due to a toxin despite its name. It is a hypersensitivity reaction.

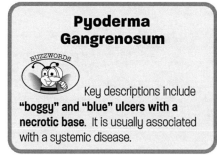

Pyoderma Gangrenosum

Key descriptions include **"boggy" and "blue" ulcers with a necrotic base**. It is usually associated with a systemic disease.

Toxic Shock Syndrome

Toxic Shock Syndrome presents with **fevers, hypotension,** and **rash**. Any kid who comes in with a **sepsis-like picture and a rash** should make you consider TSS. These patients will have erythroderma, or diffuse reddening of the skin.

Even though tampons do NOT cause most cases of TSS anymore, they may imply its use in the question (e.g., by noting the Tanner staging in an adolescent girl in septic shock) or her recent menstrual cycle.

Treatment is with **antibiotics** and **aggressive supportive care.**

Erythema Confusiosum

I always had a hard time keeping my "erythema" rashes straight. Apparently I am not alone, and this may cause confusion on the exam if all of the "erythemas" are included among the choices.

Whenever I see the word "**erythema**" *fill in the blank* "—**osum**," my eyes glaze over and everything tends to jumble together. Here is our primer for keeping it straight, so the words or pictures that go with them won't confuse you.

Erythema Multiforme

This is the one associated with Stevens Johnson syndrome. I picture Steve Johnson as someone with a BIG MOUTH who can get oral lesions, thus **Multi ORAL forme** (and that reminds me that other mucous membranes can be involved as well, e.g., anal and genital area). The **foot can also be involved**: with his big mouth, he is always **placing his foot in his mouth**. It starts with fever and other general symptoms.

Erythema Infectiosum

This is **"Fifth Disease:"** slapped cheek. Picture a giant red 5 on the face, which follows an "infection." This will be associated with Parvovirus B19. (Remember, Parvo has a **V** in it, which is the Roman numeral 5, for 5th Disease).

Erythema Chronicum Migrans

Erythema chronicum migrans (ECM) is associated with Lyme disease.

Here Lyme disease is seen as a **"CAN"**:

> **C**arditis
> **A**rthritis
> **N**euritis

The CAN "migrates all over the woods," thus chronicum migrans. The classic bullseye rash is present in 70% of cases.

Erythema Nodosum (No Doze em)

Erythema nodosum causes painful bluish lesions on the shin. (Thus, **No Doze,** because you can't sleep with painful shins). This is associated with TB, birth control pills, inflammatory bowel disease, and fungal infections.

At least one third of cases are idiopathic. And most cases of EN are self-limited, requiring only symptomatic treatment with NSAIDs.

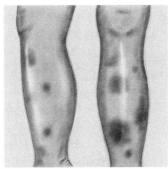

Erythema Nodosum

Erythema Marginatum

This is associated with **rheumatic fever,** and is one of the major Jones criteria. It is an erythematous macule on the trunk, which clears centrally.

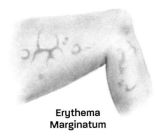

Erythema Marginatum

Pests of Life

Scabies

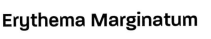

The key descriptors are intensely pruritic **linear lesions** that are **papular** or **pustular**. They will classically note **burrows which are pathognomonic** and **involvement between the digits.**

Classic scabies has burrows, is **highly contagious** and affects other family members, although other family members with lower host responses may not develop the intense reaction the index patient did and may be missed.

Diagnosis is usually clinical, but can be confirmed by identifying mites and eggs in skin scrapings.

Scabies is treated with **permethrin 5% cream (Elimite®)** applied and left overnight and washed off in the morning. All household contacts must be treated as well.

A second treatment one week later is recommended for the eggs. The itching may persist for weeks after the initial treatment and require topical steroids for symptomatic relief. Linen and clothing used in the prior 3 days should be washed in hot water.

You could be asked why the patients are still having symptoms despite adequate treatment. Your choices may be that they did not leave on the initial treatment long enough, they never did the second treatment a week later, or they're just having a hypersensitivity reaction to the dead mites and their excrement.

Scabies in **infants** can appear on the **scalp** as well as the **palms and soles**.

Head Lice

Head lice will typically be described in 1-2 children in the same family, with **intense scalp itching** and with **excoriation** on the nape of the neck and/or behind the ears. They will describe nits on the hair shafts as **white dots that cannot be removed.** Don't expect them to mention that classmates were diagnosed; that would be too easy. [2]

The primary treatment consists of **permethrin cream rinse,** which should be **repeated** a week after the first application. The house should be thoroughly cleaned, and **close household contacts should be treated** as a preventive measure. Asymptomatic classmates do not need to be treated.

Many areas of the country have lice **resistant to permethrin.** Know that there are many $300 alternatives to try if this appears to be the case, but first make sure they used the permethrin appropriately.

Even after successful treatment, itching can continue. This does not constitute treatment failure. **It represents an inflammatory reaction, and this can be treated with steroid creams.** Severe itching may also be helped with diphenhydramine or hydroxyzine.

Those Amazing Lice

Facts about lice you might actually be expected to know:

- They can last 36 hours without a blood meal
- Fresh eggs on hair shafts can hatch 10 days later
- Despite their name, pubic lice can also exist in other locations, such as on facial hair[4]
- Pubic lice are much slower moving than head lice
- Pubic lice impact all races equally, while head lice rarely infest African-Americans.

Pertinent Points about Permethrin

Whether you are treating scabies, head lice, or pubic lice a key part of therapy involves a **second treatment** with permethrin one week after the first.

---

[2] Insert your own inappropriate or perverse joke here.

HOT TIP

Do not fall for any answer that includes "nits must be removed before kids can return to school". This is not correct, especially on the boards!

Head Lice vs. Crabs

COIN FLIP

While head lice are common in children, pubic crab lice are not. **Pubic lice is strongly suggestive of sexual abuse.**

BUZZWORDS

If they describe **maculae ceruleae (which are blue-gray macules on the abdomen or inner thigh)**, this is a clinical sign consistent with pubic lice.

TREATMENT

Treatment of choice for pubic lice is the same as head lice: permethrin.

HOT TIP

For crabs in the eyelashes, **petroleum jelly** applied three times a day for 10 days is often sufficient treatment.

Other Papular Rashes

Molluscum Contagiosum

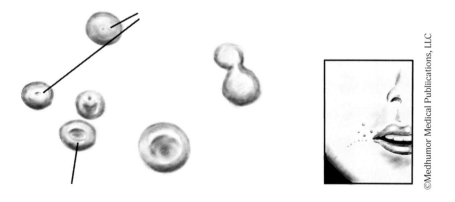

©Medhumor Medical Publications, LLC

BUZZWORDS

If they show or describe **pearly "pink or flesh-colored" papules with central dimpling**, think of molluscum contagiosum.

TREATMENT

No therapy is needed; it will clear in months to years.

Molluscum is differentiated from warts and comedones by the **central umbilication**. In addition, Wright staining will reveal **viral inclusion bodies**.

Molluscum Contagiosum is caused by the Molluscum contagiosum virus from the Pox family.

Papular Urticaria

Here they could describe or show **pink and excoriated pruritic lesions** on the **extensor surfaces** of the arms and legs. They are frequently described as **clustered erythematous papules** with a **central punctum that recur episodically, often at night, and may last up to 10 days.**

 No other family members are affected, differentiating this from scabies.

 Papular urticaria is due to **a delayed hypersensitivity reaction to an insect bite**.

Don't expect them to trace it to an individual insect bite or suggest the history of one. They won't. However, the correct answer for the best management is to **identify the causative agent** (so the family can then go about the business of eliminating the causative agent).

 They could present you with a toddler who has a 2 month history of a recurrent pruritic rash of clustered erythematous papules. They focus on the recurrent rash and its pruritic quality and throw in that "nobody else in the family is similarly affected."

It will be very tempting to pick the diversionary choice, scabies, chalking up the absence of symptoms in other family members as a deliberate attempt to throw you off track. After all, haven't we all seen cases of scabies where only one family member is affected, at least on initial history? Resist all temptations to scratch that irresistible itch, since this is the boards and no history means <u>no</u> history.

The correct diagnosis is papular urticaria.

Acne Vulgaris[3]

Sebum is produced by the sebaceous glands in response to **androgen production**, which is the case in **both males and females**.

This is the perfect environment for proliferation of the archenemy of teenagers everywhere: *Propionibacterium acnes*. And where there are bacteria proliferating, there come WBCs to fight the good fight, which leads to pustules and inflammation.

Acne vulgaris is divided into 2 major categories, which have additional subcategories. It is important to note these, since treatment is different and will separate the "haves" (passing grade) from the "have nots" (those taking the exam again). Let's go to the blackboard vulgaris.

Acne is divided into inflammatory and non-inflammatory and it is important to note that acne correlates with pubertal stage.

Non-inflammatory

Non-inflammatory obstructive lesions (comedones) are seen.

Closed Comedones

Closed comedones are "**whiteheads**", which are follicles that are covered with epithelium.

Open Comedones

Open comedones are "**blackheads,**" which have no epithelial covering.

The black color comes from oxidation of melanin, not dirt (which is a common misconception). This, like any myth, can come back to haunt you during the exam.

The appearance of comedones prior to age 8 could be a sign of **precocious puberty**. If this is presented to you on the exam, routine management of acne may not be what they are after.

Inflammatory Acne (the good, the bad, and the papule)

These are seen later in puberty and consist of erythematous papules, pustules, and nodules (cysts)

Papules

Papules are small, red, solid lesions.

Adenoma sebaceum can be mistaken for acne. If "acne" is placed in quotes, then you are likely being presented with adenoma sebaceum, which are also known as **angiofibromas**. These are small papules that are firm and may appear pink, red, or brown (or somewhere in between) in color.

---

[3] I believe this is Latin for nasty.

This is especially the case with "acne" that is resistant to treatment, often on the nose and cheeks.

 Adenoma sebaceum should have you thinking about Tuberous Sclerosis.

Pustules

 Pustules are superficial, <5 mm, and are filled with pus.

Nodules (cysts)

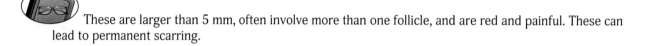 These are larger than 5 mm, often involve more than one follicle, and are red and painful. These can lead to permanent scarring.

Systemic steroids can lead to acne. This appears primarily on the trunk, and they would have to give a history of a disorder where systemic steroids would be used (in order to point you in this direction). **Anticonvulsants** such as phenobarbital and phenytoin (Dilantin®) can lead to acne as well.

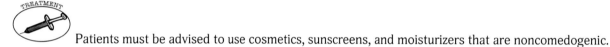 Patients must be advised to use cosmetics, sunscreens, and moisturizers that are noncomedogenic.

Patients must be made aware that, regardless of choice of therapy, treatment of acne will be a long term process requiring at least 6-8 weeks before initial improvement is seen.

Acne is not caused by poor hygiene or improper bathing habits. For psychological reasons they expect you to know that teens need to be reassured that this is a normal part of growth and development. Chocolate does not cause or accelerate acne, despite popular belief.

Vigorous scrubbing and squeezing of pimples can lead to permanent scarring.

Neonatal acne requires no treatment.

Salicylic Acid

 Salicylic acid reduces the formation of obstructive lesions and therefore is good for comedonal acne.

It is less irritating than the tretinoins but it is also less effective.

The wash is also good for large areas with acne, such as the chest and back.

Benzoyl peroxide

Benzoyl peroxide is primarily **bactericidal** and used mostly for controlling inflammatory acne but may be used for comedonal acne as well. Because it can prevent the emergence of antibiotic resistance among *P. acnes*, it may be used in patients on antibiotic therapy. It can be irritating to the skin, but this can be reduced if the right formulation is used.

Benzoyl peroxide may not be applied at the same time as tretinoin because then tretinoin will not work.

Topical antibiotics

Topical antibiotics, in addition to being **bactericidal**, are also **anti-inflammatory** so clearly these are great for treating inflammatory acne.

Tretinoin

Tretinoin, derived from vitamin A, can play an important role in **preventing acne** by halting the process that plugs hair follicles. This is therefore the best treatment for noninflammatory (comedonal) acne.

Topical tretinoin can result in an "initial flare-up" of acne 2-3 weeks after treatent is begun. Unlike isotretinoin, there have been no reports of malformations in infants of women who have used tretinoin during pregnancy.

Oral Antibiotics

Like topical antibiotics, oral antibiotics have **anti-inflammatory qualities**. The use of oral antibiotics is reserved for **moderate to severe inflammatory acne**. It is particularly effective against acne on the trunk. The most commonly used oral antibiotics are **tetracycline** (unless pregnant or under age 9)**, doxycycline,** and **minocycline**.

Bacterial resistance is a problem, and therefore continued use would not be appropriate. The condition can be controlled, but oral antibiotics do not "cure" acne.

Patients on OCPs who start oral antibiotics must be counseled to use back up contraception because of a theoretical decrease in efficacy of the OCPs.

Oral Contraceptives

Because of the anti-androgenergic effects combined oral contraceptives containing both estrogen and progestin may improve acne.

This of course should only be used in female patients. Therefore, check the gender of the patient in the question. Picking OCPs for males would be a careless, costly error indeed.

Long acting progestin implants and depot medroxyprogresterone may worsen acne.

Isotretinoin (Accutane®)

This powerful agent does it all:

- Antibacterial
- Reduces sebum production
- Anti-inflammatory
- Destroys comedones
- Some have claimed it even clears the cache on your computer and blocks spyware.

Isotretinoin is now used often in combination therapy (often alongside benzoyl peroxide), especially in patients with with multiple inflammatory lesions (since it helps reduce the formation of new lesions).

Check the wording of the question to see if there is a history of steroid use. This can sometimes worsen symptoms when taken at the same time. Remember to "rule out pregnancy" when Isotretinoin (Accutane®) is prescribed. **Pregnancy should be ruled out before, during, and after treatment.**

Side effects to be aware of include: dry lips, dry skin, dry eyes, nosebleeds, and headaches.[4] Rarer side effects may include elevated triglycerides or liver enzymes.

Alopecia Hairpecia

You need to identify different hair loss patterns. This is Pediatrics, so unless the question is about the funny Canadian on *Whose Line is it Anyway*, "male pattern baldness" will not be one of the correct choices. There are only a limited number of alopecia patterns you need to know.

Tinea Capitis

Black dots or **broken hairs** are common descriptors. Additional descriptions would include **kerions**, which are tender boggy areas of induration. **Fungal culture** is the gold standard for diagnosis. Tinea capitus will often have associated **occipital adenopathy**.

The treatment of choice is **oral griseofulvin** for 6-12 weeks. If alternatives like **fluconazole, itraconazole,** and **terbinafine** are listed, they are also acceptable.

Routine labs prior to using griseofulvin are *not* necessary.

Tinea Capitis

Annular lesions

Widespread breakage at scalp

Small patches of erythema or scaling

Salt-and-pepper appearance

Bye Bye Ketoconazole

UPDATED & NEW
BREAKING NEWS
INFORMATION Oral ketoconazole should no longer be prescribed for any dermatomycosis because of the risk of hepatotoxicity.

---

[4] Similar to the side effects of studying for the Boards in dry, poorly aerated rooms.

Alopecia Areata

This is easy to pick out because there will be **no inflammation** described or shown. The cause of alopecia areata is unknown. The hair follicles of alopecia areata may be described as an exclamation point with a narrow base and normal upper shaft!

Alopecia Areata

Patches of complete hair loss — Normal scalp

Short, easily-pulled hairs at margins

Nail pitting can be seen in patients with alopecia areata.

CASE STUDY

You are asked to evaluate a child with areas of "complete hair loss," with no scalp lesions noted. Other than the alopecia just described and nail pitting, the rest of the physical exam is negative. The hair is tightly braided. What is the most likely diagnosis and treatment?

THE DIVERSION

You will be very tempted to pick "hair braid alopecia" (aka traction alopecia) as the diagnosis and "unbraid the hair" as the correct treatment. If you do, you will be pulling your own hair out, because you just blew another easy question.

ANSWER REVEALED

The correct answer, especially given the nail pitting, would be alopecia areata, and the management would simply be reassurance. If your reassurance doesn't cure it, the next step would be corticosteroids.

Telogen Effluvium

DEFINITION

This is the **sudden loss of large amounts of hair** during routine activities such as washing and brushing the hair. It is often triggered by **stressful events** like a febrile illness, surgery, or emotional stress.[5]

BUZZWORDS

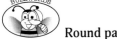

Round patches, **well defined**, and **complete areas of hair loss** are your buzzwords.

COIN FLIP

This is distinguished from other forms of hair loss in that there is no inflammatory reaction and the "telogen bulbs" can be seen under shedded hairs on microscopic exam.

Traction Alopecia

DEFINITION

This hair loss is caused by tight pulling, like hair in braids, or by **trichotillomania** (a habit of pulling on one's own hair).

---

[5] Might be the explanation for any hair loss you may be currently experiencing.

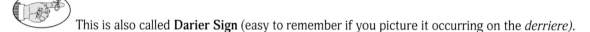

Irregular patches of hair loss or **incomplete patches of hair loss** may be described. **Hair shafts of different lengths** is an important characteristic they might include, which would differentiate this from other forms of alopecia.

Mastocytosis

Mastocytosis refers to a group of **non-inherited disorders** with excess mast cell degranulation and mast cell accumulation in various tissues.

Urticaria Pigmentosa

This is the most common form of mastocytosis.

They may present this to you as mastocytomas, **pigmented lesions usually red-brown in color that flush or turn into hives** and develop **blisters,** particularly with rubbing or scratching. It is typically described in an infant during the first 6 months of life.

This is also called **Darier Sign** (easy to remember if you picture it occurring on the *derriere).*

This is **pathognomonic for the presence of mast cells within the lesion** but don't try this in the office because it may trigger a generalized flush and urticarial attack!

Other than antihistamines to reduce itching, no treatment is needed.

However, if they ask, these infants should **avoid narcotic pain relievers, radiocontrast material, and NSAIDs.**

Histiocytosis syndromes

Langerhans Cell Histiocytosis

Langerhans cell histiocytosis (LCH, formerly Histiocytosis X) has several typical features that will be included in the presenting history. Once these features are committed to memory, the answer will jump out while you are reading the question.

Patients may present with:

❑ Persistent scalp or diaper seborrheic rash
❑ Chronic ear drainage or chronic mastoiditis

❑ Lytic lesions in the skull or vertebral collapse

❑ Excessive urination[6]

LCH is diagnosed by **skin biopsy** and **electron microscopy** which will show tennis racket-shaped "Birbeck granules".

Pigmentation Variations

Pityriasis Versicolor[7]

The classic description is **hypopigmented patches** that get **worse with exposure to the sun**. A **fungus** causes it, and **KOH prep** confirms the diagnosis.

Treatment is with **astringents** (to strip the superficial layers that are primarily involved) or **topical antifungal creams**. It can take a few months of sun deprivation to get rid of it. This is mortifying news for sun worshipping coastal teens.

Fluconazole, and itraconazole are also considered appropriate in certain situations and could be the correct answer they are looking for. **Topical selenium sulfide** is also acceptable.

Look at both Pityriasis versicolor and ash leaf spots side by side in your atlas and know the distinguishing characteristics. With ash leaf, they will very likely include the other characteristics of tuberous sclerosis. Versicolor will fluoresce with Wood's lamp.

Incontinentia Pigmenti

This is an **X-linked dominant condition** that is usually **lethal in males**.

The skin lesions present in 4 stages:

1. Erythematous papules and vesicles in crops **along the lines of Blaschko** that last 1-2 weeks.
2. Then come **swirls of warty growths**.
3. Then come streaks of **hyperpigmentation** in a **marble cake pattern**.
4. And finally **hypopigmentation** sets in.

Kind of catchy don't you think... Blaschko crops... warty growths... marble cake... fade away. Okay, maybe not.

---

[6] Both from diabetes insipidus and from pituitary involvement.

[7] Yes another thing that has changed, no longer known by its former name Tinea versicolor.

Vitiligo

An acquired **autoimmune destruction of melanocytes** leading to **depigmentation**. The exact cause is unknown but appears to have a genetic component.

Treatment includes **topical steroids** and **tacrolimus/ pimecrolimus**. Most cases are slowly progressive, but some exhibit spontaneous repigmentation.

Pityriasis alba

Post-inflammatory hypopigmentation seen in atopic skin.

Pityriasis alba will have **hypopigmentation**, but vitiligo will have **complete depigmentation**.

Neurocutaneous Syndromes

Sturge Weber

Characteristics could be associated with Mikhail Gorbachev of the old Soviet empire.

- ❏ Port wine stain (aka "nevus flammeus") in a trigeminal distribution
- ❏ Developmental delay (former Soviet Union)
- ❏ Seizure (of power)
- ❏ Hemiplegia (half as powerful as before)
- ❏ Vision problems/calcification/glaucoma

Glaucoma occurs on the same side as the port wine stain. The **focal seizures** occur on the contralateral side.

The port wine stain is often associated with a **venous leptomeningeal angiomatosis,** which needs to be identified by **MRI.**

The size of the port wine stain **does not correlate** with the extent of CNS involvement of the lesion. In fact, **one can have a venous leptomeningeal angiomatosis even when there is no skin lesion.**

The port wine stain itself is merely a cosmetic concern and can be treated by **tunable dye (pulsed dye) laser.**

Genodermatoses

Genodermatoses are inherited single-gene disorders with skin manifestations. They include:

- Neurofibromatosis
- Ataxia telangiectasia
- Incontinentia pigmenti
- Gardner syndrome
- Peutz-Jeghers
- Xeroderma pigmentosum
- Epidermolysis bullosa

Klippel Trenaunay Weber syndrome can also present with a port wine stain. However, the associated features are quite different.

Only 8% of those with a facial port wine stain lesions have Sturge Weber syndrome. Clearly, this is higher if the port-wine stain is distributed along the **branches of the trigeminal nerve** and those children require and **immediate referral to Ophthalmology**.

Neurofibromatosis

Neurofibromatosis is a disorder with skin, CNS, and orthopedic manifestations. There are two types - think of Type 1 as more peripheral and mild, and Type 2 as central.[8]

Neurofibromatosis Type 1: Von Recklinghausen Disease

Like a mix and match menu, two (2) of the following seven (7) criteria make the diagnosis of NF1:

❑ Café au Lait Spots (6 or more, which may appear after birth).
The spots must be >5 mm wide in kids >15 mm post pubertal

❑ Lisch Nodules (2 or more) (iris hamartomas[9] – which may not show up until adulthood[10] and can only be seen on slit-lamp exam)

❑ Neurofibromas (typically do not show up until after the onset of puberty)

❑ Optic Nerve Glioma

❑ Inguinal and Axillary Freckling (Crowe sign)

❑ Tibial pseudoarthrosis

❑ Family History of NF1 (first-degree relative)

Remember, **2 out of 7 makes the diagnosis**. However, for patients with a single clinical finding, there is a genetic test that can be confirmatory. But the mainstay of diagnosis remains clinical.

Remember this is **autosomal dominant on chromosome 17**, and an affected parent has a 50% chance of transmitting this to any one child. The other 50% of cases are due to spontaneous mutation.

You might remember that NF 1 is on Chromosome 17 from Step 1 studying because "Von Recklinghausen" has 17 letters. But that would also require you remember how to spell Von Recklinghausen!

Despite the name, **neurofibromas** have nothing to do with the brain;[11] they are skin lesions that appear either on the surface (and are easily seen) or deep in the skin (and can only be found by palpation).

---

[8] In fact, Type 2 is also sometimes known as central neurofibromatosis because of the higher incidence of meningiomas and acoustic neuromas.
[9] Remember Iris is an "old" name, so these do not show up until adulthood.
[10] You can remember this because Iris is an old fashioned name
[11] You, of course, knew that already, right?

Kids with NF1 can get **pheochromocytoma** and **renal artery stenosis,** and need to be monitored often for **hypertension**. This is a concept that can be tested on the exam.

Change neurofibromatosis to **"Nero Finds a Toaster"** which rhymes with "Neurofibromatosis".[12]

❑ Picture Nero in a giant toga. He is playing the fiddle and drinking 6 cups of coffee
    (**Café au Lait Spots).**
❑ The reason he can do so much at once is that he has bones shaped like giant platters
    (**Bony Defects).**
❑ He keeps playing and he can't see the fire because he has an **Optic Glioma.**
❑ Everyone leaves and the fire rages, working its way up so his skin begins to burn
    (beginning with **axillary freckling).**
❑ The freckles get bigger and bigger until they look like "Fish Nodules" – to remind you of
    "Lisch Nodules." These fish are zoological wonders since their bodies are giant eyeballs
    (to remind you that **Lisch nodules occur in the eye**).
❑ This "Hot" situation is how Nero finds a "toaster."

Look this over 5 times, writing it down (some of you might like to draw this to help keep this in long-term memory), and you will have this association locked in. Even though this is a bit convoluted it is more efficient than rote memory.

Neurofibromatosis Type 2

Remember, this is the subtype with the **acoustic neuroma**, also known as **schwannoma**.

One way to remember this is by imagining the **N** in Neuroma as the number **2** on its side. It is also associated with **chromosome 22**.

Patients usually present with **hearing loss** or **tinnitus** related to their acoustic neuromas. However, **ocular symptoms** may dominate due to **cataracts** or **hamartomas of the retina**.

Remember that **NF2** is associated with **chromosome 22** and gives you trouble with your **2 eyes** and your **2 ears**. You can imagine giant #2s replacing your eyes and ears if that helps.

Definitive diagnosis can be made by bilateral cranial nerve VIII masses on **CT or MRI**.

---

[12] Nero, the Roman leader who played the fiddle while Rome burned.

Tuberous Sclerosis

I like to think of this as the "potato" disease since potatoes are tubers (which is how this was named in the first place).

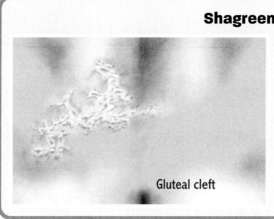

Shagreen Patch

The drawing depicts the shagreen patch associated with tuberous sclerosis

The features include the following:

- Firm yellowish-red or pink area of nodules

- Orange peel or cobblestone texture

- In patients with tuberous sclerosis the shagreen patch is nearly always found on or around the lumbar region of back

Gluteal cleft

Once again, we use a mix and match menu, which is why there is often confusion with the other neurocutaneous syndromes.

Diagnosis is made by the presence of **two (2) or more** of the following features:

- ❏ More than 3 **Ash Leaf Spots**
- ❏ **Periventricular/Cortical Tubers**
- ❏ **Sebaceous Gland Hyperplasia**
- ❏ **Shagreen Patch**
- ❏ **Sub/periungual Fibroma**
- ❏ **Cardiac Rhabdomyoma** –
   will develop in half the cases – especially seen in infants
- ❏ **Retinal nodular hamartomas**
- ❏ **Renal angiomyolipoma**

PERIL

The adenoma sebaceum can often be mistaken for acne (vulgaris) and they will try to trip you up with that. Therefore, look for tuberous sclerosis hints in the question.

Leather and Leafs

It is important to remember the typical findings, since they will be described or shown on the exam and their more formal terms will not be used.

Ash Leaf Spots – Hypopigmented skin (as in "ash" colored), also known as hypomelanotic macule. This is often the earliest sign but may not be visible without a Wood's lamp.

Sebaceous Gland Hyperplasia These are really adenomas, and is usually described or shown on the face.

Shagreen Patch – Cobblestone appearing skin; shagreen is actually a type of leather that has an orange peel appearance. It would have been infinitely less confusing had they called it an orange peel patch, but confusion, not clarification, seems to be the order of the day

Periventricular/Cortical Tubers – These typically present and manifest as seizures.

Ectodermal Dysplasia (ED)[13]

DEFINITION

A group of **inherited** disorders that involve developmental abnormalities of the **skin** as well as the **teeth, nails, hair** and **sweat glands**.

Ectodermal dysplasia

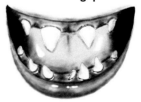

- Peg-shaped, pointed, or missing teeth
- Defective enamel
- Dentures as early as two years of age

---

[13] Not to be confused with Erectile Dysfunction ED.

Epidermolysis bullosa (EB)

A group of **inherited** disorders that manifest as epithelial fragility.

Suspect EB in infants and children presenting with **recurrent blistering of the skin and mucosa after minor trauma** as well as **nail changes**.

ED and EB both involve the skin and nails.

Ectodermal dysplasia is developmental; it presents as bad skin, teeth, and nails and they stay bad.

Epidermolysis bullosa starts out normal and blisters on and off until the skin, nails, and mucosa scar.

Hemangiomas

A hemangioma is a benign neoplasm made up of proliferative and hyperplastic vascular endothelium.

Infantile hemangiomas

Infantile hemangiomas, previously known by their fruity moniker, **strawberry hemangiomas,** are usually present at birth or shortly thereafter, gradually get larger, reaching their maximum size **by 6-9 months of age**, and then slowly involute over the years.

Treatment is usually required for complicated hemangiomas that may interfere with a vital structure or function. For example, ones that could **interfere with breathing, eating, hearing**. In addition, watch for ones that are at **increased risk for ulceration, scarring, and disfigurement**. Otherwise monitoring without active intervention could be appropriate.

An important recent development that can definitely make its way onto the exam would the use of **oral beta blockers, specifically propranolol**. This is now the first line treatment for complicated cases.

Kasabach-Merritt syndrome

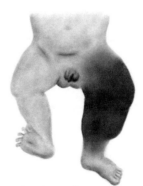

This is a hemangioma that enlarged rapidly due to the **sequestration of platelets** into the lesion, resulting in **low platelet counts** and a **vulnerability to bleeding**. Psst...these kids can have a consumptive coagulopathy, ya know, DIC.

Kasabach-Meritt syndrome

Sun, Skin, and Melanoma

You may be questioned on skin lesions that should be investigated further. See box below for indications that warrant further investigation.

Congenital melanocytic nevi are at risk for transformation into melanoma. **Giant congenital nevi** have the greatest risk for later transformation to melanoma.

Malignant Melanoma

The risk for melanoma is **cumulative**, with more **sun exposure over time** resulting in higher risk for malignant melanoma and other forms of skin cancer. Other risk factors include **family history** and **fair complexion**.

Although sun exposure is a risk factor for melanoma, melanoma can appear in any part of the body, even those that have never and should never see the sun.

Relearning the alphabet

The traditional ABCDs of melanoma included:

> **A**symmetry: two halves do not look the same
>
> **B**orders: that are irregular, rough or notched
>
> **C**olors: that are unusual or change
>
> **D**iameter: larger than 6mm

And recent studies have recommended adding an E:

> **E**volution, recent change, new appearance

As a matter of fact, an entirely new alphabet has been devised for children since they rarely follow the above rules for adults!

> **A**melanotic: may be pink or red and even resemble warts
>
> **B**leeding, bump: May not be flat and may ulcerate
>
> **C**olor uniformity: not varied
>
> **D**e novo, any **D**iameter: may not arise from previous lesions, and may be smaller than 6mm

Chapter 30

Rheumatology: Rheum with a View

Ankylosing Spondylitis (AS)

Ankylosing spondylitis (AS) mainly affects the **sacroiliac joints**, and may eventually lead to fusion of the spine. The **HLA-B27 antigen is positive over 90% of the time.** It affects **males** primarily (3:1), can involve the **eye** (iritis, uveitis), and is known to be associated with **inflammatory bowel disease**.

Look for the **bamboo spine** on the plain film in a teenager with **night pain** and **morning stiffness relieved by exercise. Pain of large joints, such as the knee,** could also be a part of the presentation.

Ankylosing spondylitis can also present as a **leg and back pain**, which is **increased when bending over**. Systemic symptoms, including a **low grade fever and weight loss**, can be part of the presentation.

Picture a **Giant Eye** replacing the sacroiliac joint to remember to associate AS with **uveitis** and **iritis**.

A good way to differentiate the pain of AS from mechanical low back pain is that the pain of AS should **improve with activity and get worse with rest** – the opposite being true of mechanical low back pain.

In ankylosing spondylitis, ANA and RF should be **negative,** with a normal or mildly elevated **ESR**.

Enthesitis related Arthritis (ERA)

Enthesitis related arthritis (ERA) is a new player in the field here. **Juvenile ankylosing spondylitis is a subset of this type of arthritis.** Therefore it is associated with human leukocyte antigen(HLA)- B27 antigen.

Important physical findings to watch for would be uveitis and sacroiliac joint inflammation. This could be described as hip pain, and lower back stiffness especially in the morning. Watch for description of pain especially at the insertion of tendons.

In case you didn't know it before, enthesitis is inflammation of the entheses, the insertion sites of tendons and ligaments to the bone surface.

Juvenile Dermatomyositis (JDM)

They can describe a school-aged kid, **younger than 10 years,** with a **rash on the face** similar to that found in lupus, as well as tight **shiny or scaly skin** on the **extensor surfaces of the extremities or over the interphalangeal joints (Gottron's sign).** The rash can be very itchy and, if on the scalp, may cause hair loss. They may also describe with **periungual red bumps** which are really nail fold telangectasias.

The Malar Rash

When you see a malar rash, think

- **Juvenile Dermatomyositis** (in toddlers and preschoolers)
- **Systemic Lupus Erythematosus** (in teenagers)

Other causes include viral illnesses and sunburn.

The rash might be described as a **heliotrope,**[1] **violaceous, or "butterfly" discoloration of the malar region and/or eyelids.**

HOT TIP

Consider this diagnosis strongly if they present you with a patient who is now having **difficulty getting dressed, raising her arms above her head, or climbing steps,** is **clumsy,** or presents with **voice change** or **difficulty swallowing,** because these are signs of **large proximal muscle weakness** classic of the "myositis". There is a 2:1 female to male predominance.

The heliotropic rash coupled with proximal muscle weakness is a slam dunk.

> **CPK everywhere**
>
> Of course creatine phosphokinase (CPK) may be elevated in other muscle disease (ie. DMD), but lucky for you, JDM hardly ever presents in children without the rash.

CASE STUDY

Suppose they present you with a patient with the typical findings of dermatomyositis. You read through the entire question written in 0.0001 helvetica font and you are astute enough to make the diagnosis. Your diagnosis is confirmed when you complete the hellish task of reading through to the end of the novel, which they call a "question," when they give away the diagnosis and ask you for the most appropriate <u>initial</u> step in evaluating the patient.

THE DIVERSION

You are down to 3 perfectly logical and seemingly correct choices: EMG, MRI, and creatine kinase (CPK) levels. Which one is the most appropriate initial step?

ANSWER REVEALED

You know that the diagnosis is based on clinical findings, but here you are forced to choose an initial test. EMG is a bit invasive and, therefore, not the correct initial choice. MRI is not an appropriate initial test. The most appropriate initial study, that is relatively non-invasive and readily available, is the **creatine kinase level which is often elevated**. The ALT and AST will also be elevated but not the GGT.

If you are presented with a case that is clearly JDM and asked what labs should be ordered, creatinine kinase, lactate dehydogenase, and/or aldolase levels would be correct choices.

Henoch Schönlein Purpura (HSP)

There are always several questions on HSP on the exam, so here are some critical points to remember:

DEFINITION

HSP is the most common systemic vasculitis in children and involves the skin, GI tract, joints, and kidneys. The etiology is unknown, but it often has **an antecedent bacterial or viral infection**. Boys are affected slightly more often than girls.

---

[1] Heliotrope means "sun-turning" after the plants that turn towards the sun or the sun worshippers on 90210.

The rash of **palpable purpura** (usually on the **lower extremities and buttocks**) is present in all cases of HSP but it may not always be there as the first sign. The **colicky abdominal pain** is also found in most cases, sometimes with **heme positive stools**. Often **intussusception** is the cause of the abdominal pain. **Renal disease**, presenting as hematuria, proteinuria, azotemia or hypertension is common, as is **arthritis/ arthralgia.**

There is no laboratory test diagnostic of HSP, but an elevated BUN ; stool, and a urinalysis with hematuria are suggestive of HSP in the right clinical scenario.

Remember, there is **no thrombocytopenia** to accompany all these "bruises" all over the legs, so look for **a normal platelet count. The PT/ PTT will also be normal.** This is often misdiagnosed as abuse; however, HSP would be apparent from the remaining history.

There is no specific treatment – **care is supportive only** and most cases resolve without sequelae.

If there is mild proteinuria (not in the range of nephrotic syndrome) and mild hematuria, weekly UA checks is all that is indicated.

A referral to a nephrologist would be indicated for hypertension, high levels of proteinuria or labs consistent with acute renal insufficiency.

> ### IgA vasculitis AKA HSP
>
> HSP is also referred to as IgA Vasculitis because it is an autoimmune vasculitis associated with IgA deposition.
>
> A UA needs to be performed on ALL patients with HSP looking for hematuria and proteinuria. The findings on renal biopsy in HSP are identical to those found in IgA nephropathy.
>
> In most cases, the hematuria and proteinuria are transient and resolve in a few months without permanent kidney damage. The risk of long-term renal disease is increased in patients presenting with nephrotic-range proteinuria, elevated creatinine, hypertension, and in females.

The rash of HSP can be mistaken for **erythema marginatum (seen in rheumatic fever).** Since they both also have joint pains, distinguishing them can be difficult.

The joint pain seen in rheumatic fever is more severe and a more prominent feature. In all fairness, they will have to present you with other signs consistent with **rheumatic fever** or HSP to allow you to make the correct choice. However, you need to know what these features are to answer correctly.

A salmon-colored evanescent rash can be seen with **JIA**; however, you won't typically see abdominal pain, and the rash will not be purpuric.

Juvenile Idiopathic Arthritis (JIA)

Juvenile Rheumatoid Arthritis has now joined the disease witness protection program and is now known as Juvenile Idiopathic Arthritis or JIA. JIA is the most common rheumatologic disease of childhood. It is basically a diagnosis of exclusion, and other diseases in the differential must be ruled out first.

JIA typically presents with **morning stiffness, joint redness, swelling, pain, and limited range of motion.**

The age of onset must be **less than 16 years of age**, and symptoms must be present for **at least 6 weeks in at least one joint.**

Remember to consider Acute Rheumatic Fever and Lyme disease in your differential diagnosis.

Large joint involvement is more common than involvement of small joints. **ANA is often positive**.

Girls are affected much more often than boys except for systemic onset, in which the gender ratios are equal and in a rare one called IBD-related enthesitis JIA, which is more common in boys.

Rheumatoid factor (RF) would seem like the perfect lab to order, but don't be fooled. The RF is seldom positive. In addition, since there are loads of false positives.[2] RF in and of itself is of no help in diagnosing JIA.

The following are the characteristics of the specific subtypes of JIA:

1. Polyarticular

5 or more joints are affected in the first 6 months of disease.

- Usually small to medium joints, symmetric disease
- Systemic disease is uncommon in polyarticular JIA.

2. Oligoarticular

4 or fewer joints are affected during the first 6 months of disease.

- Usually medium to large joints, asymmetric disease
- Oligoarthritis is an **ANA-positive** disease in **toddlers**.
- These are the kids that get bad **chronic uveitis**, which is the main morbidity of this otherwise mild subtype.

This is the reason ophthalmologic consultation is required for all children with chronic arthritis. **Chronic uveitis is the #1 treatable cause of blindness in children.**

3. Systemic JIA

Systemic Onset JIA (formerly known as **Still's disease**).

- Systemic-onset JIA affects **males and females equally**.
- **Extraarticular involvement** is common.
- Most JIA **deaths** involve systemic JIA.
- It is an important consideration in evaluation of **fever of unknown origin**.

> ### NO ANA NO!
> ANA is NOT a screen. Once JIA is diagnosed, only then an ANA is checked.

> ### The minor leagues of JIA
> There are 3 smaller players in the JIA games called the Juvenile Spondyloarthropathies:
>
> 4. **Psoriatic arthritis:** may have a positive family history of psoriasis and may have nail pitting and dactylitis. It is more common in girls despite association with HLA B-27.
>
> 5. **IBD-related arthritis:** involves sacroiliac tenderness and HLA B-27. This is the only arthritis more common in boys. Watch for acute anterior uveitis.
>
> 6. **Undifferentiated arthritis:** a wastebasket for any one that does not fit criteria of another chronic arthritis.

---

[2] The most common reason for a child to make RF is infection.

Systemic manifestations may precede joint manifestations by several months. Presenting symptoms include:

- **High fever to over 39°C** with **shaking chills** and quick return to basline of at least 2 weeks' duration that is documented as **"quotidian"** which means "daily" for at least 3 days.
- **Leukocytosis** as high as **30-50,000**
- **Rash** – small, salmon-colored macules with central clearings which coalesce and are **evanescent** "come and go" which occurs usually at the peak of the fever.
- **Hepatosplenomegaly**
- **Lymphadenopathy**
- **Pleuritis/pericarditis/serositis**

Uveitis is rare in systemic JIA. Both **ANA** and **RF** are usually **negative.**[3] Most of the systemic manifestations are **self-limited.**

JIA vs. Leukemia

When leukemia presents with musculoskeletal symptoms in addition to the hematologic findings, it can be difficult to distinguish from JIA. Here is what you should focus on in the question in order to make the distinction:

JIA	Acute Leukemia
Morning stiffness, spiking fevers, and rashes are typical.	The musculoskeletal pain is more likely to **awaken the child at night** and will present as **bone pain that does not involve a joint**.
Symptoms of JIA are periodic and waxing and waning.	Symptoms should be persistent and worsening.
Hematologic abnormalities are milder.	Hematologic abnormalities tend to be more severe than those found in JIA.

Lymphadenopathy, leukocytosis, anemia, fatigue, and hepatosplenomegaly are typical of both disorders, so **will be of no help**; therefore, you can filter these out if you are trying to decide between JIA and ALL.

Treating JIA

Treatment includes:

1. PT and OT
2. anti-inflammatory meds
3. psychosocial support.

JIA in the Long Run

Long-term consequences of JIA include:

- leg-length discrepancy
- joint contractures
- permanent joint destruction
- blindness from chronic uveitis

50% of children with JIA continue to have active disease into adulthood.

---

[3] ANA is only positive about 10% of the time.

1st line treatment is NSAIDs, most commonly **indomethacin, ibuprofen, and naproxen.** Children with JIA on NSAIDs are at risk for all known side effects of NSAIDs, including GI bleeding and elevated LFTs.

2nd line treatment (if NSAIDs don't work) are steroids and immunosuppressive meds.

Methotrexate (MTX) may be necessary in children with aggressive disease. MTX is a **folate-antagonist.** Side effects are mainly **gastrointestinal distress** and **pulmonary toxicity.** Since children on MTX are **immunosuppressed,** they are at risk for infection and need to **avoid live vaccines.** Children on MTX are also at risk for **lymphoproliferative malignancies.** Despite these risks, MTX is considered the **"gold standard"** therapy for children with JIA.

Driving Arthritis

Typically when you think of arthritis in children, you think JIA. However, there are other conditions that cause arthritis. If you consider how difficult it would be to perform surgery with a thick leather glove, it will be easy to remember the mnemonic **GLOVE.**

Causes of Arthritis in children

GC (Gonorrhea), Genetic Syndromes
Lyme disease
Osteomyelitis
Viral (Toxic Synovitis)
Evasive infection (i.e. septic arthritis)

Don't forget that GC can manifest as arthritis. This is easy to forget.

Monoarticular disease: Can all be remembered as **beginning with L**

Lyme and other infections

Legg-Calve-Perthes disease

Leukemia and bone tumors

Polyarticular disease: Remember the word FIRE CAM

Fabry and Farber disease

Infections, IBD

Reactive arthritis (post strep, rheumatic fever, or serum sickness)

E lupus = SLE

Connective tissue disease: sarcoidosis, and vasculitis

And

Malignancy

Kawasaki Disease (KD)

Kawasaki disease should be considered anytime you are presented with a child with a fever of unknown origin (FUO). It's formal name is Mucocutaneous Lymph Node Syndrome, but MCLNS seems harder to remember than KD.

Kawasaki Disease typically presents in children **younger than 4 years, most commonly around age 2.** It is more likely to present in the **winter** and **spring**. It is more common in **males** and in patients of **Asian (most specifically Japanese)** descent.

The diagnosis requires **acute high fever of at least five days' duration.** In addition, **there must be at least four of the following of the five criteria**:

1. Cervical lymphadenopathy (1.5 cm or larger)
2. Oropharyngeal findings (red fissured lips, strawberry tongue, red oral/ pharyngeal mucosa)
3. Bilateral conjunctivitis (without exudate)
4. Diffuse rash (macular papular/erythema multiforme like)
5. Erythema/ Edema Hands/ Feet (periungal desquamation can be described)

Additional features that can be seen but are not required for diagnosis include:

- Sterile pyuria[4]
- CNS symptoms such as seizures and aseptic meningitis
- Polyarthritis that is migratory
- Hydrops of the gallbladder
- Thrombocytosis

Think of a giant (30 ft) 2 year old riding a Kawasaki motorcycle without a face shield. The result is **conjunctivitis** and **fissured lips.** His **hands desquamate** from turning the accelerator grips, and his **feet desquamate** from trying to brake using his feet while **turning sharp corners.** In addition, he is going so fast that he develops a **high fever** and has an **elevated platelet count.**

Lab Findings

You will be expected to know the important laboratory findings in Kawasaki disease. Keep in mind the following:

Thrombocytosis by the **5th day** of illness.[5] **Leukocytosis** by the **12th day** of illness.

Normocytic anemia consistent with chronic illness is also part of the laboratory findings.

Acute phase reactants such as **C-reactive protein, ESR,** and **alpha-1 antitrypsin** remain high for **4-6 weeks.**

Sterile pyuria is present in 80% of cases.

Lipid panels are abnormal with **decreased levels of total cholesterol and HDL.**

ANA, RF, and **circulating anticoagulant** will **not be elevated in Kawasaki disease.**

---

4 White cells in the urine.
5 Remember to write the word in the margins when presented with a very high platelet count, since you are remembering descriptive terminology which is hard to pick out of a sea of numbers.

Kardiac Manifestation

The primary concern in Kawasaki disease is **vasculitis of the coronary arteries.**

When the diagnosis is suspected, prompt treatment is essential. If the diagnosis is clear, start treatment even BEFORE getting a cardiac echo.

In ALL cases of suspected KD, a 2-dimensional **cardiac echo** must be done to look for coronary artery aneurysms.

Even kids with no coronary findings need a follow up echo one year after the illness.

KD is treated with:

- An initial dose of IVIG, 2 g/kg (over 12 hours)
- **Aspirin** is given **initially** at very high doses (80 mg/kg/day until the fever subsides)
- **Aspirin maintenance is** then given at a lower dose (5 mg/kg/day for 2 months)

> ## Achey Breakey Heart
>
> Kawasaki disease is the leading cause of **acquired heart disease** in developed countries.
>
> Rheumatic heart disease is the leading cause in developing countries.

> ## IVIG and vaccines
>
>
>
> Measles and Varicella-containing vaccinations must not be given for 11 months after IVIG.

KD or not KD

When you are presented with a patient with Kawasaki disease, you will also be given choices in the differential that can easily be confused for Kawasaki disease. However, if you pay attention to the following fine details, you will be well prepared to make the important distinctions:

Hypersensitivity reactions (such as drug reactions and Stevens-Johnson Syndrome) – This will be tempting, especially if they present a patient on antibiotics who has not responded to treatment and has developed a macular papular rash. However, in a drug reaction one would not expect high fever or the other clinical criteria associated with Kawasaki disease.

JIA/Systemic Type – This will also present with fever and rash, as well as adenopathy. However, the **fever will not be acute**, and the rash will be described as an **evanescent, reticular rash** that appears when the **fever peaks.** They would also have to describe other signs of JIA, including hepatosplenomegaly, pleural effusions, or cardiomegaly.

Cardiomegaly is not a sign of Kawasaki disease.

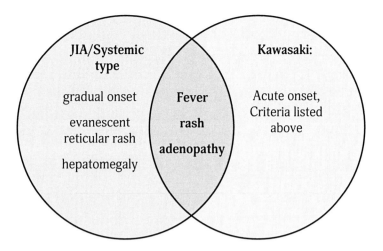

Measles – Both measles and Kawasaki present with fever and conjunctivitis; however, **measles presents with an *exudative* conjunctivitis.** The **rash starts at the hairline and progresses downward to the extremities.**

Scarlet Fever – The rash in scarlet fever is seen primarily in **flexural areas** of the extremities and of course will have a positive *Strep* test.

Other infections and toxin mediated diseases that might look like KD include viral infections such as **EBV** and **enteroviruses, Rocky Mountain spotted fever** and **Leptospirosis, Staph scalded-skin syndrome,** and **toxic shock syndrome.**

Lyme Disease

This is a topic that is full of myths and misconceptions. Here are some important points to remember:

Lyme disease is caused by infection with the spirochete *Borrelia burgdorferi* and the body's immunologic response to this infection. The spirochete is carried by the **Ixodes deer tick**, for those interested in entomology!

> ## Checking Ticks
>
> Deer ticks need to feed at least 36 hours to transmit Lyme disease.
>
> Therefore **frequent tick checks** are the best way to prevent Lyme disease.

Hitting the ECM Rash Bullseye

The classic "Bullseye" rash is called **erythema chronicum migrans** (ECM).

The rash does not appear in 25% of cases. Therefore, its absence in the clinical history does not rule out Lyme disease. You will most likely be presented a patient with lyme arthritis **without a distinct history of ECM rash or deer tick bite.**

Progression of the Disease

First Two Weeks	**Erythema chronicum migrans rash** at the site of the tick bite.
	Very vague flu-like symptoms with **severe arthralgia** and **extreme fatigue.** Even though malaise and fatigue are such common early signs, their non-specificity often leads to a delay in diagnosis.
Several Months	The second stage of Lyme disease is characterized by **CNS, cardiac, and arthritic disease.**
	Here you *can* picture the symptoms "migrating" (to remind you that the rash is called "migrans") as a "lime in a **CAN**" where CAN stands for Carditis, Arthritis (pauciarticular), and Neurological Signs (CNS). This also includes **Bell's Palsy** (a common finding).
Years	Progression of some of the "CAN" symptoms in stage 2, especially arthritis.

Lyme Arthritis

The **Arthritis** is **pauciarticular,** involving **large joints** (especially the knee).

While the knee may be tender and appear swollen, the pain is not unbearable (as it will be with other forms of acute arthritis, such as septic arthritis) so you might even see these kids **walking around with a huge knee.**

Lyme, Labs, and Limbo

Lab confirmation is no easy task with Lyme disease. **Remember that detectable levels of serum antibodies don't build up until 4-6 weeks, so false negatives are common,** especially initially.

If treatment is implemented early, immunologic response is blunted, and lab results are unreliable. In addition, **false positives with other disorders are common.** This includes autoimmune diseases like **SLE, dermatomyositis,** and other **rickettsial** diseases.

The most commonly seen tests are antibody-based, but these can be confusing. The current recommendations first call for a **Lyme enzyme immunosorbent assay (EIA) titer or fluorescent antibody (FA) test and if that is positive or equivocal, then a confirmatory Western blot test is indicated to confirm.**[6]

Treatment is with **doxycycline** for those 8 years and older. For those younger than 8 years of age, **amoxicillin** is recommended (or **cefuroxime** in the case of penicillin allergy). Watch for the age of the patient in the presentation. The typical treatment course is **14 to 21 days,** with maximum duration of therapy 4 weeks.

---

[6] Western blot is more sensitive but not more specific.

Exploding Lymes

If they tell you about a child treated for bona fide Lyme disease who then develops chills and fevers and possibly hypotension with a sepsis-like picture, they are describing the **Jarisch-Herxheimer reaction**, which is the result of **lysis of the organism** and the **release of endotoxin**.

Reactive Arthritis

Any arthritis that follows infection but not infection of the joint itself. This is also known as toxic synovitis.

Watch for a history of an unrelated illness several weeks prior to the current symptoms that could include the classic triad of **arthritis, uveitis** and **urethritis**.

Reactive arthritis[7] falls under the category of **"seronegative spondyloarthropathy,"** which is just a fancy way of saying that, like anklylosing spondylitis, the **ANA and RF factors should be normal**.

Just like ankylosing spondylitis, reactive arthritis also can be **associated with HLA-B27** in up to 90%. The male to female ratio is 4:1.

The following mnemonic can get you an easy point:

With reactive arthritis, you hurt at your **knee** (arthritis), where you **see** (uveitis), and where you **pee** (urethritis). Just remember "can't see, can't pee, and can't climb a tree."

Reactive arthritis often occurs post-infection with either **enteric** *(Yersinia, Shigella, Campylobacter or Salmonella)* or **venereal** *(Chlamydia and gonorrhea)* organisms Post-Strep disease is NOT Reactive Arthritis. Obviously, most cases in children will be post enteric, while postvenereal is a consideration for sexually active teenagers.

> ### IBD and Arthritis
> Remember to think of inflammatory bowel disease when presented with a child with arthritis.

> ### Chlamydia Arthritis
> The most common cause of reactive arthritis in the US is *Chlamydia trachomatis*.

Treatment is **supportive**, with NSAIDs and antibiotics.

Sarcoidosis

Sarcoidosis presents with **history of weight loss and fatigue**, with **hilar adenopathy**. They may mention **chronic cough** or describe it in the absence of any respiratory symptoms. It is seen more 4 times more frequently in **African Americans** than Caucasians.

---

[7] Reiter's syndrome is now called reactive arthritis. Panush, RS, Wallace, DJ, Dorff, RE, Engleman, EP. Retraction of the suggestion to use the term "Reiter's syndrome" sixty-five years later: the legacy of Reiter, a war criminal, should not be eponymic honor but rather condemnation. Arthritis Rheum 2007; 56:693.

Noncaseating granulomas is the hallmark. Additional findings include **bilateral periobronchial cuffing on chest x-ray**.

Watch for an otherwise healthy **afebrile** child who **fatigues easily** during sports sometimes to the point of quitting the sport.

The granulomas actually secrete a form of Vitamin D, which causes **hypercalcemia** and **hypercalcuria**. This results in **renal disease** and **eye disease**.

Sarcoidosis often **involves the heart**, and the presentation of an EKG with a rhythm disturbance could help distinguish a diagnosis of sarcoidosis from tuberculosis. **A negative TB test will be your clue that you are not dealing with tuberculosis.**

> **Triad of Sarcoidosis**
> 1. arthritis
> 2. rash
> 3. uveitis

So if it looks like TB and acts like TB and sounds like TB but it's not TB, then it's sarcoidosis.

Depression and other problems can also explain fatigue and a child dropping out of a sports program. They will have to give you a sign of sarcoidosis, such as a **chronic cough**, if that is the answer they are looking for. Asthma would also include cough, but not fatigue.

Scleroderma

Scleroderma results in a thickening and tightening of the skin, often with induration. Literally, this means "hard skin." **Females** are affected much more frequently than males.

There are two main forms of scleroderma.

Localized Linear Scleroderma

The localized form of scleroderma will begin as a **linear hyperpigmented patch** that becomes more and more fibrotic. It only involves skin and adjacent subcutaneous tissue. Initially, patches of skin are painful and tender. Additional descriptions might include **shiny hypopigmented skin with a brown border**. This is sometimes referred to as **morphea**.

The active lesions can also be described as having a red border with a white waxy center. As they become inactive they could be described as hyper or hypo-pigmented.

Localized scleroderma is more common and has a better outcome than the systemic form. The localized form requires minimal treatment and is self-limited.

Treatment of the localized form consists of topical lubricants and, occasionally, **photochemotherapy**. In the presence of widespread progressive disease, other treatment modalities could include **steroids, antimalarials, and immunosuppressives.** This would include **methotrexate** and **penicillamine,** among other agents.

Systemic Scleroderma

The systemic form is rarely seen in children, but just in case it does pop up on the boards. The systemic form involves the nervous system and visceral organs.

The systemic form may also present with **sclerodactyly,**[8] **pulmonary fibrosis**, and **reflux/dysphagia from lower esophageal sphincter incompetence**.

Most people present with **Raynaud's,** and almost everyone has this at some point in their course. **ANA is almost always positive.**

Systemic Lupus Erythematosus (SLE)

SLE is caused by **the formation of antigen-antibody complexes in a variety of tissues. It is almost always found in women,** though the gender ratio is more equal in younger children. It is much more common in **African Americans, Hispanics,** and **Asians,** than in Caucasians.

Most patients present with **rash, fever**, and **arthritis**. Other common symptoms at presentation include **fatigue, weight loss, lymphadenopathy** and **hepatosplenomegaly.**

A diagnosis of SLE is suggested[9] when **4 or more** of the following features present over time.

- Malar rash
- Discoid lesions
- Photosensitivity
- Oral ulcerations
- Arthritis and serositis
- Hematological abnormalities
- Renal abnormalities (common)
- The presence of anti-ds-DNA, anti-DNA and anti-Smith antibodies.
- Psychosis or other neurologic abnormalities including headaches and depression
- Positive ANA

Name that Antibody

Antibodies to double-stranded DNA **(anti-ds-DNA)** are very specific for SLE since positive results are rarely seen in other patients, including those with other rheumatological disorders.

---

[8] Localized scleroderma of the digits.
[9] With 96% accuracy, which is close enough for the exam.

Severity of disease flareups can also be tracked via anti-ds-DNA levels, which fluctuate accordingly. The severity of disease can also be traced via C3 and C4 levels, which are inversely proportional to disease severity. C3 and C4 levels go down in more active/acute disease states.

Anti-Smith antibodies are also very specific to SLE, but remain elevated regardless of disease activity so they are not useful for tracking disease. It is only useful for identifying disease.

Clinical Disease

Polyserositis affects any organ that has a **pleural covering**, which includes primarily the heart (pericarditis) and lungs (pleurisy).

Renal disease is an important component of SLE. Look for signs of nephritis along with other signs of lupus presented in the question.

Cerebritis is a result of areas of **microischemia and vascular disease**. It results in **seizures**.

Neonatal Lupus

When neonatal lupus does occur, there are usually no clinical signs; however, without clinical signs there would be no board exam, just blank pages.

The signs on the Boards to look for are **rashes on the trunk** and, **most importantly, 3rd degree heart block**. A newborn presenting with **bradycardia** should tip you off that they could be alluding to a diagnosis of neonatal lupus-which could also be associated with **hydrops fetalis**. The heart block can lead to cardiac failure, and the baby may need a pacemaker.

Heart block would be the most likely explanation for death in an infant born to a mother with SLE.

Most newborns born to women with SLE do NOT develop neonatal lupus. If presented with a neonate with heart block or low heart rate, they will almost certainly not mention a history of lupus in the mom. In fact, in many cases the mom doesn't know she has SLE.

Smoothly rowing your boat to diagnosis

Anti-SSA antibody is closely associated with neonatal lupus. Notably, most infants with congenital heart block have mothers who test positive for anti-SSA or anti-SSB antibodies.

> **Pick a fact-ANA facts**
>
> The ANA is an extremely sensitive screening test (negative rules it out) – it will be positive in almost all SLE, but it is also positive in many other inflammatory disorders.
>
> If the *ANA* is negative, it is very unlikely to be lupus (because it is a highly *sensitive* test).
>
> On the other hand, the *dsDNA* test is very *specific*. Positive rules it in.
>
> Remember – a sensitive test is how you screen for a disease. A specific test is how you secure the diagnosis.

> **Raynaud Triad**
>
> Raynaud Triad (Raynaud's Phenomenon) can be **a part of Lupus**.
>
> The triad consists of the following, which I remember with the **white**, **blue**, and **red** of the French Flag. Raynaud was French, wasn't he? The fingers have:
>
> ❑ Ischemia **(white)**
> ❑ Cyanosis **(blue)**
> ❑ Coldness **(red)**

Synovial Fluid

They will give you Synovial Fluid to look at, and based on the findings you may have to mix and match. Here are some Guidelines:

SYNOVIAL FLUID	COLOR	VISCOSITY
Normal Synovial Fluid	Yellow or clear	Normal or slightly increased viscosity; WBC less than 200
Arthritis secondary to Trauma	Clear or bloody	Increased viscosity; WBC less than 2,000
Lupus	Yellow or clear	Normal viscosity; WBC 5,000 and LE cells
Rheumatic Fever	Yellow-cloudy	Decreased viscosity; WBC 5,000
JIA	Yellow-cloudy	Decreased viscosity; WBC 15,000-20,000
Reactive arthritis	Yellow-opaque	Decreased viscosity; WBC 20,000
Septic Arthritis	Yellow	Variable viscosity; WBC 50,000-300,000 and low glucose and bacteria
White Zinfandel Wine	Light amber hue	Viscosity - light on the palate with a hint of oak

Chapter 31

The Eyes Have It

Spelling Counts !

Remember, ophthalmology is spelled with 2 Hs and we cover much of it in other sections. Here we pick out some important pieces of information on which they can test you.

Vision Development

You will be expected to be familiar with the visual capabilities of infants. The following will help you "track" these facts in order to keep them straight on the exam.

Ability to Fixate – begins at 6 weeks of age.

 Infants can **Fix** at **Six** weeks of age

Color Perception develops at 2 months of age.

Binocular vision with convergence ability develops at around 3 months of age.

Picture a pair of binoculars that are a giant "3," which is the shape of binoculars.

Preference for patterns, including faces, occurs at 4 months of age.

Baby Eyes

HOT TIP The visual acuity of a newborn is around 20/200. By 1 year of age, this improves to 20/30.

Checking Vision

By age 3, the best assessment of visual acuity is by Lea Symbols® or HOTV letters since the kids are preliterate.

Allen figures and Tumbling Es and Lighthouse symbols are not standardized and are no longer recommended.

The Rhythm of Nystagmus

You could very well be called upon to identify a variety of forms of nystagmus and try to keep them straight until you actually experience pendular nystagmus yourself. What's pendular nystagmus? Follow the bouncing eyeballs and we will explain.

Optokinetic Nystagmus

If you can spell this without vertical nystagmus and vertigo on flat land, you are almost there. This merely refers to the ability to see a moving target, follow it, and then return to the original gaze. This is one of the **earliest reflexes**; infants develop this in the first few months of life.

Pendular Nystagmus

Pendular nystagmus is equal velocity movements in both directions (to and fro). It is often a sign of an underlying disorder such as **multiple sclerosis** or **spinocerebellar disease**.

Jerk Nystagmus

Jerk nystagmus is characterized by a slow phase back to the central position with a quick gaze laterally.

Jerk nystagmus can be normal when a child gazes far upwardly or laterally.

Orbital Alignment

Ophthalmologists, in addition to having the most frequently misspelled specialty, have a language that only they and Kenny from *South Park* understand.

First some definitions in the following table:

Eye-speak	What it means to you and me
Esotropia / Esophoria	Inward turning eye (a form of strabismus). Tropia is constant; Phoria comes and goes
Strabismus	Misalignment of one eye in relation to the other.
Exotropia / Exophoria	Outward turning eye.
Hyperopia	Hyperopia is farsightedness where parallel rays are focused behind the retina, distant objects are seen more distinctly than near ones . Most children normally have mild hyperopia. This is the refractive state most likely to be seen in a 3 year old.
Anisometropia	Difference in visual acuity between the eyes (ie. 20/20 in one and 20/200 in other)

Instrument Screening

The primary goal of instrument based vision screening in young children is to identify risk factors for vision loss. It does not replace vision screening.

A Benign Nod

Spasmus nutans is a benign, transient disorder without known cause that is characterized by **pendular nystagmus, intermittent head tilt, and nodding or head bobbing**.

It can be mistaken for muscular torticollis. It self resolves.

Amblyopia

Amblyopia is the permanent loss of visual acuity due to active cortical (brain) suppression of vision of the non-dominant eye when it's vision has been limited. Before age 3, strabismus is the most common cause. Between ages 3 and 6, anisometropia and strabismus are equal risk factors.

Amblyopia is more successfully treated when identified earlier, and becomes impossible to treat after age 7-9.

Let's discover the "cover test"

- The child is asked to look at one particular spot

- **The eye with strabismus deviates instead of fixating on the object.**

- Then one eye is covered

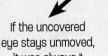

If the uncovered eye stays unmoved, it was always " paying attention", ie. good eye.

If the uncovered eye moves, it was deviated, ie. bad eye.

If a child has vision loss and you **attempt to cover the good eye**, he will resist your doing so (because he won't be able to see.) This is ripe for a trick question.

The corneal light reflex test (Hirschberg test) is used to elucidate eye malalignment.[1] **Here you shine a penlight on both eyes and expect a symmetrical light reflex and if the light reflex is different in one eye than the other, there is malalignment.**

Screening for strabismus is crucial, and they want you to know that. **Untreated strabismus may result in amblyopia.**

Port Wine and the Eye

Remember that infants born with Sturge Weber are at risk for **glaucoma** on **the same side** as the port wine stain, so if they describe a child born with a port wine stain, it is the glaucoma that should be addressed first.

Violaceous discoloration is another way of describing a port wine stain.

The Strawberry of my Eye

These, in general, resolve without any intervention unless they are on or near the eyelid **and are interfering with vision**, in which case they may need to be dealt with early on.

Glaucoma

Congenital glaucoma presents with persistent **tearing** "**lacrimation**", photophobia, blepharospasm (excess blinking), corneal clouding, redness, edema, and **progressive enlargement of the eye**.

This requires prompt referral to an ophthalmologist to measure intraocular pressure and perform surgery if necessary.

---

[1] It is pretty much a simple test named after the famous doctor and sushi chef.

Cataracts

Watch for the description of a child who is "clumsy," spills liquids more than the average child, and runs into objects due to faulty depth perception.

If you are presented with an infant with congenital cataracts, **rubella, CMV,** and **galactosemia** are the important associations to know.

They may also be hereditary, associated with other infections (TORCH) and metabolic/genetic syndromes (parathyroidism, Smith-Lemli-Opitz), or associated with other ocular malformations.

> ### Cataract Family
>
> The first step in the evaluation of an infant with **congenital cataracts** is the evaluation of the parents for cataracts, since 50% are inherited as an **autosomal dominant** condition.

Things that go Bump in the Eye

Styes

Styes are also known as "external hordeolum," and result from acute infection (usually *Staph*) of sebaceous glands in the eyelid. Most commonly at or near an eyelash follicle.

Warm compresses and possibly topical antibiotics are the mainstay of treatment. Incision and drainage might be needed if there is no improvement, but oral antibiotics will **not** be the correct answer. **Usually tender/ painful.**

Chalazion

Chalazion is a lipogranuloma, caused by a blocked oil gland (Meibomian or Zeis). It is due to **chronic inflammation,** not bacterial infection, and is **typically painless**. Most commonly above the eylashes on upper eyelid.

> **You are presented with a patient with a 4-month history of a painless nodule on her upper eyelid. What is the appropriate treatment?**
>
> If you read this question quickly and didn't note that this is a chronic painless nodule, you might have mistaken it for a stye and quickly picked topical antibiotics and warm compresses. In the blink of an eye you would have chosen the incorrect answer.
>
> When answering a question about a nodule on the eyelid, pay careful attention to the details of the history. If you are dealing with a chronic painless nodule, "referral to ophthalmology for surgical excision" is the correct answer. Once again, ophthalmology is the one specialist referral that is often a correct choice.

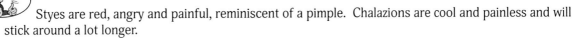

Styes are red, angry and painful, reminiscent of a pimple. Chalazions are cool and painless and will stick around a lot longer.

"Cool as a clam-azion".

Nasolacrimal Duct Obstruction

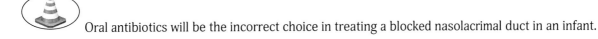

The initial treatment is **massaging the duct** 2-3 times a day. If there is evidence of eye infection, then **topical antibiotic** treatment is indicated.

Oral antibiotics will be the incorrect choice in treating a blocked nasolacrimal duct in an infant.

If blocked duct is not resolved by 12 months of age, then ophthalmological consultation would be in order.

You are evaluating a 2-month-old with excessive tearing of the left eye and mucoid discharge. When you evaluate the crying infant, you notice that the tears pool on the left eyelid and cheek. The parents note that child has nasal congestion and coughs occasionally. The pregnancy and delivery were unremarkable.

What is the appropriate management?

You could be presented with several diversionary choices here, including systemic treatment with antibiotics for a presumed diagnosis of chlamydia. In addition, you will be presented with the option of prescribing topical antibiotic drops for a presumed diagnosis of bacterial conjunctivitis.

None of these would be correct. Noting the nasal congestion is a diversion. Even the occasional cough is a diversion. For a diagnosis of chlamydia pneumonia, they would have to describe a more persistent staccato cough or chest x-ray findings (neither of which are noted in the vignette). For chlamydial conjunctivitis, they would have to describe bilateral eye discharge.

The correct diagnosis is a blocked nasolacrimal duct, for which the appropriate management would be conservative measures, i.e., massage and warm compresses. Topical antibiotics would only be indicated when erythema and other signs of infection are described.

Planetary Cellulitis

Even though they both present with **edema and redness around the eye**, you will be expected to distinguish between a patient with orbital and periorbital cellulitis.

Orbital Cellulitis

Since this is an infection invading the eye itself, it is the more serious of the two.

The key buzz words in the description which should tip you off are **compromised vision, proptosis**, and **decreased extraocular movement**. Watch for **pain exacerbated by eye movement**.

This can be caused by spread of **skin infections**, including **insect bites** and from **sinusitis, upper respiratory infection**, and **dental infections**.

Staph aureus is the most common pathogen when the infection is caused by initial skin infection. Other bacteria that spread from the respiratory tract or sinuses include *Strep pyogenes*, Peptostreptococcus, Bacteroides, and nontypeable *H. flu*.

Since *H. influenza* **type b** can cause this, pay particular attention if they describe a patient who has **incomplete immunizations**. If they note the patient **immigrated from a developing country**, this means they are assumed to be unimmunized.

CT may be needed to differentiate between orbital and periorbital cellulitis and is indicated to document the extent of involvement in orbital cellulitis.

Children with orbital cellulitis need to be **admitted to the hospital for IV antibiotics**, and **Ophthalmology** needs to be consulted.

Periorbital Cellulitis (a.k.a. preseptal cellulitis)

Periorbital cellulitis is the less serious of the orbiting twins. It may be treated with **oral antibiotics** that cover typical **skin and respiratory flora**.

Remember that periorbital cellulitis can spread to become orbital cellulitis. If they describe **decreased EOM or proptosis**, they are more likely describing orbital cellulitis.

If they describe a red swollen periorbital area which is described as being itchy/pruritic rather than painful, then you're probably dealing with an insect bite or an allergic reaction rather than an infection.

Corneal Abrasions

The presentation of corneal abrasion on the exam will likely include **photophobia, tearing,** and **intermittent sharp pain**. They might also describe an **irregular red reflex** or a **dulled corneal light reflex**. Positive **fluorescein staining** of the cornea would be a slam dunk, but that is unlikely to be included in the description.

Remember to include a corneal abrasion in the differential of an **irritable infant**.

After confirmation with fluorescein, all that is needed is **antibiotic ophthalmic drops or ointment**.

In the past, eye-patching was considered to be routine, but this is now contraindicated, as are anesthetic and corticosteroid eye drops.

If you are presented with a patient with symptoms of corneal abrasion following mild trauma, the first thing to do is **fluorescein stain the eye**, not prescribe topical antibiotic.

Keep Your Eyes on the Retina

It is very likely that you will be presented with at least one funduscopic view of the retina. In this section, we include black and white illustrations of the retina.[2]

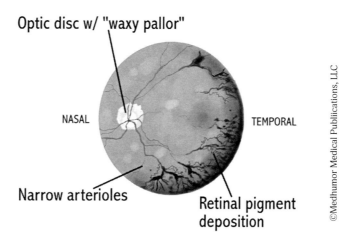

Retinitis pigmentosa

Optic disc w/ "waxy pallor"

NASAL

TEMPORAL

©Medhumor Medical Publications, LLC

Narrow arterioles

Retinal pigment deposition

With **Retinitis pigmentosa**, look for the following:

- Pallor in the center of the optic disc.
- Narrow arterioles coming off the optic disc.
- Retinal pigment deposition on the periphery.

---

[2] "Pictures Worth 100 Points" contains color drawings of several funduscopic views of retinal diseases.

Retinal
hemorrhages

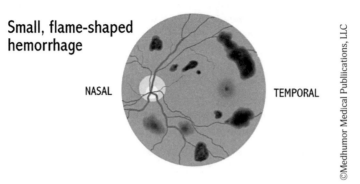

Small, flame-shaped
hemorrhage

NASAL   TEMPORAL

©Medhumor Medical Publications, LLC

For **retinal hemorrhages**, look for flame-shaped hemorrhage

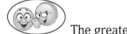 This is typically seen where **child abuse** (ahem, "non-accidental trauma") is suspected or, on the boards, where it is hinted at in the history.

Roping In ROP

Which infants should be screened for ROP?

- Birthweight less than 1500 grams or GA less than 32 weeks
- Birthweight 1500 - 2000 grams with an unstable clinical course, judged to be at risk

When to screen? 31-34 weeks postconception or 4 -6 weeks after birth, **whichever is later**.

The greatest risk factor for developing ROP is **prematurity**, with a gestation less than 28 weeks.

If presented with an infant greater than 37 weeks gestation on oxygen, the risk for ROP is very low, since retinal vascularization is almost complete at that gestational age.

CASE STUDY **You are presented with an infant who has developed retinopathy of prematurity. You are asked to select from several choices the** *most likely risk factor for ROP.*

THE DIVERSION This is a question where you need to put on the brakes before picking the answer that was previously consistent with conventional wisdom. In this case, when the oxygen fastball is thrown down the middle, you want to be caught looking, looking at the correct answer, that is.

ANSWER REVEALED The correct answer in this case is *very low birth weight or prematurity.* Studies have shown that exposure to oxygen or the maintenance of oxygen saturations above 95% over time does not influence the progression of ROP. The incidence of ROP is inversely proportional to birthweight and gestational age.

Retinopathy of Prematurity

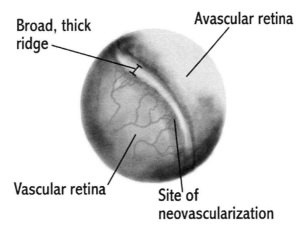

Broad, thick ridge

Avascular retina

Vascular retina

Site of neovascularization

©Medhumor Medical Publications, LLC

Ophthalmia neonatorum

DEFINITION

This is the term for conjunctivitis in the **first 4 weeks after birth**. The most frequent causes in the U.S. include *S. aureus, S. epidermidis, S. pneumoniae,* and *M. catarrhalis*. It may also be caused by *C. trachomatis, N. gonorrheae,* and *herpes simplex* virus (HSV).

BUZZWORDS

N. gonorrhea **neonatal conjunctivitis** is a much more severe infection than chlamydia. It presents as a **hyperacute hyperpurulent conjunctivitis 24 to 48 hrs after birth.**

Chlamydial conjunctivitis typically develops 5-14 days after delivery with a watery discharge that progresses to a mucopurulent discharge.

> ### Neonatal prophylaxis
> GC and Chlamydia conjunctivitis may both be prevented by erythromycin ointment prophylaxis at birth.

PERIL

50% of infants with chlamydial conjunctivitis have coinfection in other sites and may progress to pneumonitis. Therefore, chlamydial conjunctivitis needs to be treated with systemic, not topical, antibiotics. The treatment of choice is **oral erythromycin for 14 days.**

TREATMENT

Treatment is with **IV ceftriaxone** and frequent saline lavage. These infants also need to be evaluated for disseminated GC disease.

BUZZWORDS

Neonatal HSV conjunctivitis may present 1-2 weeks after birth. Classic skin vesicles are often absent. These infants **require admission to the hospital** and consultation with an ophthalmologist.

TREATMENT

Treatment is with **IV Acyclovir** whether HSV is disseminated or not.

Don't Shoot if you see the Red in their Eyes

BUZZWORDS

Conjunctivitis presents with **erythema** of the conjunctiva resulting in **pink eye** or **red eye** with **discharge** that may be clear to purulent and may cause **eye matting**. Symptoms may include a **foreign body sensation, itching, burning,** or **photophobia.**

PERIL

If you are presented with a patient with "red eye" who is **wearing contact lenses**, pause and read the question carefully. In this case, **referral to ophthalmology** for definitive care would be the correct answer.

CASE STUDY

An 18-year-old girl presents with a red irritated right eye. The symptoms have persisted despite removal of her contact lenses 9 hours ago. On physical examination, there is marked conjunctival irritation, with difficulty keeping her eye open. Her funduscopic exam is normal and her pupils are equal and reactive with no discharge noted. There is diffuse uptake of fluorescein stain, with no focal uptake noted. What is the most appropriate next step in managing this patient?

THE DIVERSION

You will be tempted to take the diversionary path and assume that the diffuse uptake of stain represents a corneal abrasion. You will not be fooled into applying an eye patch with topical antibiotics. However, you could be very easily lulled into choosing to prescribe antibiotic drops rather than refer to an ophthalmologist.

ANSWER REVEALED

Well, you would have been deceived into believing that a corneal abrasion is the correct choice – however, if the correct diagnosis were a simple corneal abrasion, they will describe *a focal uptake of stain*. Diffuse or multifocal uptake in a patient wearing contact lenses could represent a gram-negative infection and/or ulceration of the corneal epithelium. These conditions require urgent follow up and management by an ophthalmologist. This is one of the rare occasions where referral to a specialist will be the correct answer on the boards.

Bacterial Conjunctivitis

Acute bacterial conjunctivitis may be caused by *S. aureus, S. epidermidis, S. pneumoniae, M. catarrhalis*, and *Pseudomonas*. In those **underimmunized**, make sure you remember *H. influenzae type b* as a possibility.

TREATMENT

In most cases, acute bacterial nongonococcal conjunctivitis is benign and self-imited. Topical antibiotics may be used to hasten resolution and limit spread to others.

PERIL

Hyperacute presentation, where the infection has a very rapid onset, may be caused by *N. gonorrheae* or *N. meningitidis*. Watch for **severe extremely purulent discharge** with **pseudomembrane formation**. Urgent ophthalmology referral is recommended along with admission and IV antibiotics.

Viral Conjunctivitis

Adenovirus is the most common cause of viral conjunctivitis.

Red Eye, Red Flags!

PERIL

Watch for any of these in the red eye as red flags:

- severe eye pain
- ciliary flush
- photophobia
- irregular corneal light reflex
- persistent blurred vision
- corneal epithelial defect
- proptosis
- pupil unreactive to light
- reduced ocular movements
- worsening after 3 days of treatment
- compromised host: neonate, immunocompromised, contact lens wearer

Symptomatic relief is accomplished with **artificial tears** and **cool compresses**. Topical antibiotics are not recommended, and **steroid drops are contraindicated**. If resolution does not occur as expected within 2 weeks, referral to an ophthalmologist is warranted.

Viral conjunctivitis is **highly contagious** and patients should avoid touching their eyes, shaking hands, and sharing towels. They should be advised to **wash hands frequently**.

> **From the Eyes to the Ears**
>
> Conjunctivitis-otitis syndrome is caused by *H. influenzae type b* and is treated with amoxicillin-clavulanic acid.

Allergic Conjunctivitis

Eye itching and **watery or mucoid discharge** are usually present.

Intense itching is what will help you differentiate it from bacterial infection. Presence of other **atopic conditions** like allergic rhinitis and atopic dermatitis will help you identify it.

Viral conjunctivitis is also more likely to start in one eye, while allergic conjunctivitis usually **starts in both eyes simultaneously** upon exposure to the allergic trigger.

Systemic Diseases

Remember systemic conditions when presented with conjunctivitis

- **Kawasaki disease** involves a **non-purulent** and **bilateral** conjunctivitis with **perilimbal sparing**.
- **Measles** presents with an **exudative** conjunctivitis.
- The uveitis of **Juvenile Idiopathic Arthritis** may be confused with conjunctivitis.

> **Zero Steroid Tolerance**
>
> Any test answer that involves applying eye topical steroids will be the WRONG CHOICE.
>
> Topical eye steroids need to be prescribed by an ophthalmologist.

Eye Trauma

In most cases the **"don't refer out to a specialist" rule will not apply here**. The following are the buzzwords indicating referral to an ophthalmologist: **pupil irregularity** and/or **significantly reduced visual acuity**. You also want to watch out for wording that would imply a serious orbital fracture and/or decreased extraocular eye movements.

Hyphema

A hyphema is a **collection of blood** between the cornea and the iris, usually following eye trauma. On the exam the presentation will be a child struck in eye by an object (baseball, bat, etc.).

Treatment would be immediate opthalmology referral, eye shield and topical cycloplegics. If that isn't one of the choices then the correct answer would be methods that decrease intraocular pressure: bed rest in reverse trendelenburg at 30 degree angle, antimemetics and aggressive pain control.

Patching the eye would not be appropriate; a **shield** should be used.

Blowout Fracture

 A patient with a blowout fracture has an **inferior orbital wall fracture**.

The typical history would be a patient who sustains **blunt trauma** to the eye, has **double vision/ diplopia** when looking to one side, and limited upward gaze secondary to inferior oblique/inferior rectus muscle entrapment. Pupillary reflexes will usually be intact. It is diagnosed by CT.

The following table will help you differentiate a variety of clinical ophthalmological vignettes you could be presented with on the exam.

Diagnoses	Clinical presentations
Corneal abrasion	Severe pain and **tearing**, with no diplopia or dysconjugate gaze
Hyphema	Presents as **blood in the anterior chamber**, with possible visual impairment, without *diplopia*
Traumatic iritis	Pain and **severe photophobia** without diplopia.[3]
Detached retina	Visual deficit in the peripheral field, described as **curtain-like**. No dysconjugate gaze.

Sports Clearance

 Vision worse than 20/40 in one eye corrected is considered functionally a 1-eyed athlete because trauma leading to vision loss in the better eye would lead to significant disability.

Activities considered High Risk for eye injury include:

- baseball
- basketbal
- hockey
- lacrosse
- racquet sports

And eye protection would be indicated for 1-eyed athletes.

---

[3] Sounds like the beginnings of a nice ophthalmology song parody.

UPDATED & NEW BREAKING NEWS INFORMATION Since there is no eye protection available for wresting, and wrestling has recently been identified as high risk for eye trauma, 1-eyed athletes should not participate in wrestling.

Chapter 32

See No Evil, Hear No Evil, Speak No Evil: ENT

Upper respiratory disease is a big part of a general pediatric practice; therefore, ENT is an important section that is highly represented on the exam. Distinguishing the profound from the insignificant will be the key to getting the questions correct on the exam as well.

Ears

Quick review of the structures of the ear - it helps to keep everything straight going forward:

- outer: external ear and ear canal.
- middle: tympanic membrane, ossicles
- inner: cochlea, Eustachian tube, semicircular canals

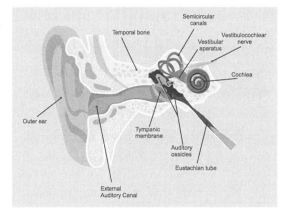

Hearing Loss

BUZZWORDS

In infants and toddlers, suspect hearing loss when they describe **speech delay.** In older children, clues would include **ignoring commands** and **increasing of the television or music volume.**[1]

Hearing loss is broken down into **conductive** and **sensorineural**.

> ### Listen to the Early Bird
>
> Early intervention is needed to help facilitate language development in children with all forms of hearing loss.

Conductive Hearing Loss

DEFINITION

This occurs when **sound fails to progress to the cochlea.** Obstruction can occur anywhere along the way from the external canal to the swinging ossicles.

HOT TIP

The most common cause of conductive hearing loss is an **effusion**. By definition, the effusion is present in the **absence of inflammation**.

> ### More than Meets the Ear
>
> If they present you with a patient with an external or middle ear malformation, watch for hints that there are also craniofacial, renal, or associated **inner** ear malformations.

PERIL

It is important to note that you will not always be completely deaf with conductive hearing loss. You can typically hear sounds loud enough to be conducted through bone. So don't let that fool you! If you are presented with a patient who is hearing sufficiently it does not mean that conductive hearing loss has been ruled out!

---

[1] Assuming one does not live in a subway station.

Causes of Conductive Hearing Loss	
Inner and outer ear malformations	This causes the **most severe** degree of conductive hearing loss.
Trauma	Larger **perforations** result in significant hearing loss. In addition, post-traumatic hearing loss is usually associated with **disruption of the ossicles themselves**.
Tympanosclerosis	We have all seen this (basically scarring on the TM), usually after several bouts of OM. They could very well show this to you; remember that this results in **minimal hearing loss**.
Chronic OME (OM with Effusion)	This is the most **common cause** of conductive hearing loss.
Cholesteatoma	This is the result of **keratinization of the epithelial cells in the middle ear**.

Sensorineural Hearing Loss (SNHL)

Sensorineural hearing loss can be blamed on **malfunction of the cochlea** and/or **auditory nerve**. It may have toxic (drugs), infectious, genetic, or traumatic (physical or acoustic) causes.

Medications

Furosemide (Lasix®) and ethacrynic acid may cause temporary hearing loss.

Picture a Loop earring piercing the cochlea, causing sensorineural hearing loss.

Remember that **aminoglycosides** like **gentamicin** and **tobramycin** can lead to hearing loss.

Salicylate results in **reversible sensorineural hearing loss**. Hearing can return to normal within a week. A **high-pitched tinnitus** is what they could describe.

Infectious (Intrauterine and perinatal)

Cytomegalovirus (CMV), toxoplasmosis, rubella, and syphilis are common in utero causes of sensorineural hearing loss.

Among **acquired** infections, **bacterial meningitis** is the most common cause of childhood sensorineural hearing loss. It tends to occur early in the illness (usually in the first 24 hours). This is an important concept that can be tested on the exam.

Viral Labyrinthitis

Viral labyrinthitis could be described as a **sudden onset of bilateral sensorineural deafness**. Prognosis for recovered hearing is variable and there is no treatment, just watchful waiting.

Turn Down the Volume

Repeated exposure to loud sounds, including pounding music through AirPods® headphones, can lead to high frequency sensorineural hearing loss. The same applies to the loud sound produced by power tools.

CMV Hearing Loss

Congenital CMV is the most common cause of **sensorineural hearing loss**.

These infants may even pass the newborn hearing screen and have **profound hearing loss by one year of age**.

It is very important that all children who have meningitis have a **hearing test as soon as possible**. If the meningitis doesn't get you, the antibiotics will (see above).

It is not related to the severity of the illness, the age of the patient, or when antibiotics were started.

Other causes of acquired hearing loss are **varicella, measles, mumps,** and **influenza**.

Genetic

More than 500 causes of **syndromic and nonsyndromic genetic hearing loss** have been reported.

Alport syndrome is most commonly an X-linked dominant condition that results in defective type 4 collagen so it affects eyes, kidneys and **ears**. They have bilateral sensorineural hearing loss and hematuria. So all boys with sensorineural hearing loss (SNHL) need an UA.

Mitochondrial and neurodegenerative disorders are another significant cause of genetic hearing loss. Other common genetic conditions for SNHL are Jervell & Lange-Nielson Syndrome and Waardenburg Syndrome.

> ### Syndromic Hearing Loss
>
> *HOT TIP*
>
> Hearing loss is associated with **CHARGE syndrome** and and other syndromes that involve **cleft lip and palate**.

Grab Bag

Other risk factors for sensorineural hearing loss include issues associated with **prematurity**, such as **prolonged ventilation, hyperbilirubinemia, low birth weight, Rh factor, maternal diabetes,** and **neonatal depression**.

Head trauma, noise exposure, toxin exposures like alcohol, and **radiation therapy** for head and neck tumors are additional risk factors.

Age Appropriate Hearing Tests

Newborn Hearing Screening

HOT TIP

Initial testing should be done by 1 month of age with the goal of identifying hearing loss by 3 months of age, and intervention **before 6 months of age**.

There are two screening tests for newborns in the nursery:

> ### Did I hear you right?
>
> A completely DEAF infant will have "normal" language development until about 9 months. That's because cooing and babbling do not depend on hearing.
>
> It's the cutting off the "mamamama" and "dadadada" into "mama" and "dada" that requires hearing, and that typically occurs at about 9 months.

1. Auditory brainstem response (ABR)

Auditory Brainstem Response (ABR) uses electroencephalographic waveforms to determine the child's perceptual threshold, i.e. it tests the vestibulocochlear nerve's response to sound.. This test requires the patient be asleep, so children older than six months of age may require conscious sedation for an ABR.

2. Otoacoustic emissions (OAE)

Otoacoustic emissions (OAE) test measures sounds that are made by the cochlea in response to clicking sounds, ie it tests the hair cell function.

Behavioral Observation Audiometry (BOA)

BOA is used for **infants who are less than 6 months of age**. This is **only a screening test**, and infants who **fail this must then undergo ABR testing**. In this test, the infant is **awake**, and the infant's behavior is observed in response to sound.

Visual Reinforced Audiometry (VRA)

Visual Reinforcement Audiometry (VRA) is **best for ages 6 to 24 months**. This tests for **bilateral hearing loss** so that intervention to prevent language development impairment can be started.

If a patient fails a hearing screen or has equivocal results, he/she needs a referral to an audiologist. If you are given a patient that has physical, cognitive, or behavioral concerns that may interfere with administration of the screening, referral to an audiologist would be the correct choice.

Play Audiometry

This is best for children **2-4 years of age**.

Conventional Pure-Tone Audiometry Screen

The conventional Pure-Tone Audiometry Screen is appropriate for children who can cooperate with commands (typically age **4 and above**). This can **test each ear independently**.

Tympanometry

Tympanometry results can invariably be shown or described on the exam. Often, the results are either normal or abnormal due to technique.

An example of poor technique includes the probe being wedged against the external canal; this may cause abnormal results.

> **Targeted Intervention**
>
> Politics aside, infants with significant congenital sensorineural hearing loss should receive "targeted intervention" by 6 months of age.
>
> This means using either external (hearing aids) or implantable (cochlear implants) devices to allow them to hear, and thus develop as their peers.

Tympanometry does not measure hearing sensitivity. Instead, it simply evaluates the **middle ear function** by measuring its response to changes in air pressure. You *can* have a normal tympanogram with significant sensorineural hearing loss. On the other hand, a patient can have an abnormal tympanogram and still have normal hearing.

Tympanogram

This is a graph of the tympanometry results. Take a minute to look up examples of the types below. Knowing the differences between each type and what causes it can score you easy points.

Type A: **a normal result**. If hearing loss is present, it will be SNHL.

Type A$_s$: same shape as Type A but has shallower amplitude (hence the 's'). Due to **TM scarring**, **otosclerosis** or **ossicular fixation**.

Type A$_d$: same shape as Type A but has a higher amplitude. It is associated with **ossicular disarticulation** (hence the 'd').

Type B: There is no peak and it is more like a flat line. It can be low amplitude - think of a stiff membrane due to middle ear fluid or an obstructed tympanostomy tube. Or it can be high amplitude due to continuity between the middle and outer ear with a perforated TM (trauma, tubes). More buzz words to recognize are that it **reflects an absence of pressure or the absence of mobility**.

Type C: a peaked graph that is left shifted and represents **eustachian tube dysfunction**. *Conductive hearing loss is likely.*

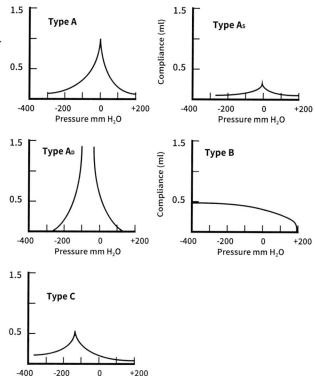

Otitis Media

"Otitis media" encompasses the diagnoses of acute otitis media (AOM) and otitis media with Effusion (OME). They will both present with fluid behind the TM and are both best diagnosed with pneumatic otoscopy.

Three criteria are needed for acute otitis media (AOM):

1. recent abrupt onset (< 48 hours)
2. bulging TM with effusion
3. erythema of TM

Otitis media with effusion (OME) refers to inflammation of the middle ear with effusion but without signs or symptoms of infection.

Erythema of the TM is not enough by itself to hang your diagnostic hat on since it's likely to be there whenever kids have a fever.

The most common bacterial culprits in acute otitis media are:

- *Streptococcus pneumoniae*
- *H. flu* (non typeable)
- *Moraxella catarrhalis*
- *Streptococcus pyogenes* (Group A Strep)

Chronic Suppurative Otitis Media (CSOM)

To break down this long title - it simply means there is >6 wks of purulent ear drainage.

CASE STUDY

You are presented with a 4 year old child with chronic purulent drainage through his perforated left tympanic membrane. The best treatment for this would be:

THE DIVERSION

There are two potential diversions here. One is cholesteatoma and the other is acute otitis media. What is being described here is *chronic suppurative otitis media*, which is defined as purulent otorrhea for 6 weeks or longer. The absence of keratinized epithelial tissue rules out cholesteotoma. The "chronic drainage" rules out acute otitis media. You now have to pick an antibiotic or recognize the most common cause.

ANSWER REVEALED

The most common cause is *pseudomonas* and therefore the treatment of choice is *topical/otic ofloxacin* with daily suctioning of the canal to allow antibiotic to reach the infection. In addition to *pseudomonas*, chronic suppurative otitis media can be caused by *Staph* and *Fusobacterium necrophorum*.[2]

Cholesteatoma is a keratin-producing squamous epithelial lesion:

- Cholesteatoma can be the result of chronic suppurative otitis media, or chronic Eustachian tube dysfunction.
- Cholesteatomas develop behind the mid anterior quadrant of the TM.
- Cholesteatomas can dissolve tissue and bone and reach into the CNS.

CASE STUDY

You are presented with a 9 year old boy who has purulent discharge from his right ear over several months despite several courses of antibiotics. On physical exam you note retraction of the tympanic membrane and squamous debris. What do you do next?

THE DIVERSION

You might be tempted to pick higher dose antibiotics or other more conservative measures.

ANSWER REVEALED

This is the description of a **cholesteatoma**, and, therefore, this is one of those rare times when referral to a specialist will be the correct answer. Although cholesteatomas are technically benign, they expand and destroy bone so they need to be removed surgically. Late recognition remains a major cause of permanent hearing loss.

---

[2] No, we did not make that one up.

If they describe a **"foul smelling discharge despite treatment of a perforated TM,"** it is a clue to a diagnosis of cholesteatoma.

Cholesteatomas require urgent ENT referral for surgical management. Recurrent rates are as high as 50%.

Otitis Media and the CNS

If they describe a child who is being treated for OM but **not responding** and returns with classic signs of meningitis, then it is not a trick question, and workup and treatment for meningitis would be indicated.

Although intracranial suppurative complications of otitis media only occur 1% of the time, the incidence is higher on the boards.

Watch for subtle clues in the history, including **fever, irritability,** and **lethargy.** More specific signs would include **headache, double vision,** and **vomiting.**

Withholding antibiotics

Keep the following in mind when answering questions on basic garden variety otitis media that for infants over 6 months with unilateral otitis and nonsevere symptoms and for toddlers over age 2 with nonsevere symptoms even with bilateral disease, withholding antibiotics for 48-72 hours to see if symptoms resolve may be the best option.

80% of the time, otitis media will resolve without antibiotics.

Close follow up must be ensured or a "safety net" prescription may be provided in case the child worsens.

Antibiotic Selection

Initial antibiotic choice is **high dose amoxicillin (90 mg/kg/ day)**. Amoxicillin clavulanate as a first line therapy is indicated only if a patient has failed treatment with amoxicillin in the last 30 days or if the patient has a concomitant purulent conjunctivitis (due to its association with resistant strains of bacteria). If a patient fails to have symptom improvement in 2-3 days on amoxicillin, then it is indicated to switch to amox-clav to complete the antibiotic course or IM ceftriaxone x3d.

When the child has a Type 1 allergy to **penicillin, 2nd or 3rd generation cephalosporins like cefuroxime, cefdinir,** and **cefpodoxime** are acceptable alternatives.

Resolving Recurrent Otitis

Prophylaxis with antibiotics is no longer recommended for the prevention of recurrent otitis media. Antibiotic prophylaxis is now considered to be a risk factor for colonization with resistant pneumococcus.

Tympanostomy tubes are now the treatment of choice for recurrent otitis media.

Confusion over Effusion

Chronic otitis media with effusion (OME) may result in hearing loss and language delay.

There is an increased risk of OME in patients with allergic rhinitis, adenoidal hypertrophy, and eustachian tube abnormalities.

The appropriate management would be monitoring over time, with periodic checks of TM mobility.

If OME leads to recurrent acute OM or hearing loss, then tympanostomy may be indicated.

Conditions associated with recurrent otitis media

- **A**ge <2 years
- **A**topy
- **B**ottle and pacifier prolonged use
- **C**iliary dysfunction
- **C**raniofacial abnormalities
- **C**hild Care attendance
- **I**mmunocompromising conditions
- **S**inusitis, **S**moke exposure
- **N**o breastfeeding
- **F**eeding laying flat
- **C**ertain ethnic groups/ Native Americans
- **S**ome hereditary risk

MYTH

Mothers want it, advertisers hawk it, and pediatricians often give in to the pressure[3], but antihistamines, decongestants, and other over-the-counter cold remedies as treatment for and/or prevention of acute otitis media have no proven value. So remember: Just Say No To (over-the counter cold remedy) Drugs included in the choices.

PERIL

Oral decongestants should not be used in children younger than 6 years of age, especially in those presenting on the boards. Nasal decongestants may be harmful in infants younger than 6 months of age, since rebound nasal congestion may impact respiratory function (infants are nasal breathers).

Otorrhea

Remember: otorrhea can still occur after the tubes are in place. This is because even though they equalize pressure, they **do not prevent upper respiratory tract infections**.

NonEar Ear Pain

Watch for indications that the patient might have TMJ dysfunction, cervical spine abnormality, or a sore throat as the source of the otalgia.

CASE STUDY

A 5 year old with tympanostomy tubes presents with 3 days of bloody otorrhea as well as nasal congestion. In addition to a copious amount of bloody discharge, the physical exam reveals a large erythematous mass. What is the most likely cause of the bloody otorrhea?

THE DIVERSION

With the mention of a large erythematous mass, you are probably inclined to think this is a tumor that can result in bloody otorrhea including a *rhabdomyosarcoma* or *eosinophilic granuloma* (both typically occurring in the middle ear). You might be inclined to diagnose a good old-fashioned ear infection, or perhaps you will pick the diversionary choice of *cholesteatoma*.

ANSWER REVEALED

However, the correct answer (given the mention of the presence of tympanostomy tubes) would be *tympanostomy tube granuloma*, which is a common complication of tympanostomy tubes.

External Ear

UPDATED & NEW BREAKING NEWS INFORMATION

Newborns with isolated ear pits or preauricular skin tags with no other congenital anomalies or risk factors do **not** require renal ultrasounds to screen for renal anomalies.

These infants do have a 5-fold higher risk of permanent hearing loss compared to the general population, so they require careful monitoring.

Foreign Body

BUZZWORDS

They might give you a hint as to why a child might place a foreign body in his ear, such as **developmental delay**. Presentation may involve **pain on movement of the pinna** (just as there would be with otitis externa, described below). **Otorrhea** might also be described.

---

[3] Pardon the pun!

Otitis Externa

"Pain when the pinna is manipulated." Swimming may often be described, since this is also known as "swimmer's ear".

They may even describe purulent discharge, which can also be consistent with otitis externa. *Pseudomonas* is the usual cause.

Treatment is with **antibiotic/steroid drops**. If there is a question on preventing swimmer's ear, this can be accomplished by acidifying the ear canal with OTC boric acid or acetic acid solutions (before and after swimming).

Hematoma External Ear (Cauliflower Ear)

If you are presented with a patient with **swelling and deformity of the external ear following blunt trauma**, the correct management would be ice packs and pressure initially and then evacuation of the hematoma immediately by needle aspiration to prevent potential cartilage loss.

Mastoiditis

Mastoiditis is **the most common suppurative complication of acute otitis media**.

Postauricular swelling and **erythema** is the typical description of mastoiditis. **Tenderness over the mastoid** and **outwardly displaced pinna** are other important clues to the diagnosis.

The bacteria most commonly causing mastoiditis in children include:

- *Streptococcus pneumoniae*
- *H. flu* (non typeable)
- *S. pyogenes*
- *S. aureus*

Diagnosis is confirmed by **CT** and **tympanocentesis** with **culture**.

However, a negative culture would not rule out the diagnosis, especially if they note the patient was already started on antibiotics.

Treatment of mastoiditis consists of **IV antibiotics** and **surgery**.

Benign Paroxysmal Vertigo of Childhood (BPVC)

Consider this diagnosis in a 1 - 4 year old patient with an acute onset of self-limited **vertigo** in the **absence of vomiting or loss of consciousness**. The episode is brief and typically recurrent. In addition, **nystagmus** will be described, as well as **pallor**.

If the vertigo lasts hours or days, then benign paroxysmal vertigo is unlikely. If **hearing loss** is also part of the history, then **labyrinthitis** is the more likely diagnosis.

Your Nose Knows

Rhinitis

The most common causes are **allergy, sinusitis, polyps, cystic fibrosis,** and **foreign body**.

In pediatric practice, you see lots of runny noses and FACES

> **F**oreign body
> **A**llergies
> **C**ystic Fibrosis
> **E**xtra tissue (**Polyps**)
> **S**inusitis

They sometimes describe nasal congestion in an adolescent as a clue that cocaine use is a part of the picture.

> **The Es Have It**
>
> A nasal smear with lots of **eosinophils** is more likely seasonal allergic rhinitis than anything else.

Choanal Atresia

Bilateral choanal atresia presents with **cyanosis while feeding** and **resolution with crying**.

50% of cases have associated anomalies, such as CHARGE syndrome.[4]

Evaluation is by inability to pass a 6-Fr catheter through the nares.

> **Pop Goes the Nasal (Polyp)**
>
> Cystic fibrosis is the most common cause of nasal polyps in children.
>
> Other causes include:
> • Aspirin sensitivity
> • Asthma
> • Allergic rhinitis
> • Chronic/recurrent sinusitis
>
> Therefore, if you are given a patient with nasal polyps and are asked which study to order next, the correct answer will be a **sweat chloride test**.

---

[4] Let's review, shall we? "C" for coloboma, "H" for heart defects, "A" for atresia choanae, "R" for retardation of growth and development, "G" for genitourinary problems, and "E" for ear abnormalities.

Sinusitis

In pre-adolescents, sinusitis will present as **persistent URI**, and **not necessarily facial pain** as seen in teens and adults.

Acute Sinusitis

This would be described as **persistent nighttime cough** and/or **foul breath** with **persistent nasal congestion** symptoms, typically longer than 7-10 days. If they present a patient with a **toothache, sore throat,** or **poorly controlled asthma,** the underlying diagnosis could be sinusitis.

Which Organisms are to Blame?

Most sinus infections are caused by **pneumococcus,** *H. Flu* **(non typeable),** and *Moraxella catarrhalis.*[5]

Since these bugs are similar to those that cause OM, the first line of antibiotic should be **amoxicillin.** However, if they present you with a patient who was recently treated with amoxicillin and/or attends daycare, then **amoxicillin/clavulanate** or **IM ceftriaxone** would be indicated.

Sinusitis is usually **a clinical diagnosis.** Sinus Xrays are NOT a good method to diagnose sinusitis because they cannot distinguish between URI and sinusitis.

Orbital cellulitis is a direct result of **ethmoid sinusitis.** This is easy to remember when you recall that Eye and Ethmoid both start with an E.

Brain abscess may result from frontal sinusitis (a **frontal assault**). Therefore, any trauma involving a **fracture of the frontal sinus** requires **surgical consult** and repair to **avoid CNS infection.**

Neither nasal swab cultures nor throat cultures correlate well with cultures of sinus aspirates, so ignore that data if they give it to you. Oral decongestants, nasal steroids, and antihistamines do not provide significant help for acute sinusitis.

Timing of Sinuses

You could be tested on when the various sinuses develop.

Here is your program guide:

Maxillary – At birth
Ethmoid – At birth
Frontal – 5-6 years of age
Sphenoid – 5-6 years of age

An easy way to remember this is to think that I have ME at birth (maxillary, ethmoid).Then frontal and sphenoid correlate with five and six.

Chronic Sinusitis

Chronic sinusitis, like acute sinusitis, will present as **chronic nasal congestion,** along with **tenderness over the sinuses** in a **febrile** child. An important component will be **nighttime cough.**

---

[5] Previously known as *Branhamella catarrhalis* and also known as Freddy the dysmorphic acrobat.

The predisposing factors for chronic sinusitis all make sense logically: **allergy, exposure to tobacco smoke, recurrent viral URIs, GER, anatomic abnormalities, immune deficiency, primary ciliary dyskinesis (immotile cilia syndrome),** and **cystic fibrosis.**

CT would be the study of choice for chronic recurrent sinusitis. **MRI** would only be indicated if an intracranial complication were suggested in the history.

 Antibiotics (and surgery when necessary) are the treatments of choice. Resolution may require 2-3 months of treatment.

> **Nasal Foreign Body**
>
> This is often described as unilateral, usually blood-tinged, nasal discharge. **Foul odor** will be your other clue.

Epistaxis

- Epistaxis is usually **due to dry air** and treatment is largely supportive.

- However, read the history carefully and watch for suggestions of a **foreign body** or **vascular anomalies**.

- Watch for signs of **bleeding disorders** in the family history or **bleeding/bruising elsewhere**.

- **Nasopharyngoscopy** would be indicated to locate a posterior bleeding source (anterior bleeding sources are often visible on exam).

> *CASE STUDY*
>
> **You are presented with a 13 year old boy with recurrent epistaxis. The bleeding is increasing in frequency and severity and takes more time to stop. What is the next step in managing this patient?**
>
> *THE DIVERSION*
>
> You will be tempted by many diversionary choices, such as saline nasal spray or gels, or even more invasive options, such as coagulopathy studies.
>
> *ANSWER REVEALED*
>
> When presented with a patient with a history of worsening epistaxis on the boards, it is real. It is not the subjective description by a parent. Therefore, the next step would be a CT scan to rule out a posterior nasopharyngeal mass such as a *nasopharyngeal angiofibroma*. On the boards they should note the presence of a mass, but even if they do not, consider the CT for worsening epistaxis.

Throat

Strep Pharyngitis[6]

Group A beta hemolytic strep is the most common cause of pharyngitis in children who have fever and sore throat **in the absence of URI symptoms**. Other symptoms may include headache, abdominal pain, nausea, a scarlatiniform rash.

On exam, patients may be mildly ill-appearing, and have throat erythema with tonsillar hypertrophy, palatal petechiae and cervical lymphadenopathy.

Other causes of pharyngitis include EBV, *Neisseria gonorrhoeae*, and adenovirus. The diagnosis is made by **culture and/or rapid strep**.

The treatment of choice remains **penicillin**, and waiting for culture results does not affect treatment outcome. If you are asked, treatment shortens the course *and* prevents the development of complications, including rheumatic fever and abscesses.

A *negative rapid strep* still requires a throat culture because of the high rate of false negatives.

If they present a patient with recurrent symptoms following treatment, the patient should have another culture done. A chronic carrier state is a possibility. The symptoms may also be indicative of a second infection (possibly due to another strain of Group A Strep), or noncompliance is always a possible explanation for poor response to treatment.

Infectious Mononucleosis[7]

Mono is caused by Epsten-Barr virus (EBV). Symptoms include **malaise, anorexia,** and **chills** followed by **pharyngitis with exudate, fever, palpable cervical lymph nodes, fatigue** and **hepatosplenomegaly**.

They may describe the symptoms in conjunction with treatment with **amoxicillin** or **ampicillin** along with subsequent development of a **rash**. The rash described above is not penicillin allergy, which is awaiting you as the decoy (and, of course, incorrect choice).

> ### CMV and EBV
> **CMV** can cause a mononucleosis-like illness with very similar symptoms.

This infection is usually **asymptomatic in preschool children**. The incubation period is **2 to 7 weeks**.

---

6 Additional information on strep in the corresponding section of the ID chapter.
7 Additional information on infectious mononucleosis can be found in the corresponding section of the ID chapter.

In differentiating strep pharyngitis from Epstein Barr (EB) mono, know that both can have pharyngitis with exudate, enlarged tonsils, and fever. **Hepatosplenomegaly will only be found with mono.**

CASE STUDY

You are presented with a 3 year old child with high fever, swollen lymph nodes, and other signs suggestive of mono. They then note that the monospot is negative. What is the next step?

THE DIVERSION

The diversion here is that the monospot screen is frequently negative in young children. All of the diversionary choices including repeating the monospot and others (i.e., treatment with penicillin), will be incorrect.

ANSWER REVEALED

The correct answer will be to obtain EBV IgM/IgG titers.

Monospot Limitations

❏ The "monospot" is **not as sensitive in children younger than 4**.

❏ Patients who are negative initially **can become positive 2-3 weeks into their illness**.

❏ Antibody titers can be detectable **for up to 9 months** after the onset of illness, so a positive monospot test does not necessarily mean active/current illness.

HOT TIP

Viral-specific IgM should be done for children younger than 4 who have negative monospot tests but still have symptoms consistent with mono. Lymphocytosis and thrombocytopenia are other lab signs.

TAKE HOME MESSAGE

IgM antibodies, rather than isolation of the virus, make for a definitive diagnosis.

TREATMENT

Treatment is supportive with **restricted** activity if the spleen is enlarged.

PERIL

Steroids are not indicated for uncomplicated disease but one week of oral prednisone (1 mg/kg/day, max 20 mg) may be considered in complicated cases with significant tonsillar enlargement with risk or airway obstruction, massive splenomegaly, myocarditis, and hemolytic anemia. Read the question carefully !

Gee Whiz, GC Pharyngitis[8]

The typical presentation of gonococcal (GC) pharyngitis would be a sexually active teenage whom they should specifically note has had sexually transmitted diseases in the past. The physical exam will be noteworthy for **erythematous patches**.

You will be expected to test the patient for gonococcal pharyngitis **and other sexually transmitted diseases as well**.

Peritonsillar Abscess (PTA)

Peritonsillar abscess is typically described as a patient experiencing **dysphagia**, with **difficulty opening their mouth**. Once the mouth is opened (a very common occurrence on the boards), they will have **unilateral swelling around the tonsil**, and **deviation of the uvula to one side**, along with some **exudate**.

Additional buzzwords include "**trismus**" (whatever that is)[9], "**drooling**," a muffled "**hot potato**" voice, and **cervical adenopathy**.

The etiology is usually wide and varied, including **group A Strep and anaerobes** found in the mouth. The choice of antibiotics should reflect this. The following would be correct antibiotics:

- Ampicillin/sulbactam
- Clindamycin
- Amoxicillin/clavulanate

Management

Diagnosis is made by **CT**. In addition, the **WBC will be elevated** on CBC.

Needle aspiration and drainage is critical to protect the airway and to provide symptomatic relief.

Retropharyngeal Abscess (RPA)

Classic presentation involves **enlarged lymph nodes** in a young child with **high fever**, **difficulty swallowing**, and **refusal of feedings**. The diagnosis should be **confirmed on CT**.

The patient's neck may be **hyperextended or held stiffly**, and he/she may demonstrate **drooling** and/or **respiratory difficulties**. If they mention a lateral neck film with **widening of the retropharyngeal space or of the paravertebral soft tissues**, take your gift and run.

Go for the T&A

Indications for tonsillectomy include the most obvious: repeated throat infections (7/one year, 5/year in the last 2 years, or 3/year in the last 3 years), airway obstruction, and malignancy.

Indications for adenoidectomy include chronic sinusitis and/or adenoiditis, as well as obstructive sleep apnea.

 Velopharyngeal insufficiency would present with a hypernasal voice, and is a complication of tonsillectomy and/or adenoidectomy.

---

[8] Additional information can be found in the corresponding secion of the Adolescent Chapter.
[9] Actually, trismus is the inability to open one's mouth.

You may need to differentiate RPA from **epiglottitis**. With epiglottitis, children appear more toxic and scared and **they lean forward** instead of hyperextending their necks or holding their neck stiffly. Epiglottitis was and is typically caused by **H. flu type b**. Watch for a history of **unknown immunization** record, **parental vaccine refusal**, or a patient from a **developing country**. This will suggest vulnerability to H. flu epiglottitis.

A retropharyngeal abscess is a surgical emergency. **Needle aspiration under general anesthesia** is the best approach.

Typical causes include *Strep viridans*, group A *Strep*, and *Staph aureus*, as well as anerobic bacteria. The best choices for antibiotics would include **clindamycin** or **ampicillin/sulbactam**. Throat swab culture is not likely to be helpful.

You will very likely be called upon to differentiate retropharyngeal from peritonsillar abscess. **Retropharyngeal abscess is more common in patients younger than 4 years of age**. This should be easy to remember since "retro" means to go back to an earlier age in time.

Epiglottitis

Epiglottitis is a supraglottic stenosis, and presents with **biphasic stridor.**

Epiglottitis, although now rare thanks to the Hib vaccine, is still fair game on the Boards.

Epiglottitis will be presented as a 4 - 5 year old with acute and rapidly progressive sore throat, dysphagia and high fevers leading to stridor, which can be inspiratory or biphasic. A key differentiating description will be their refusal to lay down, leaning forward while "tripoding" and drooling.

Lateral neck film will emphasize the **"thumb sign,"** which is the enlarged epiglottis.

Cough will not be included in the description.

5 Ds: Instead of the thumb sign, picture the swollen epiglottis as a **Giant Swollen D:** Drooling, Dysphagia, Dysphonia, Distress, and Deafening (and frightening) stridor.

They may throw in a parental refusal of all immunizations, or that the child is from another country. The implication here is that the Hib vaccine was not given.

Until you are ready to take the child back to the the OR for full immediate assessment, the child should be allowed to stay in the parents' arms as unannoyed as possible.

When epiglottitis is suspected, it is **a medical emergency** that requires rapid attention. Evaluation is done with all equipment for intubation, including having the **anesthesiologist** (with tacky shower cap and shoe covers) on standby in the room.

CBC and blood culture should be obtained, unless the airway is already obstructed or at risk of becoming obstructed momentarily. A **third-generation cephalosporin** (e.g., ceftriaxone, cefotaxime) directed at *H. flu* should be started empirically.

What About the Mouth?

We cover this extensively in the GI chapter, but here are some other bits and pieces to chew on.

All Those Oral Lesions

Here's how to keep all those oral lesions straight.

Coxsackievirus Group A

Coxsackievirus Group A **herpangina** often presents as several days of **fever, fussiness,** and **decreased appetite**, with **4-5 mm ulcers** in the **posterior** oral cavity on the posterior oropharynx and buccal areas while sparing the gums and tongue. If they throw in the term **vesiculopapular lesions on the hands and feet**, then this becomes the classic **hand-foot-and-mouth** and you've got the answer.

Herpes Simplex Virus (HSV)

Herpes simplex gingivostomatitis are cold sores typically described as **vesicles** on the **vermilion border** of the lips, and possibly in the **anterior** mouth, gums, and tongue. There is impressive mucosal **pain, fever,** and **adenopathy**.

Aphthous Ulcers

Aphthous ulcers are your classic canker sores, the kind you don't want to have when you are drinking lemon juice straight up or on the rocks (or with gin if you prefer).

They will be described as having a distinctive **grayish-white coagulum surrounded by a thin rim of bright erythema**. These resolve on their own over a week or so.

Cold-Induced Panniculitis

Cold-induced panniculitis can appear on the boards and be described as follows:

An infant **less than a year old,** with **tender red nodules on the cheek,** afebrile with good PO intake. **Sleeping with a water-filled pacifier** or something else very cold is the cause. They are described, or will be shown, as **deep-seated plaques and nodules**.

Make sure to look up pictures of this. It is very distinctive and makes for a prime picture question.

Remember, no treatment is necessary; the lesion clears within weeks, with no scarring. Counsel parents to avoid giving cold rings or toys for extended periods to prevent recurrence.

"Popsicle panniculitis," as it is also called, helps you remember the appearance and cause.

Playing Dentist

Delayed Eruption of Teeth

Up to 16 months is the "normal" waiting time for the first tooth to erupt. In the absence of other findings, reassurance without intervention would be correct.

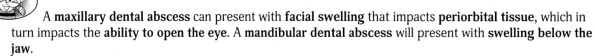

You can remember the common causes of delayed eruption of teeth as the **4 Hs plus Rickets**:

> **H**ypothyroidism
>
> **H**ypopituitarism
>
> **H**ypoplasia (ectodermal)
>
> **H**ypohidrosis (decreased sweating)
>
> **Rickets**

Tooth Avulsion

If you are presented with a child with an **avulsed permanent tooth**, know that if it is placed back in its socket within 5 minutes, there is an excellent chance it will survive.

The tooth should reimplanted by any capable adult. If it needs to be reimplanted by a dentist, the tooth should be transported in saliva (preferably the child's, of course) or milk. *Chilled milk* is preferred.

If you are presented with a child with an **avulsed baby/deciduous tooth**, replacing it can cause damage to the incoming permanent tooth, and is therefore contraindicated.

Dental Abscesses

A **maxillary dental abscess** can present with **facial swelling** that impacts **periorbital tissue**, which in turn impacts the **ability to open the eye**. A **mandibular dental abscess** will present with **swelling below the jaw**.

For both, they will likely provide some information hinting at dental disease.

Appropriate treatment would be with **penicillin**. If the patient were penicillin-allergic, then **clindamycin** or **erythromycin** would be appropriate.

Cleft Lip and Palate

The following are some important facts regarding cleft lip and palate that you will be expected to know for the exam.

Clefts are most common in **Native Americans** and **Asians** and least common in African Americans.

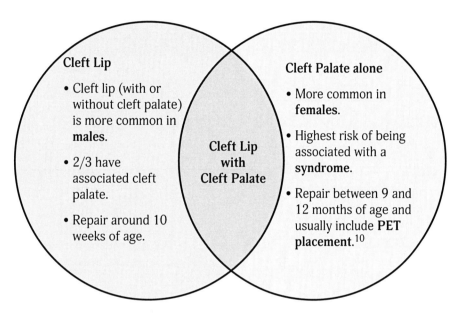

Cleft Lip

- Cleft lip (with or without cleft palate) is more common in **males**.
- 2/3 have associated cleft palate.
- Repair around 10 weeks of age.

Cleft Lip with Cleft Palate

Cleft Palate alone

- More common in **females**.
- Highest risk of being associated with a **syndrome**.
- Repair between 9 and 12 months of age and usually include **PET** placement.[10]

Any newborn with a cleft should be **evaluated by a geneticist**.

Cleft palate puts children at risk for eustachian tube dysfunction as well as vision, hearing, dental, and speech complications. Initially, special nipples are required for feeding.

To help remember some of the other syndromes besides Pierre Robin associated with clefts, consider the following mnemonic:

CAT: picture a Giant Lip, parting like a Curtain and a CAT appearing. **CAT** stands for:

Crouzon syndrome
Apert syndrome
Treacher Collins syndrome

---

[10] No, this does not mean faciliating adoption of a Clumber Collie looking for a home. PET refers to **pressure equalizing tubes**.

Upper Airway Obstructions

Obstructive Apnea

DEFINITION

When airflow ceases because the upper airway is occluded, this is obstructive apnea.

BUZZWORDS

Diagnosis of obstructive sleep apnea (OSA) requires both sleep disordered breathing (SDB) as evidenced by snoring, labored breathing, or hyperactivity, sleepiness, as well as an abnormal polysomnogram.

Clues in the presented history on the exam may include **dysmorphic facies, persistent mouth breathing, hyponasal speech,** and **cleft palate**.

PERIL

If untreated, obstructive sleep apnea can lead to **cor pulmonale** and **death**.

PERIL

Laboratory tests are not usually helpful is assessing OSA. **Polycythemia, respiratory acidosis** with **compensatory metabolic alkalosis** and **RVH on EKG** are only seen in the most severe cases.

TREATMENT

Adenoidectomy is the treatment of choice for OSA.

Adenoid hypertrophy

Obstructive sleep apnea is often due to *adenoid hypertrophy.*

PERIL

Beware that the standard examination of the oropharynx might be negative, since the adenoids are **not** typically visible on routine exam.

Extreme OSA

PERIL

If the obstructive apnea is complete (e.g., complete laryngeal atresia, severe web), treatment consists of *tracheotomy.*

Some cases, such as severe subglottic stenosis and complete vocal cord paralysis, will require permanent tracheostomy.

CASE STUDY

You are presented with a patient who is post-op from adenoidectomy and tonsillectomy, and is experiencing respiratory distress. They note a history of severe obstructive apnea. You will be asked for the most likely explanation of the acute respiratory distress.

THE DIVERSION

You might be tempted to pick pulmonary hemorrhage or hemothorax. Other diversionary choices could include tension pneumothorax, since this would likely be post extubation.

ANSWER REVEALED

The correct answer in this setting would be pulmonary edema, which is a postoperative complication in patients with severe obstructive apnea.

Sleep apnea

Sleep apnea is common in children. It is important to know that symptoms occur both at night and during the day. Night time symptoms include snoring, apnea, and enuresis.

If they provide you with a history of sleep apnea at night and ADD or ADHD complaints during the day / school then sleep apnea is likely what they are looking for. Treatment for ADHD will not likely be correct in this context.

Stridor Cider

Stridor is due to **turbulent flow** through a **narrowed** segment of the respiratory tract.

All that glitters is not croup and epiglottitis. The key again is in the wording, and in the specifics that differentiate similar clinical presentations of stridor.

Fortunately, you can answer questions on stridor correctly just by becoming familiar with the buzzwords in the following sections. On the other hand, you could be the best on-site diagnostician, but get these questions wrong if you do not know these buzzwords cold. This is typical for written Board exams, as clinical skills and test taking skills are different.

If you are presented with a patient with stridor, just noting the age should help narrow down the correct answer if you are asked for a diagnosis.

Inspiratory Stridor

Inspiratory stridor is caused by **extrathoracic** (above the thoracic outlet) obstruction.

All the "structures" above the thoracic outlet are soft and collapse inward with the pressure of inspiration, and that makes for the inspiratory stridor. Extrathoracic includes supraglottic, glottic and subglottic areas (see below). Inspiratory stridor will always be more prominent, but as you get lower, the chances of also having expiratory stridor increase.

Inspiratory stridor is associated with swelling and inflammation of the tonsils and adenoids, as well as pharyngeal and **hypopharyngeal masses**.

It is easy to remember the causes of **inspiratory stridor** with the following mnemonic (**INSP**):

> Immobile Cords (Paralyzed)
>
> Noid (Adenoid) and tonsil enlargement
>
> Soft cartilage (laryngomalacia)
>
> Pharyngeal and hypopharyngeal masses

Stridor Through the Ages

From 4 to 6 weeks - laryngomalacia or tracheomalacia

1 to 4 years - croup, epiglottitis, foreign body aspiration

Older than 5 years - vocal cord dysfunction, peritonsillar abscess, or anaphylaxis

---

Laryngomalacia

Laryngomalacia is a condition in which the tissues at the entrance of the larynx collapse into the airway with inspiration.

Laryngomalacia is **the most common cause of congenital stridor.**

Infants with laryngomalacia feed without difficulty and gain weight. If you are presented with an infant who is failing to thrive, laryngomalacia is not the correct answer.

Typical descriptions of laryngomalacia include:

❑ **Suprasternal and subcostal retractions**
❑ In an infants under 1 month of age with stridor, you may see **"worsening with agitation"**
❑ Stridor that **worsens with the infant in the supine position**
❑ Symptoms **improve with expiration** (pressure from below with expiration, "stents" the floppy airway open)
❑ Symptoms do **improve with time** as the cartilage becomes firmer

Vocal Cord Paralysis

A **blunted inspiratory loop** on spirometry correlates with vocal cord paralysis, rather than asthma. Other associations with vocal cord paralysis include: recent viral upper respiratory tract infection, exposure to chemicals, fumes, or cold air, and gastroesophageal reflux disease (GERD).

Vocal cord paralysis is the **second most common cause of extra-thoracic airway obstruction** and stridor in infancy. It is usually due to **traumatic injury of the recurrent laryngeal** nerve at the time of birth, or to an impairment of the central nervous system such as a posterior fossa tumor/abnormality (Arnold Chiari malformation) or hydrocephalus.

The cry will be described as **weak** and the stridor will be described as **high pitched**.

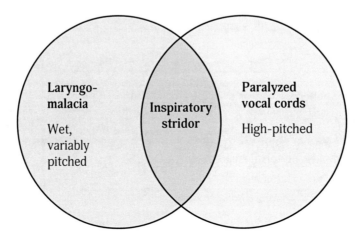

Unilateral vocal cord paralysis would be described as **persistent hoarseness**.

Vocal Cord Nodules

Vocal cord nodules are typically described as being characterized by **progressive hoarseness**, which is less severe in the morning, **without stridor or dysphagia**.

Most cases of **chronic hoarseness** in children are caused by vocal cord nodules. They occur more often in males, and tend to improve with puberty.

Vocal Cord Dysfunction (VCD)

You may be presented with a patient who has what seems to be asthma, but is actually vocal cord dysfunction. **Hoarseness** may follow endotracheal extubation, so watch for that in the history if you are asked to determine a cause. **Laryngoscopy is often required to diagnose laryngeal and vocal cord disorders.**

No need to lose your voice or sleep over all of this if you note the following:

As opposed to asthma, a patient with vocal cord dysfunction will have a **normal pulse oximeter reading**. They will note clear lung fields on physical exam and **no response to bronchodilator treatment**.

In vocal cord dysfunction, **inspiratory stridor**, rather than expiratory wheezing, will be problematic.

A classic presentation will be a teenager in sports who starts "wheezing" during activity. A history of anxiety is not uncommon.

Treatment for VCD includes referral to ENT and/or speech therapy for speech and behavior therapy along with respiratory exercises and anxiety counseling as needed.

Expiratory Stridor

Lesions **below the thoracic inlet** cause expiratory stridor. Tracheomalacia and bronchomalacia are classic examples.

Tracheomalacia

Tracheomalacia is a rare condition, in which weak tracheal wall rings **collapse during expiration**. In addition to expiratory **stridor**, extrinsic tracheal compression can also cause fixed wheezing. Infants with tracheomalacia can therefore present with **wheezing**. This can also be the result of neonatal **prolonged ventilator support**, so watch for this in the presenting history.

With laryngomalacia, symptomatic relief is noted during expiration, which is not the case with tracheomalacia.

A child who has had a TE fistula repair will frequently present later on with expiratory stridor due to tracheomalacia.

Another cause of "extrinsic compression" is the **vascular ring** (that wraps around the trachea AND the esophagus). A hint that vascular ring is the problem is **feeding difficulties** in addition to **expiratory stridor**.

"Biphasic" (Inspiratory and Expiratory) Stridor

Both congenital and acquired **subglottic stenoses** (i.e., subglottic hemangiomas) straddle both sides of the anatomical fence (intra-thoracic and extra-thoracic) can result in biphasic stridor.

How They Are Assessed

Subglottic stenosis	Direct laryngoscopy and bronchoscopy (the latter to assess the patency of the subglottis adequately)
Vocal cord function	Flexible nasolaryngoscopy or direct laryngoscopy, plus CXR and barium swallow
Vascular ring	Barium swallow study

If you are presented with an infant with "noisy breathing," the initial step is to obtain a thorough birth history and observe the breathing patterns in different positions.

The Scoop on Croup

Viral croup is synonymous with **laryngotracheobronchitis**. It will be described as a toddler, usually in fall and winter, who has a harsh, nonproductive **barking cough**, with a **low grade fever** and **URI symptoms**.

With worsening of the narrowing, they will either describe an **inspiratory stridor** or a **biphasic** (inspiratory and expiratory) stridor.

They may describe or show an AP chest x-ray depicting the steeple sign with croup, which is narrowing of the subglottic trachea. Make sure you can recognize this and differentiate it from epiglottis, which will be a lateral neck x-ray with + thumb sign.

Treatment for mild croup includes **humidified air, fever reduction, oral fluids,** and **exposure to cold night air**.

More severe croup, characterized by **stridor at rest or retractions,** may require a single dose of **dexamethasone, nebulized racemic epinephrine,** and even possible **intubation.**

Racemic epinephrine may be readministered every 15 to 20 minutes as needed. Children who have received racemic epinephrine require a minimum **3 to 4 hours of observation** before they can be discharged home.

Measles (rubeola) can also cause croup. **Watch out for children who may not have been immunized**, including children of parents who do not like immunizations, and recent immigrants, especially from developing countries, whose immunization status is unknown.

Spasmodic croup may also be described as a **"barky nonproductive cough"** and may be due to **allergies or psychological factors**. However there will be no URI or fever.

> ### Croup Who Done It?
>
> **Etiology: R**SV, Influenza, or **P**arainfluenza (RIP).
>
> To help remember **RIP**, think of a dog with a bark-like cough RIPping apart the viruses that cause croup.

Bacterial Tracheitis

This is also known as **"pseudomembranous croup,"** or **"membranous laryngotracheitis."** It is usually caused by *S. aureus*, but can also be caused by *Moraxella catarrhalis*, nontypeable *Haemophilus influenzae*, or oral anaerobes.

Bacterial tracheitis might occur several days into a bout with viral croup. Watch for **rapid deterioration** of a patient diagnosed with viral croup.

The patient will typically be described as being **toxic-appearing.** Bacterial tracheitis presents with **thick, purulent secretions** which can cause airway obstruction, and, in severe cases, cardiopulmonary arrest. They could include a neck film, described as a **"ragged air column" or "subglottic narrowing."**

With epiglottitis, the child will be described as leaning forward and drooling. In bacterial tracheitis, they will be more comfortable staying in the supine position.

Since you will likely be presented with a patient who deteriorates rapidly, it is important to know that often **intubation** is required, as well as **clearing of purulent secretions**. Broad spectrum **antibiotics** that provide coverage for *Staph* are also indicated.

Neck Masses

Sometimes, the happy little lymph nodes that live everywhere doing their job peacefully behind the scenes, become too big to be ignored. Sometimes, those lumps and pains in the neck are not lymph nodes at all. Here's what you need to know to deal with questions that include those little troublemakers.

Cervical Adenopathy

Most cases of cervical lymph node enlargement in children are **reactive**, ie. due to infection. The nodes will likely be described as **mobile and tender**, but will **not** be described as being erythematous or warm to touch. In a few days or weeks, the swelling will decrease.

> **Preauricular Nodes**
>
> The classic presentation of **adenovirus infection** would be the combination of **preauricular adenopathy** with **conjunctivitis**.

If the lymphadenopathy is **unexplained or persists**, checking for **HIV and TB** could be the correct choices.

Lymphadenitis

If the node itself is infected (rather than reactive), in addition to being **tender**, it will also be **red** and **warm** to touch.

Acute viral cervical lymphadenitis is generally **bilateral**. **Bacterial lymphadenitis**, on the other hand, is usually **unilateral**, with **more local inflammation**.

The most common organisms causing cervical adenitis are *Staph aureus* and group A strep, but remember to consider TB, nonTB mycobacteria, and cat scratch disease, if there is a subacute course with nontender nodes.

If they do not provide you with the following labs, then ordering them could be the correct answer: CBC, ESR, blood cultures, PPD, DNA, and DWI.[11]

Treatment of choice is antibiotics that can fight the beta lactamase-producers. **Amoxicillin/ clavulanate** and **clindamycin** are good choices. **Erythromycin** would be a good choice when penicillin allergy is a factor.

Atypical (NonTB) Mycobacteria

Atypical mycobacteria will typically result in persistent submental and submandibular lymph node swelling and a **PPD reaction** of 10 mm or less (less than what is expected for TB infection), and a negative interferon-gamma assay test in 1-5 year olds. They may describe an overlying **violaceous (purplish) hue**.

The best treatment is to **leave it alone**. If antibiotics are utilized, consider clarithromycin or azithromycin, plus rifampin.

---

[11] Just kidding on DWI; just making sure you are still with us.

Surgical lymph node excision can sometimes be necessary <u>depending on the history</u> they present you with.

Needle excision is never the correct answer for atypical mycobacteria lymphadenopathy because it will drain forever and the parents will hate you. You will also hate yourself for answering the question incorrectly.

Mycobacterium tuberculosis

Mycobacterium tuberculosis might be what they are after if they present a patient with **cervical adenitis who is not responding to antibiotics**. They would also likely present other risk factors for tuberculosis.

Remember that both TB and nonTB mycobacteria will turn a PPD positive. The only good way to differentiate between the two would be to **check an IGRA** (Quantiferon or T-spot blood test) which is positive in TB and negative in nonTB.

> **Infant Adenitis**
>
> With infants, *Staph* is an important cause of **acute cervical lymphadenitis**. Surgical drainage may be necessary.

Neoplasm

If a lymph node is malignant, it will be **nontender, firm,** and **non-mobile/fixed** and will **not shrink in size** over time like reactive nodes tend to do. Other clues are weight loss, fever, and other lymph nodes enlarged.

Remember if the mass is around the thyroid, that thyroid carcinoma is a possibility and a very bad thing to miss.

> **Branchial Cleft Remnants**
>
> Branchial Cleft remnants arelocated anterior to the sternocleidomastoid muscle.

Thyroglossal Duct Cyst

This is the #1 congenital cyst in the neck.

Unless there are other signs shown to you, **any midline lesion on the anterior neck** should be assumed to be a thyroglossal cyst; it should have a "Do Not Remove" sign (as in "No Surgical Excisions") hanging over it, until it has been cleared of functioning thyroid tissue.

They will describe the lesion as **moving upward with swallowing or sticking the tongue out**. There could be communication with the skin potentially leading to recurrent infections or drainage.

Even though thyroglossal duct cysts are congenital, they are rarely recognized at birth. They usually present at 3-10 years of age.

Cystic hygroma

A cystic hygroma is **a mass of dilated lymph vessels**. They might be described as being a large soft neck mass. In fact, they can be so large that they can compress surrounding structures. It may be associated with Turner syndrome.

Branchial Cleft Remnants

These remnants are located anteriorly to the sternocleidomastoid muscle. The second branchial cleft remnants are the most common.

They may present when they drain from a sinus tract get infected.

Treatment is with antibiotics or surgical excision.

Muscular Torticollis

Presentation includes a palpable fibrous mass within the body of the sternocleidomastoid muscle.

The right side is affected 75% of the time.

Dermoid Cysts

Congenital subcutaneous lesions that may or may not be noticed at birth. They are usually asymptomatic.

They may be seen anywhere in the body, but are common in the head (scalp and eyebrow edge) and neck region. In the neck, they are typically midline and may be confused with thyroglossal duct cysts.

Ultrasound is indicated. Because they grow slowly and steadily, they should be resected while small, especially if in undesirable areas (cosmetically or potentially obstructive).

Parotitis

You are expected to know the different causes of parotitis and their presentations as outlined in the following table.

Cause of Parotitis	Presentation
Viral parotitis	Presents in a preschool or school-age child with parotid swelling and **vague symptoms**, including weakness and fever.
	There will be swelling and erythema around the opening of **Stensen's duct**, but typically **no pus can be expressed** with parotid massage.
	HOT TIP There will be **no erythema** of the overlying skin.
	If the child is **unimmunized**, consider a diagnosis of mumps.
	HIV infection must be a consideration if the presenting history supports the diagnosis.
Bacterial parotitis	Occurs **before the age of 10**. The child will be described as **toxic-appearing**, with a **very high temperature**.
	Staph aureus is the most common cause of bacterial parotitis.
Salivary gland stone	This will present as **recurrent swelling of both parotid glands**.

CASE STUDY **You are presented with a patient from a developing country who has parotid swelling of a few weeks' duration which is resistant to antibiotic therapy. There is no information on the biological parents. You are told that the patient received multiple vaccines, although it is not well-documented. You are asked for the most appropriate study to help establish the diagnosis.**

THE DIVERSION You would, of course, realize that this is most likely viral parotitis, since this child most likely did not receive an MMR vaccine. Therefore, picking a study such as mumps titers to establish mumps as the correct diagnosis would be automatic.

ANSWER REVEALED You would have automatically picked the wrong answer. An important part of the history is the lack of knowledge about the biological parents. This, coupled with the information that some vaccines were given, should make you suspicious for HIV infection.

Chapter 33

Adolescent Medicine and Gynecology

Adolescent Cognitive Development

The 3 main areas of cognitive development that occur during adolescence are:

1. Develop reasoning skills, ie. explore consequences both hypothetical and logical
2. Think abstractly, ie. love and spirituality
3. Start thinking about thinking, ie. think about their feelings and how others see them

Adolescent Psychosocial Development

The 3 major tasks of adolescence are:

1. Establishment of autonomy, ie. become independent of the parents
2. Develop a sense of identity, ie. who the youth is, what he's good at, and his self-worth
3. The ability for future orientation, ie. career as well as moral, religious and sexual values

Separation from family

It is crucial that parents accept separation and even some rebellion as a healthy step in their teen's development.

The **peer group** is very important in a young adolescent's separation from the family.

During **early adolescence** (12-14 years), the peer group is same-sex and teens are most concerned about how they appear to their friends, frequently changing clothing and hairstyle to fit in.

During **middle adolescence** (15-17 years), the peer group is mixed-sex and finding a mate becomes important.

During **late adolescence** (18-21 years), adolescents move away from peer groups and into relationships.

Teens who do not not identify with any peer groups ("loners") have significant psychological difficulties during adolescence.

Changing bodies and self-esteem

Rapid body changes have a significant effect on an adolescent's sense of self.

Early maturing boys in high school are often perceived as older and more responsible, do better at sports and tend to be more popular, but if it happens much earlier, they may develop hostility and distress symptoms.

Early pubertal maturation in girls puts them at higher risk for conduct problems, depression, early substance use, poor body image, pregnancy, and early sexual experimentation.

Risk-taking teens

Teens DO perceive risk, but it does not keep them from partaking in the risk-taking behavior. They seem to gain significant emotional satisfaction from engaging is such behavior.

The concrete thinking adolescent (12-14 years) is more concerned with how he looks to his peers than the risk of the behavior. They lack the ability to link cause and effect.

> ### Weight/High and Low in Adolescent Females
>
> If they present you with a question regarding an adolescent girl with a weight issue then the answer they want is to "ask her what she thinks about her weight". If it's an adolescent boy the same would apply.

> ### Teen Deaths
>
> **Motor vehicle accidents (MVA)** remain the leading cause of morbidity and mortality among 16-20 year olds.
>
> Risks are increased by inexperience and risk taking behavior (speeding, not wearing seat belts, drugs and alcohol use, texting and other distractions).
>
> **Homicide** and **suicide** are the other two major causes of death in this age group.

Adolescent Behavioral Health

Eating Disorders

Anorexia Nervosa (A.N.)

The hallmark of A.N. is the **inability to maintain a healthy body weight**.

In order to make the diagnosis of anorexia nervosa the following criteria must be met:

1. Distorted body perception
2. Restriction of energy intake leading to significantly low weight in the context of age, sex, developmental trajectory, and health
3. Intense fear of gaining weight with restriction of energy intake

> ### Anorexa Nervosa Mortality
>
> Anorexia nervosa has the **highest fatality rate** of any mental health disorder.

CASE STUDY You might be given several signs and symptoms consistent with an eating disorder and will have to pick the one that is *most* important in making the diagnosis.

THE DIVERSION Many of the choices will seem correct because they do occur with anorexia nervosa, including *excessive exercise, depression, dieting over several months, and/ or taking diuretics.*

ANSWER REVEALED These are all diversionary answers since the correct answer is that the patient "thinks" they are fat, despite their weight being normal. This is the most important criteria for making the diagnosis. The other choices are too non-specific.

Indications for hospital admission with anorexia

- Weight <75% of ideal body weight
- Acute weight decline and refusal of food
- Hypothermia
- Hypotension
- Bradycardia
- Orthostatic changes in BP or pulse
- Electrolyte abnormalities
- Arrhythmia
- Suicidality
- Failure to respond to outpatient treatment

ARFID

DEFINITION ARFID is not a new species of insect. It stands for Avoidant/ Restrictive Food Intake Disorder, a new category of eating disorder including conditions in which there is a disturbance in eating without fear of gaining weight.

UPDATED & NEW BREAKING NEWS INFORMATION ARFID may lead to a failure to gain weight appropriately, a significant nutritional deficiency, a dependency on enteral feeding, or a marked change in psychosocial functioning.

Bulimia Nervosa

DEFINITION An important feature of bulimia nervosa is **binge eating**, which is the consumption of an amount of food larger than most people would eat in one sitting. This is coupled with **a compensatory mechanism such as vomiting, diuretic/laxative use, or excessive exercise.**

BUZZWORDS Some of the physiologic and lab findings may be a result of vomiting, including:

- Salivary and/or parotid gland enlargement
- Dental enamel erosion
- Bruises or calluses over the knuckles from forced gagging (Russell's sign)
- Low potassium
- Low chloride
- Metabolic alkalosis
- Elevated amylase

Indications for hospital admission with bulimia

- Syncope
- Hypothermia
- Arrhythmia
- Electrolyte abnormalities
- Intractable vomiting
- Boerhaave syndrome
- Suicidal ideation
- Failure of outpatient treatment

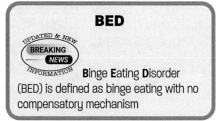

BED

Binge **E**ating **D**isorder (BED) is defined as binge eating with no compensatory mechanism

Achalasia must be distinguished from bulimia. Key information in the history would include **involuntary** vomiting soon after food is ingested.

Adolescents and Consent

Ethical Legal Issues

Even though thankfully this isn't the bar exam, you must know some basic legal issues as they pertain to minors.

Parental Consent

Invariably, a question or two will come up on the exam regarding parental consent, including when parental permission is required and when it is not.

Parental Consent is *not* needed:

- Life threatening emergencies (also sexual assault services)
- Medical care during pregnancy (also family planning)
- Treatment for sexually transmitted diseases (also HIV testing)
- Treatment for substance abuse

Confidentiality must be maintained in these situations if the patient requests it. However, the exception to this rule would be where the patient is a danger to himself or others.[1]

Emancipated minors do not need parental consent to receive treatment.

An emancipated minor is defined as a person under legal age who is no longer under their parent's control and regulation and who is managing their own financial affairs.

A "mature minor" is one that you clinically feel is able to understand the medical issue presented and can help in his or her decision making. It is not a legal term.

In cases where parental consent is not required, informed consent is still required. In such cases the minor is allowed to give informed consent instead of the parent.

Parental consent *is* required for:

Virtually all other medical and surgical procedures, including blood donation.

---

[1] This is the case for most states in the US, and therefore, would be correct for purpose of the Board exam.

Adolescent Physiologic Development

You say Tanner; I say SMR

What was once called Tanner staging is now known as Sexual Maturity Rating. The names have changed, but the stage is the same.

MALE

	SMR 1 Prepubertal	SMR 2 Beginning of puberty	SMR 3	SMR 4	SMR 5
Pubic Hair	Absent	Fine hair appears	Coarse, curly, and pigmented	Denser and curled, but less abundant than adult	Extends to the inner thigh, adult-like
Phallus Size	Childlike	No change	Increased phallus size	Closer to adult male	Adult size
Testicular Size	Volume < 2.5 mL	Increased size and volume; scrotum more textured	Increased size		Adult size

Female

	SMR 1 Prepubertal	SMR 2 Beginning of puberty	SMR 3	SMR 4	SMR 5
Pubic Hair	Absent	Hair along the labia	Coarse, curly, and pigmented	Denser and curled, but less abundant than adult	Extends to the inner thigh, adult-like
Breast	No glandular breast tissue	Small breast buds with glandular tissue	Breast tissue extends beyond the areola	Enlarged areola and papilla form a secondary mound	No longer a separate projection of the areola from the remainder of the breast

Menstruation Issues

Menarche

- The onset of menses will occur, on average, two years after thelarche (at approximately age 12 or 13).
- The first few cycles only last 2-3 days and may occur only every 2-3 months.
- The **peak height velocity occurs before menarche**. One would expect a girl to be at SMR stage 3 or 4 at the onset of menarche.

HOT TIP

Menstruation that persists beyond 10 days is abnormal and requires a workup.

However, infrequent menstrual periods during the first 2 years post menarche do **not** generally require a workup beyond reassurance and followup.

After menarche, girls are within 4cm/2inches of adult height.

Physiologic leukorrhea

DEFINITION

Physiologic leukorrhea is a white, odorless, mucoid discharge that precedes menarche by 3-6 months and can continue for several years.

It requires no intervention.

CASE STUDY

You are presented with an 11 year old girl who is SMR stage 2 and has bloody vaginal discharge. You have to determine the etiology.

THE DIVERSION

One of the diversionary answers could be reassurance, using the logic that this may be the onset of menses, or menarche.

ANSWER REVEALED

However, if you realized that the onset of menses occurs at SMR state 3 or 4, you would have been spared the indignity of answering this question incorrectly. The correct answer would be another explanation, such as vaginal foreign body, which is a common occurrence in girls this age (i.e., small pieces of toilet paper causing local irritation and mild bleeding).

Pregnancy

Fertile Facts

- The most likely reason for not using contraception is a desire to become pregnant
- 1/2 of all pregnancies occur within 6 months of the first time experiencing intercourse
- 1/5 occur during the first month

Contraceptives

Combined Hormone Contraceptives (CHC)

- There are other indications and advantages of combines hormone contraceptives besides its descriptive calling card.

- They **decrease the risk for ovarian cysts, uterine and ovarian cancers**, and even **colorectal cancer** and **osteoporosis**.

- They help **reduce free testosterone levels** and **decrease hirsutism**.

- They **reduce the risk for salpingitis** and **ectopic pregnancy**.

- They provide some protection against **acne** and **iron deficiency anemia**.

- CHCs would be indicated for **dysmenorrhea, dysfunctional uterine bleeding, PCOS, irregular menses**, and/or **menorrhagia**.

Oral contraceptives may not be ideal for teens because difficulty with adherence may lead to unintended pregnancy and breakthrough bleeding. They also may lead to nausea and small increased risk of venous thromboembolism.

The transdermal contraceptive patch works just like oral contraceptives but is a patch applied to skin and changed weekly.

Absolute Contraindications

- ❏ Migraine headache with aura or neurologic changes
- ❏ Pregnancy or <21 days post-partum
- ❏ Uncontrolled hypertension and certain significant heart conditions
- ❏ Liver disease
- ❏ Breast cancer
- ❏ History of CVA
- ❏ A history of deep vein thrombosis
- ❏ A history of pulmonary embolism
- ❏ Known Factor V Leiden mutation or other thrombophilic condition
- ❏ Major surgery with prolonged immobilization
- ❏ Complicated solid organ transplant

> COC have not been associated with weight gain.

> **Hold the Estrogen!**
> Progestin-only pills methods are ideal for patients who have contraindications to COCs and since they tend to suppress periods over time, they are also indicated for patients with catamenial (SAT word for menstrual-associated) symptoms such as migraines and epilepsy and to suppress periods in patients with physical and mental disabilities.

Depot medroxyprogesterone acetate (DMPA)

BUZZWORDS

"Depot Provera" injections are effective for contraception 3 months at a time. Other benefits include decreased blood loss and decreased cramping because of suppressed ovarian cycling.

Limitations of use include quarterly visits for injection, irregular bleeding, and the most dreaded teen side effect of all... weight gain, so it must be used with caution in obese patients.

> *HOT TIP*
> All contraceptive methods are associated with fewer health risks than pregnancy and delivery.

Long Acting Reversible Contraceptives (LARCs)

IUD

The newer IUDs are considered to be safer than in the past, without the increased risk for PID or infertility down the road and are currently advocated as the preferred method of contraception for all women regardless of age and parity.

Etonogestrel Subdermal Implant

Also known as Nexplanon, this progestin-only implant is preferred by many teens due to ease of use. Some hesitate due to fear of the procedure. Main side effect is irregular bleeding but it tends to subside and periods may eventually stop.

Pap Smear Timing

Current guidelines recommend a screening Pap smears start at age 21, regardless of age of first intercourse.

Primary Amenorrhea

DEFINITION

By definition, primary amenorrhea is the **lack of menses by age 15**, or 3 years following breast development.

If you are presented with a teenager with primary amenorrhea, keep the following diagnoses in mind:

> **Before the period !**
>
> Don't miss it! The #1 cause of amenorrhea you need to consider is PREGNANCY, even if they swear up one side and down the other that they've never had sex. A girl may become pregnant even before her first menstrual period, in which case it would present and be described as "primary amenorrhea".

Androgen insensitivity Syndrome[2]

BUZZWORDS

This condition was formerly known as **testicular feminization** and will present with **normal breast development** in the **absence of pubic hair and menstruation**.

Turner Syndrome

BUZZWORDS

A typical presentation would be an **amenorrheic girl** with breast development limited to **breast budding** and **no pubic hair development**.

Watch for other features of Turner syndrome in the history. These could include **short stature, a low hairline** and **low set ears**, as well as a **heart murmur, hypertension**, or **lymphedema of the hands and/or feet**.

HOT TIP

A **karyotype** study would be indicated.

---

[2] Covered in detail in the Endocrinology chapter.

Secondary Amenorrhea

3 months of amenorrhea AFTER the onset of menarche.

The most common causes of secondary amenorrhea are **pregnancy, PCOS,** and **exercise-induced amenorrhea.**

It can also occur in **anorexia nervosa**, with amenorrhea **preceding** weight loss. In such a case, in all fairness, they would have to provide you with other signs suggestive of anorexia nervosa.

Polycystic ovary disease

Polycystic ovary disease should be suspected in any female adolescent who, in addition to **amenorrhea or dysfunctional uterine bleeding**, presents with **obesity, hirsutism** and **acne.** Lab findings often include **elevated testosterone levels.**

It is a clinical or biochemical diagnosis.

One would think that the ovarian US would be a slam-dunk if you saw many cysts. But imaging is not a method of diagnosis because ovarian morphology is very varied in adolescents.

Treatment would include **diet and exercise** first. **Low-androgen oral contraceptive pills medications** would be second-line agents. **Spironolactone** would be an example of an anti-androgen medication **Metformin** is an option in obese patients.

While obesity is a common association, it isn't always present, and therefore lack of obesity doesn't rule out polycystic ovary disease.

Exercise-induced amenorrhea

The typical presentation is a teenager who is involved in **heavy athletic training** whose menstrual cycles gradually become lighter and then stop. Lab values would include **low serum estradiol (E2)** levels, which increases their risk for **low bone density and osteoporosis.**

These patients are at **increased risk for eating disorders**, including anorexia nervosa.

> The Female Athletic Triad:
> 1. Amenorrhea
> 2. Osteoporosis
> 3. Disordered eating

Management would include:

1. Increase caloric intake
2. Reduction in the intensity of athletic training
3. Calcium supplements

In the unlikely event they are smoking, they need to stop since this increases the risk for stress fractures

Hormone replacement ie, OCPs to regulate periods, would **not** be the correct treatment.

Dysmenorrhea

Primary Dysmenorrhea

Primary dysmenorrhea is **crampy lower abdominal pain and pelvic pain** that occurs **with menses** and is **not due to other pelvic pathology**. It is due to prostaglandins produced during the ovulatory cycle.

Treatment is with **prostaglandin inhibitors** such as NSAIDs, including ibuprofen or naproxen. **Oral contraceptives** are only indicated when the NSAID treatment fails.

Primary dysmenorrhea is a significant cause of teens missing or modifying school, work, sports activities, and social engagements.

Dysmenorrhea is more common in girls who have **early menarche**, **heavy menses**, and a **family history of dysmenorrhea**. Teens who **exercise regularly** are less likely to experience dysmenorrhea.

Secondary Dysmenorrhea

In teens whose dysmenorrhea is not responding to NSAIDs and OCPs, remember to rule out **NON GYN causes** of pelvic pain (like irritable bowel syndrome) and consider referral to rule out **endometriosis** as correct answers.

Dysfunctional Uterine Bleeding (DUB)

Consider this diagnosis for menstrual bleeding **beyond 10 days**.

The most common cause of dysfunctional uterine bleeding is **anovulation** during initial onset of menarche.

> **TB and DUB**
>
> In developing countries, TB is a common cause of DUB.

If you are presented with a patient with dysfunctional uterine bleeding, consider the following **underlying etiologies**:

- Tubal Pregnancy/ Threatened abortion
- PID
- Thyroid disease
- Medications
- Bleeding disorder
- PCOS
- Trauma
- Systemic disease (diabetes, lupus, kidney disease).

> **Menorrhagia, Metrorrhagia, and Mind Blowing Nomenclature**
>
> **Menorrhagia**, or hypermenorrhea: heavy or prologed bleeding at regular intervals.
>
> **Metrorrhagia**: irregular vaginal bleeding.
>
> **Menometrorrhagia**: heavy vaginal bleeding at irregular intervals.
>
> **Polymenorrhea**: frequent vaginal bleeding more often than every 21 days.

Treatment is medical with **reassurance** and sometimes **NSAIDs**. **OCPs** are a good alternative for persistent cases.

The possibility of **iron deficiency anemia** should be considered.

> **Painless Bleeding**
>
> In cases of heavy menstrual bleeding without pain, consider Chlamydia.

GYN at all Ages

Neonatal Vaginal Discharge

Pink vaginal discharge in an otherwise healthy newborn is most likely due to the influence of maternal estrogen withdrawal; no intervention is necessary in that case.

Vitamin K deficiency would **not** be the cause unless they describe other signs such as petechiae.

Labial Adhesions

Vaginal adhesions are commonly seen during infancy and in pre-school girls. They are similar to the adhesions seen in the foreskin in males, and usually resolve spontaneously.

In cases of dysuria or secondary bacterial infection, treatment with **estrogen cream** would be indicated.

Imperforate Hymen

Imperforate hymen will present in a girl who has reached full sexual maturity in the absence of menarche. Additional findings will include **cyclical abdominal pain, midline abdominal mass, and/or bluish bulging hymen.**

Another condition to consider and differentiate from imperforate hymen is **tubo-ovarian abscess.** Tubo-ovarian abscess can also present with intermittent abdominal pain; however, the abscess is usually not palpable midline.

Hydrometrocolpos is the collection of fluid in the uterus, in this case due to imperforate hymen and retained menstrual fluids.

If they present you with a patient with signs and symptoms consistent with imperforate hymen and/or hydrometrocolpos, and ask for the **most appropriate step** in the patient's evaluation, the correct answer will be **physical examination of the external genitalia.**

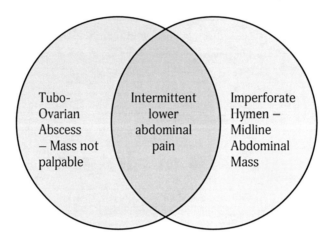

Vulvovaginitis

Vulvovaginitis presents as **vaginal irritation, pain,** and **pruritus.** It can also present as **dysuria.**

Vulvovaginitis can be due to **non sexually transmitted diseases**, including:

- *Enterobius vermicularis* (pinworms)
- Group A beta hemolytic Strep
- *Staph*
- *Candida*

Sexually transmitted causes include:

- Gonorrhea
- Chlamydia
- Trichomonas Vaginalis
- Herpes Simplex

Most vulvovaginitis that will present on the boards is not due to sexual activity in teens or sexual abuse in children. Usually it will be **non-specific** due to poor hygiene, chemical irritants such as bubble bath, or tight clothing.

- Vaginitis can also be due to a **foreign body** (such as toilet paper), which may also include **discharge** and a **foul odor**.
- **Candida infection** could be seen in a pre-pubescent girl if there is a history of recent antibiotic use.
- *Neisseria gonorrhea* will typically include a description of **green discharge**. A **beta hemolytic strep infection** could present similarly.

Candida vaginitis

Candida vaginitis may be described as some variation of **milk curd discharge** that is **itchy**.

Treatment is with **topical clotrimazole**.

Bacterial Vaginosis (BV)

Bacterial vaginosis includes *Gardnerella vaginalis, Ureaplasma,* and *Mycoplasma hominis.*

It is not considered an STI, but is often associated with sexual activity.

A malodorous **fishy** = amine odor is diagnostic. Diagnosis can be made by the **"Whiff Test,"** which is testing for the presence of amines after the addition of potassium hydroxide.

"Clue cells" are vaginal epithelial cells covered by bacteria so the cell walls are not visible.

Most women with BV are asymptomatic. If symptomatic, treatment includes metronidazole, tinidazole, or clindamycin.

Male sexual partners do not need to be treated, but same-sex female partners should be offered testing and treatment.

Recurrences occur often.

> **The diagnosis of Bacterial Vaginosis requires 3 out of 4 symptoms/ signs.**
>
> 1. copious grey-white vaginal discharge
> 2. vaginal pH >4.5
> 3. clue cells under microscopy
> 4. presence of fishy odor when discharge contacts 10% KOH

"Classic" STIs

Condyloma acuminata (Venereal Warts)

Condyloma acuminata appear as **flat papular lesions**, which are often **pedunculated** in the genital and/or anal mucosa. Transmission in adolescents and young adults is almost always **via sexual contact**.

Venereal Warts are caused by the **human papillomavirus (HPV)**. The lesions are **non-tender** and will **bleed with minor trauma**. Anogenital warts are often asymptomatic in males, and this could easily be a question on the exam.

It is a risk factor for the development of **cervical cancer**.

Anogenital warts have a high spontaneous resolution rate. Therefore, it may be a reasonable option to observe for 1-2 years before treatment.

Medical treatment would be with chemical cauterization with **podophyllin** or **podofilox. Surgical excision** is another alternative. But most importantly, observation is the initial management. **Vaccination** would still be recommended since the vaccine would protect against strains other than the one contracted by the patient.

The Dopplegangers

You will be expected to differentiate condyloma acuminata from similar genital lesions as follows:

Molluscum contagiosum differ in appearance, location, and size. Molluscum is much smaller, is rarely genital, and will be described as **smooth and flesh colored**, with **central umbilication**.

Bartholin cysts are large and tender; and may present as a fluctuant mass on vaginal wall.

Condyloma lata is part of secondary syphilis, and will be described as **whitish-gray papules that have coalesced** in the genital area. They are flatter than condyloma acuminata, and will also present with **systemic symptoms**, including fever.

The words **condyloma lata** and **condyloma acuminata** can look alike at first glance, and this is something that will definitely be taken advantage of on the exam. Even though they are clinically dissimilar, they will both appear among the choices in any given question since they both have condyloma as their first names.

Herpes Simplex

The **primary lesion** (initial infection) will be **painful,** and usually they will describe **tender inguinal nodes**. It, and all subsequent lesions, will be described as ulcerative.

Treatment of primary HSV infection is oral **acyclovir**. Other correct treatment choices could include **famciclovir** and **valacyclovir**.

CASE STUDY

You are presented with a patient with a history of unprotected sexual intercourse several weeks ago who now has several vesicular lesions on the penis. What would be the *best diagnostic test to do initially?*

THE DIVERSION

You very astutely recognize that this is a herpes lesion. One of the choices you are given is a Tzanck test, which you know is associated with diagnosing herpes, so you lock into this answer. If you do this, you have locked into the wrong answer, and you and the patient described in the vignette both should be more careful and less impulsive.

ANSWER REVEALED

The correct answer is **viral culture for herpes simplex**. The Tzanck test does detect multinucleated giant cells, but its sensitivity is less than 50%. In addition, it does not differentiate herpes from varicella. Therefore, when it comes to herpes viruses, "Tzanck you but I don't know **HSV** from the next "**ella**."

Pediculosis Pubis

Pediculosis pubis, or as it is known in less lofty circles — "crabs" — will have a classic presentation described below.

BUZZWORDS

Patients with pediculosis pubis will present with **red, crusted suprapubic macules**. They could also be described as **blue-gray dots**, which are *maculae ceruleae*.

HOT TIP

Some important points regarding pediculosis pubis that you might be tested on include that they are **slow moving** and **sluggish**, which is why they spread primarily by close contact, especially sexual contact. They can last 1-2 days without a meal, which for them is blood. In addition to the **pubic area**, they can infest **anal hairs** as well as **facial hair**, including **eyelashes**.

PERIL

Finding of pubic lice **in any child** should raise the suspicion of **sexual abuse**.

TREATMENT

If you are asked for the correct treatment for pediculosis pubis, the correct choices would include **permethrin 1% or 5%, pyrethrin with piperonyl butoxide,** and **malathion**. For the eyelashes, application of **petroleum jelly** several times a day for 10 days is sufficient.

Lindane is considered a 2nd line treatment, but not in neonates or pregnant women.

Trichomonas Vaginalis

Trichomoniasis is estimated to be **the most prevalent nonviral STD in US teens.** It is **NOT reportable,** so the "true" numbers are not known.

Trichomoniasis is often **asymptomatic in males,** and this could easily be a question on the exam.

Symptoms in women are **burning, itching, abnormal vaginal odor,** and **dyspareunia** (pain during intercourse). The key words here are **flagellated organisms** on wet mount, **frothy yellow discharge,** and **strawberry cervix** because of the petechiae on it.

Well, we will have to revert to something off color here. Because the organism is **"flagellated,"** picture an organism that carries a "whip" and **whips the cervix,** which explains the petechia and the **"strawberry cervix."**

Treatment is either **tinidazole** or **oral metronidazole** a.k.a. **Flagyl®,** which is easy to remember since it treats **flagellated organisms.** Alternatively, envision a bunch of flagellated organisms riding the metro/subway.

Patients should be advised to abstain from sexual activity until both partners have been treated and are without symptoms.

Because the recurrence rates are so high, repeat testing 3 months after the initial testing is recommended.

Neisseria gonorrhoeae (Gonococcus; G.C.)

Gonorrhea is most commonly asymptomatic.

Gon-ARTH-rhea - Gonorrhea may be associated with **arthritis.** So consider this with any case of arthritis in an adolescent.

Also remember GC can lead to **pharyngitis** presenting with sore throat, fever and cervical adenopathy.

> ## Who's More Popular?
>
> *Chlamydia trachomatis* is the most common *reportable* STD.
>
> *Neisseria gonorrhoeae* is second.

GC In Males

Gonorrhea in males presents as **dysuria** and **discharge.** Infection can progress to **epididymitis,** with **unilateral pain and swelling of the scrotum.**

GC in Females

Females get **urethritis** and **cervicitis**, along with **dysuria** and **malodorous discharge**. Infection may ascend to any part of the female reproductive tract, and may lead to **peritonitis** or **peri-hepatitis** (Fitz-Hugh-Curtis syndrome).

Disseminated gonococcal infection

Disseminated gonococcal infection occurs in about 1%-2% of GC cases.

Local symptoms are not usually present once dissemination becomes apparent. Instead, **fever, arthritis** and **rash** are more common. Also possible are **meningitis** and **endocarditis**.

Diagnosis is aided by the gram stain showing **intracellular gram-negative diplococci**. A culture is the gold standard, but **empiric treatment** is often indicated prior to culture results.

 Partners need to be treated.

 Patients being treated for gonorrhea should also receive treatment for chlamydia.

> ### Treat all you can!
>
> Unless otherwise noted, **Expedited Partner Therapy (EPT)** applies and you are expected to choose, treatment and educational material for all sexual partners in the last 60 days, and the most recent sexual partner even if it has been more than 60 days.

Chlamydia

For uncomplicated **chlamydia genital infections**, doxycycline for 7 days or azithromycin in a single 1 gram PO dose are acceptable.

Pelvic Inflammatory Disease

Minimal criteria for diagnosis include lower abdominal or pelvic pain along with uterine, adnexal, OR cervical motion tenderness.

Additional criteria to be sure:

- WBC in vaginal secretions
- Temp > 38.3°C
- Elevated ESR or C-reactive protein
- Lab evidence of GC or chlamydia
- Abnormal cervical or vaginal mucopurulent discharge

Watch for an adolescent with **lower abdominal pain** and a **shuffling gait** who may very well deny sexual activity. The pelvic exam may be significant for an extremely painful **cervical motion tenderness** known as the **chandelier sign**.

During a pelvic exam for PID, in addition to obtaining **chlamydia and GC cultures**, you are also expected to obtain specimens for microscopic examination of vaginal discharge for **trichomoniasis** and **bacterial vaginosis**. In addition to GC and chlamydia, PID can be caused by anaerobes and gram-negative rods.

Patients with PID also need **testing for syphilis and HIV**. PID is a risk factor for **ectopic pregnancy** and **infertility**.

You would be expected to look for evidence of **human papillomavirus**. In addition, you will be expected to counsel on the **HPV vaccine**.

> ### STI Screening
>
> They may present you with an **asymptomatic** sexually active female and ask for the most appropriate STI screen. The correct answer will be **urine PCR for chlamydia** or **gonorrhea** along with appropriate blood tests for **HIV** and **syphilis**.
>
> **Syphilis screening** is also indicated in pregnancy, high risk populations, trans-actional sex,[3] and correctional facilities.

Treating PID

Because it is difficult to make a rapid diagnosis and the consequences of missing PID are potentially devastating, the CDC recommends **empirical treatment** for all sexually active females at risk for STIs who present with lower abdominal or pelvic pain and meet them minimal criteria above.

> ### Continued PID Pain
>
> If **pain persists** after treatment, **abdominal ultrasound is indicated** to look for **tubo-ovarian abscess**.

Outpatient Treatment

For Gonococcal infections, single dose Ceftriaxone is the preferred regimen.[4]

Presumptive treatement of Chlamydia with doxycycline is warranted if Chlamydia hasn't been ruled out.

Treat for both unless Chlamydia was specifically ruled out !

The CDC recommends that all patients diagnosed with PID be rechecked within 72 hours of starting therapy.

Patients must also **notify the partner** so they can be treated at the same time, and abstain from intercourse until both are treated.

---

3 According to Wikipedia: Transactional sex is a superset of prostitution, in that the exchange of gifts for sex includes a broader set of (usually non-marital) obligations that do not necessarily involve a predetermined payment or gift, but where there is a definite motivation to benefit materially from the sexual exchange.

4 IM 500 mg for < 150 Kg. and 1 Gram for > 150 Kg.

Inpatient Treatment

Hospitalization is required if follow-up is not assured (as in most teenagers) or symptoms don't improve in 48 hours. Hospitalization is also indicated for patients who can't tolerate outpatient management, are severely ill, have tubo-ovarian abscess, or are pregnant.

Fitz Hugh Curtis

Here is some important additional information (and source of potential diversion) you need to know about regarding Fitz Hugh Curtis syndrome.

HOT TIP

Fitz-Hugh Curtis can be due to **chlamydia** as well as **gonorrhea**.

CASE STUDY

You are presented with a female teenager with right upper quadrant pain along with nausea and vomiting. They will note that oral contraceptive pills are the only medications she is taking. You will be asked for the best initial step in making the correct diagnosis.

THE DIVERSION

Since you will be focusing on the right upper quadrant pain, you may ignore the fact that she is on oral contraceptives – you have been diverted away from thinking it is important, because they noted them as the "only" pills she is taking. Therefore, you will be tempted by all the diversionary choices, including serum amylase, lipase, abdominal CT or ultrasound, plain abdominal film, serum LFT levels or even a surgical consult.

ANSWER REVEALED

By falling for all the diversions, you probably would have dismissed the correct answer, which would be cervical cultures. Whenever they mention the "only medication" a patient is taking, you should read it as a "very important" medication that reveals a part of the history. Putting this together, you have a sexually active female with right upper quadrant pain, which would be consistent with Fitz Hugh Curtis, which is perihepatitis - a manifestation of gonococcal and chlamydial infections.

TREATMENT

Treatment would be the same as for PID. The right upper quadrant pain due to perihepatitis should resolve within two days after treatment

PERIL

Remember that "Fitz-Hugh-Curtis" is **peri-hepatitis,** not hepatitis. LFT values will therefore be normal, as noted below.

Pelvic pain is not necessarily due to PID. Additional causes of pelvic pain to keep in mind are as follows:

Ovarian Cyst

 They will typically present you with a teenager with **unilateral abdominal "discomfort,"** typically mid-cycle. They will probably throw in a positive ultrasound showing a **fluid filled cyst on the ovary**.

The question will focus on management. Here size is important.

- Cysts smaller than 6.0 cm will only require follow-up ultrasound
- Cysts greater than 6.0 cm or those that are causing significant symptoms beyond discomfort would require laparoscopic cyst aspiration.

Ovarian Torsion

Ovarian torsion will present as **sudden lower abdominal pain which radiates to the back, side, or groin/leg on the same side,** with nausea and vomiting.

Diagnosis is confirmed with Doppler ultrasound, but this should not delay **surgical consultation** if ultrasound access is not immediately available.

Sexual Abuse

This will most likely occur by someone **close to or known by the family**, so look for clues in the question to this effect. They may also describe something that is not abuse, and parental reassurance is the correct answer.

The description of a child who acts out by describing **explicit adult sexual behavior** should be a strong indicator that the child may have observed or experienced inappropriate sexual behaviors.

Hymenal Damage: Since the hymen can be damaged in other ways (like falling on a balance beam), the appearance of the hymen alone is not a good way to assess sexual abuse or molestation. It needs to be evaluated in the context of the history.

A common hymen variant lacks tissue above the 3 and 9 o'clock positions. If presented with this information, know that it is too nonspecific in and of itself to confirm sexual abuse.

Urethral prolapse often presents in African American girls, ages 3-8 years, as a hyperemic doughnut-shaped mass. Treatment is warm sitz baths and follow-up with an urologist.

"Foreign body," such as toilet paper, might be the answer they are looking for, especially if they describe a foul odor from the vagina.

There will be a clue in the question indicating suspicion of abuse if that is the road they want you to travel down.

Vaginal discharge in a child on antibiotics is usually just a yeast infection when no other information is given.

White discharge can be due to **physiological leukorrhea.** It is due to the desquamation of epithelial cells under the influence of estrogen, typically in a girl around 11 (or just prior to menarche.)

Congenital condyloma acuminata

One mode of transmission of anogenital warts is through a contaminated birth canal.

While anogenital warts can be transmitted through the birth canal, this will usually manifest by age one. Some would argue that it can be attributed to perinatal transmission up to age 3. Therefore, if they present a child with new onset of condyloma genital warts **after age 3, it is likely due to child abuse**.

Gender Dysphoria

Gender dysphoria is defined as an incongruence between an individual's experienced gender and gender assigned at birth (primary/secondary sexual characteristics). It must be present for 6 months.

You may be called upon to differentiate different subtleties relating to gender. If you remember the following definitions, these should be easy points:

Gender identity refers to an innate sense of one's gender. If they say a patient "feels that they are a woman", or are a "boy trapped in a girl's body", this is most likely getting at the concept of gender identity.

Gender expression refers to one's public display of their gender. This can include clothing, makeup and affirmed pronouns, to name a few.

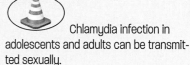

Culture Positive for Sexual Abuse

Neisseria gonorrhea infection on genital, rectal, and pharyngeal secretions cultures should be strongly considered a result of sexual abuse.

Since chlamydia and *Neisseria gonorrhea* are often linked, it is tempting to link them here as well.

Chlamydia infection in adolescents and adults can be transmitted sexually.

Chlamydia can also be vertically transmitted during the birth process and persist in positive cultures for months.

However, rectal and vaginal chlamydia infection transmitted at birth should not persist past 18 months of age.

However, sexual abuse should be considered in any prepubertal child beyond infancy who they present with vaginal, urethral, or rectal chlamydia infection.

Chapter 34

Sports Medicine and Physical Fitness

Conditioning programs

It is important to note that **conditioning is encouraged**, but know that the following caveats could make their way onto the exam.

The most important factor is the encouragement of increased physical activity **modeled by the parents. This is more important than simply decreasing screen time**.

For preschool age children this takes the form of less organized activities. For example, using balls and other toys that require physical activity. Taking walks in parks or the the zoo.

Children should be encouraged to be active. Children with developmental or coordination issues should be referred to physical therapy to accomplish this.

For children 6-17 years of age, correct answers would include:

- Aerobic 60 minutes of "moderate to vigorous" bone strengthening activities 3x per week (running, jumping, etc.), and
- muscle building activities 3x per week (climbing, push-ups, etc.).

In the days before there was an internet, this was called "getting out and playing with your friends."

Weight Training

You need to distinguish **weight training** from **power lifting programs**. **Weight training** involves many reps with low resistance. This is safe for preadolescents. **Power lifting** is not considered to be safe for preadolescents because of the risk of apophyseal avulsion fractures.

Weight training should begin with low resistance until until proper technique is learned. Supervision is important.

Overuse Injuries

For anyone who has been involved in organized sports it seems like every parent thinks their kid is getting ready for a D1 scholarship. The result is overuse injuries for which there are no scholarships available.

Participation in a variety of sports with time off to recover is a key to preventing overuse injuries.

Sports, Fluids, and Electrolytes

Water is generally the appropriate first choice for hydration **before, during, and after sport participation**. Water rather than sports drinks is the fluid of choice.

Correct choices will include language that emphasizes drinking adequate fluids, before, during and after athletic activities. Keeping the urine light colored is one way to gauge successful hydration.

HOT TIP It is important that young athletes be reminded by staff to keep up with fluid intake; left to their own devices, they will not do so.

COIN FLIP **"Energy drinks"** tend to contain stimulants such as caffeine and guarana and have no place in the diet of children.

Wrestling with Weight Control in Athletes

It is common for competitive wrestlers to try to lose weight to qualify for a lower weight category, thinking they will be more competitive.

PERIL It is important to keep in mind that the weight loss, especially weight loss that occurs in a short period of time, is primarily **water weight loss**. Dieting behaviors to alter weight are not limited to females.

Cardiac Findings in the Athlete

The following findings would warrant **referral to a cardiologist** prior to clearing for participation in sports:

- Syncope, near syncope, or chest **pain on exertion**
- **Palpitations** at rest or irregular heart rhythm
- Excessive **shortness of breath** or fatigue with **routine activities**
- **Family history** of Marfan syndrome, cardiomyopathy, long QT syndrome, or clinically significant arrhythmias or premature death
- Weak or **delayed femoral pulses** consistent with coarctation of the aorta
- Any of the following on cardiac exam: fixed split second heart sound, a systolic murmur graded 3/6 or greater, or **any diastolic murmur**
- A patient with **Turner syndrome** with any **chest pain**. Turner syndrome is associated with coarctation of the aorta, bicuspid aortic valve, aortic stenosis, etc.

> ### During Exertion Don't Delay
>
> Syncope or collapse **DURING** exertion is more concerning than **AFTER** exertion. Any child who experiences syncope during exertion should be witheld from similar activity until cleared by a cardiologist.

Any of the following are **contraindications to sports participation**:

- **Pulmonary vascular disease** with cyanosis and large right-to-left shunt
- **Severe pulmonary hypertension**
- Severe **aortic** valve **stenosis** or **regurgitation**

- Severe **mitral** valve **stenosis** or **regurgitation**
- Cardiomyopathies
- Vascular form of Ehlers-Danlos syndrome
- Anomalous origin of the right coronary artery
- Catecholaminergic polymorphic ventricular tachycardia
- Acute pericarditis
- Acute myocarditis (within 6 months of onset)
- Acute Kawasaki disease (initial 8 weeks)

CASE STUDY

They can, and will, present you with a healthy — in fact a very healthy — athletic teenager with findings that would be abnormal in another teenager, but are normal for an athletic teenager. This is an important concept you could be tested on.

THE DIVERSION

In certain athletes like long distance runners, modest **left ventricular hypertrophy** is a normal finding. Another typical finding is a **low heart rate**, typically in the 60s.

ANSWER REVEALED

No sports restriction will be the correct answer in both of these situations if the rest of the history and exam are normal.

Specific Considerations

Hypertension

Monitoring and restricting sports activities has made its way onto the boards and there are a variety of scenarios you can be tested on. The following factors should help you navigate those waters successfully !

Hypertension and Athletic Participation

Based on the definitions in the callout box the following caveats should help guide you through questions on clearing athletes for sports participation in the face of hypertension

Hypertension Stage 1

These athletes can participate in all sports without restriction unless they have end organ disease. The most important example would be left ventricular hypertrophy.

Stage 1 Hypertension - BP in the 130s / high 80s

Stage 2 Hypertension - BP 140 / 90 or higher

First some important definitions:

 Dynamic Activity – this is really aerobic activity. As you can imagine this results in an increase in systolic BP. It also results in a decreased diastolic BP and decreased peripheral resistance.

Static Activity - the classic example is weight lifting. This results in an increase in both systolic and diastolic BP with no decrease in peripheral resistance.

 Static activity are those that involve straining.

Hypertension Stage 2

Athletes with Stage 2 hypertension should take steps to lower their BP first before engaging and/or have their risk evaluated.

HOT TIP Those with hypertension Stage 2 can **continue with aerobic / dynamic activity and conditioning**. They cannot participate in high static activities. Wrestling and weight lifting would be considered to be high static activity.

TAKE HOME MESSAGE If you are presented with a patient with stage 2 hypertension they can continue with aerobic workouts but no static exercise until the BP is under control. Competitive sports would need clearance.

The Diabetic Athlete

You may be tested on the concept of exercise in the diabetic patient.

While exercise is encouraged, keep in mind the following caveats.

TAKE HOME MESSAGE In general, kids with Type I Diabetes may play ANY sport as long as proper diet, fluid, and insulin therapy are maintained. Pay extra attention to sustained activities.

During periods of exercise, **increased caloric intake** or **decreased insulin dose** will be needed to avoid hypoglycemia. There could be a **delayed response to exercise** hours later resulting in hypoglycemia. Keep this in mind if presented with a question involving this scenario.

During episodes of poor control, especially with ketosis, vigorous exercise should be deferred.

Atlantoaxial Instability / Down Syndrome

Children with Down syndrome are at risk for atlantoaxial instability(AAI) Prevalence is approximately 15%.

UPDATED & NEW BREAKING NEWS INFORMATION Routine cervical spine x-rays before participating in sports are no longer indicated. This has been replaced by annual neurological screening. If a myelopathy is identified on screening, then a cervical spine film would be indicated.

Seizure Disorders

Children with a **well-controlled** seizure disorder may participate in all sports. If the seizure disorder is **not well-controlled**, they will need to avoid contact sports as well as certain noncontact sports like archery, riflery, swimming, and sports involving heights.

Marfan syndrome

Avoid sports that carry a risk of bodily collision. What are low-collision sports you ask? We are glad you did. Some of these are bowling, golf, tennis, and track.

Crucial Cardiac Cautions

Since children with Marfan syndrome are at risk for aortic enlargement and/or aortic dissection, you need to know which physical restrictions are appropriate. They should refrain from activities that involve muscle straining, such as weight lifting, as well as contact sports.

> **CASE STUDY**
>
> **You are presented with a 18 year old coming in for a sport physical. He has answered NO to all the clearance questions and has been playing basketball with no issues at all.**
>
> **On the physical, you note a normal S1 and S2 and no murmur until he does his duck walk, and then you hear a 3/6 harsh systolic murmur at the left lower sternal border.**
>
> **You   A. diagnose an innocent murmur and clear him for basketball**
>
> **B. suspect a pathologic murmur and proceed with a work up**
>
> **C. clear him for now so he doesn't start the beginning of the season but have him return in one month to recheck the murmur if he's still alive**
>
> **THE DIVERSION**
>
> Clearly, C is not wise. You need to decide, good murmur vs bad murmur. Just remember: murmurs that you hear supine but go away on sitting or standing are good, and you can let those kids walk on out of your office. Murmurs that get louder on sitting or standing are bad.
>
> **ANSWER REVEALED**
>
> In this case, this teen is at risk for Hypertrophic Obstructive Cardiomyopathy (HOCM), previously known as Idiopathic Hypertrophic Subaortic Stenosis (IHSS) and needs a full workup.
>
> HOCM is the #1 cause of sudden death in US athletes. These patients do not die from the obstruction, they die from ventricular arrhythmias, especially ventricular fibrillation. 90% will have an abnormal EKG. The echocardiogram is a highly sensitive and specific test for HOCM.

The Heat is On

Heat illness includes both **heat exhaustion** and **heat stroke**, and you need to be able to distinguish between the two.

Heat Exhaustion

Heat exhaustion is the milder form of heat illness. These patients will present with mild dehydration and a **core temperature less than 104°F (40°C)**. They may present a child who has a **headache** and is **thirsty, nauseated,** and possibly **vomiting**. This is due to uncompensated fluid losses.

Patients in heat exhaustion will be sweating and have normal mentation; those in heat stroke will not be sweating and have altered mental status.

Patients with heat exhaustion simply need to **stop exercising** and **drink fluids**.

Heat Stroke

Heat stroke is based on the following:

- **Temperature > 104°F (40°C)**
- Flushed, with hot, **dry skin** (not sweating)
- **CNS depression** (confusion, vertigo, syncope, and lethargy)
- Severe dehydration

Heat stroke can lead to **end organ damage** because of the release of **endotoxins** and **cytokines**. Therefore, dehydration is only part of the problem.

Heat stroke is a medical emergency. Stop the activity, remove the child from the heat, and decrease the core body temperature. Rehydration is **via IV fluids only**, with use of vasopressors to maintain BP if needed.

Evaporative cooling which is the spraying of cool water (~15°C/59°F) on a patient while using fans pointed at them is more appropriate than the application of ice and just as effective.

Oral rehydration would be inappropriate given the CNS depression seen in heat stroke. Cooling **below 101-102°F** could lead to **hypothermia and is inappropriate.**

Neurological signs such as delirium, coma, and seizure marks an important distinction between heat exhaustion and heat stroke.

Additional complications could include, ARDS, renal failure, hepatic injury, DIC, rhabdomyolysis as well as a variety of electrolyte abnormalities.

Seizures in the context of heat stroke are managed with benzodiazepines.

Sprains, strains, and pains

You are expected to understand what defines different degrees of ligament sprain as follows:

Ankle Injuries

Most ankle injuries are inversion injuries involving the lateral ligaments, especially the **anterior talofibular ligament.**

The single leg hop is a good test for gauging whether physical therapy and/or other intervention is the correct answer.

Strains and sprains

DEFINITION

Sprain - injury of ligaments

Strain - injury of tendons or muscles

Most injuries that occur in the knee and ankle are due to *incomplete healing of a previous injury,* which may not have received appropriate medical attention. This is especially true with the ankle and a frequently tested topic. Physical therapy and clearance before returning to activity would be a correct choice.

Ankle Sprains

The **immediate treatment** of an ankle sprain would be the **application of ice**. This should continue for 20 minutes at a time over the first 36-48 hours.

Angling for a Return to Action

Invariably, you will be called upon to answer the question regarding when a child can return to sports after an ankle injury.

 The correct answer will be one or all of the following:

- Full range of motion
- Full strength
- No swelling
- No pain
- No joint instability

Pain over a bone **physis in a pre-adolescent child** should be assumed to be a Salter Harris I fracture, **even if the x-ray is normal**, and will require splinting to protect the bone for Salter Harris Type 1.

If you are presented with a child who "recovers" from an ankle injury, returns to competitive sport, and then sustains another more severe injury in the same ankle, what is the most likely cause?

The diversion (and implication) is that the child has sustained a new injury, since they tell you he has "recovered" from the previous injury before returning. However, this is often in quotes, or should be in quotes, since the child probably never fully recovered from the initial injury.

The most likely answer will be reinjury because the child returned to competitive play too soon. They should only return when normal strength, balance and range of motion of been recovered.

Compartment Syndrome

CASE STUDY

You are presented with a child who was running in on a fast break while playing basketball. He was stopped by an opponent who was completing his 7th year of high school varsity ball, and who stepped on his ankle and lateral leg. You note no deformity, just a bruise and marked swelling. The foot has a strong dorsal pulse, with some diminished sensation to pinprick and light touch. What is the most appropriate next step?

THE DIVERSION

You might be tempted to choose ice, since that is the most appropriate immediate step in an ankle sprain. There is no deformity or evidence of a displaced fracture, and pulses are intact, so getting the swelling down would be top priority. What could be wrong with ice? Probably nothing, except it would be the wrong choice on the boards for this question.

ANSWER REVEALED

The signs and symptoms described , bruising with marked swelling and decreased sensation, with compartment syndrome, and therefore **obtaining compartment pressures** would be the correct choice. The presence of a pulse and lack of paralysis simply means that it is in the early stages, and does not rule out compartment syndrome.

MNEMONIC

The signs and symptoms of compartment syndrome can be remembered as the 5 Ps

    Pain (with passive stretching)

    Paresthesias

    Pallor

    Paralysis

    Pulselessness

The last two are late findings in compartment syndrome and their absence as in the case above does not rule it out.

PERIL

Ice won't help, and a compression dressing will make it worse. These will, of course, be among the diversionary choices you might be given.

Knee Troubles

Subluxation of the Patella

This is typically due to **indirect trauma**. Usually from a non-contact twisting injury. Subluxation is a partial dislocation. Watch for a description of a **"pop"** after a **change in direction off a pivoted knee**. On physical exam they will describe **pain over the lateral aspect** of the patella, with possible **deformity over the medial aspect**. This may represent patellofemoral instability.

Developing and maintaining quadriceps and hamstring strength, as well as flexibility, is the appropriate treatment.

Patellar Dislocation

Treatment

The treatment of of patellar dislocation after proper reduction would include immobilzation, NSAID, x-ray to rule out avulsion fracture and physical therapy.

Patellofemoral syndrome

Presents as **anterior knee pain** in adolescents involved in **jumping, running,** and **squatting** sports due to **patellar maltracking**. It affects **females** more commonly due to the higher Q-angle between the femur and the tibia.

Diagnosis is made **clinically**. Xrays are not helpful.

Knee bracing, patellar taping, and NSAIDs are helpful, as are quad strengthening exercises. Referral to Orthopedics would be appropriate if the condition does not improve after 4-6 months of these interventions.

> ### Knee Effusion Confusion
>
> Any Knee effusion causes confusion and therefore imaging studies will likely be the correct answer
>
> An effusion with locking or catching, osteochondritis dissecans is the most likely diagnosis. Meniscal tears are unusual in children and will likley be an incorrect choice !

> ### Giving away to ACL
>
> Any athlete with a history of the knee "giving way" with activities, needs further evaluation, especially for an anterior cruciate ligament (ACL) tear, which is 3-4 times more common in females than in males.

Knee Injuries

ACL Tear

- More common in female athletes (4.5 to 1 ratio)
- Common in football, basketball, skiing, and soccer athletes
- Secondary to a non-contact pivoting injury
- Can be associated with meniscal tears, as well as other ligamentous injuries

---

- Symptoms: knee pain, swelling, hemarthrosis
- Exam: Lachman sign is the most sensitive test
- Anterior drawer sign
- Imaging: MRI
- Treatment: NSAIDs, rest, ice, physical therapy, operative reconstruction

MCL Injury

MCL sprains can be usually treated with bracing and rehabilitation.

Meniscal Tear

- Medial tear is more common than lateral tear
- Knee pain, locking/clicking of the knee, knee swelling
- Imaging: MRI
- Exam: Apley Compression Test
- Treatment: rest, ice, NSAIDs, physical therapy, surgical repair

Under the Knee

Medial Collateral Ligament Sprain (MCL)

This is diagnosed with pain when **valgus** stress is applied. MCL strain is treating with bracing ahd physical therapy.

Thigh Injuries

PERIL

If you are presented with a patient who develops a **large area of swelling** over his thigh after blunt trauma, do not assume you are being presented with a fracture or an incidental discovery of a lytic lesion. In the absence of other hints, this is likely a **soft tissue hematoma**, which can be large due to the substantial blood supply to the quadriceps.

TREATMENT

Other than NSAIDs, ice, and rest, there is no other necessary treatment. If severe, the blood loss may be significant enough to cause a drop in hematocrit, resulting in **fatigue and dizziness**. In this case, more significant interventions may be necessary.

It's all in the Wrist

 If you are presented with a patient who has pain over the **"anatomical snuffbox"** (which will likely be described as pain over the dorsum of the hand near the base of the thumb), the most likely diagnosis is **scaphoid fracture**. This is the case even with a negative Xray. In fact, a negative Xray is quite common. Scaphoid fractures have a poor prognosis.

Treatment consists of splinting and follow-up with orthopedics.

> **You are asked to evaluate a 12-year-old gymnast who has had left wrist pain which has gotten progressively worse over 3 months. However, she does not recall injuring the wrist. On physical exam, there is no swelling, normal range of motion, and no pain noted over the wrist joint itself. Point tenderness is limited to the distal radius.**
>
> **What is the most likely explanation for the wrist pain? What is the most appropriate management? What would you expect to see on x-ray?**
>
> Among the diversionary x-ray findings, you could be presented with scaphoid bone fracture. For diagnosis, you will be tempted to pick wrist fracture or wrist sprain. Regarding management, diversionary choices could include "cease all training," or "continue all physical activity."
>
> Since there is no pain over the wrist joint, scaphoid fracture and/or wrist sprain are not likely. The presentation is consistent with distal radial epiphyseal injury. If the girl were to continue her current training, she is likely to disrupt the growth plate. Therefore, the correct answer would be to rest and splint the wrist until it is healed. **However, this would not mean stopping all training**. She can still engage in training activities that don't involve her wrist, such as running, which would help maintain her stamina.

Elbow Drama

Supracondylar humeral fractures typically occur in a boy age 5-8 years falling on an **outstretched arm** which is hyperextended at the elbow.

A supracondylar fracture of the humerus will impact the vasculature. There may be no external signs of trauma. **Therefore, if trauma to the elbow is mentioned in the question, watch for a description consistent with neurovascular compromise and consider this diagnosis.**

Double Bubble Trouble

Bilateral xrays are often needed to diagnose physeal injuries of the elbow.

Pain Management

There is a tendency to undertreat pediatric patients for pain.

You may be tested on this, and it is best to pick choices that manage pain more, rather than less, aggressively.

The risk for respiratory depression with opiates is lower than commonly believed, so a correct answer might include a choice of titrating up on the dose to manage pain appropriately.

HOT TIP

In addition to obvious signs — such as pallor and cyanosis of the distal extremity — watch for **pain on passive extension of the fingers.** A nondisplaced supracondylar fracture might not be obvious on x-ray.

Little Leaguer's Elbow

DEFINITION

Medial Humeral Epicondyle Apophysitis.

BUZZWORDS

A child who participates in a sport where they are throwing overhand in an exaggerated fashion for example baseball, football or tennis is at high risk.

The history will describe medial elbow pain that worsens with throwing.

The description of the physical exam will note swelling and tenderness with palpation over the medial epicondyle and olecranon process.

PERIL

The X-ray can be normal or show apophyseal avulsion fractures of the medial humeral epicondyle

TREATMENT

Supportive including physical therapy.

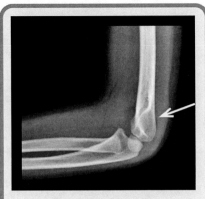

Posterior Fat Pad

PERIL

A **posterior fat pad sign** is seen on lateral elbow XR and is indicative of an **effusion** associated with a **fracture**, which may or may not be visible on Xray.

An **anterior** fat pad is usually a _normal_ finding and not suggestive of a fracture. Bilateral x-rays are usually needed, unless it is accompanied by a positive "sail sign".

Bilateral x-rays are usually needed for comparision.

CASE STUDY

You are presented with a patient who has an elbow injury. They note that there is decreased grip strength and decreased radial pulse. You correctly diagnose supracondylar fracture of the distal humerus.

THE DIVERSION

The choices you will be presented with won't be very humerus at all. You will need to decide if this is a result of direct vascular injury or a transient neurological deficit.

ANSWER REVEALED

The correct answer will be transient neurological deficit. This is because the absent radial pulse is likely due to compression of the radial artery, and not direct trauma to the artery. This will resolve with reduction of the fracture. The neurological deficit, manifested as decreased grip strength, is also transient.

Other elbow injuries to watch out for on the exam and their differentiating characteristics are as follows:

Elbow Injury	Distinguishing Characteristics
Dislocation of the elbow	Age 11-15; fall on an outstretched arm which is **supinated** with the elbow **partially extended** - <u>not hyperextended</u>. However, these too can be associated with **neurovascular compromise**.
Epiphyseal Fracture	Older children due to direct impact with the arm **laterally rotated** on impact. Neurovascular compromise less likely.
Lateral condyle fracture	Forearm is supinated, neurovascular compromise very unlikely.
Annular Ligament Displacement (Nursemaid's Elbow)	Nursemaid's elbow will not present with elbow swelling and tenderness. If patient has tenderness/swelling, consider fracture and obtain an XR. If he doesn't and history is concerning for nursemaid's, then perform reduction with supination/flexion versus hyperpronation at the elbow. Of note, hyperpronation technique found to be more successful.

Pulling over to the Shoulder

Even though this is not the orthopedic or sports medicine boards, you are still expected to shoulder the burden, if you will, of distinguishing between subtle differences in the differential diagnosis of shoulder injuries.

The following table outlines the typical buzz words and the injuries they are associated with.

Mechanism of injury / Physical findings	Diagnosis they are looking for
Pain and swelling over the distal clavicle.	Acromioclavicular injury
Direct force to the posterior shoulder. Pain over the sternoclavicular joint, with respiratory discomfort.	Posterior sternoclavicular dislocation
Shoulder and upper arm pain in the absence of asymmetry.	Proximal humeral fracture HOT TIP CT imaging of the chest should be obtained due to concern for surrounding structure injury (esophagus, great vessels, trachea, pneumothorax).
Shoulder pain with elevating and lowering the arm, without any deformity. In addition, this will present as chronic pain, most likely in the absence of acute injury.	Rotator cuff injury HOT TIP Proper training regarding throwing technique is crucial to prevention of injury.

HOT TIP
The diagnosis of **shoulder dislocation** is clinical, but x-rays are indicated for confirmation and assessment of other injuries, including fractures. Neurovascular integrity is re-evaluated post-reduction. In addition to immobilization with a sling, you must also fill the space between the arm and body with a pillow or blanket.

CASE STUDY
You are asked to evaluate a teenage baseball player who sustained a shoulder injury. He has pain over the distal clavicle, with point tenderness over the superior aspect. He cannot raise his arm above his head. X-ray is negative for clavicular fracture, shoulder fracture, and dislocation. What is the most likely injury?

THE DIVERSION
You will be dazzled with lots of tempting diversionary answers, including a variety of tempting "occult" fractures, such as "occult clavicular fracture" and "occult proximal humerus fracture." Another diversionary choice would be a shoulder separation.

ANSWER REVEALED
The correct answer in this scenario would be acromioclavicular separation. Children younger than 13 are more prone to sustain a fracture of the distal clavicle. In children older than 13, such as the teenager in this vignette, an acromioclavicular separation is more likely. This patient had point tenderness. The typical pain of a shoulder separation would be more diffuse.

HOT TIP
Evaluation for neurovascular compromise would be appropriate.

Clavicular Injuries

BUZZWORDS
Clavicular fracture occurs with a **fall on an outstretched arm or directly on the shoulder**. The child will be holding the arm with the opposite hand.

TREATMENT
Most clavicular fractures will heal without much intervention other than an arm sling.

PERIL
However, **medial clavicular fracture with anterior or posterior displacement will require an evaluation for possible displacement of the trachea or mediastinal structures.**

PERIL
Other reasons to refer to orthopedics include completely displaced fractures (more than one bone width), comminution, and shortening of clavicle.

Acromioclavicular separation can be distinguished from a clavicular fracture by the presence of tenderness directly over the AC joint and a **palpable step-off** of the anterior shoulder joint **in the absence of crepitus**.

AC joint separation will occur in older "skeletally mature" teenagers with a history of a fall or direct blow to the superior or lateral aspect of the shoulder with the arm adducted.

Treatment for AC joint injuries include rest, ice, and slinging for immobilization.

In younger children a clavicular fracture is more likely, so note the age of the child presented in the question.

Concurring on Concussion

It is important to know the definition of a concussion, which is **an alteration in the <u>level</u> of consciousness — not necessarily a loss of consciousness**.

Immediately after sustaining an injury and developing symptoms consistent with concussion, the patient **must be kept out of the game or practice**.

There are many changes and updates in the diagnosis and management of concussion that are likely to be tested on the exam.

The standard protocol for concussion treatment **was** to basically cacoon with physical and cognitive rest until full resolution of symptoms. The protocols are now based on the vestibulo-oculomotor signs described below.

Concussion PRE - Screening

Most contact sports now require assessment and documentation of neurocognitive function PRIOR to sports participation which serves as a baseline test used to compare with post traumatic results.

These tests are not diagnostic for concussion. They do not determine treatment.

it is not diagnostic for concussion, and does not inform treatment choice in patients who are still symptomatic. The tests are most useful when there is a preinjury baseline result for comparison with results obtained after complete resolution of concussion-related symptoms.

Vestibulo-oculomotor (VO) Signs

Some of the clues in the history would include, as you can guess, vestibuolo-oculomotor deficits including, dizziness, persistent headache, and fogginess especially with reading. Oculomotor signs would include diplopia and/or blurry vision.

It will be important to watch for a history of suggestive of a vestibulo-oculomotor concussion. These are considered signs that predict prolonged recovery. Dizziness in particular is ominous sign for prolonged recovery. Early identification and treatment is crucial.

There is a **brief VO screen** that can be done in the **office** and this could be a correct choice to a question regarding initial diagnosis.

Patients with signs of VO disturbance on the initial in office screen should be referred for specific vestibular rehab treatment. In the absence of V/O signs prolonged periods of physical rest might prolong recovery. Return to contact sports is to be be a gradual process with specific benchmarks leading up to it.

Beware Prolonged Rest

Prolonged periods of physical rest after a routine, non VO concussion, is no longer considered to be beneficial.

Relative rest is encouraged rather than complete cacooning. This is followed by gradual return to play including moderate non contact physical activity.

However the gradual return to play is now:

> Moderate, non contact physical activity is okay.

Return to **contact sports** can occur after

> A) No concussion associated signs or symptoms at rest
> B) No recurrence of symptoms with exercise
> C) Return to baseline cognitive function and academic performance.

If the symptoms recur, at any step, the patient must rest for 24 hours before returning to the process.

The trainer typically serves as a liaison between coaching and medical staff.

Concussion Risky Sports

Concussion Rates By Sports:

> 1. Boys' Tackle Football -- still highest
> 2. Girls' Soccer
> 3. Boys' Lacrosse
> 4. Boys' Ice Hockey
> 5. Boys' Wrestling
> 6. Girls' Lacrosse
> 7. Girls' Field Hockey

Pains in the Neck

Answering questions regarding the management of neck injuries and neck pain, can itself be, uh, a pain in the neck. However, we can help you avoid exam score-threatening injuries with the following important points.

In answering a question regarding an acute injury, you should follow the ABCs of CPR, **while keeping the neck in a stable position.** In a football player with a neck injury, breathing can be assessed by placing the hand beneath the shoulder pads and jersey to assess chest expansion. If the patient is prone, then the correct step is to **log roll them while maintaining neck stability.**

Removing shoulder pads and/or helmet on the field **is never correct**. If airway management is needed, you are supposed to **leave the helmet on** and remove the face guard only.

The most common sports-related cause of neck injuries is **football**, not diving. However, diving is an important mechanism for cervical spine injury, and could be presented as such on the exam.

Even if the c-spine film is negative, the patient can only return to sports **when there is no pain with motion or palpation** of the cervical spine, **all neurological tests are negative**, and there are **no description of tingling sensation in the extremities**.

Mouth Guards

They could present you with a list of sports and ask which ones require a mouth guard. One of the choices could be "all of the above," or choices can contain a "yes" for some but not all.

Collision sports like football, soccer, basketball, hockey, and wrestling are obvious. However, if you are presented with non-collision sports such as *shot putting* or *discus throwing*, you might be inclined to think to yourself or perhaps even aloud in the exam room, "Discus throwing? Shot putting? There is no contact there! Are these even sports?" You would then pick choices with no mouth guard needed. If you did, you just shot put away a point!

Both shot putting and discus throwing require a mouth guard to —believe it or not — protect from dental injuries secondary to teeth clenching. In fact, children with braces are recommended to wear a mouth guard during *any* sport.

Speaking of which, perhaps a mouth guard would be required for NY Jets fans, who have clenched their teeth watching their team supposedly play football over the past few years.

Know that mouth guards significantly **lower the risk of trauma to teeth**, but do very little to reduce concussion risk.

Sports Clearance

You will be expected to determine if patients with various conditions are eligible to participate in specific sports. It is important to note that **children with fevers cannot participate in sports.** Children with **carditis** and acute **hepatosplenomegaly** (which could include children with mono) cannot participate in high contact sports.

Exercise induced asthma - can play sports, but should take prophylaxis albuterol prior to exercise.

HOT TIP

Rather than list each sport's categorization, we will note some of the ones which may **not** be as obvious. For example: **Handball, baseball, squash,** and **volleyball** are **not** considered limited contact sports. **Water polo,** on the other hand, is considered to be a contact sport.

The following conditions mandate that a child **refrain from participating in contact sports:**

- Splenomegaly
- Hepatomegaly
- Repeated concussions

PERIL

The single organ rule only applies to kidneys. Children with a single ovary or testicle can participate in contact sports. Children can wear protective equipment to safeguard most other single organs.

Keep your Eye on the Ball, Or Not

Special consideration is given to eye protection. **Baseball is the leading cause of sports-related eye injuries,** mostly in children younger than 14, often by being hit with a pitched ball.

Therefore, all children younger than 14 should be wearing a face guard when at bat. In addition, children with only one functional eye (corrected vision less than 20/50) need to wear protective goggles when in the field.

Children with corrected vision lower than 20/40 need additional ophthalmologic evaluation before being cleared to participate in collision sports.

CASE STUDY

You are presented with a patient with mono and asked for the best management of this patient with regards to sports clearance. They will include choices involving medications such as steroids and IV immunoglobulins.

THE DIVERSION

The diversion is that you may focus on the medical condition and treatment because you are so proud that you figured out the patient had mono and possibly splenomegaly.

ANSWER REVEALED

You would be prouder if you realized that the question is really about knowing that ANY splenomegaly precludes participation in contact sports. The correct answer regarding management would be **avoiding contact sports until the splenomegaly is resolved.**

Most recommendations suggest rest for 3 weeks after acute mononucleosis prior to resumption of activity.

The Juice on Steroid Use

If a teen is suspected of using performance-enhancing substances, a good interview is an important part of making the diagnosis. You won't know unless you ask.

The Side effects of Anabolic Steroid Use

The side effects can be **renal, hepatic,** and **psychological**.

Those who use needles are at risk for **HIV** and **hepatitis**.

In **females** you can see:

- Hirsutism and low voice
- Early closure of epiphyseal plates
- Clitoromegaly
- Decreased menstruation
- Breast atrophy

In **males** you can see:

- Severe acne
- Irreversible gynecomastia
- High-pitched voice
- Hypogonadism[1]

Steroids can result in **violent behavior**. Therefore, if you are presented with a teenager who is experiencing a **sudden change in mood**, withdrawal from steroids could be the cause. **Hypertension** can be seen in both males and females.

Arrhythmias and seizures are *not* signs of steroid use. Cross them out if presented as choices on the exam.

Lab Findings with Steroid Use

Common lab findings they might present you with include:

- Elevated LFTs or signs of cholestasis with transient jaundice
- Lower HDL
- Increased LDL
- Oligospermia and azoospermia[2]

Trolling for Roids

You will need to know the timing of steroid detection, specifically:

PO Steroids – remain in the urine days – weeks

IM Steroids – remain in the system 6 months or more

Sneaky Growth Hormone

Growth Hormone enhances athletic ability and due to the short half life of 4 hours it is NOT detected in current drug testing, which accounts for its increasing popularity.

Brachial Plexus Injuries (aka "Burners" "Stingers")

 This is an injury that results from the stretching of the brachial plexus.

 The typical context is a football injury. There will be pain and numbness shooting down the arm to the thumb.

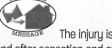 The injury is self limited and after sensation and strength return to normal they can return to regular activity.

Recurrent "burners" needs to be evaluated for possible cervical stenosis or other underlying cause.

---

[1] Yes small testicles and a high pitched voice is an easy image to remember, and one that can probably be used to discourage steroid use among grunting, weight lifting athletes.

[2] If the part about the high-pitched voice and small testicles doesn't discourage steroid use, then this certainly should.

Dietary Supplements

Studies show that protein supplements and creatine are not helpful in young athletes to enhance performance.

It may actually be harmful in endurance sports They are unnecessary when a solid diet is adhered to and good hydration practices are followed.

> **Flipping the Jersey Finger**
>
> *DEFINITION*
>
> A torn flexor tendon of the finger is called a "Jersey finger".
>
> *BUZZWORDS*
>
> Will typically involve the 4th finger, which gets caught in another player resulting in pain in the distal finger with swelling. They will describe an inability to flex the finger.
>
> *TREATMENT*
>
> Here referral to a specialist will be the correct answer. This requires urgent intervention with a hand surgeon within one week.

Chapter 35

Toe, Knee, Chin: Musculoskeletal System

Much of this chapter includes orthopedic conditions. "Strong as an ox and twice as smart" is the old adage about our orthopedic colleagues.

They have to be strong in order to lift the words that describe the geography of bones in diagnosing musculoskeletal disorders. With words like varus, valgus, Las Valgus, and Las Vegas, it is easy for the uninitiated to get confused. Before embarking on the specifics of what you will need to know for the Boards, here is a glossary of terms from the orthopedic cabinet.

Picture the "valgus" as a "gust" of wind blowing out the distal portion of the deformity, everything else will flow from there.

For example, you would know that **Genu Valgum** is "knock-kneed" since the distal part of the leg is pointed outward. Or you can picture "gum" keeping the knees stuck together.

Orthopedic definition of Heart: Pumps nafcillin to the bones. Also a 1970s band from Seattle.

In general monitoring every 6 months should be sufficient. In children older than 7 years, x-rays would be indicated if the intermalleolar distance (with the knees lightly touching) is greater than 8 cm.

Defining Orthopedics

Physeal/Physis: Growth plate.

Metaphyseal/Metaphysis: The end of the long bone, adjacent to the growth plate or physis. It is separated from the epiphysis by the growth plate. In adults it is no longer separated from the rest of the long bone.

Metaphysical: Having to do with the non-physical world.

Varus/Varum: When the distal part of the deformity points towards the midline.

Valgus/Valgum: When the distal part of the deformity points away from the midline.

Epiphyseal/Epiphysis: It is the rounded end of a long bone. During bone development it is separated from the long bone. Once the growth plate closes it is of course a part of the long bone.

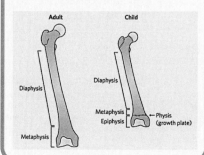

Genu Varum (Bow Legged)

VARUS AND VALGUS KNEE DEFORMITY

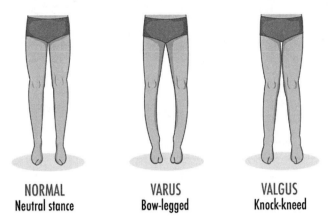

NORMAL	VARUS	VALGUS
Neutral stance	Bow-legged	Knock-kneed

With few exceptions, genu varus is a normal condition, requiring only reassurance.

  Genu Varum would be bow legged. The distal portion of the leg points inward or medially. You can think of how you would sit on a motorcycle which makes the sound VARUUUM!

  Intervention would be required with abnormal findings, such as **when it is unilateral, worsens after age 1, or does not resolve after age 2**. X-ray findings of physeal and epiphyseal distortion would also indicate the need for intervention.

If genu varus is present **after age 2,** then more significant causes, such as **rickets or Blount's disease,** should be considered. When this is the case, there will be something in the history to tip you off.

Blount's Disease

In Blount's disease, there is actual pathology of the proximal tibial physis and epiphysis. There are 2 types:

Infantile Blount's Disease

Infantile Blount's disease is seen in **African Americans** and **shouldn't be confused with rickets.** Note that rickets can also occur more frequently in African Americans due to decreased absorption of UV light. **No treatment is needed** for infantile Blount's disease.

If they are referring to rickets, then other signs of the disorder will need to be presented.

Adolescent Blount's Disease

The adolescent is **usually overweight**. As is the case with infantile Blount's disease, adolescent Blount's disease also occurs **more frequently in African Americans.**

Here treatment is some form of intervention, ranging from **bracing to surgery.**

Breaking Bad

Salter Harris Fracture Classifications

Being familiar with the Salter Harris classification of growth plate fractures will surely come in handy on the exam.

There are five types.

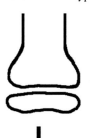

Type 1

This is identified by **separation of the epiphysis and metaphysis.** The fracture is directly through the physis. **X-ray may be negative, with tenderness being the only sign.**

Casting is needed for 2-3 weeks.

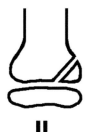

Type 2

Here, **a piece of the metaphysis splits, as well as some physis.**

It is managed by **closed reduction casting** for 3-6 weeks.

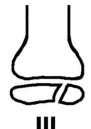

Type 3

This fracture involves **the growth plate and extends to the epiphysis.**

Open reduction may be necessary.

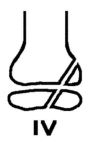

Type 4

There are cracks through everything, **all layer**s.

Type 4 requires reduction in the OR to avoid growth disruption.

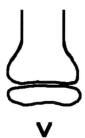

Type 5

This is a **crush type injury/compression fracture** causing **microvascular compromise**. It is associated with a high rate of **poor growth after the injury.**

Greenstick Fracture

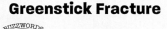

A Greenstick fracture typically occurs following a fall on an outstretched hand with a cortical break on one side of the bone and intact periosteum on the opposite side.

FOOSH = **F**all on **O**uts**t**retched **H**and

The break is not through the bone – one side is broken and the other bent. Like a "Green stick" – get it?

Adding Salt and Pepper

MNEMONIC

One way to memorize the Salter Harris classification is as follows:

S Type 1   **S**traight through growth plate, separated

A Type 2   **A**bove the growth plate

L Type 3   **L**ower-through the epiphysis (lower portion)

T Type 4   **T**otally through the metaphysis, growth plate and epiphysis

R Type 5   c**R**ush to remember this is a compression fracture.

Osteogenic Picture Imperfecta

OI- collagen defect from mutation in **COL1A1** and **COL1A2**, leads to fractures and blue or gray sclera.

BUZZWORDS

Important physical findings should be an important hint that a diagnosis of osteogenesis imperfecta is the diagnosis include gray/ blue sclera, triangular face, macrocephaly with a large anterior fontanelle, as well as pectus excavatum or carinatum.

OI Type I

HOT TIP

Osteogenesis Imperfecta (OI) Type 1 is **the most common** form and is the **classic nondeforming** form. It is inherited in an **autosomal dominant** fashion and is the one with the really **blue sclerae. Fractures occur during the preschool years. Rarely are they born with fractures**.

PERIL

They can even develop fractures during regular hip exam, so even the Ortolani and Barlow are contraindicated. Instead, hip ultrasound is used to monitor their hip joints.

HOT TIP

The majority will develop **hearing loss** by the time they are adults. Hearing loss (both conductive and sensorineural) is considered to be a major feature of OI type 1. They end up with **normal lifespan** and **normal height**.

OI Type II

This is the **most severe form** of the disease, and is **usually lethal** at less than one week of age.

OI Type 2 is inherited as either a **dominant new mutation** or "**germinal mosaicism**".[1]

BUZZWORDS

Children with OI Type 2 are **born with multiple fractures** and are sometimes described as having a "**bag of bones**" appearance. They are usually **stillborn** and rarely live past the postnatal period.

---

[1] Germinal mosaicism is when the defect exists in germinal cells but not in regular somatic cells. Therefore, it can be transmitted as a dominant trait, but appear to be recessive since it is not an expressed phenotype in the parents.

OI Type III

Type 3 is known as the **progressive deforming type**. Children with OI Type 3 are **born with fractures** and the deformities are **progressive**.

They have **wormian bones** in the skull and **codfish vertebrae**. The adult height is **extremely short** (around 3 feet). The **intellect is normal**, but **hearing is affected** because of fractures of the middle ear bones after puberty.

OI Type IV

Kind of like Type 1, but the **sclerae are white**, not blue.

OI Type V

Have **progressive calcification** in the interosseous membranes and no blue sclera.

OI Rhyme Time

- OI1 is won (the best)
- OI2 is TOO bad
- OI3 is worse to be
- OI4 is blue no more
- OI5 is calcified

OI Treatment

Goal is to improve quality of life by minimizing pain and disability while optimizing mobility and function.

Craning Your Neck

Torticollis

Cause of Neck Tilt	Distinguishing Characteristics
Muscular Torticollis	Muscular torticollis usually results from **positioning** or **trauma**, such as bleeding into the sternocleidomastoid muscle after birth or after an injury in older children.
Paroxysmal Torticollis	This is a **migraine variant** that may even manifest in infants. Children present with repeated attacks of head tilting, which **only last for minutes at a time**. These require no intervention, and are often accompanied by **vomiting, irritability, and pallor**.
Vertebral anomalies	These will obviously present from birth and be diagnoseable by XR.
Posterior fossa tumor	Head tilt secondary to a brain tumor will include physical findings consistent with an upper motor neuron process, including **increased deep tendon reflexes**. This would require an MRI to establish a diagnosis.

Congenital Torticollis

Typical description would be an infant with **a mass in the sternocleidomastoid muscle** with **head tilted** to the ipsilateral side, chin pointing to the opposite side and/ or **facial asymmetry**.

Congenital torticollis requires **daily stretching and physical therapy**. If this therapy is not implemented or is not effective after one year, surgical intervention will be necessary.

Congenital torticollis can be associated with **developmental dysplasia of the hip**.

Klippel-Feil Syndrome

Klippel-Feil syndrome is due to **fusion of the cervical vertebrae** and may present as congenital torticollis. Additional findings include **short neck** and **low occipital hairline** resembling Turner syndrome. Associated findings include:

- scoliosis
- spina bifida
- renal problems (missing one kidney)
- Sprengel deformity
- deafness

"Clipper File" syndrome. Picture a file of hedge clippers instead of a neck - now THAT would be one stiff neck. You can also picture the clippers delivering a bad haircut, resulting in a "low occipital hairline."

Sprengel Deformity

Sprengel deformity results from **failure of the scapula to descend to its normal position during fetal development**.[2] The affected side of the neck will seem broader and shorter.[3] Therefore, it **mimics torticollis**.

Picture a "scapula made of sprinkles on someone's neck."

Developmental Dysplasia of the Hip (DDH)[4]

The reason for the name change from "congenital" is to acknowledge that it is a progressive problem. The number one cause is improper positioning, either in utero or postnatally.

---

[2] Typically there is an abnormally high and medially rotated position of the scapula.
[3] Of course, there is a scapula sitting there.
[4] Formerly known as CDH (Congenital Dislocation of the Hip) but now known as DDH since joining the witness protection program for diseases that cooperate with the FBI.

Risk Factors for DDH

Risk factors for DDH in the newborn include:

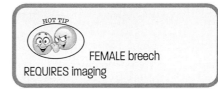

HOT TIP

FEMALE breech REQUIRES imaging

- Female (#1 risk factor)
- Breech positioning
- Family history of DDH in first degree relative (parent or sibling)
- Improper swaddling methods

Other conditions frequently associated with DDH include **torticollis, metatarsus adductus**, and **calcaneovalgus** [a.k.a. club] foot.

DEFINITION

- **Barlow** is the part of the exam done with knees adducted and with downward pressure to try to dislocate the hip. Unstable hips may be normal and this may resolve in the first few weeks of life.
- **Ortolani** is the attempt at relocating a dislocated femoral head. This is the most important clinical test for detecting DDH at 0-3 months.

MNEMONIC

Remember "Barlow **out**" is when you cause the dislocation by pushing the hip **out** of socket. "Ortolani" starts with an O (for "out") and ends with an "I" (for "in") so this is when you reduce the dislocation.

PERIL

The Ortolani and Barlow maneuvers will **not be reliable after 3 months of age**. Do not use these maneuvers for suspected OI patients as you can cause fractures- only screen for DDH with Ultrasound.

Abduct vs Adduct

Abduct is to "take away", like when a person is abducted from their home.

Adduct is to "bring together" like when you add insult to injury.

TAKE HOME
MESSAGE

After 3 months of age, **limitations in hip abduction** will be the most common sign of DDH. **Unequal knee height** [Galeazzi sign] may also be present. They might also show or describe **asymmetric gluteal folds**, but this is a nonspecific and common finding in infants.

Waffling on Waddling Gait

COIN FLIP

While a waddling gait is a typical description of a child with uncorrected DDH, there are other causes you should consider, depending on the context they give. For example:

COIN FLIP

If they describe a "click" on Boards, you can safely dismiss it. But you should always work up a "clunk".

Diagnosis is made by **real-time U/S with manipulation** in the first 4 months of life and by **AP and frog leg Xray** after that time.

In infants with risk factors but a normal exam, waiting until 6 weeks of age to get the hip US may reduce false positive results, but imaging should delayed beyond 6 months of age.

PERIL

Do not image in first 2 weeks of life, the false positive rates are too high.

Rickets can be the correct answer if they describe leg bowing and other findings consistent with rickets.

Legg-Calvé-Perthes disease could be described as a patient with a waddling gait and a limp. This would likely be described in a child around age 7.

Slipped capital femoral epiphysis could present this way; would likely include knee pain in an overweight young adolescent.

Treatment is with the **Pavlik harness**, which holds the hips in a position of abduction, flexion, and external rotation. This is more reliable than double or triple diapers. Complications of treatment include avascular necrosis of the femoral head and femoral nerve palsy.

Watch for the presentation of a child with a **waddling gait** or **leg length discrepancy**. These are the consequences in a child whose DDH was not corrected.

Leg Tilt

BREAKING NEWS

Leg length discrepancies are usually asymptomatic, but should be monitored for worsening during growth.

If you are presented with a child with a leg discrepancy of 2 cm or more, then a referral to an orthopedist would be the appropriate next step.

Less than that, monitoring would be appropriate.

Muscle, Joint, and Bone Infections

Viral Myositis

Typical presentation is with **weakness and tenderness** localized to a muscle, most often the calf muscle. Neurological exam will be unremarkable. Lab findings would include **elevated creatinine kinase**. They will likely include a history of a **recent respiratory illness or influenza**. No treatment is necessary.

Metabolic myopathies due to mitochondrial dysfunction might present with a similar picture; however, there will also be **rhabdomyolysis** (described as dark urine) noted in the history.

Toxic Synovitis (Transient Synovitis)

Toxic synovitis is a misnomer, since it is not that toxic at all. Look for the following in the history: **recent URI** (usually within 1 month prior to presentation), **hip pain or limp**, some **passive ROM, normal ESR,** and **normal or slightly elevated temperature** in a well-appearing child. If joint aspiration is done, the gram stain will be negative.

The cause is often viral and culprits include Parvovirus B19, influenza, hepatitis B, rubella, Mr. Ebstein-Barr virus, and possibly every other known and unknown virus in the universe.

No matter how severe the pain, "toxic" synovitis is benign and requires nothing more than NSAIDs and supportive care. It is a **diagnosis of exclusion** after other more serious infections are ruled out.

B19 Bomber

Parvovirus B19, the "B 19" bomber, seems to cause anything and everything. Besides hip pain, they might describe flushing of the cheeks to suggest Fifth disease.

Septic (a.k.a. Pyogenic) Arthritis

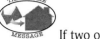

Evaluation of a child suspect of having a septic joint should include a CBC with differential, sedimentation rate, C reactive protein, and a blood culture.

If two or more of the following are present, Orthopedic Surgery should be consulted immediately:

- fever > 38.5° C,
- refusal to bear weight,
- sed rate >40,
- elevated WBC,
- elevated C reactive protein.

Septic arthritis usually presents in children under age 2, is much more serious, and requires aggressive intervention. It is usually due to **hematogenous spread**.

Look for the following in the presentation: **fever, "won't walk" or "won't move it", high WBC and sed rate, positive gram stain,** and **increased joint space on x-ray.** The joint will likely be **warm, red,** and **swollen** and the child will **fight you** touching or moving it.

In general imaging is not necessarily the definitive way to to diagnose and treat septic arthritis.

- If septic arthritis of the hip is suspected then the most appropriate next would be ultrasound.

- If an effusion is detected then a diagnostic aspiration is indicated.

- If it is suspected then immediate drainage, irrigation and empirical antibiotics to cover Staph is indicated.

The key steps are **joint aspiration and initiation of IV antibiotic therapy**. Rapid intervention plays an important role in prognosis. IV antibiotics should be started pending culture and sensitivities. Once there is clinical improvement, oral antibiotics can be continued for another 3 weeks.

In general, the septic hip is the most difficult joint to diagnose. If the history suggests a septic hip, then choose antibiotics and treatment. **Treatment should begin even before the diagnosis is confirmed.**

Septic Arthritis Organisms

The most common pathogen overall is *Staph aureus*.

In neonates, *Group B Strep and E. coli* must be considered.

In infants and children, remember *Strep pneumo*, group A beta hemolytic Strep, and *H. Flu.*

In teenagers, *N. gonorrhea* must be considered.

What's Groin on ?

If you are presented with a teen with groin pain it very likely represents femoroacetabular joint pathology of the hip.

The proper next step would be xray or arthrography.

MRI would not be correct since it is not a good method to visualize the acetabular labrum.

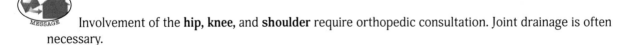

CASE STUDY You are presented with a patient who recently immigrated from a developing country. He presents with a sore ankle that is painful to both passive and active movement, red, and mildly swollen. This was preceded by similar symptoms in the knee yesterday (which is better today). There is also a diffuse macular rash. You are asked for a diagnosis to explain the presentation.

THE DIVERSION You might be tempted to pick several diversionary choices including meningococcemia, septic arthritis, or even post-infectious synovitis.

ANSWER REVEALED However, the key here is their noting that the patient is a recent immigrant. This usually means an infectious disease that is either 1) rare due to immunization, or 2) an oldie but a goodie, a disorder that is not seen very often. In this case, a migratory arthritis involving large joints coupled with a rash should lead you to the correct diagnosis of rheumatic fever.

Staph aureus is the most common cause of septic arthritis in all age groups. It occurs through hematogenous spread. Therefore any empirical treatment should provide for Staph coverage.

TREATMENT The treatment of choice for empiric antibiotics for septic arthritis depends on the age and the suspected bug.

- **Neonates** - ampicillin
- **Infants through 3 months** – cefuroxime or cefotaxime
- **Children** – cefazolin or ceftriaxone
- **Adolescents** - must add azithromycin to ceftriaxone or cefixime in order to cover for GC

HOT TIP For children with **sickle cell disease**, you must extend coverage for *Salmonella*, using cefotaxime.

PERIL If the question hints that **MRSA** is prevalent, vancomycin should be included in the correct choice.

TAKE HOME MESSAGE Involvement of the **hip, knee,** and **shoulder** require orthopedic consultation. Joint drainage is often necessary.

Osteomyelitis

DEFINITION Osteomyelitis is **infection of the bone**, as opposed to septic arthritis, which is infection of the joint.

It begins with **localized tenderness** over the metaphysis, as well as **pain on weightbearing**.

Osteomyelitis results either from **direct** injury or infection, like stepping on a nail, or via **hematogenous spread**, getting a free ride in the blood to get to a site even far away from the initial injury or infection.

Diagnosis is made by **direct aspiration** of the metaphysis, which is sent for culture and sensitivity.

Who done it?

Just like in the game *Clue*, where the culprit was Colonel Mustard in the kitchen with a rope, the questions here are Who, When, Where, and Why?

Staph aureus is the most common cause of acute hematogenous osteomyelitis in all ages.

The Neonatal Period

In neonates, the infection usually results from hematogenous spread, and often affects the **femur and tibia**. Besides *S. aureus*, group B streptococci and *Escherichia coli* are common causes.

Although it is typically contracted via hematogenous spread, **a septic joint** is present 50% of the time among neonates with osteomyelitis.

Beyond the Neonatal Period

A septic joint is rarely seen with osteomyelitis beyond the neonatal period. Besides *S. aureus*, other etiologies include Group A strep (a.k.a. *Strep pyogenes*), *Kingella kingae*, and *H. flu* type b.

In children with **sickle cell disease**, the most common cause of osteomyelitis is *Salmonella*.

In children who **step on a nail**, a common cause of osteomyelitis is *P. aeruginosa*.

Initial treatment of osteomyelitis is always IV, and the choice of antibiotic obviously depends on who you think the guilty party is.

Team Bone Scan or Team MRI?

Bone scans are useful early, when the exact location of the infection needs to be identified and the infection is too early to be detected on plain film. Bone scan can pick up abnormalities within 3 days of onset. X-ray findings in osteo do not generally appear until 10 to 14 days after infection.

MRI with contrast is much more specific and can distinguish infection from other causes of inflammation. For example, if you are presented with a child who has sickle cell disease, the distinction between infarction and infection would be identified on MRI, not bone scan.

Bone scans are better at "where is there trouble?" while MRIs are better at "what is the trouble?"

Unable to Shake the Pelvis

Pelvic osteomyelitis is prone to abscess formation; read the question carefully to determine if this is what they are alluding to.

Pelvic osteomyelitis is seen more frequently in boys around age 8, and is typically right sided. The cause is *Staph aureus*.

The pain is often referred to the hip or thigh. It can present as **abdominal pain**. WBC will be normal, and plain film may be negative. MRI and bone scan would be the studies of choice.

Treatment should continue for 4-6 weeks as follows:

Etiology of Osteomyelitis.	Treatment of Osteomyelitis
Staph aureus / Group A strep	Oxacillin / Nafcillin 1st / 2nd generation cephalosporin Clindamycin (for patients who are pen allergic)
H. flu	2nd or 3rd generation cephalosporin
Children with sickle cell	Have to assume **Salmonella** is highly likely, and starting with a 3rd generation cephalosporin would be the correct initial course until culture and sensitivity back
Concurrent puncture wound	Would need to cover for **pseudomonas** and/or **anaerobic organisms**.

Children may be sent home on oral antibiotics when

1. There is **a good response to IV meds,** and a **specific organism is identified,**
2. A trial of PO antibiotics and **good serum levels** are documented while still in the hospital,
3. You have **compliance assured (parental reliability)**

HOT TIP

The most common complication of osteomyelitis is recurrence. Surgical intervention might be required with chronic infection, especially when an abscess is suspected.

Non Infectious Limps and Pains and Umpa Lumpas

Legg–Calvé–Perthes Disease

DEFINITION

Legg Calve Perthes Disease is **avascular necrosis of the femoral head.** It usually presents as **hip pain** and/ or **limp** in children (usually **boys**) with a peak at ages **4-10 years**. They could show the classic x-ray, **with one femoral head being smaller than the other**.

PERIL

Remember, **hip pain can frequently be referred to the knee or groin.** This means that they say their knee hurts, but the cause is really in the hip. Physical exam will show limited hip motion with internal rotation and abduction.

TREATMENT

These children should be made **nonweight-bearing** and referred to ortho for **splinting** and **possible surgery**.

> Trivia: Young **Forrest Gump** had Legg Calve Perthes in the movie.

Slipped Capital Femoral Epiphysis (SCFE)

A SCFE is essentially a Salter Harris I fracture of femoral capital epiphysis

A teenager (usually male and obese), with **a limp** and **knee pain**. The knee pain is actually **referred hip pain**. They may describe the leg as **extended and externally rotated**.

Since SCFE is diagnosed by Xray, it could show up on the board exam as an x-ray. If you look at this once, it will be obvious on the exam. One hip will be normal and the other will look like an ice cream scoop falling off the cone. The ice cream scoop is the acetabular head.

SCFE can occur with various endocrinopathies. Keep this in mind when there are any lab values included in the history, especially those that are endocrine-related.

Keep hip pathology in mind with any description of knee pain on the Boards.

SCFE is treated with **immobilization, no weight bearing**, and **stabilization** with pins and/or bone grafts.

Osgood-Schlatter Disease (OS) (AKA-Tibial Tuberosity Apophysitis)

Osgood-Schlatter disease is typically described in an **athletic adolescent** who presents with **pain just below the patella**.

The pain may be exacerbated by running, jumping, and kneeling. On exam, they present with tenderness at the tibial tuberosity and may report pain with trying to extend the knee against resistance.

Osgood-Schlatter disease is the result of stress from **excessive activity** at the **insertion of the patellar tendon at the anterior tibial tubercle**. The tibial tuberosity is the location of a specialized growth center called the **apophysis**. This is the site where the quadriceps muscle attaches via the patellar tendon. This is why adolescents are prone to this "overuse injury", or "apophysitis", during the period of rapid growth.

Treatment consists of a couple of weeks' **rest** with gradual resumption of activity, **ice**, and **NSAIDs** for pain and inflammation. A patellar strap may help by reducing the tension caused by this tendon pulling on the tuberosity. Stretching and strengthening the quadriceps may also help.

Sever's Syndrome (calcaneal apophysitis)

Sever's syndrome is like the Osgood-Schlatter of the heel.

It presents as heel pain in young athletes, especially those doing soccer, basketball, gymnastics and running. It is somewhat more common in boys than girls and peaks at 8-12 years of age.

It is especially common in sports that require cleats.

Just like OS, treatment is with rest, ice, NSAIDs, and wearing shoes with proper cushioning.

Observing the Occult

You could very well be presented with a patient with an occult fracture.

The history will imply or clearly note that there are no systemic symptoms, no recent viral illness, no signs of infectious etiology, and no history that would lead you to suspect a trauma that was missed.

A **"toddler's fracture"** can occur during the course of learning to walk. It may not be apparent on x-ray. On physical exam there will be **point tenderness**, and this could be the only clue in the question pointing to this diagnosis.

Since ligaments are stronger than underlying bone in children, a sprained ligament will not likely be the correct answer. Force strong enough to cause a ligament tear in a child would more likely result in a fracture.

Bone Cysts

Unicameral bone cysts, or **simple bone cysts**, are fluid-filled cysts (usually seen prior to skeletal maturity) that are typically found at the proximal humerus or femur. These are *not* precancerous.

These typically are asymptomatic and are diagnosed as pathological fracture after minor trauma.

Aneurysmal bone cysts are typically seen on the tibia or femur. These present with pain, which can be in the absence of swelling. They can be associated with underlying bone tumors and may require orthopedic referral if this is on the exam.

If present on vertebrae, can have signs of nerve compression.

Ehlers-Danlos Syndrome

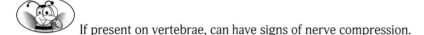

Typical presentation is skin that **stretches** and joints that are **hypermobile** like Spongebob Squarepants. These kids also have **poor wound healing,** so keep this diagnosis in mind if poor wound healing is included in the question.

Because the hypermobile joints can become painful, these children often end up in the Orthopedist's or the Rheumatologist's offices.

Most types of Ehlers-Danlos Syndrome have a **normal life expectancy.**

"Elbow Dancing syndrome."

> ### Growing Pains
> This will be described as being "bilateral," "worse at bedtime," and "joint pain without swelling."

Because of **easy bruisability**, Ehlers-Danlos can be mistaken for child abuse. Watch for the presentation of a child with multiple bruising and other manifestations of Ehlers-Danlos syndrome, to avoid being tricked into assuming child abuse.

Hypermobility: This will be described as "loose joints" (we're not talking about the kind of people with pinky rings at a Saturday night slam) in people who get injured and sustain sprains easily. They need to be counseled to stretch before sports and to be vigilant in the sports they play. No other intervention is needed.

Back Anomalies

Scoliosis

Besides knowing when to hold'em, when to fold'em, when to walk away and when to run,[5] with scoliosis, you will need to know when treatment is needed and when observation alone is okay.

They might describe **"asymmetry of the hips, shoulders** and/or **scapula"** on the physical exam, without coming right out and telling you it is scoliosis.

Congenital Scoliosis

Patients may present in infancy or much later, depending on the degree of curvature. Causes include **malformation of the spinal column or ribs**.

Although congenital scoliosis is often associated with other malformations, most cases are *not* hereditary.

For congenital scoliosis, bracing is not helpful as primary treatment. However, it would be the correct answer for post-op treatment.

Children with congenital scoliosis should be screened with **renal ultrasound** and **cardiac echo**, due to the high association with renal and cardiac disease. Spinal MRI would also be indicated, since there is also a high association with spinal abnormalities.

Chromosome analysis, ophthalmologic evaluation, and head ultrasound are **not** routinely indicated.

Secondary Scoliosis

There are instances where scoliosis is associated with an underlying condition or syndrome. Watch for signs of delayed pubertal development, neurological deficits, or dermatologic lesions. **Neurofibromatosis** is an example of a disorder where scoliosis may be more commonly seen.

---

5 In case you're going to spend the next 45 minutes trying to remember where that's from, it's Kenny Rogers' *The Gambler*.

Neuromuscular or paralytic scoliosis is seen in children with conditions such as muscular dystrophy, myopathies, cerebral palsy, tethered cord syndrome, spinal muscular atrophy, DDH, OI, Klippel-Feil syndrome, connective tissue disorders like Marfan syndrome and Ehlers-Danlos syndrome, spina bifida, or those who have sustained a spinal cord injury. The degree of curvature tends to progress.

Idiopathic Scoliosis

Idiopathic scoliosis is an isolated scoliosis with no identified cause. This represents 80% of the cases in practice, but not necessarily 80% of the cases on the boards. These tend to worsen by 1 degree per month during the growth spurt, until skeletal maturity.

If the degree of curvature increases by more than 1 degree per month during the growth spurt, then this may be more than just idiopathic scoliosis, warranting an MRI, orthopedic consultation, bracing, and possibly surgery.

- ❑ **Curvature of less than 25 degrees requires observation only.**
- ❑ If there is **more than 2 years of growth still expected (child is still growing), bracing** is required for curvature **between 25-40 degrees.**
- ❑ Surgery will be **needed for a lumbar or thoracic curvature greater than 40 degrees.**
- ❑ Young premenarchal patients with large initial curves are at risk for the highest degree of progression.

If they describe interventions such as "manipulation" or "electrical stimulation," it will be the wrong answer. (Rolfing, mud therapy, and aerobic psychotherapy have not received FDA approval yet either.)

Kyphosis

Kyphosis is the convex alignment of the thoracic spine in the sagittal plane (also known as the side view).

The normal range is 20-40 degrees; therefore, don't be intimidated into thinking this is abnormal.

For kyphosis less than 60 degrees, no intervention is needed other than follow-up. Pulmonary function studies would not be indicated in an asymptomatic patient unless kyphosis is well above 60 degrees.

CASE STUDY You are presented with a teenage patient who "can never stand up straight" and has chronic upper back pain. You note kyphosis on physical examination along with a "distended abdomen." You are asked for the most likely diagnosis.

THE DIVERSION Among the diversionary choices will be chronic poor posture, scoliosis, spinal tumor and vertebral osteomyelitis.

ANSWER REVEALED The combination of "bad posture, kyphosis and back pain" in a teenager should lead you to a diagnosis of **Scheuermann disease**. Scheuermann disease is a "fixed kyphosis" which presents at puberty. Treatment is primarily with NSAID medication, physical therapy and observation over time. Surgery is sometimes required.

Milan Lucic currently of the Edmonton Oilers has this condition.

Back Pain

By now, if you have been sitting long enough reading through all of this, your back is probably killing you.

If scoliosis and kyphosis are not the answer, you must sit at the table listed below to answer these questions correctly.

Main Categories	Subcategories	Associations
Infectious	Diskitis	Usually caused by *Staph aureus*
	Spinal Epidural Abscess	
	Vertebral osteomyelitis	
Developmental	Spondylolysis	
	Spondylolisthesis	Progression of spondylolysis, leading to stress fractures and subluxation of vertebral bodies
Traumatic Causes	Herniated disc	
	Vertebral Stress Fracture	
	Overuse syndrome	
Tumors	Osteoid osteoma	Night pain relieved by NSAIDs
	Osteoblastoma	Osteoid osteoma greater than 1.5 cm
	Aneurysmal bone cyst	
	Osteosarcoma	
	Ewing sarcoma	

Elbowing the Problem

Annular Ligament Displacement

BUZZWORDS

This has been classically known as "Nursemaid's elbow".[6] The typical description is of a child that was **pulled by the arm**, is now **not using the involved arm**, and was brought in by an hysterical relative. Usually young child (1-4 years old) holding arm close to their body with elbow flexed and forearm pronated.

PERIL

If there is no swelling, point tenderness, or discoloration, **x-rays will not be necessary**.

TREATMENT

The "best way to manage" the problem will be to reduce it, **but only after checking for other injuries**.

The Skinny on Fat Pads

HOT TIP

Should they mention the visibility of the **posterior** fat pad on x-ray of the elbow, it suggests fracture and accumulation of fluid. However, an **anterior fat pad is a normal finding**.

MNEMONIC

Regarding fat pads, remember **P** = **P**oor (**P**osterior) and **A** = **A**ll right (**A**nterior) fat pad.

Hand Issues

Polydactyly

Although polydactyly can be associated with various syndromes, it is usually an isolated **autosomal dominant trait**. In fact, if you encounter such a patient in real life, you will often note that the parents had an extra digit surgically removed.

You are expected to know the basic management of polydactyly. With simple postaxial polydactyly (which occurs off the 5th finger/toe and amounts to little more than a skin tag), ligation until it falls off is usually sufficient.

For more complicated cases involving bone, soft tissues, and tendons, **referral to a hand surgeon** may be necessary.

Club Foot

For those who prefer Latin, Club Foot[7] is called *Talipes Equinovarus*. Simply put, the **foot is internally rotated and the Achilles tendon is contracted**.

TREATMENT

Urgent referral to Ortho is indicated. Treatment consists of stretching, serial casting, and possible surgical release of the tendon late in the first year of life.

Toe Walking

Although toe-walking can be a normal phase, it is an issue when it persists **after age 2-3 years**, or when kids are **unable to put their heels down at rest**.

---

[6] This was formerly known as Subluxed Radial Head.
[7] Club Foot is also a Mediterranean vacation spot for tired podiatrists, and would be correct if it were one of the choices.

The most common cause of toe-walking is **idiopathic** and it tends to present right when kids learn to walk, but other conditions such as **cerebral palsy, spinal cord tumors**, and **neuromuscular problems** such as **tethered cord** need to be considered and ruled out.

Children who initially walk normally and develop toe-walking later must be evaluated for conditions like **muscular dystrophy, Charcot-Marie-Tooth disease**, and other **hereditary neuropathies**.

Correct initial treatment is **foot dorsiflexion exercises** several times per day to maintain full range of motion at the heel cord. Gently remind the child to put the heel down when walking.

Children who persist in toe-walking or who develop heel-cord contractures with no other known musculoskeletal conditions should be referred for orthopedic evaluation and possible short-term casting to break the habit.

Intoeing

There are 3 causes of intoeing

1. Metatarsus adductus in infancy

2. Tibial torsion in toddlerhood

3. Femoral anteversion in early childhood (child will sit "W style" with hips turned in and knees turned out)

Tibial torsion and femoral anteversion almost always resolve spontaneously by school age[8], which is the answer they are seeking on the boards.

The use of bars and other devices has not been shown to correct natural "in-toeing."

Neither Dennis Browne bars, sleeping on the back, sleeping in bars, Buster Brown® shoes, nor the dog that lives in the Buster Brown® shoes[9] is the answer they are looking for.

---

[8] Our podiatry colleagues vacationing at Club Foot state otherwise, but they aren't writing Pediatric Board questions.
[9] Most of you are too young to remember Buster Brown shoes. Google it.

Chapter 36

SUDS and SUD
Substance Abuse Disorder[1]

Overall Use[2]

Alcohol, tobacco, and marijuana are among the substances most frequently used by adolescents.

ALCOHOL: 50% of students have tried alcohol by 10th grade; despite this, use has reportedly declined to a record low.

TOBACCO: 35% of 12th graders have tried cigarettes; again, use has reportedly declined a record low.

MARIJUANA: use is stable with 45% of all 12th graders saying they have tried it at least once.

Where there's smoke, there's more smoke. Use of **more than one drug** is more common than single drug use in this population.

Initial age for experimentation is around middle school.

The earlier a child starts using a drug, the more likely it is that they will develop dependency.

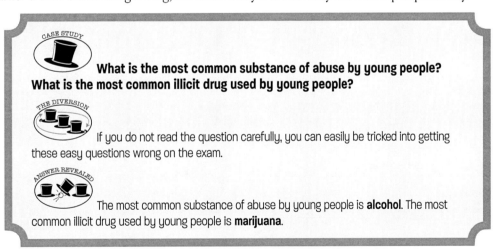

What is the most common substance of abuse by young people? What is the most common illicit drug used by young people?

If you do not read the question carefully, you can easily be tricked into getting these easy questions wrong on the exam.

The most common substance of abuse by young people is **alcohol**. The most common illicit drug used by young people is **marijuana**.

More ER visits are due to the ill effects of marijuana (and/or drugs that might be mixed in with it) than for alcohol use.

---

[1] New DSM-Diagnosis: Maladaptive pattern of use despite significant substance-related problems.
[2] According to the 2015 National Survey on Drug Use and Health (NSDUH)

Risk factors

Risk factors that increase the risk for adolescent drug use include:

- Low self esteem and poor coping skills
- Alienation from conventional norms
- Homosexuality
- The use of performance-enhancing drugs
- Parental use/abuse of drugs
- Child abuse
- Inconsistent parenting
- Drug use among close friends
- Early academic failure
- Disconnect from family, school, and community
- Early behavior problems (ADHD, ODD, mood and disruptive behavior disorders)
- Depression, conduct disorders, and antisocial personality disorders

Studies show that the media play a powerful role in influencing adolescent behaviors related to alcohol and tobacco.

TAKE HOME MESSAGE Protective factors toward substance use include a sense of connectivity to school, family, community and faith.

Anticipatory Guidance

You will likely be questioned on appropriate anticipatory guidance. Keep the following in mind when answering questions on this subject.

Parents should be encouraged to discuss and help their teenagers understand the circumstances under which they will be pressured to try drugs.

HOT TIP Appropriate actions by the **pediatrician** would include universal screening, ie. using standardized questionnaires and asking open ended questions in confidence, as well as questioning the adolescent about his/her attitude in general regarding drug and alcohol use. Screening does not mean drug testing.

UPDATED & NEW BREAKING NEWS INFORMATION An example of one screening tool is the CRAFFT which is a questionnaire for teens assessing their risk for substance abuse. **CRAFFT** stands for **C**ar **R**elax **A**lone **F**orget **F**riends **T**rouble.

PERIL **Casual use** should not be dismissed. The transition from casual use to dependence may occur much more quickly in adolescents than adults.

In addition to identifying which drugs are being used by teens, it is important to identify **how often** and **the context** within which they are being used.

Drug Abuse and Psychiatric Disorders

Psychiatric comorbidity, especially conduct disorder, is common in children who use drugs.

The psychiatric disorder often preceded the use of drugs, and often worsens after onset of drug use.

HOT TIP In the case of ADHD, children who are appropriately treated are less likely to abuse drugs than those with ADHD who aren't treated.

Drug abuse can both mimic and/or worsen psychiatric disorders. For example, the use of alcohol or cocaine (or both together) can induce depression (or it can happen the other way around, with depression leading to substance abuse). These substances may also cause psychosis or mimic anxiety disorders.

There is a higher likelihood of physical trauma being reported by children who are abusing drugs.

Birds of a Feather

One of the strongest predictors of substance use is hanging around peers who use substances.

Obtaining information from the school and/or law enforcement is considered appropriate.

Declining school performance may be a red flag that the problem is substance abuse.

Drug Screening

In general, urine drug screens have high sensitivity, are relatively inexpensive, and reflect substance use **within the previous 48 hours**. Marijuana (THC), however, can be detected in urine drug screens for several weeks.

Urine specific gravity and the **creatinine concentration** impact the validity of drug tests. Therefore, if these values are provided in a question that includes a positive urine tox screen, factor them in when answering the question.

Urine tox screens are just that, screens. Therefore, **positive screen results must be confirmed** by gas chromatography and mass spectrometry.

When indicated, urine drug screen specimens should be collected **under direct observation**.

Hair testing can evaluate for substance or chronic exposure (typically weeks to 2-3 months earlier), but it is difficult to collect proper samples and is prone to external contamination.

Blood testing (whole, serum, plasma) is fairly accurate, but invasive, slow, and expensive.

Confidentiality

The one exception to strict confidentiality would be if the adolescent is **at risk of harming him/herself or others**.

Know that when an adolescent is placed in a drug treatment program, the pediatrician is expected to track progress.

Random drug screening is not recommended. If the parents request a drug test, obtaining it will be the wrong choice on the exam. The correct answer will be to do a **thorough history and physical exam** and addressing the risks and concerns.

Asking the parents for their own mental health and drug use history, could be a correct answer on the exam, although that might be a tough one in the real world.

Pick Your Poison

Inhalants

 Inhalants are among the most commonly used drugs by adolescents.

Commonly used inhalants include volatile hydrocarbons such as **toluene paint thinner, gasoline, kerosene, cleaning fluids, aerosols, lighter fluid, organic solvents, glue,** and **spray paint** as well as nitrite compounds such as nitrous oxide and amyl nitrate.

Aerosols are usually sprayed into a bag and then inhaled from the bag. **Liquids** are usually poured unto rags and placed against the mouth and nose.

Immediate effects

 The immediate effects of inhalant abuse would include **decreased inhibition,** followed by short lived **drowsiness** and **lightheadedness**. This leads to **ataxia** and **disorientation**.

Effects are noticed **within seconds** and last 5 to 15 minutes. Therefore drug testing is very difficult.

On exam, **sluggish pupillary responses** and **bradycardia** may be noted.

You may also note an eczematous "glue-sniffer's rash" around the nose and mouth.

Intoxication

Inhalant intoxication may be characterized by **generalized muscle weakness, confusion, hallucinations, ataxia, delirium, nystagmus,** and/ or a **lack of coordination**. Ultimately, they may experience a **hangover** similar to an alcohol hangover.

Asymptomatic patients would require only observation for 6 hours.

Symptomatic patients May require oxygen, bronchodilators, and other supportive care, including intubation.

Morbidity and Mortality

The fatal effects of inhalants may include

- Asphyxia ➜ death
- Cardiac Arrhythmia ➜ death
- Aspiration ➜ death

Hydrocarbon ingestion

A child who inadvertently got into these substances would likely present with:

- oropharyngeal/ gastric irritation
- nausea/ vomiting
- cough/ wheezing
- tachypnea

They may provide you with evidence of hypoxemia and/ or diffuse bilateral ARDS-like infiltrates on CXR.

The **most common** *fatal complication* is cardiac arrhythmias.

The adolescent will present with **mental status changes**, but the result of both **head CT** and **urine tox screen** will be **negative**.

The presentation can be similar to **alcohol intoxication**: agitation and ataxia. It can also be similar to **PCP** intoxication. However, they will have to give you a clue. First, they might note that the tox screen is negative, and then they will have to note something consistent with the diagnosis, such as **abnormal smell on their breath**.

Long term use of inhalants can lead to **liver and kidney damage, neuropathies, neurophychiatric disorders, encephalopathy, dementia,** and **bone marrow suppression.** Gasoline sniffers can develop **lead toxicity**.

Urine assays are available to detect urinary metabolite of specific hydrocarbons.[3]

Marijuana

Present-day marijuana is much more potent than that from decades ago.

Highly concentrated inhaled products (waxes, dabs, budders)and edible products can contain high amounts of THC, the most psychoactive cannabinoid in marijuana.

Physiologic consequences

Acute effects

All of the acute effects of marijuana begin with a **D**. You can remember this because it'll be the grade they'll be getting in most of their classes.

The acute physiologic effects of marijuana include

- Dry mouth
- Dilated pupils
- Drowsiness
- Distortion of time

Couch Potato Pot Head !

Chronic cannabis Syndrome aka Amotivational Syndrome has been seen with heavy chronic use. It is characterized by difficulty concentrating, withdrawal/moodiness, and loss of interest in previous activities or anything other than using marijuana.

---

[3] Reference *Common Substances of Abuse*, PIR, Vol 39, No 8, AUG 2018.

If you are asked how to monitor discontinuation of marijuana use, the correct answer would be serial measurements of **urine THC: creatinine ratio**, which should decrease as marijuana use is discontinued.

Additional physiological consequences may include **compromised immune function** and **decreased sperm count.** The latter is reversible, and should serve as motivation to discontinue use.

Impaired coordination can be seen in adolescents using marijuana regularly.

After marijuana use, teens may experience **tachycardia** (lasting up to 3 hours), along with **increased blood pressure** because of catecholamine release.

Chronic effects

- **Pulmonary** - Just like tobacco smoke, there are carcinogens in marijuana smoke, and significantly more of them.
- **Cardiovascular** - Tachycardia and poor stamina
- **Gastrointestinal** - Cannabis hyperemesis syndrome is seen after chronic inhalational use and presents with severe abdominal pain, nausea, and vomiting, and is often relived by long hot showers or baths.

 Gynecomastia is a consequence of chronic marijuana use.

Psychological consequences

Teens using marijuana may experience **learning problems**, deficits in **problem-solving skills**, and **memory impairment** (which may last up to 1 month after they last used marijuana).

Symptoms of underlying **personality disorders, depression,** and **anxiety** can worsen, as well as increased risk for chronic marijuana use in adolescence has been associated with adulthood psychotic disorders as well as illicit drug use and drug addiction.[4]

Not surprisingly, **school performance is generally worse** in children who use marijuana, and chronic marijuana use in adolescence is correlated with lower high school graduation rates.

Withdrawal

Characterized by **irritability, insomnia, tremors,** and **nystagmus.** Withdrawal peaks within 4 days and can continue for 2 weeks.

Effects begin **within seconds** after inhalation and fall rapidly over then next 30 minutes, but the drug and its metabolites are **lipid-soluble** so they are stored in fatty tissue and released slowly. Tests may remain **positive for a month.**

Alcohol Use and Abuse

Alcohol is **the most common substance of abuse** by young people.

---

[4] Reference *Common Substances of Abuse*, PIR, Vol 39, No 8, AUG 2018.

Acute Alcohol Intoxication

They may describe a teenager presenting to the ER with **dizziness, ataxia, slurred speech, visual disturbance, nausea,** and **vomiting.** In addition, you need to look for:

- **sluggishly reactive pupils**, but normal pupil size
- **lower body temperature**
- **low heart rate and BP**
- **hypoglycemia**

With higher doses, look for **irritability, stupor, respiratory depression,** and **even coma.**

Ethanol (Ethyl Alcohol) Toxicity

Alternately, especially on Boards, you could be presented with a **toddler** who got a hold of **drinks left over after a party the night before and parents found him unresponsive.**

The table below outlines blood alcohol levels, expected clinical consequences, and management strategies (mostly symptomatic).

Blood Alcohol Level	Clinical Presentation	Management
Mild < 0.1 g/dL 100 mg/dL 0.1% Blood Alcohol Content (BAC)	Euphoria, lowered inhibitions, and impaired coordination	Hide the car keys and the kitchen spoons and forks, and follow closely to the bathroom
Moderate 0.2 g/dL 200 mg/dL 0.2% BAC	Slurred speech, ataxia, impaired judgement, and mood swings	Monitor until sober or until given a VH1 reality TV show, "Backstage Binging" co-hosted with Justin Bieber featuring a Britney Spears comeback tour, whichever comes first
Severe > 0.3 g/dL 300 mg/dL 0.3% BAC	Confusion and stupor	Consider joining the White House Press Corp
Greater than 0.4 g/dL 400 mg/dL 0.4% BAC	Coma, respiratory depression and death	Potentially lethal you don't want to go there
Beyond 0.45 g/dL 450 mg/dL 0.45% BAC	Charlie Sheen	Currently on tour

If presented with a patient with ethanol toxicity, **monitoring for hypoglycemia and electrolyte imbalance is important.** You should also be aware that ethanol intoxication **can mask the toxicity of other drugs.**

The presentation of ethanol toxicity might not be obvious. Remember, ethyl alcohol might be present in items other than a liter of Absolut Citron®. Ethyl alcohol is also **present in mouthwash, cough and cold preparations, elixirs,** and even **colognes** and **perfumes**.

Chronic Alcohol Abuse

The medical effects of alcohol abuse are **primarily GI**, including **esophagitis, gastritis,** and **peptic ulcer disease**.

Adolescents have not been using alcohol long enough to have the other effects seen in adults such as cirrhosis of the liver. Therefore, do not be tricked into picking any answer that includes that as an effects of alcohol abuse.

The primary consequences of alcohol use and abuse in teenagers are from **physical trauma** and **overdose**.

The majority of adolescents who **binge drink** are not at risk for becoming alcoholics as adults. They are at risk, however, for having **preexisting depression**.

Alcohol Withdrawal

Symptoms begin 5-24 hours after reduction of intake and may last up to a week. They include

- increased heart rate and blood pressure
- fever and sweating
- tremors and seizures
- vomiting and diarrhea

Amphetamine Abuse

Amphetamines are **stimulants**, just like cocaine, and they primarily have **sympathomimetic effects**.

Short term physiological signs of amphetamine toxicity would be adrenergic, including **tachycardia, high blood pressure, sweating, agitation,** and **fever. Hyperthermia** can be part of the presentation as well. Ophthalmological findings would include **dilated pupils with slow reaction to light**. The perception that **insects are crawling on one's skin** may be a sign of amphetamine toxicity. **Nystagmus would not be a finding with amphetamine use.**

Cognitive changes can occur including anxiety, aggression, paranoia, memory impairment.

If higher doses of amphetamines are ingested, it can lead to **fatal arrhythmias**.

State of Drunkenness

The definition of legally drunk varies from state to state.

A BAC of 0.08% is considered legally under influence in most states.

By the way, the unit g/dL is interchangeable with the BAC %. To convert to mg/dL from g/dL you multiply by 1000.

Therefore a BAC of 0.08% corresponds to 0.08 g/dl or 80 mg/dL.

OTC D&D

Dextromethorphan and Diphenhydramine are popular OTC drugs of abuse, especially by preteens.

Dextromethorphan is found in cold and cough medications and should be suspected in cases of abrupt changes in behavior with tachycardia, mydriasis, and diaphoresis, gait disturbance, and euphoria or hallucinations. Common street names are Orange Crush, Skittles, Vitamin D, Dex and Robo.

Diphenhydramine, a common anti-allergy and sleep aid, presents with dry flushed skin.

Treatment of Amphetamine Overdose

Treatment focuses on the specific symptoms, as well as **decontamination** with gastric lavage and activated charcoal. Remember to check the **ABCs** first, including airway protection.

Monitor and treat specific **arrhythmias**.

Benzodiazepines are used to treat **high blood pressure**, as well as the associated **agitation**. Patients may require **haloperidol for psychosis**.

Patients with **hyperthermia** require a **cooling blanket**.

Hemodialysis may be required.

> ### Rapid In, Rapid Out
> Stimulants may be detected in blood and urine only for 48 hours after the last dose due to their rapid metabolism.

> ### Cocaine Every Which Way
> Besides the usual pill form, methamphetamine, like cocaine, may be inhaled nasally and taken intravenously.
>
> Smokeable forms of cocaine "crack" and meth "ice" have instant and extremely intense but short-lived euphoria or "rush".

Cocaine Abuse

Cocaine, like amphetamines, is a stimulant.

Cocaine Toxic Effects

At Lower Doses – euphoria and overconfidence, irritability, insomnia, tremors, tachycardia, hypertension, hyperreflexia, diaphoresis, dilated pupils and flushing.

At Higher Doses - aggressive and violent behavior, hypertensive crises, dysrrhythmias, seizures, coma, **myocardial infarction**, stroke, cardiovascular collapse, and possible renal complications including renal failure, and death.

With chronic abuse, one can see **choreoathetotic movements**, due to depletion of dopamine storage.

> MNEMONIC
> I always have a hard time keeping Miotic and **Mydriatic** straight. These are too close to the terms used to describe cell division. Think:
>
> Miotic
> (The **o** is pinpoint pupil.) vs.
>
> Mydriatic eyes
> (Picture the **d** propping the pupil open. Also, note that my**d**riatic and **d**ilated have a **D** in them.)

Nasal septal perforation or chronic rhinorrhea can be seen with chronic use and would help differentiate cocaine abuse from other stimulants.

Death secondary to cocaine ingestion is *not* dose-dependent.

Since they are all stimulants, treatment of cocaine overdose is treated the same as amphetamine overdose.

Withdrawal

Acute withdrawal symptoms can be severe, earning the title of the 'crash,' and includes severe depression with suicidal ideation. Otherwise, milder symptoms such as increased appetite and sleep, fatigue, and problems concentrating can last up to 14 days

Narcotic and Opiate Toxicity

BUZZWORDS

The typical presentation of opiate toxicity would be a comatose teenager in the ER who is responsive to painful stimuli, with **pinpoint (miosis) but reactive pupils, cyanosis, and respiratory depression**. Additional "depressions" include **decreased shallow respirations, bradycardia, hypotension, and low temperature**.

HOT TIP

"Narcotic bowel syndrome" is abdominal pain, nausea, constipation, seen in patients who keep increasing their opioid doses.

PERIL

Opiates are effective analgesics but have significant potential for dependence, abuse, potential, and overdose. Dependence may occur with as little as 3 weeks of use.

When possible, alternative pain control should be considered, and if opiates are the only option, the lowest dose and the shortest duration possible are recommended. Appropriate disposal of medication is also crucial.

BUZZWORDS

Abrupt withdrawal of opioids in a dependent patient may lead to agitation, rhinorrhea, tearing, joint and muscle pains, nausea, vomiting, and diarrhea. Fever, tachycardia, tachypnea, and hypertension may also occur.

COIN FLIP

Other conditions with **decreased levels of consciousness**, and how they differ from opiate toxicity:

Conditions with depressed level of consciousness	How it differs from opiate toxicity
DKA	Dehydrated with **rapid** deep breathing, pupils are not constricted
Organophosphate toxicity	Does have **constricted pupils**; however, also presents with **profuse sweating, tearing, abdominal pain, wheezing,** and **respiratory distress**
Major head trauma	**Dilated pupils**, which are nonreactive

TREATMENT

Treatment of opiate toxicity consists of the antagonist **naloxone**, which can also cause patients to go into withdrawal symptoms if they are dependent.

Hallucinogen effects

Sympathomimetic

Sympathomimetic effects include tachycardia, hypertension, and increased reflexes

Cholinergic

Cholinergic effects include miosis, flushing and diaphoresis

Cerebellar

Cerebellar effects include *vertical and horizontal nystagmus, ataxia*, and lack of coordination

Psychological

A feeling of disinhibition and euphoria and, in large doses, may produce a psychosis that may look like schizophrenia.

Barbiturates

Barbiturates are *sedatives*. Signs and symptoms of barbiturate overdose (including phenobarbital) would include the brady twins (**bradycardia** and **bradypnea**), and the hypo triplets (**hypotension, hypothermia,** and **hypoactive bowel sounds**), as well as their hypo cousin (**hyporeactive pupillary reflex**).

Pupil size will be normal. Therefore, if they describe miosis or pinpoint pupils, they are more likely describing opiate overdose rather than barbiturate overdose.

Initial symptoms of **slurred speech, unsteady gait, impaired judgement,** and **poor impulse control** look a lot like alcohol intoxication. **Clues to barbiturates will include nystagmus.**

Benzodiazepines

These are medications used for anxiolysis. Toxicity would result in slurred speech, ataxia, miosis, and AMS. Overdose can present in a coma-like state **but with normal vital signs since respiratory depression is rare.**

Withdrawal can be **life-threatening** due to abrupt cessation causing very difficult to control seizures. Therefore, it is best to start a patient on long-acting benzo then slowly taper.

Other signs of withdrawal include elevated HR and BP, sweating, flu-like symptoms, confusion, insomnia, and severe anxiety and/or agitation.

Hallucinogens

Hallucinogens include **mescaline** (peyote cactus), **psilocybin** ("magic mushrooms"), **jimsonweed, LSD, PCP, ecstasy** (a derivative of amphetamine), and dextromethorphan (DXM) OTC. All hallucinogens are taken orally.

The following presentations are consistent with hallucinogen use:
- **Distortion of body image**
- **Paranoia**
- **Agitation**
- **Auditory and visual hallucinations**
- **Distortions of time**

Is it Schizophrenia or Hallucinogen Use?

This distinction is difficult to make acutely, because the acute effects of hallucinogen use can be similar to those seen in schizophrenia. The patient should preferably be evaluated **after they are off all drugs for 2-4 weeks.**

The absence of a family history of schizophrenia and the absence of symptoms when the patient is drug-free point away from a diagnosis of schizophrenia.

Visual hallucinations are common with hallucinogen ingestion. However, **auditory hallucinations** and **completely disorganized, delusional thinking** is more consistent with schizophrenia than hallucinogen ingestion.

Mega Hallucinogen

LSD is the most potent hallucinogen.

PCP

They will likely describe someone who is **wide-eyed (mydriatic)** and **violent**. Unless Charlie Sheen is one of the choices, PCP ingestion will be the correct answer. PCP would also result in **anasarca** and **asymmetric pupils**.

Look for muscle rigidity and hyperreflexia to differentiate it from other ingestions.

MDMA (3,4-methylenedioxymethamphetamine)

Also known as ecstasy or molly. Classically, the rave drug. It is a stimulant *and* hallucinogen.

Intoxication is classically described as profuse diaphoresis, hyperthermia, hypertension, bruxism, and feelings of euphoria.

A classic description on the exam could be a **seizing** patient who has been at a party dancing all night. They want you to **connect MDMA with seizures from hyponatremia** that result from profuse sweating and excessive water intake.

It is different from other stimulants/hallucinogens because it is structurally similar to serotonin. A patient on medications like an SSRI that takes MDMA may present in serotonin syndrome.

Treatment of hallucinogen intoxication

In general, treatment of hallucinogen intoxication is supportive with **a calm environment and dim lighting** while trying to talk the teen back into reality discussing familiar things in a reassuring tone.

A **cooling blanket** will help alleviate the risk for seizures, hypertension, and hyperthermia. In addition, haloperidol, chlorpromazine, or lorazepam may be helpful.

Combative Confusion

A patient presenting to the ER who is combative could be under the influence of a variety of drugs. Pay close attention to the details for a diagnosis of the specific drug.

Invisible Ecstasy

Ecstasy will <u>not</u> show up in most drug screens unless very high quantities were ingested, in which case the test will be positive for amphetamines.

New(ish) kids on the block

Bath salts: synthetic cathinones that are stimulants plus hallucinogen.

Can present with severe anxiety, agitation, paranoia and combative behavior.

Spice, K2: Synethetic canabinoids. Similar to marijuana but also have a hallucinogenic effect that is relatively short lived.

Highly Important Hallucinogens

A few drugs to mention that are unlikely to be heavily tested but you might see them as answer choices.

- **Gamma-hydroxybutyrate (GHB, roofie):** is a very potent CNS sedative that results in anterograde amnesia. It produces eurphoria and feelings of increased sexuality.

- **Flunitrazepam (Rohypnol):** a benzodiazepine that is not FDA approved in the US (likely because it is extremely potent). It has the same effects as GHB.

- **Ketamine (Special K):** hallucinogen that results in distorted perception and out of body experience.

Combating the confusion of the combative patient.

Drug	Characteristics	Distinguishing Features
Cocaine	Tachycardia, tremulousness	Hypertension, mydriasis
Alcohol	Combative behavior and agitation	Tremulousness is not a common feature in a teenager
Inhalants	Characterized as a "quick drunk" with disinhibition and agitation	Hallucinations, generalized muscle weakness, and nystagmus
Opiates	Can present with agitation	Tremulousness and tachycardia are not part of the profile
Amphetamines	Combative, tachycardia, mydriasis	Nystagmus is not part of the profile.
PCP	Combative	Both vertical and horizontal nystagmus

Tobacco Use

Physiologic effects of nicotine

The short term physiologic effects of nicotine include:

- Increased alertness
- Muscle relaxation
- Enhanced memory and alertness
- Decreased appetite
- Decreased irritability

One can see the attraction of nicotine physiologically, and why it can be so addicting.

The **adverse effects of nicotine** include **peptic ulcer disease.** Nausea and vomiting are common *initial* effects that wear off quickly.

Smoking Cessation

Smoking cessation is difficult because of the discomfort caused by withdrawal, rather than the absence of pleasurable symptoms. For example, **increased appetite** is one of the more important adverse effects of withdrawal.

> ### Up In Smoke
>
> In 2016, 20% of high school students admitted to using a tobacco/nicotine product (inhaled, oral, or dermal) in the last 30 days.
>
> While smoking cigarettes seems to be decreasing, the use of electronic cigarettes seems to be increasing.

> ### Chewing Tobacco
>
> Teens are often unaware of the potential immediate risks of chewing tobacco. The nicotine in chewing or smokeless tobacco can cause **early fatigue during sports**. It can also cause **tachycardia** and **vasoconstriction**.

The 5 As for Brief Intervention in smoking cessation include

1. **Ask** about tobacco use: in every patient at every visit
2. **Advise** to quit: in a clear strong personalized manner
3. **Assess** willingness to attempt quitting: is now a good time?
4. **Assist** in quit attempt: counseling, referral, pharmacotherapy
5. **Arrange** follow-up: preferably within the first week of quit date

Scare tactics about long term ill effects rarely work with adolescents, who view themselves as being immortal.

Chapter 37

Critical Care

Acute Respiratory Distress Syndrome

Acute respiratory distress syndrome (ARDS) used to go by the name "adult respiratory distress syndrome" until it was discovered that it can also occur in children and on the pediatric board exam.

ARDS is the most severe form of lung injury and the result of some "insult". The most common etiologies in children are sepsis, pneumonia, aspiration, trauma, and near downing episodes.

The prognosis is better if it occurs in the context of trauma.

ARDS includes 3 clinical features:

1. parenchymal lung disease with infiltrate on chest X-ray
2. hypoxia
3. respiratory failure not due to cardiac cause or volume overload

You could be presented with a patient who is relatively asymptomatic following the initial triggering insult. Don't be fooled. It **can take several days** for symptoms of ARDS to present.

The lungs are only the opening act. The headliners include liver, kidney, brain, and bone marrow dysfunction. This **multi-organ involvement** is the actual cause of death, not the respiratory failure.

Near Drowning

Homeward Bound?

If the patient is asymptomatic with **no loss of consciousness** and required **no resuscitation in the field**, the patient can be observed for 6-8 hours in the ED and if vital signs, including pulse oximetry, are all normal and chest XR is clear near the end of the observation period, they may be safely discharged to home.

Hospital Bound?

Children rescued from near-drowning episodes can look quite **stable** upon **arrival to the emergency department**, and **then go downhill and require advanced life support**.

Duration of asphyxia is the key to prognosis. **The duration of time from submersion to restoration of adequate respiration determines the extent of the damage.**

Any one of the following predicts **risk for future deterioration** and warrants continued medical supervision:

❏ A history of **apnea and CPR in the field**.

❏ **Neurological signs** (seizure or disorientation) or **respiratory failure** from aspiration.

❏ **Arterial desaturation** and/or **tachypnea** (specifically, this might be a warning sign of aspiration pneumonia or acute respiratory distress syndrome. See previous section.)

Unfavorable signs that may **worsen prognosis** include:

• Submersion > 25 minutes

• > 25 minutes of CPR at the scene

• Apnea or coma at admission

• Need for cardiac meds to establish perfusing rhythm

• Initial arterial pH of <7.1

Flail Chest/Hemothorax

With respiratory symptoms following blunt trauma to the chest, they want you to know that the **MOST important procedure to perform initially**[1] **to determine management of this child is physical examination of the chest.** Physical examination is almost always going to be the correct answer to any question if it is one of the choices.

You will want to examine the chest even if[2] there are no signs of respiratory distress and tachycardia.

What you are looking for in this case is **flail chest**, which is defined as **2 or more rib fractures in 2 or more locations.**

This results in **paradoxic chest wall movements**, with the underlying lung being pulled into the chest cavity during chest expansion and pushed out during chest wall relaxation.

If you are presented with a history of flail chest with respiratory distress and tachypnea, the most appropriate next step is **placement of a chest tube** (to decompress the hemothorax and/or pneumothorax).

> ## Very Bad Chest
>
> Major thoracic injuries that are immediately life-threatening:
>
> • tension pneumothorax
>
> • massive hemothorax
>
> • flail chest/ pulmonary contusion
>
> • pericardial tamponade

---

[1] Once a stable airway and breathing have been confirmed or included in the history.

[2] Make that "especially if".

The ABCs of Pediatric CPR

Remembering a few important points regarding CPR will very likely score you 1-2 points on the exam.

 The most important concept is that this is now **C-A-B**, NOT A-B-C!

Take only **5-10 seconds to check for a pulse**. If you cannot find a pulse in that time, start **compressions** immediately.

The chest should be compressed at least **1/3 of the anteroposterior depth of the chest** (approximately **1.5 inches or 4 cm** in infants) or approximately **2 inches (5 cm)** in children.

Proper compression rate is **at least 100/minute** allowing for **complete chest recoil** between compressions.

One Rescuer CPR

For everyone, infants to adults, the ratio is **30 compressions to 2 ventilations**, starting with compressions.

> **First things First**
>
> Don't forget to activate EMS (call 911) and grab the AED the first chance you get!

Two Rescuer CPR

In infants and children, the ratio with two rescuers is **15 compressions to 2 ventilations**.

After **2 minutes**, switch rescuer roles.

Infant CPR

When performing 2-rescuer CPR on an infant, the **two-thumb-encircling hands technique** is preferred over the 2 fingers on the sternum technique.

> **Pulse Check**
>
> **For infants**, check the **brachial** pulse.
>
> **For children**, check **carotid** or femoral pulses.

Other CPR Considerations

 If an airway has been established during CPR, the ventilation rate should be **1 breath every 2-3 seconds for infants and children**, or **20-30 breaths per minute** accounting for age and clinical condition (new PALS 2020 guidelines). Avoid hyperventilation. Ventilation is independent of compressions, which are delivered at the same **100/minute rate** without pausing.

> In adolescents and adults, the ratio is **30 compressions to 2 respirations** regardless of the number of rescuers.

If rescue breaths are needed but not compressions in infants and children, give **a breath every 2-3 seconds** (about 20-30 breaths per minute).

Chest compressions can generally be discontinued once **spontaneous HR reaches 60**. This rule is not absolute. If there is still evidence of poor perfusion, e.g., delayed cap refill, weak pulses, or cool extremities, chest compressions should continue.

After C-A-B, consider D for Disability: consider causes for injury and altered mental status, such as check pupils, check glucose, and consider naloxone administration. Then proceed with detailed history and exam. Comprehensive post-arrest care is an area of increasing emphasis.

Automatic External Defibrillator (AED)

If the rhythm is shockable and multiple rescuers are present, the goal is to deliver the first shock **as soon as possible.** Perform CPR while awaiting the AED. If there is only one rescuer present and the arrest is unwitnessed, perform CPR for two minutes/5 cycles prior to leaving to obtain the AED.

After each shock, **immediately resume CPR, beginning with compressions**.

In non-shockable rhythms, early epinephrine administration after starting CPR is associated with increased survival.

Intraosseous (IO) infusion

This is indicated to obtain emergency access in children during life-threatening situations, including cardiac arrest, shock, burns, and status epilepticus. Consider placing an IO after **2 minutes of unsuccessful attempts** at IV access if the patient is unstable or coding.

IO may be used to infuse medications including code medications, blood products, and fluids. **It should be removed when another method of vascular access is achieved.**

The preferred sites for IO in children are **the anteriomedial surface of the proximal tibia and the distal femur**.

Malignant hyperthermia

Malignant hyperthermia is a genetic hypermetabolic state that follows the administration of halogenated inhalational general anesthesia or succinylcholine and leads to **metabolic acidosis, hyperthermia,** and **cardiac arrhythmia,** as well as a **markedly elevated creatine kinase concentration** and **myoglobinuria**. Additional findings include **tachypnea, muscle rigidity, increased carbon dioxide production**, and **fever**.

Treatment includes **immediately stopping offending agent, hyperventilation, oxygen,** and **dantrolene**.

Shock

Shock is defined as **insufficient delivery of oxygen** to meet tissue demands.

On the exam, tachycardia is often the first sign, followed by evidence of decreased perfusion (change in capillary refill, change in mental status, decreased urine output, etc). **Hypotension is a late and ominous sign.**

Types of shock: Multiple can exist in same patient!

- **Hypovolemic:** History of volume or blood loss, dehydration in the presenting history.
- **Distributive:** Most commonly sepsis, can also be anaphylaxis or spinal/neurogenic. Watch for a history of infection or high risk for infection. Distributory shock is due to systemic vasodilation resulting in decreased blood flow.
- **Cardiogenic:** Watch for non-specific presentation with vague symptoms like fatigue, abdominal pain, respiratory distress. Often "cold" shock. Look for hepatomegaly.
- **Obstructive:** Blood flow can't get though the heart and lungs. Cardiac tamponade, pulmonary embolus, tension pneumothorax in the presenting history would be your key. Narrow pulse pressure, pulsus parodoxus are additional clues for obstructive shock.

"Cold" vs. "Warm" shock

Warm Shock

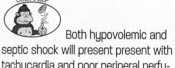

Here you have high cardiac output and low systemic resistance (SVR).

Watch for a history of warm extremities and "flash capillary refill" where you gently press the finger or toe and the refill happens briskly. Bounding pulses would be another indication that the question is about warm shock. They will also describe widened pulse pressure.

Vasoconstriction would be the correct treatment. **Norepinephrine, vasopressin** or **high dose epinephrine** would be correct answers.

Cold Shock

Here you have the opposite occuring

With cold shock you would have **high** SVR state with a **delayed** capillary refill. Thready/ diminished rather than bounding pulse with **narrow** pulse pressure

---

Septic or Hypovolemic Shock

COIN FLIP

Both hypovolemic and septic shock will present present with tachycardia and poor periperal perfusion. Both hypovolemic and septic shock will have tachycardia and poor perfusion.

Suspect **hypovolemia** in children with persistent vomiting, diarrhea, or obviously, blood loss.

Children with **sepsis** will appear more ill and may have history of fever.

Initial treatment is with **fluids.** Hypovolemic shock will respond much better to fluids than septic shock. After fluid administration, continued shock will require addressing the underlying cause of the shock.

It might seem confusing that **epinephrine** can be used and would be the correct answer for **both cold** and **warm shock**.

High dose epinephrine increases SVR. Therefore it would be appropriate for **warm shock**.

Low dose epinephrine functions as a vasodilator and is inotropic and therefore would be appropriate for **cold shock**.

You can also just remember that cold and **low** both have L's to remember that low dose epinephrine is used for cold shock.

Chapter 38

Emergency Medicine

Remember your ABCs

The first priority for any unresponsive child brought to the ER is to go right to the ABCs (Airway, Breathing, and Circulation).[1] What should you do first? **Establishing an airway** is always the answer they are looking for, regardless of the reason the patient is unresponsive.

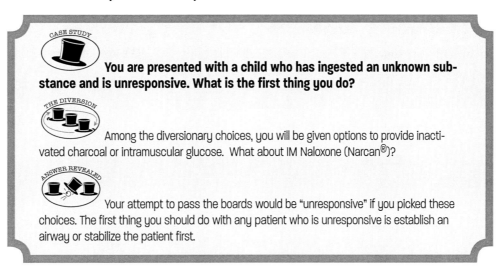

CASE STUDY You are presented with a child who has ingested an unknown substance and is unresponsive. What is the first thing you do?

THE DIVERSION Among the diversionary choices, you will be given options to provide inactivated charcoal or intramuscular glucose. What about IM Naloxone (Narcan®)?

ANSWER REVEALED Your attempt to pass the boards would be "unresponsive" if you picked these choices. The first thing you should do with any patient who is unresponsive is establish an airway or stabilize the patient first.

Endotrachel Intubation

Indications for endotracheal intubation include

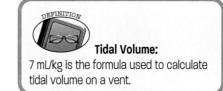

DEFINITION
Tidal Volume:
7 mL/kg is the formula used to calculate tidal volume on a vent.

- inadequate oxygenation or ventilation (respiratory failure)
- inability to protect or maintain airway
- potential for deterioration (as in transport)

ET Tube Size

The child's age divided by 4, plus 4, determines ET tube size. A four year old would be 4/4 plus 4, which would be a size 5 ET Tube.

HOT TIP If an **intubated** patient experiences **sudden deterioration**, consider DOPE

- **D**isplacement of the ETT
- **O**bstruction of the ETT
- **P**neumothorax
- **E**quipment failure

---

[1] Apparently this is now known as CABs since circulation is now checked first. Regardless stabilization comes first before all else.

Meds that can be given by ET Tube

Consider it a **LANE**:

Lidocaine
Atropine
Naloxone (Narcan®)
Epinephrine

Atropine is indicated for bradycardia, not asystole.

> ### Tubing Gone Wrong
> Potential complications of ET Intubation include:
> - gastric distention and aspiration
> - hypoxemia
> - bradycardia
> - increased ICP
> - mechanical trauma
> - pneumothorax/ pneumomediastinum
> - post-obstructive pulmonary edema

Convert Numbers to Words

Questions that deal with ER and critical care will be filled with vital signs and lab values. This is another example of where it is critical[2] to to change numbers into descriptive words. For example, if you see a temperature of 101.2, think "febrile"; if HR is 120, think "tachycardia." The pattern they are depicting will then become more evident.

Evaluation of Fever in the ED

- A temperature higher than 41° C (105.8° F) correlates with invasive bacterial infection. **Temp > 41.7 (107) suggests hyperthermia due to dehydration with fever and needs to be emergently addressed.**
- Consistently using the same method (oral, axillary, tympanic, etc.) to take the temperature is more important than the actual method used. This way it is easier to monitor for body temperature changes.
- Tactile temperature noted by parents is not considered to be reliable.

Fever by Age

Fever in **infants younger than 1 month** requires a septic workup (CBC with differential, blood cultures, lumbar puncture, cath urine, and chest XR if there are respiratory symptoms) and empiric I.V. antibiotics, pending culture results.

Infants between 1-2 months of age require a workup but not necessarily inpatient management and/or empiric antibiotics if initial studies are not suspicious for invasive infection.

From **3-36 months**, clinical judgement can play an important role. Watch the history they present. Look for identifiable sources of infection and treat as such. If they present a child that may not have been immunized against pneumococcal disease, for example, workup for occult bacteremia may be indicated.

>36 months, focus on comfort rather than temperature reduction.

---

2 Pun intended.

Of course, at any age, factor in **underlying conditions** such as **sickle cell disease** or **immunocompromised status** if this is part of the history.

Rectal temperatures are preferred in the first few years of age due to accuracy, but are **contraindicated in neutropenic patients**, since the rectal trauma may lead to bacteremia.

> **Before Going Viral**
>
> Remember to have a very low threshold for checking the urine in an infant and toddler girl with high fever without a source before calling it viral.

CASE STUDY

They may present a variety of 5 year-old children with fever. They will list a few underlying diagnoses and ask which child is in the MOST need of fever-reducing agents (also known as antipyretics).

THE DIVERSION

Among the choices will be a child with a history of febrile seizures, as well as a few obviously wrong choices, like a child with an ear infection, and a couple you have to think about, like a child with encephalitis and a child with congestive heart failure. Whenever an answer seems obvious, like, "a history of febrile seizures," you have to assume for at least a moment it cannot be the correct choice. In this case, that would be a wise move.

ANSWER REVEALED

The child with a history of febrile seizures that is now 5 years old is just about out of the age of risk, so a febrile seizure is not a high priority. The child with encephalitis needs treatment directed to the encephalitis, and, of course, otitis media is not a priority. However, a child with congestive heart failure would need to have the fever reduced to reduce oxygen demand and subsequent cardiac output demand.

Sudden Infant Death Syndrome (SIDS)

When to reassure and when to be concerned will be tested in several questions. Here is what you need to know.

Risk factors for SIDS

Infants are most vulnerable for SIDS between the second and fourth month of life.

Intrinsic (prenatal):
- non-white race
- male gender
- prematurity <37 wk gestation
- prenatal maternal smoking and/or alcohol use

Extrinsic (postnatal):

- prone or side sleep position
- sleeping on adult mattress, couch, playpen, or soft bedding
- bed-sharing
- upper respiratory infection
- maternal smoking after birth

> **Pacifying Anxiety**
>
> Pacifiers may be protective against SIDS, and the AAP actually now recommends "considering" them at naptime in the first year of life (after the first month for breast-feeders, so as not to interfere with successful breastfeeding).

 99% of SIDS infants have one of these risk factors.

Obviously, once the infant is born, only the extrinsic factors can be manipulated to prevent SIDS.

Apnea Monitoring

 There is no evidence that apnea monitors are useful in reducing the risk of SIDS.

The only indication for a home apnea monitor is for an infant with bonafide **apnea of prematurity** that responds to stimulation when experiencing apnea.

Brief Resolved Unexplained Event (BRUE)

BRUEs were previously known as ALTEs (Apparent Life Threatening Events) and involve an episode in which the infant has:

- ❏ a sudden alteration in breathing
- ❏ cyanosis or pallor
- ❏ a change in tone
- ❏ an altered level of responsiveness
- ❏ and recovered successfully with no medical condition to explain the event.

 A 2-month-old boy suddenly is found **limp, cyanotic, and apneic**. He is revived with mouth-to-mouth resuscitation. When he is seen in the emergency room, findings on **physical examination are normal**.

While the physical exam may be normal on presentation, it is the **history that is alarming**.

 BRUEs may be further classified into low or high risk.

Low risk BRUEs include:

- age > 60 days
- gestational age 32 weeks or more and postconceptional age 45 weeks or more
- occurrence of only one BRUE episode (no priors or repeats)
- duration of episode one minute or less
- needed no CPR by trained medical provider
- no concerning history or physical findings

High Risk:

- If ANY of the low risk criteria are not met

BRUE and SIDS are completely separate entities. Don't be misled into choosing an answer that states that apnea or BRUE precedes or is a risk factor for SIDS.

Management on a low-risk BRUE involves only optional (1-4 hour) observation in ED with reassurance and family education regarding BRUEs. Offer CPR training and arrange follow up check with medical provider in 24 hours. No other tests are indicated unless there are findings on history or exam.

Bites, Fights, and What's Right

Inevitably, kids will bite each other and get close to animals that will bite them. Here is what you need to know:

Dogs and Cats

Cats bite deeply and make little puncture wounds; therefore, **cat bites are worse than dog bites**.

The most important first step is extensive irrigation under mild to moderate pressure with sterile normal saline, sterile water or tap water – not prophylactic antibiotics.

Antibiotics would be indicated when you foresee a problem.

> ### Wound Shapes
>
> Should you have to distinguish this on the picture section, human bites would be **half-moon** shaped; dog bites are **tears**; and cat bites, are **punctures**.

CASE STUDY You are asked to evaluate a child who sustained a cat bite the day before. He presents with tenderness and swelling of his right index finger. The patient is penicillin allergic and you are asked to pick the appropriate treatment.

THE DIVERSION Included in the choices will be amoxicillin, penicillin, and/or amoxicillin/clavulanate. These should be easy to eliminate since they mention the patient is penicillin allergic. However, you might also be fooled into believing this is Cat Scratch Disease and pick "supportive care only" or "surgical excision." If you do, you will be scratching your head while petting your cat when you realize you got this question wrong.

ANSWER REVEALED If you are presented with a patient who develops cellulitis at the site of an animal bit within 24 hours, the likely etiology is *Pasteurella multocida*. You must cover for *Staph* as well as *Pasteurella multocida*. If the patient weren't penicillin allergic, amoxicillin/clavulanate would be appropriate. In this case, the appropriate medications include cefuroxime, cefpodoxime, doxycycline, azithromycin, or trimethoprim-sulfamethoxazole. If age appropriate, fluoroquinolones would be a correct choice to cover Pasteurella. If you choose one of these answers, you will be well on your way to "pasteurelling the boards."

MNEMONIC The problems start with "C":

> Contaminated (ie. dirty wounds)
> Cats, Canines (dogs), and Crazy humans
> Crush injuries
> Cartilage involvement
> Cuticles (hands and feet)
> Compromised (Immunocompromised)
> Cute faces (and not-cute faces too)
> Concealed areas (genitalia)

HOT TIP Primary wound closure is usually NOT recommended for dog bites, except for bites to the face.

TREATMENT The appropriate antibiotic for cat and dog bites would be **amoxicillin/clavulanate** to help protect against both *Staph aureus* and *Pasteurella multocida*.

An alternative for penicillin-allergic patients is **clindamycin plus trimethoprim-sulfamethoxazole**.

Dog and cat bites are not considered to be at risk for tetanus unless they are contaminated with soil, but may need to be evaluated for rabies.

Human Bites

Like cat bites, human bites have high risk of infection.

Remember to consider the possibility of child abuse and transmission of infections such as HIV and Hepatitis B.

Amoxicillin-clavulanate is preferred for prophylaxis and infected human bite wounds to cover for *viridans streptococci*, *S. aureus*, and anaerobes.

Human bites ARE at risk for Tetanus.

Human Bites not on the face should only be sutured if:

- Clinically uninfected
- <12 hours old
- Not on the hand or foot

Child Bites

Most dog bites to young children occur in the home.

Spider Bites

There are two primary spider bites to be concerned about creeping up on the boards.[3]

Brown Recluse (Loxosceles reclusa)

The presentation is usually a **target lesion** consisting of a red circle surrounding a white ring. This is different than the target lesion associated with Lyme disease, and appears within hours (as opposed to weeks with Lyme disease).

A bite that becomes **necrotic** is more likely to be a brown recluse bite than a black widow spider bite.

Although systemic symptoms can be part of the presentation, this is a rare presentation. The reaction is typically a **self-limited** local painful lesion that requires no additional treatment, but it may be severe.

The Black Widow (Latrodectus mactans)

Often the bite is nothing more than a **puncture wound that is barely noticed**. However, **systemic symptoms** can present within 8 hours, including:

- **Muscle aches**- involving the abdomen, lower back, and chest, as well as the extremities
- **Hypertension**

Treatment consists of **local wound care** and **pain control**.

Parenteral **benzodiazepines** are indicated in the case of severe muscle spasms, and **tetanus prophylaxis** may be indicated.

Antivenom is only used as a secondary option if these supportive measures do not work, or in small children, and in those with severe symptoms.

Wound excision, steroids, hyperbaric chambers, dapsone, and/or watching the movie *The Fly* in rewind mode would not be correct management choices for black widow spider bite on the exam.

Snake Bites

You will need to know if they are describing a snake bite by a venomous or non-venomous snake.

Fortunately you will not be examining a live snake, only a live board question, which can be dangerous and fatal to a passing grade only.

---

3 Pun intended.

If they describe, or show you a picture, a snake with a **triangular head and fangs**, or obviously a rattler, it is likely venomous (insert your favorite lawyer joke here). If they describe a snake with a **round head**, it is probably not venomous.

The one exception is if they describe a **red and yellow snake** with a round head. As you recall "red and yellow killed a fellow."

Since this is not the herpetology board exam, they will more likely describe the wound itself rather than the snake. If they describe **fang marks**, assume it is a venomous bite.

Initial signs of venomous bites are **local erythema and swelling**, followed by **enlarged lymph nodes** and **bullae**.

If the wound appears to be from a **non-venomous snake**, **wound cleaning** and **tetanus** status verification are all that is needed.

If the wound is **venomous**, the first step in the field are the **ABCs** of stabilization. Then **immobilize the limb** and **let it hang** at the patient's side.

> **ANTIVENOM**
>
> Antivenom (Crotalidae Polyvalent Immune Fab) might be appropriate for cases of coagulopathy, hypotension, systemic collapse, or local tissue injury.

Applying a tourniquet, applying ice, and/or sucking the venom out of the wound are appropriate on episodes of *MacGyver* and even *MacGruber*, but would be incorrect on the boards.

MacGyver might be able to help transport the patient to an appropriate facility, and this would be a correct choice.

Scorpion Stings

Scorpion stings are most common in the southwestern US and the sting contains neurotoxins which lead to mild to moderate pain, paresthesia, sympathetic, parasympathetic and neuromuscular symptoms.

Effects are most severe in children younger than 5 who can progress to tachycardia, hypertension, increased secretions, opisthotonus with muscle twitching and fasciculations, roving eye movements and nystagmus.

Most stings can be treated with just oral pain medications, wound care and tetanus prophylaxis. Consider antivenom in severe cases.

Head Trauma

The clinical impact of increased intracranial pressure can be gradual. In particular, remember that **papilledema is often absent initially**.

Subdural Hematoma

The presentation is usually gradual with nonspecific signs like **irritability, increasing head circumference, pallor and anemia** in infants and persistent **headache, vomiting,** and **drowsiness** in older children.

"Shaken Baby Syndrome" often involves **subdural**, hematomas. In addition, children with shaken baby syndrome may also present with **retinal hemorrhages** and/or **bulging fontanelle**.

The **CT** picture of blood in the subdural space due to tearing of the intracranial bridging veins is diagnostic. The first and second hours are the most critical.

Severe head injuries, especially those associated with a subdural hematoma, can **lead to SIADH**. Pay particular attention when they describe a recent head injury and provide you with electrolytes and urine osmolality values.

Subarachnoid Hemorrhage

Results from the tearing of the small vessels of the pia mater in significant blunt trauma and hearing forces.

Symptoms include loss of consciousness, severe headache, and signs of meningeal irritation.

Epidural Hematoma (EH)

This is typically an **arterial bleed**, but may also be venous, and occurs between the skull and the dura mater.

 They can describe a child sustaining **blunt head trauma,** most likely from a fall but also from being hit by a baseball or baseball bat. Possibly with **pupillary findings** (ipsilateral, dilated and unreactive pupil) and/or with **loss of consciousness**, who then goes through a **lucid period** of improvement, **only to deteriorate later**.

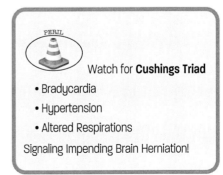

PERIL

Watch for **Cushings Triad**

- Bradycardia
- Hypertension
- Altered Respirations

Signaling Impending Brain Herniation!

HOT TIP

Remember, this can result in a **bloody atraumatic LP**, so if they describe an "atraumatic" tap with lots of red cells in the question, epidural hematoma is a possibility (as is herpes).

HOT TIP

On CT, epidermal hematoma appear as lens-shaped bleeds that DO NOT cross suture lines. Epidural hematomas require **emergent surgical intervention**.

Retinal Hemorrhages

TAKE HOME MESSAGE

They have shown retinal hemorrhages in a picture. A vague reference to retinal hemorrhage with no suggestion of abuse in the history might be the only hint you will get.

Any child with **inexplicable mental status change**, even with no history or external signs of head trauma, should be evaluated for retinal hemorrhage.

BUZZWORDS

In cases of abusive head trauma, watch for a toddler who is **afebrile** and **irritable**, with or without bruises, and consider **non accidental trauma**.

HOT TIP

Whenever the concern for abuse is there, the correct answer will be to **obtain a head CT**, an **ophthalmologic exam** for retinal hemorrhages, and **a skeletal survey**.

Work-up of Head Trauma

PERIL

MRI is useful in determining the age cause, and extent of head bleeds. It is not useful in emergency settings where the immediate diagnosis of a head bleed is necessary.

PERIL

The presence or absence of physical signs is never the sole deciding factor in deciding whether to obtain a head CT scan following head trauma.

Abuse and the History

PERIL

The most highly predictive historical feature for abuse in head trauma is having no history of trauma.

Therefore if they mention no history of trauma the opposite may be true.

Also be alert for changes in history, delay in seeking care, and blaming the injury on a sibling.

Subdural hematoma, rib fractures and retinal hemorrhages = Child abuse.

For children <u>over</u> age 2y

a head CT is indicated for:

- history of LOC
- history of vomiting
- severe headache
- high risk mechanism of injury
- concern for inflicted injury
- abnormal behavior or neurological examination

For children <u>under</u> age 2y

a head CT is indicated for:

- non-frontal scalp hematomas
- a palpable skull fracture
- history of LOC
- severe mechanism of injury
- not acting normally per parents
- abnormal neurologic exam
- concern for inflicted injury

Suspicious?

TAKE HOME MESSAGE

As mandated reporters, health care providers are legally required to report to local child protective services any suspicion of abuse, even while the work up is underway.

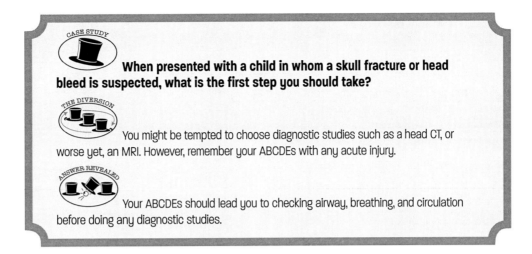

CASE STUDY When presented with a child in whom a skull fracture or head bleed is suspected, what is the first step you should take?

THE DIVERSION You might be tempted to choose diagnostic studies such as a head CT, or worse yet, an MRI. However, remember your ABCDEs with any acute injury.

ANSWER REVEALED Your ABCDEs should lead you to checking airway, breathing, and circulation before doing any diagnostic studies.

Skull Fractures

Linear fractures

These are the **most commonly occurring skull fractures** in children. They most often occur in the **parietal region**.

15-30% of linear skull fractures have underlying **intracranial injury**.

> **Paging Neurosurg!**
>
> Neurosurgical consultation is necessary for all depressed skull fractures, basilar skull fractures, and skull fractures with associated intracranial injury.

Infants are at higher risk for skull fractures than older children because of their thinner skulls, and infants can suffer skull fractures from falls as short as 4-5 feet.

BUZZWORDS Linear skull fractures are usually associated with **scalp hematomas** and the physical findings are identical in accidental and intentional injuries, so the history is critical.

Inflicted injury should be suspected if the history is not consistent with the clinical findings, if the mechanism reported is not consistent with the child's developmental abilities, if no history of trauma is given, if there has been a delay in seeking treatment, or if there are other inconsistencies or changes in the history by the caregivers.

TREATMENT Most heal without complication without specific therapy other than pain management.

Temporal Bone Fracture

BUZZWORDS A child with a temporal bone fracture will be described with a combination of the following: **visible bleeding from the ear** or **hemotympanum**, along with **hearing loss** and possibly **facial paralysis**. CSF **otorrhea** may also be described or hinted at.

Basilar Skull Fracture

They could describe "clear rhinorrhea," and "clear otorrhea" which are really **CSF**. Another important sign is the **Battle sign**, which is **ecchymoses behind the ear**. One can also see **raccoon eyes**, which is **periorbital ecchymoses**. It can also involve the **abducens and facial nerve palsy (6th and 7th cranial nerves)**.

They have increased risk of meningitis.

> ### Hematoma alert!
>
> Scalp hematomas (non-frontal) are predictive of skull fractures in infants under 1 year.

> Diagnosis of skull fracture is by CT, not skull XR.

Coma Status

The higher the number, the better the prognosis. 15 is normal; a score **less than 8 is a severe coma** and an indication to intubate. Prognosis is inversely related to the index and **length of time of coma**.

Remember, "Coma score down to 8, time to stop and intubate."

Poor prognostic signs include **cerebral bleeding, brain edema**, and a **coma lasting longer than 6 hours**.

The Glasgow Coma Scale[4] is only useful for head trauma; it is not useful in assessing metabolic coma.

> ### Increased ICP
>
> The Glasgow coma scale runs from 3 to 15. There is no ZERO!
>
> Mannitol and Lasix®, along with hyper-ventilation, are methods to reduce ICP.

Brain Death

Criteria for brain death:

- There must be a **known and irreversible cause of coma**
- Absence of hypotension, hypothermia, metabolic disturbance, and sedating effect of medication
- **Two brain death examinations** by different examiners done 12 and 24 hours apart confirming the absence of brainstem reflexes including the reflex to breathe
- No ancillary studies are necessary

Organ donation requires **EITHER cardiac OR brain death**.

Nose Trauma

As a general rule, "surgical intervention" is rarely the answer on boards, except when it comes to the eyes. This is another exception to that rule.

---

[4] Not to be confused with the Stupor Index while studying for the Boards.

If they describe **swelling of the nasal septum** with any degree of **obstruction**, immediate ENT consultation is indicated for drainage. If this is not done, there is a risk for significant cartilage damage with saddle nose deformity (the kind you see in hockey players, boxers, and other people who stick their noses where they are not welcomed).

Abdominal Trauma

Blunt abdominal trauma is a common unrecognized fatal injury in the pediatric population.

A FAST (focused abdominal sonography in trauma) should be used to evaluate for abdominal free fluid.

A negative FAST and abdominal exam does not completely rule out an intra-abdominal injury, but the presence of free fluid on FAST should lead you to the answer of a prompt abdominal CT with IV contrast as the next step.

If the patient they describe is hemodynamically unstable, with blunt abdominal trauma and a free fluid on FAST, then direct transfer to the operating room without further imaging would be the correct next step, if this is the presented history.

Splenic Rupture

HOT TIP

Splenic rupture will typically be presented in the context of **blunt abdominal trauma**. A few important caveats are worth reviewing. These may be worth a couple of points on the exam.

- Attention to the **ABCs** should be the first step.
- Peritoneal lavage will be incorrect, since **abdominal CT with contrast** is a safer and more effective diagnostic tool.
- Abdominal CT with contrast would only be correct for a hemodynamically stable patient.
- If there is free fluid on FAST exam, or go straight to the OR without passing go or getting any imaging.
- Baseline CBC, while useful, is not a reliable diagnostic measure.
- Surgery is indicated when there is hemodynamic instability.
- **IV fluids and blood products** are often indicated, and may be a correct choice on the exam.

Child Abuse or Decoy?

There are many child abuse imitators. Presentations that can appear to be due to child abuse but are in fact not due to abuse. If you are not careful you will be tricked into choosing the wrong answer by barking up the child abuse tree. Fixation error when presented with what **seems to be** red flags for child abuse can lead to incorrect answers. Watch for signs of alternative explanations in the history. Like the bizarre characters on Batman, these impostors are likely to make an appearance on the Boards.

When the question blatantly implies abuse, it will usually be the incorrect answer. As luck would have it, when the right answer IS abuse, the question will divert you away from choices consistent with abuse.

HOT TIP

Lesions of child abuse are **rarely symmetrical**.

HOT TIP

The most common form of abuse is neglect.

Fractures

Look for hints that they are talking about **osteogenesis imperfecta**, such as bluish coloration of the sclerae.

Other factors which can result in fractures that are not secondary to abuse are **hypophosphatasia, hyperparathyroidism, Fanconi syndrome, Menkes syndrome, and pathologic fractures.**

Research demonstrates that Vitamin D deficiency does NOT lead to increased fractures.

A **skeletal survey** should be performed in all children under age 2 when there is any concern for physical abuse. If an abused child has siblings younger than age 2, they should also have a skeletal survey performed. A repeat skeletal survey may be necessary 10-14 days after the initial one to reevaluate for fractures.

Bone scans are no longer recommended.

Fractures

Fractures occur in a small number of cases of abuse.

The following types of fractures have high specificity for abuse:

- Metaphyseal "bucket handle" fractures
- Posterior rib fractures
- Spinous process fractures
- Scapular fractures
- Sternal fractures

Fatal Blows

Abusive head trauma is the leading cause of death from child abuse. Abdominal trauma is second.

Who done it?

Only 7% of reports of abuse are for physical abuse.

In 80% of cases of physical abuse, a biological parent is the perpetrator.

You are asked to choose from a list of fractures to determine which one is most likely secondary to abuse. Included in the list are ones that are easy to eliminate; you are well-prepared and know that non-displaced linear skull fractures in an infant, clavicular fractures, and supracondylar elbow fractures can all be accidental.

After eliminating these choices, you might be down to two choices: **bucket handle** fracture and **buckle fracture of the distal radius**. Hmm... you might wonder which one is associated with child abuse — bucket handle or buckle. Well, if you don't know for sure you might have poured another question down the bucket.

Buckle fractures are not associated with child abuse. **Bucket handle fractures** are associated with abuse. You can remember this by picturing somebody getting hit by an adult holding a bucket by the handle. It's not a pretty picture – but, then again, neither is failing the Boards.

"Bruises"

There are a variety of skin lesions that imitate abuse: **Mongolian spots** (dermal melanocytosis) and **Henoch Schönlein Purpura** are a couple of examples. What will often distinguish abuse is how it progresses.

Accidental bruises tend to occur **over bony prominences** (foreheads, knees, shins, and elbows).

"Those who don't cruise, don't bruise", so a nonmobile infant (typically under 9-12 months) who **has a bruise**, no matter how "minor", must receive a **full child abuse evaluation** and a **report to Child Protective Services**.

If there is **variation in color**, this usually indicates abuse but don't forget coagulopathies, so check a PT/ PTT.

If they mention that the child is from an **Asian culture**, in particular Viet Nam or Cambodia, know that **cupping** and **coining** of the back are culturally normal and not technically abuse.

> ### Risk Assessment
>
> The most significant risk factor for abuse is the age of the child, with infants and toddlers at highest risk for serious and fatal abuse. Children with disabilities are also at high risk.

> ### Color Dating
>
> Don't let them trick you into dating bruises by colors. Because of the variation in individuals and location of bruising, trying to date bruises by colors is notoriously unreliable.

"Burns"

Stevens Johnson Syndrome could be misdiagnosed as a burn, but here distribution will be the key, and there will be something in the question to tip you off to SJS. It is the **distribution around the mouth** that is key. Remember Erythema MultiORALforme.

Dislocations

Any toddler with a history of being **"swung by the arms"** will most likely have a **subluxation of the radial head (Nursemaid's elbow)**, rather than a fracture.

Hyperpronation of the forearm or supination of the forearm with flexion of the elbow will be your answer regarding management.

Periorbital Ecchymoses

Periorbital ecchymoses can be a sign of **neuroblastoma** rather than abuse, especially on the boards.

We Didn't Start the Fire: All About Burns

Electric Burns

Most injuries involving exposure to household electrical current involve only skin.

When electric current courses through the body, it is called **arc exposure**, which results in deep tissue burns and internal organ involvement sometimes with only **minimal visible injury**. This can lead to **arrhythmias, rhabdomyolysis** and **renal failure**.

Thermal Burns

You will be expected to distinguish between **accidental** and **non-accidental** burns based on the description in the history.

Minor (accidental) burns in children must NOT include:

- hands
- face, eyes, or ears
- feet
- perineum

and they may not cross joints or be circumferential.

A **splash-like** configuration is suggestive of an **accidental** injury.

The classic **"stocking and glove" distribution** would be a dead giveaway that it is **non-accidental** cause.

Full thickness burns are rarely an accident, since children will usually withdraw before a full thickness burn sets in

Automatic administration of antibiotics is not necessary. The first step in a minor burn treatment is **debridement and irrigation**.

Minor burns should be cleaned gently with **mild soap and water**.

Watch for hints that tetanus immunization is not up to date.

Measuring Burns!

 There has been a recent change in the designation of burns.

 Burn Degrees

Superficial (first degree): only damage epidermis. Symptoms include redness and pain. Examples: sunburn and flash burns.

Partial-thickness (second degree): damage epidermis and superficial dermis. Signs include fluid-filled vesicles.

Full-thickness (third degree): destroy epidermis and dermis. Signs and symptoms include white or leathery appearance with no pain.

Burn Inhalation Injury

Inhalation of smoke and its toxins is responsible for 80% of burn-related deaths.

Signs of airway injury include facial burns, carbonaceous (black) sputum, singeing of nasal hair and eyebrows, hoarseness, shortness of breath and stridor.

Fiberoptic bronchoscopy is indicated, along with possible intubation even before the development of over respiratory distress.

Burns to go!

The following burns must be referred to a local Burn Center for treatment:

- moderate or severe burns (>10% TBSA)[5]
- any full thickness burns
- electrical burns
- chemical burns
- burns involving hands, feet, face, genitalia, perineum or major joints
- inhalation injury

---

[5] TBSA is Total Body Surface Area

[RULE OF 9s]

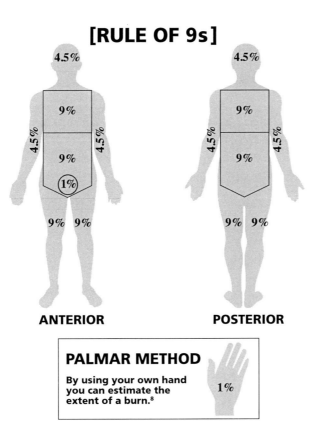

ANTERIOR   POSTERIOR

PALMAR METHOD

By using your own hand you can estimate the extent of a burn.[8]

1%

Rule of Nines[6]

If they ask you to estimate the extent of a burn as a percentage of the total body, here is the rule of 9s.[7]

Arms = 9% each (9 x 2)

Legs = 18% each (9 x 4)

Trunk = 36%   (9 X 4)

Head and neck = 10%   (9 X 1)

Perineum = 1%

Superficial burns are nor included in this calculation.

The Parkland Formula calculates the fluid deficit after a significant burn:

4ml/kg x Wt (kg) x % Body Surface Area affected

Lacerations

Infection prevention is best accomplished with **irrigation** and **debridement**. Irrigate with normal saline under low pressure (but higher pressure may be indicated in very contaminated wounds).

 Shaving hair is unnecessary.

Veering from the Vermilion border

Any laceration described as crossing the vermillion border should be referred to a plastic surgeon.

---

[6] Superficial (first degree burns) do not count towards burn size.

[7] This is not valid in all children. Typically, it is valid only in older children, some say only in those over 16 (which technically are not children at all).

[8] For a small child you would need to adjust this formula, especially if you have a large hand.

Chapter 39

Pharmacology and Pain Management

Remember hearing that "children are not just little adults"? That certainly applies here. Children's bodily functions, anatomy, physiology, etc are very different from the adults and influence the drug effects, especially on the boards!

It is important to recognize that the drug you prescribe will interact with the child and the interaction is dictated not just by the **characteristics of the drug but** also by the **characteristics of the child** (age, weight, genetics, diet, and end-organ function).

We will first walk you through the basics of pharmacology, and then cover some crucial points of several drug classes that might find their way into the test.

Volume of Distribution (Vd)

 Volume of distribution represents the theoretical volume in the body (fluids and tissues) in which the drug may be found after absorption.

The **concentration of the drug** =
Amount administered (dose) /
the volume of distribution (Vd)

or

Vd =
administered amount of drug (D) /
Drug plasma concentration immediately after dosing

Clearance

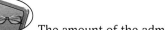 The fraction of the drug that is cleared from the body in any given unit of time.

Clearance is important because it dictates how much of the drug must be given and how often to maintain the desired concentration in the body.

Bioavailability

 The amount of the administered drug that actually reaches the blood. This can be important on the exam.

Of course, if the drug is administered IV, this would be 100%.

> **Heavy Metal Influence!**
>
> Cephalosporins and fluoroquinolones decrease the bioavailability of calcium, magnesium, iron, and aluminum compounds.

When a drug is not administered IV (is administered PO, sublingual, PR, IM, SQ etc.), both **host factors** (such as diet, illness and organ function) and **drug factors** (such as whether the drug is taken whole, crushed, made into solution, or injected intramuscularly) determines its bioavailability. Watch for these factors loaded into the question, they are loaded for a reason!

When a drug concentration is low, it may be because the bioavailability is low or because the clearance is high.

Half-life (T$_{1/2}$)

The amount of time required for the concentration of the drug to **decrease by half**.

- After 1 T$_{1/2}$, 50% of the drug will remain.
- After 2 T$_{1/2}$, 25% of the drug will remain.
- After 3 T$_{1/2}$, 12.5% of the drug will remain.
- After 4 T$_{1/2}$, 6.25% of the drug will remain.
- After 5 T$_{1/2}$, 3.125% of the drug will remain.

Therefore, after **FIVE half-lives**, approximately 97% of the drug will have been cleared from the body.

When a drug is administered at a **constant interval**, it will accumulate in the body until the amount in equals the amount out and the drug reaches **steady state**. Drug accumulation follows the same pattern as the T$_{1/2}$ clearance, so that **a drug will reach 97% of steady state after five T$_{1/2}$**.

When the dose or the dosing interval changes, another five T$_{1/2}$ are required to reach the new steady state concentration.

Absorption

The progression of the drug from the site of administration to the target sites.

Drugs administered by the oral route are especially different in children than adults because:

- neonates and young infants have an elevated gastric pH
- neonates and young infants have delayed gastric emptying
- proteins that are required for conversion from a prodrug to a drug, and also for drug transport, are expressed differently at different ages

Lipophilic Double Agents

Isotretinoin and **griseofulvin** should be taken with fatty foods because they are lipophilic agents. Their bioavailability is enhanced by these foods.

Half a Life

UPDATED & NEW
BREAKING
NEWS
INFORMATION
If there is a kidney problem or liver issue that decreases the clearance of the drug then the medication's half-life will be increased.

Dialysis can decrease a medication's half-life.

An overall decrease in metabolic rate can increase a medication's half-life.

Got Milk?

Tetracycline, doxycycline, and ciprofloxacin are chelated by dairy products. Therefore, no dairy with these three.

Antacid and Iron Man

If an antacid is administered with an iron supplement, the antacid will bind to the iron preventing its absorption and increasing its elimination in the GI tract. Watch for hints that a child is taking an antacid in the question.

Even crushing tabs into a suspension, adding flavoring, and mixing drugs with formula or juice to help young children take the medication may change the drugs absorption and ultimately the concentration.

Distribution

Distribution refers to where the drug disperses after it is succcessfully absorbed into the systemic circulation.

> **Sulfuring through Phenytoin !**
>
> Phenytoin is distributed bound to plasma proteins. When sulfa drugs are administered concurrently, the sulfa causes the phenytoin to unbind, thereby increasing its potential toxicity as well as its elimination.

The **higher percentage of total body water** and the **lower body fat stores in children** cause different distribution of drugs depending on whether they are **hydrophilic** (water-loving) or **lipophilic** (fat-loving).

The serum levels of albumin, other binding-proteins, and transporters also affect the distribution of drugs.

Metabolism

The liver is the primary organ for drug metabolism, but other organs such as the skin, kidney, GI tract, and lungs also have drug-metabolizing enzymes.

Infants have slower drug metabolism than older children and adults and are more prone to many adverse drug reactions.

The first phase of liver metabolism involves a group of oxidases referred to as **CYPs** (CYP= cytochrome P450). Different CYPs become active at different ages and the drug metabolism changes depending on the level of each CYP.

The metabolism of drugs is also affected by **concomitant drugs and herbal remedies** such as St. John's Wort, ginkgo biloba, and milk thistle, which may be ingested by the mother and transferred to the infant via breast milk. Watch for a history of a mother taking **complementary medications;** that's in there for a reason.

Coumadin is an important drug where certain medications, foods, or herbal remedies can increase or decrease the effect. For example - cranberry juice can increase the effect of warfarin and potentially cause bleeding. Keep this in mind when presented with a question that involves a child taking an herbal medication. This can be snuck in with phrasing such as "other than" fill in the blank herbal med the patient is not taking any medications.

Drugs interact to affect how other drugs are metabolized, for example:

Drugs	Impact
Erythromycin, ciprofloxacin, cimetidine, and omeprazole have **inhibitory** effects on hepatic enzymatic systems	This reduces theophylline, codeine, **beta blockers**, antidepressants, corticosteroids, warfarin, and metronidazole metabolism, resulting in **increased bioavailability and toxicity**.
Rifampin, phenobarbital, carbamazepine, and phenytoin are potent enzymatic **inducers**	So one of these drugs will cause other drugs metabolized by the same enzyme to be **eliminated quicker, requiring higher dosing** to maintain a desired concentration.

Excretion

The liver and the kidney are responsible for most drug excretion: the liver through bile and kidney through urine. Hopefully you knew that!

Excretion is dependent on the ability of **transporters** to get the drug from the circulation into the bile or urine for excretion. If one drug inhibits that transporter, then another drug may not be transported and will accumulate to toxic levels in the body.

The functional expression of these transporters is age dependent and is also affected by liver or kidney disease or injury.

So watch for their mentioning liver and kidney disease as being the clue that a drug toxicity is at play!

Elimination of drugs in infants is unpredictable, which is the reason why levels must be closely monitored.

Medications that are eliminated by the liver will not be impacted in a patient with renal disease. The same rule would apply for a medication that is eliminated by the kidney in a patient with primary liver disease.

> ### Watch the Dig levels!
> Quinidine and amiodarone may inhibit renal metabolism of digoxin, resulting in elevated levels.

> ### Why is it not Working?
> In general, if you are presented with a teenager on a given medication, **poor compliance** is often the most likely explanation for variable effect and/or unexpected drug levels.

Beta Blockers

These drugs are used for **SVT** and **hypertension** and include **atenolol, metoprolol,** and **propranolol**. They are also used to treat certain hemangiomas.

Beta blockers block the binding of epinephrine and norepinephrine to their receptors.

Side effects of beta blockers you need to be aware of include:

- **CNS** → Difficulty sleeping and subsequent fatigue. Mood changes and depression can be seen in adolescents.
- **Smooth muscle** → Bronchospasm and cold extremities.
- **Cardiac** → Bradycardia, heart block and /or hypotension.
- **GI/Metabolic** → Hypoglycemia, Hyperkalemia.

Beta blockers can also result in **sexual dysfunction**. Therefore, if you are presented with a teenager who is not improving clinically on beta blockers, e.g., for SVT, consider non-compliance as the cause.

> ### Not so Cute Drugs for Prolonged QT
> If you are presented with a patient with prolonged QT syndrome pay close attention to the medications they are taking. The following medications can cause prolonged QT ! -
>
>
>
> **A**ntibiotics (azithromycin, erythromycin, metronidazole),
>
> **A**ntifungals (azoles),
>
> **A**ntivirals (nelfinavir),
>
> **A**ntimalarials, anaesthetics (halothane),
>
> **A**ntiarrhythmics (procainamide, amiodarone, sotalol),
>
> **A**ntidepressants (amitriptyline),
>
> **A**ntipychotics (risperidone),
>
> **A**nd -- ondansetron, and some **A**DHD medications (stimulants).

Let's face it – the specter of sexual dysfunction would hardly be a motivating factor to take beta blocker medication for a member of an age group that usually feels relatively invincible and is highly interested in sexual function.

Remember that beta blockers can **exacerbate asthma** so cardioselective ones like atenolol are preferred over propranolol.

Diuretics

Acetazolamide

Acetazolamide is a **carbonic anhydrase inhibitor (CAI)**.

"**Acid Soul Amide**" will help you remember that it results in **metabolic acidosis**. It works on the proximal tubule by **preventing the reuptake of bicarbonate**, which makes for **alkaline urine**.

Furosemide/Lasix®

"**Loop Diuretics**" block the absorption of $Na+$ and $Cl-$. They also result in the **wasting of calcium and** $K+$ **and** $H+$.

Picture a giant word, "Lasix," and a giant loop of Henle. The loop changes to a **H**oop through which **H hops out**, and Lasix changes to LasiKs (which is how most patients pronounce it), a giant Lasso grabbing the **K** (**K**loride, and **K**alcium), and kicking them out. The result: **hypochloremic hypokalemic alkalosis**.

In addition, you are expected to know that **ototoxicity** and **renal toxicity** are potential **dose-related** side effects of furosemide.

Side effects of both loop and thiazide diuretics:

- Low Potassium
- High Uric acid
- Metabolic alkalosis
- Volume contraction

Thiazide Diuretics

These include **hydrochlorothiazide** and **metolazone**.

Sodium and **chloride** are lost at the distal tubule, resulting in hyponatremia and hypochloremia. Since it operates on the distal tubule, water is also lost, resulting in **contraction alkalosis**. In addition, bicarb is retained as a negative anion[1] to replace the lost chloride anion. This results in **metabolic alkalosis**.

Picture a giant "thigh" blocking fluid from re-entering the kidney.

Mannitol

Mannitol is an osmotic diuretic. It is not secreted or reabsorbed by the tubules. Through osmotic pressure it keeps water in the tubules resulting in an osmotic diuresis.

This simply exerts osmotic pressure, **pulling fluid from IC to EC space**, with no **acid base effect**. It also **blocks fluid reabsorption at the kidney level, further decreasing IC fluid levels**.

Pharmacological Cornucopia

Metformin - Used mostly in Type II Diabetes to lower glucose levels but now increasingly being used to manage significant overweight and obesity after non pharmacological means have failed.

Erosive Esophagitis related to Gastroesophageal reflux - First line treatment is Proton Pump Inhibitor.

Hypertension - Non pharmacologic methods are attempted first (diet and exercise). If needed, then first line medications include ACEI, ARBs, long acting calcium channel blockers, thiazide diuretics.

Doxorubicin - If you have a child with history of chemotherapy, see if they were exposed to anthracyclines (such as doxorubicin) as this can cause cardiomyopathy.

Spironolactone

Sodium is spiraled out and **potassium is taken in**; therefore, it is **potassium sparing**.

A way to remember that spironolactone is potassium (K) sparing, is to think of it as "spiral-no-lack-K-tone." It is a spiral that **does not lack K**.

Spironolactone can also lead to **metabolic acidosis**.

Aspirin

In addition to **Reye syndrome**, you are expected to know that the **most likely adverse effect is GI irritation**. Another adverse reaction is **tinnitus**, which is dose-related.

---

[1] Yes, we know this is a redundancy (all anions are negative), so no e-mails on that one.

Side Effect Show and Contradictions to keep in mind		
Drug Name	**Side effects**	**Contraindications**
NSAIDs (Ibuprofen)	Acute Interstitial Nephritis (How offensive! Get rid of it!	Pregnancy, Renal disease
Primaquine	Dizziness	G6PD - can cause Hemolytic Anemia
Mefloquine	Anxiety	Major psychiatric Disorder
Doxycycline[2]	GI upset, Photosensitivity	Children < 8 years of age Pregnant women
Amphotericin B	Nephrotoxicity, Hypokalemia, Hypomagnesemia	

How to be Cognizant of Conscious Sedation

You are expected to be well-versed in the changing definitions for conscious sedation and related new terminology, while remaining conscious yourself. Good luck! This is what you are expected to know

Mild sedation (formerly anxiolysis) – Minimal sedation is a drug-induced relief of apprehension with minimal effect on perception and sensorium. Consciousness is sustained

Moderate sedation (formerly conscious sedation) – The patient retains the ability to respond normally to verbal commands, and cardiorespiratory functions are unaffected. Airway reflexes and and the ability to sustain airway patency is maintained.

Deep Sedation – The patient responds to repeated or painful stimuli. With deep sedation, there is further depression of the level of consciousness. The ability to maintain airway patency independently is impaired.

General Anesthesia – Unarousable with any stimulation. There is a complete loss of consciousness and airway protective reflexes. Vital signs must be maintained and monitored.

5 Star General Anesthesia – Beyond general anesthesia, this corresponds with the level of boredom you must be experiencing at this point while trying to keep these details straight.

Despite these definitions, sedation varies from patient to patient, and you are expected to know that monitoring is required in case a patient slips into a deeper form of sedation.

---

[2] Doxycyline has recently been approved for treatment of Lyme disease in children younger than 8 in certain circumstances. This is in addition to its approval in all ages to treat Rocky Mountain Spotted Fever.

Therefore, the following are **required for monitoring** during conscious sedation:

- One staff member who is **PALS certified** must be available to monitor, without other duties.
- Patients should be monitored with **pulse oximeter** and non invasive **blood pressure monitor**. Vitals should be documented in writing every 5 minutes
- **Bag mask respiratory equipment**, as well as oxygen, should be immediately available.
- **Reversal agents** such as naloxone and flumazenil should be available to reverse the effects of opiates and benzodiazepines, respectively.

 In the absence of an underlying cardiac history, EKG monitoring is **not** routinely required.

Bibliography

1. American Academy of Pediatrics. PREP The Curriculum® Content Specifications. 2019, 2020 and 2021.

2. American Academy of Pediatrics Committee on Bioethics. Ethics and the care of critically ill infants and children. *Pediatrics*. 1996;98(1):149-152.

3. American Academy of Pediatrics Committee on Infectious Diseases. Prevention of varicella: recommendations for use of varicella vaccines in children, including a recommendation for a routine 2-dose varicella immunization schedule. *Pediatrics*. 2007;120(1):221-231.

4. American Academy of Pediatrics Committee on Infectious Diseases. *Red Book: 2018 Report of the Committee on Infectious Diseases*. 31st ed. Elk Grove Village, IL: American Academy of Pediatrics; 2012, 2015.

5. American Academy of Pediatrics Newborn Screening Authoring Committee. Newborn screening expands: recommendations for pediatricians and medical homes--implications for the system. *Pediatrics*. 2008;121(1):192-217.

6. American Psychiatric Association. *Diagnostic and Statistical Manual of Mental Disorders*. 5th ed. Washington, DC: American Psychiatric Publishing; 2013.

7. Arnold C, Davis T, Frempong J, et al. Assessment of newborn screening parent education materials. *Pediatrics*. 2006;117(5):S320-5.

8. Bonanni P, Boccalini S, Bechini A. Efficacy, duration of immunity and cross protection after HPV vaccination: a review of the evidence. *Vaccine*. 2009;27 Suppl 1:A46-53.

9. Boppana S, Ross S, Novak Z, et al. Dried blood spot real-time polymerase chain reaction assays to screen newborns for congenital cytomegalovirus infection. *JAMA: Journal of the American Medical Association*. 2010;303(14):1375-1382.

10. Botkin, Jeffrey R. "Ethical Issues in Newborn Screening." *Oxford Handbooks Online*, 2016, doi:10.1093/oxfordhb/9780199981878.013.12.

11. Brenner M, Oakley C, Lewis D. The evaluation of children and adolescents with headache. *Curr Pain Headache Rep*. 2008;12(5):361-366.

12. Bukstein O, Bernet W, Arnold V, et al. Practice parameter for the assessment and treatment of children and adolescents with substance use disorders. *Journal of the American Academy of Child Adolesc Psychiatry*. 2005;44(6):609-621.

13. Burton BK. Inborn errors of metabolism in infancy: a guide to diagnosis. *Pediatrics*. 1998;102(6):E69.

14. Centers for Disease Control and Prevention. FDA licensure of bivalent human papillomavirus vaccine (HPV2, Cervarix) for use in females and updated HPV vaccination recommendations from the Advisory Committee on Immunization Practices (ACIP). *MMWR: Morbidity*. 2010;59(20):626-629.

15. Centers for Disease Control and Prevention. FDA licensure of quadrivalent human papillomavirus vaccine (HPV4, Gardasil) for use in males and guidance from the Advisory Committee on Immunization Practices (ACIP). *MMWR: Morbidity*. 2010;59(20):630-632.

16. Centers for Disease Control and Prevention. Knowledge and practices of obstetricians and gynecologists regarding cytomegalovirus infection during pregnancy--United States, 2007. *MMWR: Morbidity.* 2008;57(3):65-68.

17. Centers for Disease Control and Prevention. Updated recommendations for use of tetanus toxoid, reduced diphtheria toxoid and acellular pertussis (Tdap) vaccine from the Advisory Committee on Immunization Practices, 2010. *MMWR: Morbidity.* 2011;60(1):13-15.

18. Cobb K, Bachrach L, Greendale G, et al. Disordered eating, menstrual irregularity, and bone mineral density in female runners. *Med Sci Sports Exerc.* 2003;35(5):711-719.

19. Daneman, A., et al. "The Radiology of Neonatal Necrotizing Enterocolitis (NEC) A Review of 47 Cases and the Literature." *Pediatric Radiology*, vol. 7, no. 2, 1978, pp. 70–77., doi:10.1007/bf00975674.

20. Dietz WH. Critical periods in childhood for the development of obesity. *Am J Clin Nutr.* 1994;59(5):955-959.

21. Duff, Raymond S. "Guidelines for Deciding Care of Critically Ill or Dying Patients." *Journal of the American Academy of Child Psychiatry*, vol. 19, no. 3, 1980, p. 539., doi:10.1016/s0002-7138(09)61074-8.

22. Friedman DI. Pseudotumor cerebri. *Neurol Clin.* 2004;22(1):99-131, vi.

23. Frush K. Preparation for emergencies in the offices of pediatricians and pediatric primary care providers. *Pediatrics.* 2007;120(1):200-212.

24. Gibbins S, Stevens B. Mechanisms of sucrose and non-nutritive sucking in procedural pain management in infants. *Pain Research.* 2001;6(1):21-28.

25. Greer F, Krebs NF. Optimizing bone health and calcium intakes of infants, children, and adolescents. *Pediatrics.* 2006;117(2):578-585.

26. Harriet Lane Handbook of Pediatrics, 21st Edition.

27. Herman-Giddens ME, Slora EJ, Wasserman RC, et al. Secondary sexual characteristics and menses in young girls seen in office practice: a study from the Pediatric Research in Office Settings network. *Pediatrics.* 1997;99(4):505–512.

28. Hull, Melissa A., et al. "Mortality and Management of Surgical Necrotizing Enterocolitis in Very Low Birth Weight Neonates: A Prospective Cohort Study." *Journal of the American College of Surgeons*, vol. 218, no. 6, 2014, pp. 1148–1155., doi:10.1016/j.jamcollsurg.2013.11.015.

29. Johnston LD, O'Maley PM, Bachman JG, Schulenberg JE, eds. Monitoring the Future. National Results on Adolescent Drug Use: Overview of Key Findings, 2005. Bethesda, Md: National Institute on Drug Abuse; 2006.

30. Kozlowski KJ. Ovarian masses. *Adolesc Med.* 1999;10(2):337-50, vii.

31. Lee, Dong Hoon, et al. "Clinical Value of Fine Needle Aspiration Cytology in Pediatric Cervical Lymphadenopathy Patients under 12-Years-of-Age." *International Journal of Pediatric Otorhinolaryngology*, vol. 78, no. 1, 2014, pp. 79–81., doi:10.1016/j.ijporl.2013.10.054.

32. Lustig D, Saeed R, Abdullah B. Fructose intolerance/malabsorption and recurrent abdominal pain in children [poster]. Presented at: American College of Gastroenterology (ACG) 2010 Annual Meeting and Postgraduate Course; October 15-20, 2010; San Antonio, TX. Abstract P400.

33. Matzke GM, Dozois EJ, Larson DW, Moir CR. Surgical management of intestinal malrotation in adults: comparative results for open and laparoscopic Ladd procedures. *Surg Endosc.* 2005;19 (10):1416–1419.

34. Nelson Textbook of Pediatrics 20th Edition.

35. Neuspiel DR. Marijuana. *Pediatrics in Review.* 2007;28(4):156-7; discussion 157.

36. Ogden C, Carroll M, Curtin L, Lamb M, Flegal K. Prevalence of high body mass index in US children and adolescents, 2007-2008. *JAMA: Journal of the American Medical Association*. 2010;303(3):242-249.

37. Rasquin A, Di Lorenzo C, Forbes D, et al. Childhood functional gastrointestinal disorders: child/adolescent. *Gastroenterology*. 2006;130(5):1527-1537.

38. Rohrschneider WK, Mittnacht H, Darge K, Tröger J. Pyloric muscle in asymptomatic infants: sonographic evaluation and discrimination from idiopathic hypertrophic pyloric stenosis. *Pediatr Radiol*. 1998;28(6):429–43429.

39. Rosen, Rachel, et al. "Pediatric Gastroesophageal Reflux Clinical Practice Guidelines." *Journal of Pediatric Gastroenterology and Nutrition*, vol. 66, no. 3, 2018, pp. 516–554., doi:10.1097/mpg.0000000000001889.

40. Rudolph's Pediatrics 23rd Edition.

41. Tormoehlen, L. M., et al. "Hydrocarbon Toxicity: A Review." *Clinical Toxicology*, vol. 52, no. 5, 2014, pp. 479–489., doi:10.3109/15563650.2014.923904.

42. Wagner C, Greer FR. Prevention of rickets and vitamin D deficiency in infants, children, and adolescents. *Pediatrics*. 2008;122(5):1142-1152.

43. Warner B. Malrotation. In: Oldham KT, Colobani PM, Foglia RP, eds. *Surgery of Infants and Children: Scientific Principles and Practice*. Philadelphia, PA: Lippincott Williams and Williams; 1997:1229.

44. Yellen ES, Gauvreau K, Takahashi M, et al. Performance of 2004 American Heart Association recommendations for treatment of Kawasaki disease. *Pediatrics*. 2010;125(2). Available at: www.pediatrics.org/cgi/content/full/125/2/e234.

45. *Common Substances of Abuse*, PIR, Vol 39, No 8, AUG 2018.

46. *In Brief*, PIR. MAR 2020 p.155.

47. *Gallbladder, Gallstones, and Disease of the Gallbladder in Children*, PIR Vol 41, No 12 DEC 2020.

48. *Index of Suspicion* Vol 41 No 10 OCT 2020.

49. In Brief "Acute Flaccid Myelitis in Children" *Pediatrics in Review* Vol 40 No 11 p 602-604. NOV 2019.

50. Cote, C. (June 2019) *Guidelines for Monitoring and Management of Pediatric Patients Before, During, and After Sedation for Diagnostic and Therapeutic Procedures*. Pediatrics 143 (6).

51. *Pediatrics In Review : Pediatric Sedation Management*. Sean Barnes, Myron Yaster and Sapna R. Kudchadkar. May 2016, 37 (5) 203-212.

52. AAP 2020 policy statement: https://pediatrics.aappublications.org/content/145/6/e20201011.

53. https://www.ahajournals.org/doi/full/10.1161/HCG.0000000000000048.

54. https://www.orthobullets.com/knee-and-sports/3020/patellar-instability.

55. https://www.orthobullets.com/knee-and-sports/3008/acl-tear.

56. https://www.orthobullets.com/knee-and-sports/3010/mcl-knee-injuries.

57. https://www.orthobullets.com/knee-and-sports/3005/meniscal-injury.

58. https://www.ncbi.nlm.nih.gov/pmc/articles/PMC6394198/.

59. Kerr, J. M., & Congeni, J. A. (2007). *Anabolic-Androgenic Steroids: Use and Abuse in Pediatric Patients. Pediatric Clinics of North America*, 54(4), 771–785. doi:10.1016/j.pcl.2007.04.010.

60. Causes of painless scrotal swelling in children and adolescents https://www.ncbi.nlm.nih.gov/books/NBK559125/.

61. Fleisher & Ludwig's *Textbook of Pediatric Emergency Medicine* 7th Edition.

62. UpToDate: Undescended testes (cryptorchidism) in children. Clinical features and evaluation.

63. *Nelson's Essentials of Pediatrics* 7th Edition.

64. Undescended testes (cryptorchidism) in children. Clinical features and evaluation (UpToDate).

Index

A

Abdominal Defects 177–178
    diaphragmatic hernia 178
    gastroschisis 178
    omphalocele 177
Abdominal Pain 147, 349–353
    acute abdominal pain 349
    appendicitis 349
    recurrent abdominal pain 350
        abdominal migraines 352
        functional abdominal pain 352
        functional dyspepsia 350
        irritable bowel syndrome 351
Abducens and Facial Nerve Palsy 704
Abducens nerve (CN VI) 488
Absence Seizures 80, 511, 515
Abuse and Neglect 93–94
Acanthosis nigricans 339
ACE Inhibitors 403
Acetaminophen 98, 144, 151, 487
Acetazolamide 489, 715
Acetic Acid Solutions 589
Acetylcholine Receptor 504
Acetylcholinesterase Inhibitor 505
Achalasia 614
Acholic Stools 375
Achondroplasia 207, 227, 331
Acid Base Metabolism 183–187
    compensatory mechanisms for:
        metabolic acidosis 184
        metabolic alkalosis 184
        respiratory acidosis 184
        respiratory alkalosis 184
Acidic Ingestions 152
Acidosis 236
ACL. *See* Anterior Cruciate Ligament
Acne Vulgaris 537–541, 617, 619, 651
    benzoyl peroxide 539
    inflammatory acne 537
        nodules 538
        papules 537
        pustules 538
    isotretinoin 540
    neonatal acne 538
    non-inflammatory 537
        closed comedones 537
        open comedones 537
    oral antibiotics 539
    oral contraceptives 539
    salicylic acid 538
    topical antibiotics 539
    tretinoin 539
Acoustic Neuroma 546
Acral Keratosis 361

Acrocyanosis 388
ACTH 325, 514
ACTH Stimulation Test 325
Actinomyces sp 290
Activated Charcoal 143, 145, 146, 149, 155, 681
Acute Ataxia 494
Acute Chest Syndrome 432
Acute Flaccid Myelitis 504
Acute Hepatic Failure 493
Acute Interstitial Nephritis 717
Acute Leukemia 433
Acute Lymphocytic Leukemia 446, 555
Acute Myeloid Leukemia 439
Acute Nonlymphocytic Leukemia 446
Acute Renal Failure 466
Acute Respiratory Distress Syndrome 687
Acute Sinusitis 591
Acute Tubular Necrosis 147, 466
Acute Urticaria 252
Acyclovir 132, 171, 294, 304, 458, 502, 521, 524, 576, 625
Acylcarnitine 232
ADA Deficiency 260
Adaptive Functioning 69
Addison's Disease. *See* Primary Adrenal Deficiency
Adenoidectomy 595
Adenoid Hypertrophy 600
Adenoiditis 595
Adenoma Sebaceum 537
Adenosine 413
Adenosine Deaminase Deficiency. *See* ADA Deficiency
Adenovirus 275, 308, 475, 577, 593
ADH (Antidiuretic Hormone) 326
ADHD 71, 223, 335, 498, 499, 714
Adolescent Cognitive Development 611
Adolescent Psychosocial Development 611
Adolescents and Consent 614
Adoption 100–101
Adrenal Crisis 324
Adrenal Disorders 321–327
    adrenal crisis 324
    congenital adrenal hyperplasia 321
    Cushing syndrome 325
    Langerhans cell histiocytosis 326
    primary adrenal deficiency 324
    secondary adrenal deficiency 324
Adrenal Insufficiency 187, 234
Adrenogenital Syndrome 208
Advance Directives 43
Adverse Events 52–57

adverse drug event 52
    detecting and reporting events 55–56
    near miss event 52
    root cause analysis 53
    sentinel event 53
AED. *See* Automatic External Defibrillator
Aggressive Behaviors 86
Airbags and Car Seats 139
Airway Fluoroscopy 384
Albendazole 310, 312
Albumin Levels 461, 462, 465, 713
Albuterol 82, 470
Alcohol 180, 673, 674, 683, 685
Alcohol Abuse 674, 678–679
    acute alcohol intoxication 679
    alcohol withdrawal 680
    chronic alcohol abuse 680
Alcohol Dehydrogenase Antagonist 147
Alcohol Intoxication 677
Aldosterone 322, 324
Alkaline Ingestions 152
Alkaline Phosphatase 116, 344, 347, 449
Alkalosis 185, 716
ALL. *See* Acute Lymphocytic Leukemia
Allergic Contact Dermatitis 525
Allergic Proctocolitis 366
Allergic Reactions 247–248, 251–254
    anaphylaxis 251
    contrast media 253
    hymenoptera stings 253
    types 1-4 247
Allergic Rhinitis 243, 248–249, 590
    perennial allergic rhinitis 248
Allergy Testing 248
Allopurinol 452
Alopecia 113, 540–542
    alopecia areata 541
    telogen effluvium 541
    tinea capitis 540
    traction alopecia 541
    trichotillomania 541
Alpers syndrome 208
Alpha-1 Antitrypsin 557
Alpha-1 Antitrypsin Deficiency 208, 376
Alpha-Fetoprotein (AFP) 484. *See* Antenatal Screening
Alpha Thalassemia 424
Alport syndrome 457, 459, 583
Alternative Medicine 48, 82
    alternative treatments 81
    complementary medicine 48